THE SOCIOLOGY OF
MENTAL ILLNESS

A Comprehensive Reader

Jane D. McLeod

Indiana University–Bloomington

Eric R. Wright

Indiana University–Purdue University Indianapolis

New York   Oxford

OXFORD UNIVERSITY PRESS

2010

Oxford University Press, Inc., publishes works that further
Oxford University's objective of excellence
in research, scholarship, and education.

Oxford New York
Auckland Cape Town Dar es Salaam Hong Kong Karachi
Kuala Lumpur Madrid Melbourne Mexico City Nairobi
New Delhi Shanghai Taipei Toronto

With offices in
Argentina Austria Brazil Chile Czech Republic France Greece
Guatemala Hungary Italy Japan Poland Portugal Singapore
South Korea Switzerland Thailand Turkey Ukraine Vietnam

Copyright © 2010 by Oxford University Press, Inc.

Published by Oxford University Press, Inc.
198 Madison Avenue, New York, New York 10016
http://www.oup.com

Oxford is a registered trademark of Oxford University Press

ISBN: 978-0-19-538171-9

Printed in the United States of America
on acid-free paper

CONTENTS

ACKNOWLEDGMENTS

This volume grew from conversations that were initiated by Claude Teweles, then of Roxbury Press, over four years ago. Claude perceived the need for a comprehensive reader in the sociology of mental illness and invited us to develop a proposal. The proposal we wrote, the reviewers' comments, and the many hours we spent searching, reading, and editing selections yielded the volume you see here. We gratefully acknowledge Claude's early contributions to the project, as well as Oxford University Press's willingness to honor our contract after it purchased Roxbury Press in 2007.

We give deep thanks to Shawna Rohrman who maintained all of the files for this volume and handled all of the copyright permissions. Without Shawna's outstanding organizational skills and calm persistence this volume would not exist. We could not possibly have done it without her.

Thanks also to the editorial team at Oxford University Press who kept production on schedule and their good humors intact despite our delays. Sherith Pankratz, the senior editor who assumed responsibility for the volume after Roxbury Press was sold, offered sage advice about the organization, content, and style of the volume, along with personal encouragement, throughout the production process. Her assistant editor, Whitney Laemmli, was equally helpful, gracious, and supportive.

Jane acknowledges the patience and support of her husband, Steve Krahnke, and her daughters, Sophie and Nell Krahnke, who maintain the homestead while she buries her head in books. She is also continually grateful for the supportive environment in which she works and for her gentle and inquisitive colleagues.

Eric thanks his family and many friends who have supported him over the years as he pursued his academic career. Their love, encouragement, willingness to listen, and critical questions have made him a more careful scholar and a better person.

We also must acknowledge the extraordinary contributions of our many professional colleagues. The corpus of scholarly work on the sociology of mental health and illness is truly impressive and continues to grow with each passing year. This treasure trove of interesting and important research made our job as editors both enjoyable and difficult. We leave this project with a renewed appreciation for the many unique insights sociologists have brought to the study of mental health and illness. Yet, we were only able to represent a small sample of this rich literature here. In some cases, we reluctantly eliminated readings in order to keep the volume to a manageable length; in a few cases, publishers were unwilling to give us permission to reproduce journal articles in this format. We edited most of the selections for the sake of concision and clarity, often deleting entire sections in order that we could include more readings. Where selections have been edited extensively, we indicate so with a †, and encourage advanced readers to seek out the original article or chapter. We are grateful to the authors and publishers for allowing us these liberties with their work, and hope that the edited readings remain true to their intent.

Finally, and most important, we must acknowledge the many people we have met over the years who struggle with and/or are affected by mental illness. We are truly grateful to them for sharing their life experiences with us. Their stories inspire us, inform our scholarship, and challenge us to help our students appreciate more deeply the ways that society shapes the lives of people with mental illness.

Jane D. McLeod and Eric R. Wright
January 2009

CONTRIBUTORS

Norman B. Anderson is the Executive Vice President and Chief Executive Officer of the American Psychological Association.

Carol S. Aneshensel is Professor in the Department of Community Health Sciences at the University of California at Los Angeles.

Evelyn J. Bromet is Professor in the Department of Psychiatry and Behavioral Science at State University of New York, Stony Brook.

Martha Livingston Bruce is Professor in the Department of Psychiatry at Weill Medical College of Cornell University, Professor in the Clinical Epidemiology Program at the Graduate School of Medical Sciences, and Associate Vice-Chair for Research in the Department of Psychiatry at Cornell University.

Giovanni Burgos is Assistant Professor in the Department of Sociology at McGill University.

Carol A. Boyer is Associate Director of the Institute for Health, Health Care Policy and Aging Research and Assistant Research Professor in the Department of Sociology at Rutgers University.

Benedict Carey is a medical and science writer for The New York Times.

Avshalom Caspi is Edward M. Arnett Professor in the Departments of Psychology and Neuroscience, Psychiatry and Behavioral Sciences at Duke University.

Peter Conrad is Harry Coplan Professor of Social Sciences in the Department of Sociology at Brandeis University.

Francis T. Cullen is Distinguished Research Professor in the Departments of Criminal Justice and Sociology, and Director of the Distance Learning Master's Degree Program at the University of Cincinnati.

Olga Demler is a PhD candidate in the Biostatistics Program at Boston University.

Mary Amanda Dew is Professor of Psychiatry at the University of Pittsburgh, and is Director of Clinical Epidemiology Program at the Western Psychiatric Institute and Clinic.

Bruce P. Dohrenwend is Professor of Epidemiology at the Mailman School of Public Health and Professor of Psychiatry in the College of Physicians and Surgeons at Columbia University.

Bradley R. Entner Wright is Associate Professor in the Department of Sociology at the University of Connecticut.

Ranae J. Evenson is Assistant Professor in the Social Science Department at Wartburg College.

Rudy Fenwick is Associate Professor in the Department of Sociology at the University of Akron.

Anne E. Figert is Associate Professor in the Department of Sociology at Loyola University Chicago.

Richard G. Frank is Margaret T. Morris Professor in the Department of Health Care Policy at Harvard Medical School.

Howard H. Goldman is Professor of Psychiatry at the University of Maryland School of Medicine.

Walter R. Gove is Professor Emeritus in the Department of Sociology at Vanderbilt University.

Allan V. Horwitz is Professor in the Department of Sociology at Rutgers University.

Thomas R. Insel is the Director of the National Institute of Mental Health.

James S. Jackson is Daniel Katz Distinguished University Professor in the Department of Psychology, a Professor in the School of Public Health, and Director of the Institute for Social Research at the University of Michigan.

David Karp is Professor in the Department of Sociology at Boston College.

Ronald C. Kessler is Professor in the Department of Health Care Policy at Harvard Medical School.

Saeko Kikuzawa is Assistant Professor in the Department of Culture and Humanities at Nara Women's University.

Arthur Kleinman is Esther and Sidney Rabb Professor in the Department of Anthropology at Harvard University, Professor of Medical Anthropology in Social Medicine and Professor of Psychiatry at Harvard Medical School.

Harriet Lefley is Professor in the Department of Psychiatry & Behavioral Sciences at Miller School of Medicine, University of Miami.

Alisa Lincoln is Associate Professor of Health Sciences and Sociology and has Adjunct Appointments at the Boston University School of Public Health and the Division of Psychiatry, Boston University School of Medicine.

Bruce G. Link is Professor of Epidemiology and Sociomedical Sciences at the Mailman School of Public Health of Columbia University and Research Scientist at the New York State Psychiatric Institute.

Donald A. Lloyd is Assistant Professor in the Department of Sociology at Florida State University.

Keri M. Lubell is Behavioral Scientist for the Emergency & Risk Communication Branch of the U.S. Centers for Disease Control and Prevention.

Fred E. Markowitz is Associate Professor in the Department of Sociology at Northern Illinois University.

Jack K. Martin is the Director of Research at the Karl F. Schuessler Institute of Social Research at Indiana University Bloomington.

Athena Helen McLean is Associate Professor in the Department of Sociology, Anthropology, and Social Work at Central Michigan University.

Jane D. McLeod is Professor in the Department of Sociology at Indiana University Bloomington.

Richard A. Miech is Associate Professor in the Department of Health and Behavioral Sciences at University of Colorado, Denver.

John Mirowsky is Professor in the Department of Sociology at the University of Texas-Austin.

Terrie E. Moffitt is Kurt Schmidt Nielsen Professor in the Departments of Psychology and Neuroscience, Psychiatry and Behavioral Sciences at Duke University.

Joseph P. Morrissey is Professor of Health Policy & Administration and Psychiatry at the Schools of Public Health and Medicine at the University of North Carolina at Chapel Hill, and is Deputy Director for Research of the University's Cecil G. Sheps Center for Health Services Research.

Susan Muhlbauer, retired from University of Nebraska Medical Center College of Nursing, is on staff at St. Anthony Regional Hospital and Nursing Home in Carroll, Iowa.

Mark Olfson is Professor of Clinical Psychiatry in the Center for Community Health Partnerships at Columbia University Medical Center.

Deborah K. Padgett is Associate Professor at the School of Social Work at New York University.

Leonard I. Pearlin is Senior Research Scientist and Graduate Professor in the Department of Sociology at University of Maryland – College Park.

Bernice A. Pescosolido is Distinguished Professor of Sociology at Indiana University Bloomington and Director of the Indiana Consortium for Mental Health Services Research.

Harold Alan Pincus is Vice Chair of the Department of Psychiatry at Columbia University, Director of Quality and Outcomes Research at New York-Presbyterian Hospital, Associate Director of Columbia's Irving Institute for Clinical and Translational Research, and Senior Scientist at the RAND Corporation.

Nancy S. Pruett is a clinical psychologist at The Neuropsychology Service.

Sarah Rosenfield is Associate Professor in the Department of Sociology, and faculty member in the Institute for Health, Health Care Policy, and Aging Research at Rutgers University.

Catherine E. Ross is Professor in the Department of Sociology at the University of Texas-Austin.

David J. Rothman is Bernard Schoenberg Professor of Social Medicine at Columbia College of Physicians & Surgeons and Professor of History at Columbia University.

Thomas Scheff is Professor Emeritus in the Department of Sociology at the University of California, Santa Barbara.

Teresa L. Scheid is Professor in the Department of Sociology at the University of North Carolina, Charlotte.

Scott Schieman is Professor in the Department of Sociology at the University of Toronto.

Joseph W. Schneider is Ellis and Nelle Levitt Professor in the Department of Sociology at Drake University.

Kathryn Schulz is a freelance writer.

Patrick E. Shrout is Professor in the Department of Psychology at New York University.

Phil A. Silva was Executive Director of the Dunedin Multidisciplinary Health and Development Research Unit, University of Otago Medical School.

Eric Silver is Associate Professor of Crime, Law, Justice, and Sociology at Pennsylvania State University.

Robin W. Simon is Associate Professor in the Department of Sociology at Florida State University.

Elmer Struening is Professor in the Department of Epidemiology at Columbia University.

William Patrick Sullivan is Professor in the School of Social Work at Indiana University Indianapolis.

Ralph Swindle is Research Clinical Psychologist for Eli Lilly.

Galen E. Switzer is Associate Professor of Medicine and Psychiatry at the University of Pittsburgh.

Mark Tausig is Professor in the Department of Sociology and Associate Dean of the Graduate School at the University of Akron.

John Taylor is Associate Professor in the Department of Sociology at Florida State University.

Brent Teasdale is Assistant Professor in the Department of Criminal Justice at Georgia State University.

Linda A. Teplin is Owen L. Coon Professor of Psychiatry and Behavioral Sciences in the Feinberg School of Medicine at Northwestern University.

Peggy A. Thoits is Professor in the Department of Sociology at Indiana University Bloomington.

E. Fuller Torrey is the founder of the Treatment Advocacy Center and the Executive Director of the Stanley Medical Research Institute.

R. Jay Turner is Marie E. Cowart Professor of Sociology and Epidemiology and a Professor of Psychology at Florida State University.

Karen van Gundy is Associate Professor in the Department of Sociology and a Faculty Fellow in the Carsey Institute at the University of New Hampshire.

Jerome C. Wakefield is University Professor, a Professor of Social Work, a Professor of the Conceptual Foundations of Psychiatry in the NYU School of Medicine, an Affiliate Faculty member in the Bioethics Program at New York University, and an Affiliate Faculty member in the Center for Ancient Studies at New York University.

Philip Wang is Director of the Division of Services and Intervention Research at the National Institute of Mental Health.

Kenneth B. Wells is Professor in Residence, Psychiatry and Biobehavioral Sciences and Director of the Health Services Research Center, in the David Geffen School of Medicine, Department of Health Services at the UCLA School of Public Health, and Senior Scientist for RAND Health Services.

Blair Wheaton is Professor in the Department of Sociology at the University of Toronto.

David R. Williams is Florence and Laura Norman Professor at the Harvard School of Public Health and a Professor in the Departments of African and African American Studies and Sociology at Harvard University.

Eric R. Wright is Professor in the School for Public and Environmental Affairs and Director of the Center for Health Policy at Indiana University – Purdue University Indianapolis.

Alan M. Zaslavsky is Professor in the Department of Health Care Policy at Harvard Medical School.

INTRODUCTION

Most of you already know something about mental illness. You may have a friend or family member who has been treated for mental illness or you may have seen depictions of mental illness in movies or TV shows. You may have read newspaper accounts about the recent increase in antipsychotic prescriptions to children or about how major cities are dealing with populations of homeless persons who have mental illness. Your knowledge is the starting point for your exploration of sociological perspectives on mental health and mental illness.

Our goal in this reader is to build on the knowledge you have by presenting a strong and balanced sociological perspective on mental illness. Many different disciplines contribute to our understanding of mental health and mental illness, including psychiatry, psychology, social work, and public health, among others. Each discipline offers unique insights into the definition, causes, treatment, and consequences of mental illness. We emphasize the unique insights of sociology in this collection. Readers who are looking for information about the efficacy of psychotropic medications or about the genetic bases of mental illness will not find readings that directly address those topics here—those are not the kinds of topics that sociologists study. At the same time, we acknowledge the importance of knowledge from multiple disciplines when developing a comprehensive model of mental illness. To that end, we introduce each section of readings by highlighting key concepts and theories that sociologists use to understand the topic.

Chances are, much of what you have learned about mental illness draws on the conceptualization of mental illness adopted by psychiatry. This conceptualization sees mental illnesses as real illnesses, and the feelings, attitudes, and behaviors associated with mental illnesses as signs and symptoms of underlying disorders. The "biological revolution" in psychiatry has led to a surge of interest in the neurochemical, physiological, and genetic origins of mental illness and to an increasing reliance on medication therapies. These features of the psychiatric conceptualization encourage us to focus on the individual when defining, explaining, and treating illness. Professional definitions of mental illness are used to help individual persons understand the problems they are facing. The causes of onsets or recurrences of mental illness are sought in the family histories and personal circumstances of individuals. Treatments are tailored to the specific symptoms and responses of individual patients.

The psychiatric conceptualization of mental illness has contributed greatly to our understanding of the causes and consequences of mental illness, and has brought much-needed relief to the individuals and families who are affected. Despite its many strengths, however, it fails to capture the full complexity of mental illness as a concept that is used to understand troubling feelings, attitudes, and behaviors; as a personal experience; and as a social problem in need of remedy. Sociological perspectives on mental illness complement the psychiatric conceptualization by emphasizing the socially-constructed nature of mental illness, the origins of mental health problems in structured social arrangements, and the complex nature of personal, community, and social responses. Sociologists do not deny the reality of profound sadness, delusions, hyperactive behavior, and other signs and symptoms of mental disorders, nor do they reject the possibility that some mental disorders have their origins in genes or brain chemistry. Rather, they contend that thinking of mental illness as an objective, biological reality limits our understanding of the nature, causes, and consequences of troubling feelings, attitudes, and behaviors.

WHAT SOCIOLOGY HAS TO OFFER

Sociologists' contributions to the study of mental illness apply what C. Wright Mills called the "sociological imagination" to this most personal of experiences. In Mills' words, the sociological imagination works at the intersection of " 'the personal troubles of milieu' and 'the public issues of social structure' " (p. 8); it is "the capacity to range from the most impersonal and remote transformations to the most intimate features of the human self and to see the relations between the two" (p. 7). The sociological imagination encourages us to search for the social world that lies behind personal experiences of mental illness: to analyze how individuals and societies understand mental illness, to identify the features of society that create personal suffering, and to view personal suffering as a social dilemma.

The readings that we have selected present sociological perspectives on mental illness as represented by the dominant theoretical paradigms of the field. These paradigms include social constructionism, symbolic interactionism, and conflict theory. Each of these paradigms offers a different sociological "lens" through which to view mental illness.

- Social constructionism aims to understand the ways that people and organizations construct shared realities. In the case of mental illness, the object of analysis is the definition of the mental illness itself.
- Symbolic interactionism draws our attention to the meanings that situations have for their participants and the implications of those meanings for human action. It is a particularly useful paradigm for thinking about how the meaning of mental illness is negotiated in interpersonal interaction and about the implications of those negotiations for how people with mental illness and the people around them behave.

- As its name implies, conflict theory emphasizes conflict among competing societal groups, the inequalities that arise, and the implications of those inequalities for individual well-being. It has been applied to topics as disparate as gender differences in mental illness and why many patients reject the clinical advice they get from treatment providers.

ORGANIZATION AND THEMES

Our reader is organized into six sections that correspond to recognizable substantive areas of research: definitions of mental illness; prevalence and patterns of mental illness; social origins of mental health and illness; stigma and the social dimensions of the experience of mental illness; the history and social organization of mental health policy and treatment; and mental illness, the family, and society. In each section, we highlight three interrelated, sociological themes.

Theme 1: Mental illness is a social construction

By this, we mean that the concept of mental illness is a social product—one among many possible ways that we could understand troubling psychological experiences—rather than a representation of objective reality. The conditions that we think of as mental illness have not always been understood in that way. Hundreds of years ago, the signs and symptoms of mental illness were understood as punishments sent by God, as evidence of supernatural possession, or as signs of moral depravity and laziness. While it is easy to dismiss these early understandings as ignorant and foolish, only 40 years ago, homosexuality was considered a mental disorder in the United States. Even now, debates continue as to the appropriateness of thinking about attention deficit hyperactivity disorder, premenstrual syndrome (PMS), road rage, extreme prejudice, and other contemporary social issues as mental illnesses rather than as problematic and troubling behaviors. The first theme of sociological research on mental illness highlights the importance of social context in how mental illness is defined and treated.

Theme 2: Experiences of mental illness are shaped by the structural and cultural contexts in which people live

The likelihood that persons experience mental illness, how they understand that experience, and how they respond are all influenced by the structural arrangements of their lives as well as by the cultural meaning systems in which they are embedded. For example, persons with low levels of income and education, and who work in low-status occupations, are more likely than other persons to feel distressed and to experience depression and anxiety. Such persons are also less likely than others to have access to effective mental health treatment; their lack of access places them at greater risk of recurrences of illness. In this way, we can see how material resources are relevant to careers of mental illness.

Yet, people's lives are shaped not only by the material resources to which they have access but also by the cultural contexts that surround them. Cultural meaning systems determine whether specific problems are viewed as mental illnesses and what responses are considered normative. For example, many of the experiences that are associated with depression in Western societies are associated with neurasthenia in China, a condition that is considered a physical illness and that is thought to have both biological and psychosocial causes. Because there is a strong stigma attached to mental illness, neurasthenia offers sufferers a more acceptable interpretation of their problems. Stigma, too, is a cultural meaning that profoundly influences the experiences of people with mental illness and how societies respond. The International Pilot Study of Schizophrenia found, for example, that clinical and social outcomes were better for patients in less-developed countries than in more-developed countries, a finding that the investigators attributed to relatively low levels of stigma in the former (Leff et al., 1992).

Finally, people's decisions about whether to seek treatment are influenced by the beliefs of persons in their social networks—whether they see the problems as serious and accept the efficacy of psychiatric treatments or whether, instead, they interpret the problems as nonmedical in nature. It is not possible, then, to fully comprehend mental illness without understanding the social context in which it is experienced.

Theme 3: Mental illness is a complex, multilevel phenomenon

We can understand mental illness as an experience of individuals, but a comprehensive approach to addressing mental illness must account for the effects of and responses to mental illness of other people, families, groups, formal organizations, and governments. The responses of these groups and organizations depend on how they conceptualize the problem, their beliefs about appropriate and effective responses, the competing demands on their resources, and preexisting organizational structures. Historically, most societies have struggled to balance the needs and rights of all of these stakeholders. Together with Theme 2, this theme asserts that mental illness can be analyzed at the level of the society, group, and individual, as well as across those levels.

OUR PEDAGOGICAL ORIENTATION

In addition to advancing substantive themes, the readings we have selected emphasize three pedagogical orientations. The first of these is the importance of theoretical and empirical debates to progress in sociological research on mental illness. While sociologists share a general orientation to the study of mental illness, their views differ in many specific ways. These differences are reflected in major theoretical and empirical debates that have shaped the development of sociological knowledge about mental illness. For example, early writings on the implications of mental illness for the self proposed that, once people are labeled as mentally ill, they become trapped in the mentally ill "role" by the expectations of others, and eventually come to enact that role, and its associated disruptive behaviors, so as to perpetuate the illness. Later writings disputed the assertion that careers of mental illness are caused by entry into the mentally ill role, but nevertheless presented compelling evidence that the expectation of rejection by others leads people with mental illness to withdraw from social interaction and, thereby, impedes recovery. The section introductions locate this and other major theoretical and empirical debates in the context of the evolving knowledge base.

The second pedagogical orientation is the centrality of empirical evidence to sociological research on mental illness. While sociology boasts many compelling abstract theories, those theories come to life in the real-world observations that are used to evaluate them. Sociological research studies incorporate diverse methods, including survey questionnaires, analysis of historical documents, in-depth interviews, and ethnographic observations. Each method offers unique forms of evidence with which to judge the usefulness of theories for explaining the nature, experience, and responses to mental illness. Our selections retain details of the investigators' research methods so that you can evaluate the evidence on which sociological claims are built.

Our final pedagogical orientation is the connections among research, policy, and practice. Although the primary goal of this reader is to assert a strong, balanced sociological perspective on mental health and mental illness, we hope that the readings will also help you develop informed opinions about major social policy and ethical questions regarding the experience of distress and the lives of people with serious mental illness. Developing such opinions will require that you engage deeply with the full range of experiences of mental illness, from the personal challenges faced by people who experience serious psychiatric symptoms to the societal challenges of balancing the needs and rights of individuals with those of their communities. These challenges urge us all to develop empathy for people who are distressed or who experience serious mental illness as well as for the family members, professionals, and policy makers who try to help them.

Reference

Mills, C. Wright. [1959] 2000. *The Sociological Imagination.* New York: Oxford University Press.

DEFINITIONS OF MENTAL ILLNESS

What is mental illness? How have our ideas about mental illness changed over time, and how have those changes shaped social responses to mental illness? Who participates in deciding what mental illness is and what happens when powerful stakeholders disagree? These questions orient us toward sociological perspectives on mental illness definitions.

Many sociologists advocate a social constructionist approach to the definition of mental illness. Social constructionism is a general theoretical orientation which contends that all knowledge, including our most basic taken-for-granted assumptions, is derived from and maintained in social interaction. According to social constructionists, mental illnesses are not natural phenomena waiting to be "discovered" but, rather, are socially-constructed interpretations of individual and social problems that vary by time and place. This orientation contrasts sharply with that of psychiatry, which assumes the existence of disorders that can be defined objectively.

Each of the six readings in this section highlights a different aspect of the social construction of mental illness. Conrad and Schneider present a historical overview of interpretations of mental illness, which concludes with the interpretation that dominates currently: the medical model. Bruce describes the main tenets of that model and what it offers to our understanding of mental illness. The two selections that follow—by Conrad and Figert—analyze the processes through which specific disorders are "discovered" and then added to the *Diagnostic and Statistical Manual of Mental Disorders*, the American Psychiatric Association's official classification system. Kleinman and Schulz direct our attention to the cultural basis of mental illness definitions. Taken together, these selections present a compelling argument against the notion that mental illnesses can be understood solely as objective, biologically-based experiences. As a society, we have choices about how to interpret troubling psychological and behavioral experiences, and those interpretations have consequences for individuals, families, groups, and for society itself.

What Is Mental Illness? Psychiatric Perspectives

Peter Conrad and Joseph W. Schneider

Medical Model of Madness: The Emergence of Mental Illness[†]

The first selection in this reader comes from a book by Peter Conrad and Joseph W. Schneider called Deviance and Medication: From Badness to Sickness, first published in 1980. Conrad and Schneider trace the history of the "medical model" of mental illness, which they define as a model that "locates the source of deviant behavior within the individual, postulating a physiological, constitutional, organic, or, occasionally, psychogenic agent or condition that is assumed to cause the behavioral deviance." Their history is long but worth reading in detail as it provides a persuasive account of how we came to think of madness as illness.

The roots of the medical conception of madness run deep. This chapter explores the historical origins of the concept of mental illness, its ascendance and expansion in Western society, and subsequent domination of the medical model of madness in modern times. The concept of madness as an *illness* has a long history in Western culture but has not been always the dominant explanation of madness. We carefully review the historical development of mental illness as it is the exemplar for medical conceptions of deviant behavior. It is literally the original case of medicalized deviance.

All societies seem to recognize certain forms of peculiar and unpredictable behavior as madness. Anthropologists have never discovered that mythical idyllic culture where no idea of madness existed. Cultures define madness differently, however. Grandiose ideas are acceptable among the Kwakiutl, hallucinations among Siberian Eskimos, and fears of persecution

Conrad, Peter and Joseph W. Schneider. 1992 "Medical model of madness: The emergence of mental illness." Pp. 38–72 in *Deviance and Medicalization: From Badness to Sickness*. Philadelphia: Temple University Press.

among the Dobu; all are seen as symptoms of madness by Western standards. The Yoruba of Nigeria identify 20 separate types of madness, the Iroquois recognized undesirable mental states but did not call them madness, and the Cochiti Pueblos do not distinguish between madness and physical illness at all (Kiev, 1964). The causes of madness are attributed variously to demon possession or spirit intrusion, witchcraft or sorcery, soul loss or divine retribution for taboo violation. What each culture views as the cause of madness is dependent on its worldview. In a society with a dominant spiritual or religious worldview, one would expect madness to be attributed to some spiritual offense or otherworldly beings. Cultures that have had no contact with Western psychiatry rarely define madness as an illness. It is by no means obvious that madness is mental illness or even a medical problem. Indeed, one of the primary purposes of this chapter is to analyze how madness became defined as a medical problem in Western society. The madness-as-illness concept is a product of 2,000 years of cultural and social development. We begin our search for roots in biblical Palestine.

SMITTEN BY MADNESS: ANCIENT PALESTINE

Madness was certainly recognized by the ancient Hebrews. The Bible's Old Testament serves as our best record of the era. For example, Saul's madness is described in detail in the first book of Samuel. He believed, as did most Hebrews of the time, that madness was inflicted by a supernatural power or by an angry deity as punishment for sin. There are several references in the Bible to madness as divine retribution. In Deuteronomy, Moses warned his people that if they "will not obey the voice of the Lord your God or be careful to obey all his commandments...the Lord will smite you with madness and confusion of mind."

Although the objective criteria for identifying madness among the Hebrews was "the occurrence of impulsive, uncontrolled or unreasonable behavior" (Rosen, 1968, 37), not all those who behaved abnormally were defined as mad. The prophets also acted in strange and sometimes bizarre ways, but in the context of their society they were not considered mad. Ezekiel, a sterling example, "was subject to frenzies in which he clapped his hands, stamped his feet, uttered inarticulate cries and shook his sword to and fro" (Rosen, 1968, 53). He experienced trances and visions, as well as claiming to speak with God.

Madness and prophecy both were abnormal to the Hebrews. The Hebrew verb "to behave like a prophet" also means "to rave" or "to act like one is beside oneself" (Rosen, 1968, 42). Both were attributed to divine intervention and socially ascribed to individuals. Although the mad person and the prophet alike engaged in peculiar and extreme behavior, the prophet's was attributed to divine inspiration and the mad person's to divine retribution.

From a sociological viewpoint, there is nothing inherently mad or prophetic in Ezekiel's behavior; the prophecy was attributed by his fellow Hebrews. Prophecy was an explanation available to the Hebrews for certain types of extreme behavior and an available social role for some deviants.

ROOTS OF THE MEDICAL MODEL: CLASSICAL GREECE AND ROME

The genesis of many of the ideas and conceptions in Western thought can be traced to classical Greece. Perhaps most significant for our discussion, the Greeks introduced an original rational view of nature and humanity. This contrasted sharply with the dominant religious-cosmological views of previous cultures and allowed for the developments of a primitive "science" and a naturalistic medicine. The Romans copied and expanded Greek knowledge, thus preserving it for future civilizations.

Most historians consider modern medicine to have begun with the Greeks. Hippocrates (460–377 BC), called the "Father of Medicine," combined the speculations of the philosophers of medicine who preceded him with detailed bedside observations. He was the first to attempt to explain consistently all diseases on the basis of natural causes. The maintenance of a skeptical insistence on rational knowledge and natural explanations, a pubescent scientific attitude, forms the basis of the Hippocratic tradition of medicine.

The Greeks had two explanations for madness. The cosmological-supernatural explanation—that madness was a possession caused by the gods or inflicted by the spirit underworld—was believed by most of the Greek populace. It made sense, since the mythological gods were considered part of everyday life. The natural-medical explanation, the first elaborated medical explanation in recorded history, which defined madness as a disease with natural causes, seems to have been adopted only by certain segments of the upper classes.

Greek medicine, early in its history, rejected the supernatural explanation, conceptualizing madness as a disease or the symptom of a disease with the same etiology as somatic diseases. The causes of madness were explained by the same general theory of disease used to explain all illness, humoral theory. The *humoral theory*, which held sway in medicine from the time of Hippocrates until well into the 17th century, was deceptively simple in its physiological explanation. The theory postulated the existence of four humors: blood, phlegm, black bile, yellow bile—bodily fluids whose proportion and balance were significant to health. The four humors were thought to enter into the constitution of the body and determine, by their relative proportions, a person's health and temperament. One's disposition and state of mind were determined by the balance of these humors. Madness was looked on as an imbalance of humors, usually as an excess. For example, melancholia or depression was caused by an excess of black bile, which was generated by the liver, a sudden flux of yellow bile from the spleen to the brain would bring on anxiety and produce a "choleric" temperament. The names Hippocrates used to depict madness are still common today: epilepsy, mania (abnormal excitement), melancholia (depression), and paranoia. Indeed, a residue of this idea of mental health is preserved in our everyday language when we refer to someone as being in a "bad humor."

As treatments follow from etiological or causal explanations, the medical treatments for madness, though relatively uncommon among the Greeks, were attempts to rebalance the humors. Both physical and what we might call psychotherapeutic methods were employed. Physicians recommended rest, a limited diet, and gentle massage, as well as bleeding and cupping. If there was no improvement, nonspecific stimulants such as irritant plasters, purges, vomitives, hot and cold baths, sunbathing, and other forms of heating were asided to the regimen. When psychological factors were thought to be the cause, mental exercises, games, and recreation were used. Occasionally extreme physical "treatments" were employed: severe physical restraint, violent purges, excessive bleeding, dunking the patient into cold water, and even whipping and beating (Rosen, 1968). The Romans practiced a form of "electroshock" treatment by using electric eels applied to the head. Variations on these remedies for madness can be found through modern times.

Madness in the Graeco-Roman era was viewed largely as a family problem to be dealt with by kin. People who could not function in society and were not dangerous to others were allowed to wander about and were cared for by family. Eventually some legal restrictions on the insane were enacted: Roman law forbade them to marry, acquire property, and to make or witness a will.

Physicians on the whole did not play a large role in the treatment of madness in ancient Greece and Rome. The pauper insane who wandered the countryside received no medical care and were ridiculed and stigmatized. Those who could afford it consulted physicians. Most people, however, either because of their belief in the supernatural explanation or because relief could not be obtained any other way, sought religious and magical treatments for madness.

In Greece and later in Rome, competing theories of madness existed side by side. In retrospect, it appears that medical theories were respected by the upper classes and intelligentsia, but supernatural-cosmological theories were the favored explanations of the masses. Greek medicine, by introducing a theory that would remain the major medical explanation for more than 15 centuries, actually laid the foundation for our present conceptions of madness. Roman medicine, influenced heavily by Galen, was more empirical and pragmatic, and expanded and synthesized the knowledge of Greek medicine. After the fall of Rome, the medical definition of madness became subordinate to another supernatural view of madness that arose in the medieval period.

DOMINANCE OF THE THEOLOGICAL MODEL: THE MIDDLE AGES

The collapse of the Roman Empire in the fifth century produced a general return to supernatural beliefs, mysticism, and mythology. Although theological institutions and theories were certainly dominant, medical conceptions of madness did exist during this period, even if they did not flourish. By the ninth century the medical school at Salerno, building on the Hippocratic as well as other medical traditions, had identified a number of types of mental disorders. They called them stupor, pheresy, epilepsy, hysteria, idiocy, mania, and melancholy. The first four were considered to be physical diseases.

The medieval physicians attributed madness to either of two causes, the passions or an imbalance of humors.

The therapeutic methods used by medieval physicians were similar to the Greek and Roman treatments, although they added herbal remedies like "lettuces" and "poppies" (opiates). The first psychosurgery appears to be the Byzantine physicians' treatment called "trepanning," or incising of the skull, "to permit compressed atoms of flesh to move apart and thus relieve the pressure on the brain, which they believed was causing these operable cases of insanity" (Neaman, 1975, 25).

The medical view was not the dominant conception of madness in medieval times, however. The dominant conception was a theological view based on dogmas of the Christian Church. The Church reached its pinnacle of power during this period and was the dominant institution in defining much of human affairs. Theological doctrines pervaded education, law, medicine, and just about everything else. In the theological view, which was based on the biblical tradition, all disease and other misfortune had three principal interpretations. Disease was God's mode of punishment for sin, specifically the sin of faithlessness; it was God's manner of testing an individual's strength, as with Job; or it was a sign warning the individual, and others, that he had better repent. Medieval conceptions of madness to a large degree followed from this. Madness was seen as a *punishment for sin*. Madness was not, as it is commonly thought, depicted as sin itself but was rather caused by and a retribution for sin. An interesting consequence of the theological view of madness was that an individual was not held responsible for any behavior committed while mad, but was for the behavior that caused him to be smitten with madness.

Theological and medical views of madness were not competing conceptions of reality; medical views were subordinate to theological ones. Most physicians agreed with the theologians that the first cause of disease was always God or the Devil. This produced a complex intertwining of the medical and theological conceptions of madness and created a delicate division of labor that enabled the two institutions to coexist and divide up the social control turf.

Witchcraft, Witch-hunts, and Madness

By the late 13th century enormous social changes were occurring in Europe, producing reactions from the powerful and conservative Church. Feudalism was beginning to crack and crumble; the Gutenberg printing revolution made self-education possible; the dogma and abuses by the Church were being attacked by the precursors of the Reformation: and severe plagues had decimated the population of Europe by nearly half. The dominance and authority of the Church were being threatened and a scapegoat was necessary around which theologian dogmatists could unite.

The most spectacular and devastating Church response was the infamous Inquisition and the organized witch-hunts, which led to the burning, hanging, and drowning of perhaps half a million people accused of being witches and agents of the Devil (Currie, 1968). Mad persons were not considered to be witches and subject to persecution until the 14th century. By the 15th century the Inquisition was a powerful social force, doggedly combating heresy and other deviance. At the peak of this period the *Malleus Maleficarum* (Hammer of Witches) was published in 1487. Written by two Dominican monks, Johan Sprenger and Heinrich Kramer, and with papal approval, it became the guidebook for the Inquisition. This handbook depicted most dissidents, mad people, deviants, and especially women, as "witches" who had made a compact with the Devil and were then in his employ. Anyone who showed psychological, behavioral, or physical deviation was labeled a witch or a sorcerer. The *Malleus* described in detail how to diagnose witches, try them in court, and handle those convicted, usually by burning. The *Malleus* contended that if organic cause could not be determined for a disease, the disease must be caused by witchcraft. Furthermore, if the reader was not convinced by the authors' arguments, it was because he or she, too, was a victim of witchcraft. A highly misogynic document, the *Malleus* points out: "All witchcraft comes from a carnal lust which in women is insatiable" (quoted in Alexander & Selesnick, 1966, 98). For the next 200 years in most of continental Europe, those considered insane were caught in the massive witchcraft net, and theological rationalizations caused many to be burned at the stake.

During the Inquisition period the medical conception of madness was largely muted. There was still an occasional strike for the medical viewpoint. Johann Weyer, a German physician, is considered a central figure in the history of psychiatry because of his methodical attempts to prove that witches were mentally ill and should be treated by physicians. A careful observer and investigator who interviewed both the accusers and the accused, Weyer collected data to support his case that the women persecuted as witches were really mentally sick. His research took 12 years, and in 1563 he published *De Praestigiis Daemontum* (The Deception of Demons), a detailed rebuttal to the *Malleus Maleficarum*. Weyer, in a respectful tone and still maintaining his belief in the existence of witchcraft, argued that the accused were melancholy old women. He wrote, "Those illnesses whose origins are attributed to witches come from natural causes" (quoted in Alexander & Selesnick,

1966, 121). This is depicted as a turning point by medical historians—the first stroke of a virtual renaissance, the new search for natural causes of madness. Weyer's immediate impact was not, however, that great. "He did not acquire a true following until almost a century after his death. In the meantime the spirit of the *Malleus Maleficarum* was still alive and active" (Zilboorg, 1941, 235).

The labeling of deviants as witches was possible because an ideology, witchcraft, and a powerful ecclesiastical and secular institution, the Inquisition, had been created and legitimized. This instrument of control had been devised to eradicate dissent and deviance and to protect the established order. The established order was changing, and new conceptions of deviance began to emerge.

THE EUROPEAN EXPERIENCE: MADNESS BECOMES MENTAL ILLNESS

The Renaissance brought a rediscovery of Greek and Roman art and science, including medicine. While the Graeco-Roman model, based on humoral theory, provided *physicians* with a basic medical conception of madness, it was not the dominant one in society, nor was it the basis for state policies for dealing with madness. In fact, physicians had relatively little to do with madness until the early 19th century.

There are several significant changes that occurred between the 16th and 18th centuries that affected the ascendance of the medical model of madness to its dominant position and the legitimation of physicians as the authorities to treat it. These include the great confinement of lunatics and other deviants; the separation of the able-bodied from the lunatics; the entrance of physicians: and the emergence of a unitary concept of mental illness.

The Great Confinement

Before the 17th century, harmless mad people roamed the roads of countryside and town. Although they were occasionally abused and driven from towns, they generally led a free-wandering existence. Responsibility for the mad was with the family and local community; only in rare circumstances were obviously disturbed individuals "hospitalized" or formally excluded from the community. Dangerous and criminal mad persons were handled directly by legal procedures. One interesting, although relatively uncommon, innovation was the *Narranschiff* (literally, "ship of fools"). Ships filled with mad people would sail the rivers and the seas, stopping at various towns to load or unload some of their cargo of lunatics. Prior to the 17th century, madness and folly were not hidden away and were part of everyday life.

By the middle of the 17th century the remnants of the feudal order were fading, and a new absolutist, capitalist order was emerging. This was a period of great changes in society; among these was a shift in the treatment of madness and other deviance. In 1656 Hôpital Général was opened in Paris by royal decree. This was not a hospital in the sense we think of hospital; there was no medical treatment and nearly no medical involvement. It was essentially a paupers' prison, constructed to rid the city of idlers and beggars and other socially useless individuals. Mad people, along with criminals, libertines, beggars, vagabonds, prostitutes, the unemployed, and the poor were confined there. At one point it held 1 percent of the Paris population, about 6,000 people. Over the course of its existence, the general hospital combined the characteristics of an asylum, a workhouse, and a hospital. From the outset, social control was a major function of the hospital. With the opening of Hôpital Général, the period of "the great confinement" of the poor and the deviant began (Foucault, 1965), and institutions for the deviant and "socially useless" emerged in all European countries. Confinement became the new way to deal with deviants.

Hôpital Général and its sister institutions were great moral and social edifices. Confinement was not for medical reasons but as an "imperative to labor" to prevent "mendicancy and idleness as a source of all disorders" (Foucault, 1965, 48). The obligation to work was predominant in these institutions; indeed, through this they served an important function for the new bourgeois society. They provided "cheap manpower in the periods of full employment and high salaries; and in periods of unemployment, reabsorption of the idle and social protection against agitation and uprising" (Foucault, 1965, 51). It is significant to point out that the emerging capitalist order needed "willing" workers, and these institutions served also to "discipline the work force," that is, inculcate people with the value of work and "proper" work habits, neither of which could be assumed in the 17th century.

Separation of the Able-bodied from the Lunatics

As the importance of a competent labor force increased, it became increasingly necessary to separate the able-bodied poor from the nonable-bodied. After all, how could discipline and good work habit be instilled if lunatics were around disrupting the order of the institution? The 18th century saw a gradual separation of insanity from other forms of dependence and deviance. This gave rise, by the end of the century, to special institutions like the almshouse, the workhouse, the madhouse, and the prison. The mad were separated from other deviants, not for the purposes of special treatment but rather to protect others from the "contagion" of madness (Foucault, 1965) and to impose order and discipline on the hospital and the workhouse.

Lunatics were segregated increasingly into special institutions. The first of these appeared in the 18th century. An extensive "trade in lunacy," private madhouses owned and operated by physicians ("mad-doctors"), developed in England (Parry-Jones, 1972). These madhouses were "frequently a lucrative business dealing with the most acutely disturbed and refractory cases" (Scull, 1977) and were the precursors to the public asylums that developed a

century later. Overall, from a sociological viewpoint, the separation and segregation of the mad from other deviants was accomplished largely for social
and economic reasons, not for medical ones.

Entrance of the Physician

As noted earlier, the early institutions for the mad were not medical institutions. Through the 18th century, physicians played a small role in the
confinement and provided little treatment. In England it was not until 1774
that a physician's certificate was required for commitment to a madhouse;
until then, the judgment of a magistrate was sufficient. It was not apparent
to the judicial and political powers or to the potential clientele that physicians had any special expertise in the area of madness. Eighteenth-century
physicians did not have any explanatory theories or curative treatments that
could have made madness and the madhouse ipso facto their legitimate turf.
How did physicians become the keepers of the madhouse and ultimately the
legitimate authorities on madness?

Certainly, if physicians could provide useful curative and rehabilitative
treatments, then it would be clear why medicine came to dominate the realm
of madness. But this does not seem to be the case. Most of the therapies
used by the 18th-century physicians were ancient ones: bloodletting, dunking, and purgation were popular treatments. Fear, restraint, starvation, and
castration were also used as treatments, as were diets and a few available
drugs. New innovations, usually physical treatments, such as the "Darwin
chair" (invented by Charles Darwin's grandfather), were introduced. "In this
chair the insane were rotated until blood oozed from their mouths, ears and
noses, and for years most successful cures were reported as a result of its
use" (Ackerknecht, 1968. p. 38). Although this primitive "shock therapy" may
have aided a few disordered people, the 18th-century physician's armamen-
tarium and ability to "cure" were limited.

There was, however, considerable optimism concerning the promise of
medicine to solve problems of human suffering and pain.

> The intellectual approach to the problems of health gave the illusion that in
> medicine, as in other social sciences, the Age of Reason would mark the begin-
> ning of a new era. (Dubos, 1959, 18)

Undoubtedly some of this optimism was transferred to the physicians who
treated madness. Although limited in therapeutic ability, by the end of the
18th century the physician had become essential to the madhouse. Since
medical certificates were required for confinement of lunatics, the physician
became the gatekeeper of madness, in change of entry.

Perhaps one of the most dramatic images in the history of the treatment
of madness is Philippe Pinel, the great humanitarian director of the French
asylums at Bicêtre and Salpêtriêtre, removing the chains of the mad and liberating them from physical bondage in 1794. In 1801 he wrote a basic text

in "psychiatry," *Traite médico-philosophique sur l' aliénation mentale ou la manie* (Treatise on Insanity). Pinel emphasized the role of heredity as the first cause of, and social and psychological factors as contributory to, the development of madness. Pinel presented a classification of mental disease: melancholia, mania, dementia, and idiocy. According to him, these were located in the region of the stomach. Of greatest importance to Pinel were the principles underlying the organization and administration of institutions, beginning with the separation of different types of patients. He rejected chains, used minimum constraints, urged the importance of studying the patient's personality, and believed in the maintenance of constant routine. He stressed the benefits of *moral treatment*, which included kindness, careful coercion, and work therapy.

A contemporary and admirer of Pinel was Englishman William Tuke, a lay Quaker who founded York Retreat. Tuke developed his own brand of moral treatment. His institution, run by lay people, represented an alternative to the ascending medical perspective. Therapy at York Retreat was much more of an educational process, a pragmatic attempt to teach moral values and self-control, to remove obstacles that impeded the "natural" recovery process. "Moral treatment actively sought to transform the lunatic, to remodel him into something approximating the bourgeois ideal of the rational individual" (Scull, 1975, 227). The rate of recovery (Tuke never used the word "cure") at York, largely due to humane and kind treatment, was probably better than at most other English madhouses.

Since moral treatment seemed to work, the medical profession had to find a way to accommodate it. Physicians presented the argument that medical and moral treatments were necessary for recovery, and since only physicians had the legitimate authority to dispense medical treatments, they were the natural ones to employ or at least oversee moral treatment also. Since the physicians were relatively organized and the moral treatment people were not, they were successful at convincing Parliament to have their position officially legislated as the dominant one. The mere fact that they had to persuade the legislators is telling.

The fact that those administrating moral treatment were already using a quasimedical vocabulary—"patients," "mental illness," "recovery," "treatment," etc.—probably made it easier. Through testimony, and one suspects lobbying, physicians were able to ensure that they themselves would regulate the madhouses by the enactment of a variety of parliamentary acts (e.g., requiring medical inspection) between 1816 and 1845. This solidified their legal position as the official controllers of madness (Scull, 1975). In a real sense they "captured" madness as their domain, and clarified and extended their "authority in this area, so as to develop an official monopoly of the right to define (mental) health and illness" (Scull, 1975). By 1830 nearly all public mental hospitals had a resident medical director. This was a coup for the medical profession, since as this point they had little better to offer in terms of treatments for insanity.

THE 19TH-CENTURY AMERICAN EXPERIENCE: THE INSTITUTIONALIZATION OF MENTAL ILLNESS

In colonial America, much like contemporary Europe, insanity was seen as a kinship or constitutional matter. The "harmless" dependent insane were dealt with like other paupers, the well-to-do insane were cared for by their families, and the violent or criminal insane were punished as criminals. Public provision for the dependent insane rarely included medical treatment. Public concern was mostly about the dangerous "lunatick," who was variously found in stocks, pillories, and jails. The colonists "conceived of the family, the church and the network of community relations as important weapons against sin and crime" and madness (Rothman, 1971, 16).

The first general hospital in America, Pennsylvania Hospital, was founded by the Quakers in 1756. There were some mad people among the sick persons admitted, although they were confined to the cellar. The treatments employed were the medical treatments for insanity common at the time. "Their scalps were shaved and blistered; they were bled to the point of syncope; purged until the alimentary canal failed to yield anything but mucus, and in intervals, they were chained by the waist or ankle to the cell wall" (Deutsch, 1949, 60). It was a local custom for townspeople to come and gaze at the lunatics for a small fee. (This actually continued in some form until 1822.) One suspects that this stigmatized the mad, at the same time providing a warning for those who psychically strayed from the straight and narrow path.

The colonial governor of Virginia became concerned with the treatment of madness and the "case of the poor lunaticks." Beginning in 1766 he appealed regularly to the legislature to construct an asylum so that lunatics need not be confined to the Williamsburg jail. In 1769 the legislature passed an act "to make provision for the Support and Maintenance of Ideots, Lunaticks and other persons of unsound Minds" (Deutsch, 1949, 70). In 1773 the Public Hospital for Persons of Insane and Disordered Minds (the Williamsburg Lunatic Asylum), the first hospital exclusively for the insane, was opened in Williamsburg. Insanity was determined by three magistrates, and no provision was made for a medical examination. The Williamsburg Lunatic Asylum was meant to be a last resort. Its primary task was to keep the peace of the community and to constrain the insane from wandering about. This remained the only public lunatic asylum for 50 years.

The confinement of the insane has three sources of *legitimacy* in the Anglo-American political system (Kittrie, 1971). These principles were first developed in English law and were adopted by the colonists and later by the founders of the Republic as the basis of American law. They serve as the legal rationale for involuntary incarceration. The first source of legitimacy is the "police power" of the state to protect the peace and ensure public welfare. This was used with the violent and the "furiously mad." The second source is *parens patriae*, the principle that the state could assume guardianship of a person who was legally "disabled" and declared incompetent and could control his or her property. The third source is the state's power over the indigent members of the pauper community. This is an extension of the English concept of the Crown's responsibility for the destitute. Most confinement in the 19th century was in the name of parens patriae, with the physician as wiseman and guardian.

Benjamin Rush is widely considered the "Father of American Psychiatry." He was a signer of the Declaration of Independence, a respected reformer, and a well-known physician when he was appointed to Pennsylvania Hospital in 1783. He was firmly convinced that "the patients afflicted by madness should be the first objects of care of the physicians of the Pennsylvania Hospital" (Deutsch, 1949, 77). Rush's own theory was that madness was an arterial disease having its primary seat in the brain. Hence his treatments of purgatives, diets, hot and cold showers, and bloodletting were aimed at affecting the circulation of blood. Actually Rush was ambivalent about therapy and punishment, often not clearly distinguishing between them. He believed that physicians had to gain complete control, authority, and power over the mad person. Some of his writings make it apparent that he viewed the insane as wild beasts who needed to be tamed with "wild and terrifying modes of punishment." At other times his writing takes on a flavor of the kindness of moral treatment. Rush's crowning achievement was the publication in 1812 of *Medical Inquiries and Observations Upon the Disease of Mind*, the first American textbook in psychiatry. This was the only American work of its kind for 70 years.

We can also consider Rush as the "Father of the Medicalization of Deviance." He had a rather broad notion of madness. In his autobiography he wrote. "Chagrin, shame, fear, terror, hunger, until for legal acts, are transient madness. . . . Suicide is madness. . . . Sanity (is an) aptitude to judge things like other men, and regular habits, etc. Insanity [is] a departure from this" (quoted in Szasz, 1970, 141). Naturally he viewed physicians as the best judges of insanity. Rush defined a variety of nonconforming and deviant behaviors as medical problems: he depicted lying, drunkenness, crime, and even opposing the Revolution as diseases (the latter he dubbed "revolutiona"). He was an early and active abolitionist, although partly basing his conviction on his belief that blacks had a disease, "Negritude," that was inherited from ancestors with leprosy and had turned their skins dark. Rush saw disease in any behavior not complying with his particular worldview. As Szasz (1970) notes, "His eyes thus beheld the world in terms of sickness and health" (140).

Asylum-Building Movements: A New "Cure" for Insanity

During the second quarter of the 19th century a virtual epidemic of state asylum building took place. In 1824 there were two state asylums, but by 1860, 28 of the 33 states had public institutions for the insane, a 14-fold increase. It seems that the asylum was an idea whose time had come; institutionalization became the treatment of choice for insanity. Why did this occur at this time in history? And how does this relate to the medical conception of mental illness?

We first need to examine the perceived causes of madness in early 19th-century America. By the third decade the old order of American society was passing and was rapidly being replaced with a new one. The Jacksonian period (1828–1836) was characterized by an increase in social mobility and political participation, increased religious and intellectual freedom and enthusiasm, and a greater geographical mobility for the population. These changes, according to David Rothman (1971), created a pervasive anxiety in America. It was believed that the old social order was vanishing and that a new, more fluid, potentially chaotic order was taking its place. Students of deviant behavior in this era thought that erosion in the discipline and order of the family was the primary cause of deviant behavior.

Insanity was viewed by physicians, and most explicitly by the medical superintendents of the new institutions, as a biological disease of the brain that was "socially caused" or at least precipitated by social forces. Such factors as lack of discipline, social mobility, disappointed ambition, or economic depression were cited frequently. Although these physicians were convinced that organic lesions existed, they, unlike their European contemporaries, had no interest in biological or anatomical research. The first cause was in the social system, not the body. Insanity was a disease of civilization; any man or woman could succumb to it. Lunatics were not considered a special breed of people. One corollary of these doctrines was that if the source of madness resided in society rather than the individual, then society had a responsibility for these people. Social measures could and should be taken to alleviate and correct the sufferer's condition.

Theories of environmental cause of insanity gave birth to a new belief that insanity was curable. All that was required was to design a proper curative environment to overcome the social order, tensions, and chaos. The needs of the insane could be met by isolating them from the community and developing a model society, which would exemplify the advantages of an orderly, disciplined routine. The physicians of insanity believed they had discovered its cure. This was the invention of the insane asylum (Rothman, 1971).

The 1830s and 1840s was a utopian era in the United States. Isolated "utopian communities" such as the transcendentalist Brook Farm and the Oneida community were founded as models of a more perfect community; the celibate Shakers lived in over a dozen flourishing settlements during this peak period. The asylum movement sprang from similar utopian ideals, endeavoring to create a model society. Those who championed it were believers in asylums as great reforms and vehicles for creating a better society. Now, the reformers said, the asylum would be the curative environment, not merely a prison for the insane.

This was an optimistic time for physicians of the insane. Reports of recovery rates from some of the early asylums were astounding. A report issued by Hartford Retreat in 1827 announced that 21 of 23 new cases of insanity, an amazing 91 percent, had been cured. The newspapers publicized the report, and this marked the beginning of a curability craze that would last nearly two decades. A "cult of curability" swept the madness world. The "asylum cure" was the rule, not the exception. Reports from medical superintendents of asylums regularly claimed 80 percent to 90 percent and even 100 percent cure rates. It was a virtual contest of figures. Interestingly, these statistics went unchallenged until 1877, when Pliny Earle, an asylum superintendent from Massachusetts, pointed out that the figures were reports of recovery of cases and not persons, and that some of the impressive cure rates represented the ratio of recoveries to patients discharged, not admitted (American Psychiatric Association, 1976). One patient had been discharged 48 times with 48 cures.

The "asylum cure" consisted of (1) removal of the insane from the community, the alleged cause of mental disease; (2) confinement in an institution that was itself separate from the community (leading to the building of asylums with big lawns on the rural fringes); and (3) creation of an order in the asylum to compensate for the fluidity and disorder in society, an American version of moral treatment. As Rothman (1971) points out, the medical superintendents designed their asylums as an attempt in reconstitute the 18th-century virtues they perceived lacking in the changing society:

> They would teach discipline, a sense of limits and a satisfaction with one's position.... The psychiatrists...conceived of proper individual behavior and social relationships only in terms of a personal respect for authority and tradition and an acceptance of one's station in the ranks of society. In this sense they were trying to recreate in the asylum their own vision of the colonial community. The results, however, were very different. Regimentation, punctuality, and precision became the asylum's basic traits and these qualities were for more in keeping with an urban, industrial order than a local, agrarian one (154).

Probably without knowing it, and certainly without intention, the physicians in the asylums were preparing their charges for an impending order, rather than restoring them to past values. In America, as well as Europe, the asylum, though humanizing the treatment of the insane, also became an institution that attempted to instill the discipline necessary for industrial capitalist labor.

The ideas of the asylum and the asylum cure needed proponents to spread the word. Dorothea Dix, an energetic former schoolteacher, was "shocked" by the conditions of the mentally ill kept in almshouses and jails. She was undoubtedly the foremost champion of separate public asylums for the insane. For many years after 1841 she toured the country, visiting institutions and lobbying with legislators for the development of state hospitals. "Her formula was simple and she repeated it everywhere: first assert the curability of insanity, link it directly in proper institutional care, and then quote prevailing medical opinion on rates of recoveries" Rothman, 1971, 132). Her success was remarkable. By 1880 there were 75 state asylums, 52 of which were founded as a direct result of her efforts.

She also popularized the medical concept of madness and championed the idea that medical psychologists, as they were called, were the proper restorers of sanity.

In 1844, 13 superintendents of insane asylums organized the Association of Medical Superintendents of American Institutions of the Insane to aid in communication of knowledge and information and set standards for treatment. This organization was the forerunner of the American Psychiatric Association (the name was changed in 1921) and served both as a political force and a professional body. They published the *American Journal of Insanity*, which became the predominant journal in its field. American psychiatry developed very much as administrative psychiatry, and in its early years the association was more interested in asylum architecture, vocational therapy, and cure rates than medical research. Nonetheless, it quickly became the authoritative voice of medical opinion on insanity. The association provided the legitimation of American psychiatry as a medical specialty. "By insisting that special skills and knowledge were required for treating mental illness, psychiatrists were able to justify the exclusion of all other persons having no formal training and instruction in this specialty" (Grob, 1970, 312).

By the 1850s the optimism began to wane. Many institutions had never reached the curability rates claimed by others; "incurables" were backlogging and overcrowding asylums, and some Eastern institutions were being flooded with immigrants who were considered by some physicians as "incurable." Many deranged individuals who had resided in almshouses were transferred to asylums. The pressures of rising admissions made moral treatment increasingly difficult. By 1852 the population of Worcester State Lunatic Hospital in Massachusetts had risen to 500 and the physician-patient ratio had dropped significantly (Grob, 1970). Moral treatment, which was possible and to some degree successful, in an asylum of 120 inmates, was impossible in an institution of over 500. Gradually most of the institutions reverted to custodial care and the use of restraints for the "incurables," with the medical directors and legislators rationalizing that it was better than jail. Drugs (e.g., sedatives) and restraints became ends in themselves, not adjuncts to a therapeutic program. Some treatment was available for those recently diagnosed insane, but if they did not recover in a reasonable time, they were deemed incurable and relegated to the custodial section of the asylum. If the hospital could not be justified in terms of numbers of cured, then the easiest way to justify appropriations and the existence of the institution to the legislature was to request funds for providing accommodations and care for the growing number of chronically insane (Grob, 1970). By the late 19th century most asylums were largely custodial enterprises, with medical superintendents serving as gatekeepers and guardians.

With the end of the cult of curability, somatic or physiological pessimism replaced the more optimistic theories of social causation espoused by early asylum superintendents. The disillusionment with the asylum cure and the rise of Darwinian theory gave credence to a new idea—the degeneration hypothesis. This hypothesis stated that there is a degeneration from the normal human type through generations, transmitted by heredity, which deteriorates progressively toward extinction (Ackerknecht, 1968). This rather pessimistic view of mental illness emerged largely in Europe, especially under the influence of Benedict Augustin Morel; but it serves well as an example of the type of medical theories of madness developed at this time. Italian physician Cesare Lombroso proposed his own ideas based on the degeneration hypothesis in his writings on the "born criminal."

In terms of the history of the medical conception of madness, the 19th century was a significant period. In the United States, as in England, madness moved once and for all into medical turf. Alienists (as physicians of the insane were called), with the aid of champions like Dorothea Dix, were able to gain a monopoly over the definition and treatment of madness. All new asylums were run by medical superintendents. Medical men did not have "scientific" evidence of mental disease, nor did their asylum qua hospital offer a medical cure. In fact, both their causes and cures were specifically social. Medicine was embraced as much for its humanitarian "moral treatment" as for any technical expertise. By the time the early optimism of asylum cures had waned, medicine had secured control over the domain of insanity. Again, we point out, this was accomplished without physiological evidence for cause and before the advent of successful "medical" treatments. In America as in Europe, medical dominance of madness was a social and political rather than a scientific achievement.

THE SCIENCE OF MENTAL DISEASE

The science of mental disease developed in the asylum. The demise of the cult of curability and the constricted morality of the Victorian era supported the pessimism among the physicians of the insane. This pessimism, along with the apparent success of medicine in controlling infectious diseases and an increasing concern about the incurable immigrant insane, led psychiatrists to abandon their environmental approaches and become heavily somatic. Physicians, armed with the microscope, looked increasingly to the brain, spinal cord, and nervous system for the cause of madness. Masturbation was viewed as a cause of insanity, but it was the weakening of the nervous system and the hypothesized organic lesions produced by such "venereal indulgence" that were believed the source of insanity (see Englehardt, 1974).

The somatic approach, with one significant exception, was not particularly fruitful. The discovery of *general paresis*, a type of madness caused by a neurological breakdown in third-stage syphilis, is considered by some as medicine's "greatest triumph in the field of behavior disorders" (White, 1964, 16), and by others as providing a rationalization for the disease concept of madness (Szasz, 1976). No doubt it was a great achievement.

It followed the discoveries of Pasteur, Koch, and Lister, which had aided in the mastery of other infectious diseases. The "symptom complex" of this disorder was first described by Esquirol as early as 1805, but actual connection with syphilis as a causal agent was not made until 1894 and confirmed through a variety of clinical and microbial studies over the next two decades. When Nogochi and Moore in 1913 found *Treponema pallidum*, the infectious agent of syphilis, in nerve-cell layers of the patient's cortex, any lingering doubts that syphilis was the cause of this type of insanity were erased. Medicine finally had empirical evidence for the cause of at least one type of insanity. This provided "proof" that the medical concept of madness must be correct. If a physiological cause for one type of insanity had been found, then modern medicine would, in time, discover the causes of all mental illness. This was undoubtedly a vindication for the medical model of madness.

Late 19th-century psychiatry took its cues from its more successful sibling, somatic medicine. Alienists or psychiatrists needed only to use more tools of somatic medicine and soon they, too, would be able to discover physiological causes for all mental disease, just as for general paresis. Emil Kraepelin, a German alienist with a gift for observation and synthesis, engaged in detailed studies of "natural histories" of asylum patients. With the publication of *Psychiatrie*, which went through several revisions between 1883 and 1913, Kraepelin changed the classification system of mental illness. His descriptions of the symptom complexes of dementia praecox and manic-depressive psychosis, the two major categories of mental disorder, are still used today. He believed that dementia praecox (literally, early senility) was characterized by progressive deterioration and that manic depression (severe uncontrollable mood swings) tended to improve and recur spontaneously. Kraepelin, fully committed to the medical model, proposed only organic etiologies for mental disorders and viewed them as physical diseases. Eugen Bleuler noted that all dementia patients do not inevitably degenerate, and in 1911 he created a modified and expanded category he called *schizophrenia*. The great concern for classification of mental illness characterizes the development of psychiatry.

Freud, Psychoanalysis, and Medicalization

In 1909 Sigmund Freud, a Viennese physician and neurologist, delivered a series of five lectures at Clark University in Worcester, Massachusetts. He presented a theory of the human mind that he had developed over the previous two decades. As a result of Freud's visit and ideas, American psychiatry has never been the name. Freud's theory, which he based largely on his work with neurotic disorders such as hysteria that are rarely seen in the asylum, appears at least on the surface to be a break with the medical concept of mental disease. He suggested that mental symptoms were intelligible but distorted results of the individual's struggles with internal impulses. He assumed these symptoms arose from conflicts between biogenic drives such as sex and aggression and sociocultural forces. These conflicts usually involved parents, occurred during early childhood, and were repressed into "the unconscious." "He perceived his patients not as examples of brain disease, not victims of hereditary nervous weakness, but as troubled human beings whose strivings, hopes, fears, daydreams, and intimate feelings were mixing them up and destroying their health and happiness" (White, 1964, 38). His method of treatment was psychoanalysis, a talking cure based on a series of conversations (an hour daily for several years) in which the patient was encouraged to "free associate," say whatever came to mind, and relive and resolve past conflicts in the safety of the relationship with the therapist. This revelation and catharsis would enable the patient to develop "insight" into his or her difficulties, understand the roots of the "illness," and hopefully have a "corrective emotional experience." He gave an entirely new understanding to human problems and substituted a psychogenic explanation for a biogenic determinism.

Freud's break with the medical conception of madness was far from complete. In fact, the Freudian model of madness was grafted onto the existing medical model with little difficulty. Freud was trained as a physician-neurologist and moved slowly from organic and physically determined theories about mental illness to psychological and, to a degree, sociocultural theories of cause. No doubt his training as a physician affected the types of theories and treatments he developed. The people he saw were "patients" and they had "illnesses," albeit psychological ones, which therapy attempted to cure. His theory located the source of problems inside the patients' heads, and his treatment was individualistic. Treatment would occur in the consulting room, with the patient on the couch and the physician present in the room but not in the patient's sight. Freud himself never abandoned the notion that all psychological illness must be attributable ultimately to neurological process and could, like somatic diseases, someday be treated with pills and injections. In practice, however, because no such treatments were available, his work and practice were carried out on a purely psychological level (Ackerknecht, 1968, 93).

Freud and his early followers (e.g., Adler, Jung, Ferenczi) did not deal with the same types of madness that Kraepelin and the other asylum alienists had. Asylum inmates were too disturbed for Freud's theory. Most Freudians were concerned with what are called neurotic disorders such as hysteria, obsessions, compulsions, and phobias that kept people from optimal functioning. Freud did not investigate severely disturbed people suffering the insanity now called psychoses (including schizophrenia and manic depression), until his later years. When he did, he found these disorders inaccessible to psychoanalysis and that these patients lacked "insight" into their difficulties. Only in the 1930s did psychiatrists like Frieda Fromm-Reichman and Harry Stack Sullivan bring psychoanalysis to the inmates of the asylum.

The effect of Freud on American psychiatry was enormous. The first psychoanalytic institute was founded in New York in 1931, and eventually there were a dozen psychoanalytic centers in major cities. No one could study psychiatry, psychology, or social work, without encountering his theories and techniques and those of some of his followers. Psychoanalysts became an elite of the American Psychiatric Association. In fact, psychoanalysis became largely the property of medical psychiatry. Freud had not wanted it that way. "He had 'only unwillingly taken up the profession of medicine'; in fact, Freud had a low opinion of physicians. They were merchants, trading in the mitigation of miseries they scarcely attempted to understand" (Rieff, 1966, 83). Freud spoke out several times in his life in support of lay (nonmedical) analysis, but American psychoanalysts created a medical monopoly and trained only physicians.[1] This further medicalized psychoanalytic theory and therapy.

Freud and his followers both muted and extended the medical model of madness. They muted it by their emphasis on the intrapsychic nature of mental symptoms and psychological illnesses and by their attention to family and childhood experiences. Yet because Freudian theory was grafted onto the existing medical model, it expanded greatly the notions of mental disease. This model of psychological illness included all deviant behavior and emotional problems that were not organic in origin: essentially all human behavior problems but general paresis, senility, and organic brain syndrome. Madness, hysteria, obsessions, compulsion, phobias, anxiety, homosexuality, drunkenness, sexual deviation, chronic misbehavior in children, and delinquency, among others, were all psychological illnesses and subject to medical-psychiatric treatment.

The psychogenic movement, led by Freud and his followers, infused psychiatry with a new sense of optimism, replacing the somatic pessimism of the late 19th century. Freud's theories and techniques for the first time made it possible for physicians to spend their time understanding the patient's psyches, rather than manipulating their bodies or creating moral environments in asylums in which they resided. The Freudian "revolution" was not, however, supported by all psychiatrists. There were, more specifically, somaticists still to be heard from. The somaticism that developed in the 1930s took three forms: "shock" therapies, lobotomies, and genetic theories of mental illness.

Reappearance of the Somaticists

Manfred Sakel, a German physician who had been using insulin to treat morphine addiction, in 1929 noticed some apparent psychological improvement in a patient following a convulsion and coma produced by an accidental overdose of insulin. He extended his research and treatments to schizophrenia and reported some success at reducing overt symptoms. Over the next two decades insulin shock therapy became a common physiological treatment

---

[1] Some of the most distinguished psychoanalysts were lay analysts who were trained in Europe; for example, Erich Erikson, Erich Fromm, and Anna Freud.

for schizophrenia (Horowitz, 1959). Insulin shock had some inherent dangers, was rather expensive and time-consuming, since patients needed continuous nursing care and observation, and yielded unreliable results. In 1938 two Italian physicians, Ugo Cerletti and L. Bini, introduced an "easier" technique, electroconvulsive therapy (ECT), or, simply, electroshock. This technique consists of applying electrodes to the patient's head and passing moderate electrical currents (70 to 130 volts) through the brain for a few seconds. The patient suffers a brief but violent convulsion, loses consciousness, and on reawakening has an amnesia (memory loss) for recent events, which lasts for several weeks or months. Shock treatments are given in a series over a period of weeks. Early medical practitioners of this method advocated it for patients with schizophrenia, but it has not proven particularly useful for this diagnosis. Some recent advocates limit its use to mood disorders such as mania and depression. This crude and violent treatment is used today and remains controversial. There is no accepted explanation of how it works.

In 1935 Antonio Egas Moniz, a Portuguese neurologist, introduced the psychosurgery known as prefrontal lobotomy to the psychiatric world. Moniz believed that the fixed ideas and repetitive behavior seen in some mental patients were accompanied by abnormal cellular connections in the brain. His theory suggested that "morbid" thoughts were a result of brain disease and hence the appropriate treatment was brain surgery.

The method that Moniz conceived of as "curative" for this supposed brain damage was lobotomy, a surgical procedure that severed some of the neural connections between the frontal lobes and other parts of the brain. Although immersed in controversy from the start, lobotomy became a common treatment, and advocates such as American neurologist Walter Freeman operated on thousands of institutionalized mental patients. Moniz was awarded the Nobel Prize in 1949 for his work. Supporters claimed cure in a third and improvement in another third of lobotomized patients (Freeman, 1959), but critics claimed the "cure" was worse than the "disease." Many lobotomized patients showed marked irreversible deterioration in personality, difficulty in generalizing and abstract thinking, and an overall passivity, and remained institutionalized; in short, they became "zombies." For this reason, and because of the availability of tranquilizing drugs, by the early 1950s lobotomy fell into disrepute. Up until that time, however, approximately 40,000 to 50,000 such operations were performed in the United States. In the late 1960s a new and more technologically sophisticated variant of psychosurgery emerged, including laser technology and brain implants, and was heralded by some as a treatment for uncontrollable violent outbursts.

To summarize briefly, the discovery of general paresis symbolized medical vindication for somatic bases of mental illness. Freud and his followers both muted and extended the medical model of madness, whereas Kraepelin and the "new" somaticists attempted to develop scientific theories and data to support medical contentions. The total effect broadened and deepened professional interest in the medical model of human problems and the commitment to medical solutions for them.

THE THIRD REVOLUTION IN MENTAL HEALTH

In the early 1950s psychiatry in the United States was characterized by a "psychotherapeutic ideology" (Armer & Klerman, 1968), based essentially on the Freudian principles that madness is a result of childhood experiences and rooted in intrapsychic conflicts. Psychotherapy, though not often available in large state mental hospitals, was considered the treatment of choice. There were somatically oriented psychiatrists as well, who maintained a physiological model of madness and whose major forms of treatment were insulin and electroshock therapies. The majority of patients in large, overcrowded state institutions received no treatment at all beyond custodial care and were warehoused on "back wards." By 1955 this all began to change.

Psychotropic Medication

The use of drugs for madness has a long history. Vomitives, purgatives, neurotics, and others were used in the 19th century. The 20th century saw the development of "sedatives" to control problem patients. But it was not until the middle 1950s that drugs became a central part of psychiatric treatment. The impact of the new psychotropic drugs on psychiatry and mental hospitals has been termed by medical historians the third revolution in mental health. (Pinel's contribution is considered the first, psychoanalysis, the second.)

In France, in 1952, a newly synthesized drug, chlorpromazine, was developed. It was the first of the psychotropic drugs: chemicals that exert their principal effect on a person's mind, thought, or behavior. They did not sedate in the traditional sense. These drugs, also called phenothiazines or major tranquilizers, were considered antipsychotic drugs because they did not impair consciousness as did sedatives. They enabled, to varying degrees, mad people to function better. The popularity of the drugs took hold slowly but soon spread rapidly, first in Europe and them in the United States.

In May, 1954, the pharmaceutical corporation Smith, Kline, & French (SKF) introduced chlorpromazine under the trade name Thorazine in the United States. It was aggressively marketed by a special SKF taskforce of 50 salespeople, who, armed with promising research reports and testimonies from psychiatrists, set out to convince state legislatures (who were responsible for the then minimal drug budgets for state hospitals) and hospital administrators of the utility of Thorazine. This extensive promotion campaign was highly successful (Swazey, 1974):

> The drug impact...was rapid and profound. Within 8 months Thorazine was given to an estimated two million patients. A stream of professional publications, now totaling over 14,000, began to describe the drug's "revolutionary" impact on mental hospitals. The mass media hailed [it]...as a "miracle drug." (160)

Thorazine was soon joined by a sister medication, reserpine (and by 1969, 830 other psychotropic drugs [Swazey, 1974, 30]). Under the directorship of

Henry Brill, an early and active supporter of pharmacological treatment, New York became the first state mental health system to introduce the drugs en masse. By 1957 the psychiatric response was enthusiastic. Wards became quieter, "delusions" decreased, and institutions ran more smoothly. Perhaps most important, more patients were being discharged from mental hospitals.

A new feeling of optimism permeated the psychiatric world. Because of the dominant "psychotherapeutic ideology," many psychiatrists in the early 1950s embraced drug treatment because they believed with the aid of medications, "now we can really do psychotherapy with the mentally ill." Mental hospital staffs developed an increased medical orientation in their work. In fact, psychiatrist Jerome Frank (1974) suggests that the greatest effect of the drug revolution was on the staff and not the patients. The staff developed a more optimistic outlook and became more willing to interact with the patients. Talk of truly therapeutic rather than custodial hospitals was legion. Within a decade, however, the notions of "really doing psychotherapy" were replaced by the reality that the dispensing of drugs, called chemotherapy, would itself be the major form of treatment for most patients.

There were some critics of drug treatment who argued that drugs only masked the symptoms and did not treat causes; others suggested they were "chemical straightjackets," merely pharmaceutical social control mechanisms. The critics of drug treatments were a distinct minority, however, and the declining populations of mental hospitals relegated their critique to gadfly status.

By the mid-1950s the psychopharmacological revolution in mental health had been proclaimed. Psychiatrists could now act like "real physicians" and dispense medications for mental ills. The drug treatment itself lent support to beliefs that madness was an illness that could be treated by drugs. A few even viewed it as a cure for mental illness. Drugs qua medications suited perfectly the rhetoric of medicine in the treatment of madness.

SUMMARY

There are a few recurrent themes in our history of the medical concept of madness. Medical theories have located the source of madness in a variety of somatic organs: the humors, the stomach, the nervous system, the brain. Every era seems to have its own reform movements that lead to an increased optimism, which several years later, after the movements fall to live up to their promise, reverts to a pessimistic view of madness. This has often taken the form of a "somatic pessimism," locating the causes of madness in the physiology (e.g., the degeneration hypothesis). Medical involvement with madness, historically speaking, emerges more as a humanitarian reform than as a biomedical accomplishment. It is worth repeating that medical concepts became the dominant conceptions of madness long before there was any evidence that madness had any biophysiological components (and this is still controversial in some circles), and before any medical treatments, other than the nonmedical moral treatment, made any impact on madness. The development of the medical model of madness was a social and political rather than a scientific achievement.

References

Ackerknecht, Erwin H. 1968. *A Short History of Psychiatry.* New York: Hafner Press.

Alexander, Franz G., and S. T. Selesnick. 1966. *The History of Psychiatry.* New York: New American Library.

Armer, David J., and Gerald L. Klerman. 1968. "Psychiatric Treatment Ideologies and Professional Ideology." *Journal of Health and Social Behavior* 9:243–255.

Currie, Elliott P. 1968. "Crimes without Criminals: Witchcraft and its control in renaissance Europe." *Law and Society Review* 3:7–32.

Deutsch, Albert. 1949. *The Mentally Ill in America.* 2d ed. New York: Columbia University Press.

Dubos, René. 1959. *Mirage of Health.* New York: Harper & Row.

Englehardt, H. Tristram. 1974. "The Disease of Masturbation: Values and the Concept of Disease." *Bulletin of the History of Medicine* 48:234–248.

Foucault, Michel. 1965. *Madness and Civilization.* New York: Random House.

Frank, Jerome D. 1974. *Persuasion and Healing.* New York: Schocken Books.

Freeman, Walter. 1959. "Psychosurgery." In *American Handbook of Psychiatry,* vol. 2, edited by S. Arieti. New York: Basic Books, Inc.

Grob, Gerald N. 1970. "The State Hospital in Mid-Nineteenth –Century America: A Social Analysis." In *Social Psychology and Mental Health,* edited by H. Wechsler, L. Solomon, & B. M. Kramer. New York: Holt, Rinehart & Winston.

Horowitz, W. A. 1959. "Insulin Shock Therapy." In *American Handbook of Psychiatry,* vol. 2, edited by S. Arieti. New York: Basic Books, Inc.

Kiev, A. 1964. *Magic, Faith, and Healing.* New York: The Free Press.

Kittrie, Nicholas N. 1971. *The Right to be Different: Deviance and Enforced Therapy.* Baltimore: Johns Hopkins University Press.

Neaman, Judith S. 1975. *Suggestion of the Devil.* New York: Anchor Press.

Parry-Jones, William Ll. 1972. *The Trade in Lunacy.* London: Routledge & Kegan Paul Ltd.

Rieff, Philip. 1966. *Triumph of the Theraputic.* New York: Harper & Row

Rosen, George. 1968. *Madness in Society.* New York: Harper & Row.

Rothman, David. J. 1971. *The Discovery of the Asylum.* Boston: Little, Brown & Co.

Scull, Andrew. 1975. "From Madness to Mental Illness: Medical Men as Moral Entrepreneurs." *European Journal of Sociology* 16:218–261.

Scull, Andrew. 1977. "Madness and Segregative Control: The Rise of the Insane Asylum." *Social Problems* 24:337–351.

Swazey, Judith P. 1974. *Chlorpromazine in Psychiatry.* Cambridge, MA: Massachusetts Institute of Technology Press.

Szasz, Thomas S. 1970. *The Manufacture of Madness.* New York: Harper & Row.

Szasz, Thomas S. 1976. *Schizophrenia: The Sacred Symbol of Psychiatry.* New York: Basic Books.

White, Robert W. 1964. *The Abnormal Personality.* 3rd ed. New York: Ronald Press.

Zilboorg, Gregory. 1941. *A History of Medical Psychology.* New York: W. W. Norton & Co.

DISCUSSION QUESTIONS

1. Conrad and Schneider assert that "medical dominance of madness was a social and political rather than a scientific achievement." What do they mean by that? What evidence do they provide for their assertion?

2. What advantages and disadvantages might there be to thinking of madness as an illness rather than as a punishment for sin, demonic possession, evidence of prophetic powers, or any of other frameworks that Conrad and Schneider discuss? How are our responses to madness influenced by the frameworks we use to understand it?

Martha Livingston Bruce

Mental Illness as Psychiatric Disorder[†]

The reading by Bruce describes psychiatry's approach to classifying mental disorders. She presents the assumptions underlying that approach followed by a brief description of the major types of mental disorders included in the official classification system of the American Psychiatric Association, the Diagnostic and Statistical Manual of Mental Disorders (DSM-IV). Her overview provides a basic introduction to how psychiatrists, and the discipline of psychiatry, think about mental disorders. Interested readers can find more detail about the definitions of the disorders in the manual itself.

INTRODUCTION

To the sociologist, perhaps the single most important characteristic of the psychiatric perspective is that psychiatry views mental illness as a real illness, as distinct from being a socially constructed myth. Whereas some social perspectives might argue that "mental illness" is a label applied by society or social groups to subsets of unusual, unappealing, or disruptive behaviors and feelings, the psychiatric perspective would argue that these behaviors and feelings are themselves the signs and symptoms of true underlying disease or disorder states. Psychiatry uses the term *mental illness* for a spectrum of syndromes that are classified by clusters of symptoms and behaviors considered clinically meaningful in terms of course, outcome, and response to treatment. The purpose of this chapter is to describe how psychiatry defines and organizes these syndromes.

Bruce, Martha Livingston. 1999 "Mental illness as psychiatric disorder." Pp. 37–55 in *Handbook of the Sociology of Mental Health*, edited by C. S. Aneshensel and J. C. Phelan. New York: Kluwer Academic-Plenum Publishers.

Modern psychiatry's conceptualization of mental illness as disease or disorder has found increasing support in recent years because of evidence of genetic or biological risk factors and of physiological mechanisms (as indicated by brain scans, blood levels, and response to pharmacotherapy). The medical model of mental illness has ramifications for how individuals with psychiatric disorder are viewed by others. By suffering a disease or disorder, persons with mental illness become eligible for what sociologists call the "sick role." In the sick role, individuals are not considered personally responsible for their condition. The sick role contrasts with other models of mental illness in which individuals can elicit such pejorative labels as "bad," "weak," or "immoral" (Mechanic, 1978, 1995). The power of a medical label for the public persona of mental illness is well understood by advocacy groups, such as the National Alliance for the Mentally Ill, which prefers the even more medically oriented term, *brain disorder* for psychiatric problems. At the same time, evidence of the contribution of personal behavior (e.g., smoking, exercise, sexual practice, and diet) in the risk of cancer, hypertension, AIDS, and numerous other diseases diffuses boundaries between personal responsibility and disease risk even within the medical model. From that perspective, labeling behaviorally linked conditions such as alcohol dependence or drug abuse as psychiatric disorders becomes somewhat more consistent with the current medical model of disease than sometimes argued (see below).

Psychiatry's medical model of disease by no means negates the role of social factors in the study of mental illness. First, the sociologist's task of determining how and to what extent social factors contribute to, modify, or mediate the risk, course, and outcomes of psychiatric disorders is arguably easier when biological factors are better defined and measured. Second, the medical model's classification of persons with mental illness as having a disease or disorder places an obligation on society to care for those persons, and an obligation on persons with the illness to accept the privileges and constraints of such care. Sociologists continue to investigate the extent to which the willingness and ability of social groups to provide affordable and accessible care for persons with mental illness varies by a range of social factors, including the characteristics of the group, the characteristics of the individuals with the disorder, the kinds of treatment available, and the characteristics of the disorder itself. For example, public acceptance of medication therapy for major depression has increased rapidly in the past decade with the introduction of a class of antidepressants that are easier to use and have fewer side effects. Yet, as noted later, younger adults with major depression are more likely to be treated than older adults with major depression, in part because of the public perception that depression is an expected and therefore normal consequence of aging. Finally, the extent to which a person with a history of mental illness can function in society is an inherently sociological question, as any society can choose or not choose to structure itself in such a way as to facilitate housing, jobs, and companionship for persons with a wide range of capacities and needs. For example, various social and medical trends, including the advent of more efficacious antipsychotic medications in the 1950s, the community mental health movement in the 1960s, and the rise in managed care in the 1990s, have resulted in dramatically shortened hospital stays for persons with even severe mental illness. These changes, however, have not necessarily been mirrored by the development of sufficient treatment and support services for these individuals to maintain viable and productive lives in the community (Greenley, 1990).

PSYCHIATRY'S APPROACH TO CLASSIFYING MENTAL ILLNESS

Modern psychiatry justifies its conceptualization of mental illness as a disorder or disease in great part by the extent to which reliable diagnoses are both possible and related to a specific course, etiology, and response to treatment (Mechanic, 1978; Klerman, 1989). The two major diagnostic systems are those of the American Psychiatric Association and the World Health Organization as described in the *DSM-IV*, and the International Classification of Diseases (ICD-10; World Health Organization, 1990), respectively. These systems are purposefully similar. For the most part, these systems of modern psychiatry use phenomenonology as their fundamental classification tool. Diagnoses form the major types of category and are defined, in large part, by clusters of signs and symptoms that are clinically meaningful in terms of personal distress, associated loss of functioning, or risk of negative outcomes such as death, disability, or loss of independence.

This emphasis on phenomenology, as distinct from theories of etiology or other organizing principals, represents a change in modern psychiatry, codified in 1980 by *DSM-III* (American Psychiatric Association, 1980; Rogler, 1997). The development of *DSM-III* reflected efforts of the research community to standardize diagnostic criteria. A goal of *DSM-III* and its successors has been to encourage reliability in making psychiatric diagnoses by providing operationalized criteria for both clinicians and researchers. The strength of this approach is in offering a mechanism to increase the consistency with which diagnoses are made across individual clients, clinicians, institutions, and geographic regions. Reliability does not, of course, confer validity, and the emphasis on reliability has left *DSM-III* and successors vulnerable to considerable criticism from a wide range of theoretical perspectives (see Millon, 1983; Rogler, 1997).

To the sociologist, the potential pitfalls in relying on phenomenology to make psychiatric diagnoses are quite obvious. Even if we accept the psychiatric assumption that the disorders are "real," we also know that how individuals perceive, experience, and cope with disease is based in large part on cultural explanations of sickness and expectation about illness behavior (Kleinman, Eisenberg, & Good, 1978). As culture is highly influential in shaping the subjective experience of disease, objective indicators of disease are only imperfectly related to the reported subjective experience of the illness (Angel & Thoits, 1987). The lack of objective indicators has large implications for clinical and population-based mental health research because assessment necessarily relies upon the individual's self-reported appraisal of his or her own symptoms. These self-appraisals contribute directly or indirectly to virtually all mental health measures used in studies of the risk, help-seeking behavior, treatment, and outcomes of health conditions.

The lack of correspondence between objective and subjective measures also has implications for the accuracy of diagnoses made in clinical practice. For example, group differences in the language used to express and give meaning to symptoms affect the diagnostic process. Additional, perhaps more subtle, potential sources of bias are expectations of providers based on irrelevant characteristics of the patient, such as race and ethnicity, socioeconomic status, age, or some combination of those characteristics. In the case of depression, for example, providers often believe that depressive symptoms are normal reactions to the stresses and losses associated with aging and low socioeconomic statuses. The elderly and the poor, therefore, may be underdiagnosed (and underserved) because their symptomatology is not seen as problematic. The problem arises in finding the right line between "over medicalizing" what might be a normal reaction to these events and conditions versus ignoring a debilitating yet treatable disease (NIH Consensus Development Panel, 1992).

A second potential problem in the *DSM*'s phenomenological approach is the distinction between "mental" and "physical" conditions. In introducing its classification schema, the authors of the *DSM-IV* acknowledge the problem in using the term *mental disorder* with the implication of a distinction from physical disorders:

> a compelling literature documents that there is much "physical" in "mental" disorders and much "mental" in "physical" disorders. The problem raised by the term "mental" disorders has been much clearer than its solution, and, unfortunately, the term persists in the title of *DSM-IV* because we have not found an appropriate substitute (American Psychiatric Association, 1994, p. xxi).

This problem is especially difficult for disorders such as depression with high levels of medical comorbidity and for the study of psychiatric disorders among the medically ill (Katz, 1996). There is no gold standard, laboratory test, or methodology generally accepted by the field for distinguishing symptoms of depression from those associated with medical illness.

Although differences in classification criteria do not change the phenomena, or their underlying condition per se, the label attached to these signs and symptoms has far reaching implications. From the individuals' perspective, the type of diagnosis given will affect the type and range of formal medical or psychosocial treatment offered to them and the expectations placed on them for physical, emotional, and functional recovery by clinicians, family, friends, and employers. From society's perspective, the type of diagnosis assigned will affect findings generated from research on the risk, outcomes, and potential treatment of these phenomena. These points concern not just the diagnostic decisions made in more complex situations, such as medically ill patients, but for all psychiatric diagnoses. For these reasons an understanding of the criteria currently used by psychiatry to diagnose specific types of mental illness is an essential tool for any sociological investigation of mental illness.

TYPES OF PSYCHIATRIC ILLNESS

This section briefly introduces the characteristics of the major psychiatric disorders comprised by *DSM-IV. DSM-IV* attempts to describe the full range of psychiatric conditions, referred to as diagnoses and their subtypes, using a system of mutually exclusive and jointly exhaustive categories. *DSM-IV's* categorical orientation and focus on diagnostic dichotomous boundaries have drawn thoughtful criticism (Mirowsky & Ross, 1989; Rogler, 1997). A major concern is the notion that a person either has or does not have a symptom, or that a person either has or does not have a diagnosis. Critics argue that symptoms and conditions rest on a continuum, with individuals potentially having different degrees of symptomatology. Dichotomizing psychiatric states loses information about the degree of symptomatology in both groups. Although acknowledging this criticism and admitting to the impreciseness of classificatory boundaries, the authors of *DSM-IV* also argue that the categorical approach—that is, defining diagnostic cases—is "thus far" still more pragmatic in clinical settings and useful in stimulating research (American Psychiatric Association, 1994, p. xxii). The classification system is reinforced by financial reimbursement strategies, which usually determine payment based on whether or not a patient meets diagnostic criteria for a specific disorder.

DSM-IV CRITERIA FOR MAJOR DEPRESSIVE EPISODE

A. Five (or more) of the following symptoms have been present during the same 2-week period and represent a change from previous functioning; at least one of the symptoms is either (1) depressed mood or (2) loss of interest or pleasure.

Note: Do not include symptoms that are clearly due to a general medical condition, or mood-incongruent delusions or hallucinations.

(1) depressed mood most of the day, nearly every day, as indicated by either subjective report (e.g., feels sad or empty) or observation made by others (e.g., appears tearful). Note: In children and adolescents, can be irritable mood.

(2) markedly diminished interest or pleasure in all, or almost all, activities most of the day, nearly every day (as indicated by either subjective account or observation made by others)

(3) significant weight loss when not dieting or weight gain (e.g., a change of more than 5 percent of body weight in a month), or decrease or increase in appetite nearly every day.   Note: In children, consider failure to make expected weight gains.

(4) insomnia or hypersomnia nearly every day

(5) psychomotor agitation or retardation nearly every day (observable by others, not merely subjective feelings of restlessness or being slowed down)

(6) fatigue or loss of energy nearly every day

(7) feelings of worthlessness or excessive or inappropriate guilt (which may be delusional) nearly every day (not merely self-reproach or guilt about being sick)

(8) diminished ability to think or concentrate, or indecisiveness, nearly every day (either by subjective account or as observed by others)

(9) recurrent thoughts of death (not just fear of dying), recurrent suicidal ideation without a specific plan, or a suicide attempt or a specific plan for committing suicide

B. The symptoms do not meet criteria for a Mixed Episode.

C. The symptoms cause clinically significant distress or impairment in social, occupational, or other important areas of functioning.

D. The symptoms are not due to the direct physiological effects of a substance (e.g., a drug of abuse, a medication) or a general medical condition (e.g., hypothyroidism).

E. The symptoms are not better accounted for by bereavement, i.e., after the loss of a loved one, the symptoms persist for longer than 2 months or are characterized by marked functional impairment, morbid preoccupation with worthlessness, suicidal ideation, psychotic symptoms, or psychomotor retardation.

Source: American Psychiatric Association (1994)

For each *DSM-IV* diagnosis, the criteria are defined first by the presence of a specified cluster of signs and symptoms, usually occurring together and for a minimum duration of time. Second, these signs and symptoms—individually or in combination—must reach a minimum threshold of severity, usually indicated by functional impairment or level of distress. Third, exclusion criteria are applied, so that a symptom does not count toward a diagnosis if the symptom, for example, is due to a medical illness, medication use, or substance use. Although, in a small number of cases, *DSM-IV* does not permit certain diagnoses to exist in the context of another diagnosis (e.g., major depression is not possible if a person has a bipolar disorder), psychiatric comorbidity (i.e., a person meeting criteria for more than one *DSM-IV* diagnosis) is not only possible but fairly common (Kessler et al., 1994).

Schizophrenia and Other Psychotic Disorders

Psychotic disorders, including schizophrenia, comprise a large proportion of the conditions labeled as "severe mental illness." Schizophrenia is usually described as a rare disorder affecting approximately 1 percent of the population over the lifetime, yet this 1 percent represents as many as 4 million people in the United States today (Keith, Regier, & Rae, 1991). Schizophrenia is severe because it not only brings considerable personal suffering but also because people with schizophrenia very often are unable to complete their education, maintain a job, and otherwise function as normally expected in our society. These conditions serve as a kind of mirror for the capacities needed to live successfully in our society. In addition, the kinds of lives lived by people with schizophrenia speak to the level of intolerance in our society of people who do not have those capacities.

DSM-IV uses a relatively narrow definition, with psychosis referring to delusions, prominent hallucinations (usually without insight, that is, recognition by the individual as being an hallucination), disorganized speech (an indicator of disorganized thinking), or disorganized or catatonic behavior. Delusions are erroneous beliefs that usually involve a misinterpretation of perceptions or experiences. The bizarreness, that is, implausibility, of delusions can be difficult to judge, especially across cultures (Rogler, 1996). Hallucinations are distortions or exaggerations of sensory perception, most often hearing things no one else hears, but also seeing, smelling, tasting, or feeling things that are not present. Hallucinatory experiences are a normal part of religious experience in some cultures, making the judgment of bizarreness or abnormality particularly difficult.

Schizophrenia is defined as a disturbance lasting at least 6 months and, in its active phase, including two or more of the five symptom groups: (1) delusions; (2) hallucinations; (3) severely disorganized speech; (4) grossly disorganized or catatonic behavior, or (5) negative symptoms (e.g., affective flattening, alogia/poverty of speech, and avolition/inability to initiate and persist in goal-directed activities). These negative symptoms reportedly account for much of the morbidity associated with schizophrenia because they generally interfere with social and occupational functioning.

Depression and Other Affective Disorders

The predominate feature of depression and other kinds of affective disorders is mood. The major types of disturbances, usually experienced as episodes, are characterized by either mania or depression. These episodes form the major components of the affective diagnoses, with bipolar disorder defined by episodes of mania often interspersed with episodes of depression, and major depressive disorder defined by episodes of depression without a history of mania.

DEPRESSION.   The essential feature of a major depressive episode, as defined by *DSM-IV*, is a period of at least 2 weeks during which there is depressed mood or the loss of interest or pleasure in nearly all activities. In children, the mood may be more irritability than sadness. To meet full criteria for an episode of major depression, individuals must also concurrently experience symptoms, also lasting 2 weeks or more, from at least four out of a list of seven groups: (1) changes in weight or appetite; (2) changes in sleep; (3) changes in psychomotor activity; (4) decreased energy; (5) feelings of worthlessness or guilt; (6) difficulty thinking, concentrating, or making decisions; and (7) recurrent thoughts of death or suicidal ideation, plans, or attempts. Symptoms must be entirely new or significantly worse than normal. Symptoms also must be severe, which means they are associated with clinically significant distress and/or impairment in social, occupational or other types of functioning.

MANIA.   A manic episode is defined by a distinct period (1 week or more) during which there is abnormally and persistently elevated, expansive, or irritable mood. Concurrently, an individual must experience at least three additional symptoms from a list of seven symptom groups: (1) inflated self-esteem or grandiosity; (2) decreased need for sleep; (3) increased talkativeness; (4) racing thoughts; (5) distractibility; (6) increased goal-directed activity or psychomotor agitation; and (7) excessive involvement in pleasurable activities that have a high potential for painful consequences (e.g., buying sprees, sexual indiscretions, or foolish business investments). These symptoms must be severe enough to cause marked impairment in functioning. Variations on the manic episode include *mixed* episodes (e.g., symptoms of both depression and mania for at least 1 week) and milder *hypomanic* episodes.

Anxiety Disorders

Anxiety disorders encompass a range of diagnoses characterized by excessive worry, fear, or avoidance behavior. The major forms of *DSM-IV* anxiety disorders include: (1) panic disorder without agoraphobia; (2) panic disorder with agoraphobia; (3) agoraphobia without history of panic; (4) specific phobia; (5) social phobia; (6) obsessive-compulsive disorder; (7) posttraumatic stress disorder; (8) acute stress disorder, and (9) generalized anxiety disorder.

Panic disorder,[2] which can occur with or without comorbid agoraphobia, is diagnosed by a history of two or more panic attacks. These attacks are discrete periods characterized by sudden onset of intense apprehension, fearfulness, or terror, often associated with feelings of impending doom in situations in which most people would not feel afraid. The criteria for

---

[2] Editor's note: We include only one example here. Descriptions of other anxiety
    disorders can be found in the original chapter.

a panic attack demand at least 4 out of 13 additional somatic or cognitive symptoms, for example, shortness of breath, palpitation, chest pain or discomfort, choking or smothering sensations, and fear of "going crazy" or losing control. Attacks have a sudden onset and short duration (i.e., 10 minutes or less). Panic attacks are often experienced as a heart attack or similar physical condition, resulting in exacerbated worry by the sufferer and family, as well as substantial use of medical resources (Eaton, Dryman, & Weissman, 1991).

Substance-Related Disorders

The interplay among personal behavior, societal expectations, and biology is especially obvious in the class of conditions labeled substance-related disorders in *DSM-IV*. In *DSM-IV*, "substance" refers in large part to a "drug of abuse" obtained either legally (e.g., alcohol, caffeine, nicotine) or illegally (e.g., PCP, opioids). "Substance" also refers to medications and toxins. Substance-related disorders are problematic conditions related to consuming these substances. Perhaps more than many of the diagnoses included in *DSM-IV*, the sociologist may question the reasons for including substance-related conditions as psychiatric disorders because the causes of these "problematic conditions" (i.e., drinking alcohol or using drugs) are self-induced and often (especially in the case of alcohol) socially sanctioned behaviors. The logic for their inclusion, however, is consistent with *DSM-IV*'s reliance on phenomenology rather than etiology or cause. *DSM-IV*'s criteria focus on the signs and symptoms (e.g., craving, physiological withdrawal) rather the drinking per se.

The essential feature of *substance dependence* is a cluster of cognitive, behavioral, and physiological symptoms indicating that the individual continues to use the substance despite significant problems related to its use. A pattern of repeated self-administration usually results in tolerance (i.e., need for markedly increased amounts to achieve a desired effect or markedly diminished effect for a given amount), withdrawal, and compulsive drug-taking behavior. *Substance abuse* is less severe than substance dependence and is characterized by a maladaptive pattern of substance use, manifested by recurrent and significant adverse consequences (e.g., repeated failure to fulfill role obligations, use when physically hazardous, or multiple legal, social, and/or interpersonal problems). Compared to substance dependence, the symptoms of substance abuse tend to be defined by social rather than biological or psychological problems.

Disorders in Childhood

Although children suffer from a number of psychiatric disorders that are also common among adults (e.g., depression and anxiety), an additional set of disorders is defined by onset during childhood. Among these are mental retardation, learning disorders, pervasive developmental disorders, and attention deficit hyperactivity disorder (ADHD).

Of these, ADHD is both relatively common (prevalence of approximately 3–5 percent) and very disruptive to the life of the affected child and family. In *DSM-IV*, ADHD is characterized by persistent inattention and/or hyperactivity in more than one setting (e.g., home and school) at a level greater than normally observed in children at a similar developmental stage. To meet diagnostic criteria, at least some ADHD symptoms must appear before age 7. In addition, a child needs to demonstrate six or more maladaptive symptoms lasting six months or more related either to *inattention* (e.g., careless mistakes at school, difficulty sustaining attention in tasks, not listening, not following through on instructions, difficulty organizing tasks, avoiding tasks that require sustained effort, losing tools needed for a task, being easily distracted or forgetful) or *hyperactivity/impulsivity* (e.g., fidgeting, leaving one's seat inappropriately, leaving the room inappropriately, difficulty playing quietly, being always on the go, talking excessively, blurting out answers prematurely, having difficulty waiting one's turn, interrupting others). In ADHD, these symptoms result in considerable impairment in family, school, and social groups, and children with ADHD are often disruptive to these settings. Because many of these symptoms mirror the normal behaviors of very young children, these symptoms cannot be easily evaluated or identified until at least age 4, an age at which children are developmentally ready to pay sustained attention to tasks and more able to control their own behavior.

Dementia and Delirium

The predominant disturbance of dementia and delirium is a clinically significant deficit in cognition or memory. In both conditions, the cognitive and memory deficits represent a significant change from previous functioning, differentiating them from mental retardation. Also unlike mental retardation, dementia and delirium are disorders associated with aging and old age.

References

American Psychiatric Association. (1980). *Diagnostic and Statistical Manual of Mental Disorders* (3rd ed.). Washington, DC: Author.

American Psychiatric Association. (1994). *Diagnostic and statistical manual of mental disorders* (4th ed.). Washington, DC: Author.

Angel, R., & Thoits, P. (1987). The impact of culture on the cognitive structure of illness. *Culture, Medicine, and Psychiatry, 11,* 465–494.

Eaton, W. W., Dryman, A., & Weissman, M. M. (1991). Panic and phobia. In L. N. Robins & D. A. Regier (Eds.), *Psychiatric disorders in America: The epidemiologic catchment area study* (pp. 155–179). New York: The Free Press.

Greenley, J. R. (1990). Mental illness as a social problem. In J. R. Greenley (Ed.) *Research in community and mental health* (Vol. 6, pp. 7–40). New York: Plenum Press.

Katz, I. R. (1996). On the inseparability of mental and physical health in aged persons. *American Journal of Geriatric Psychiatry, 4,* 1–16.

Keith, S. J., Regier, D. A., & Rae, D. (1991). Schizophrenic disorders. In L. N. Robins & D. A. Regier (Eds.), *Psychiatric disorders in America*, (pp. 33–52). New York: The Free Press.

Kessler, R. C., McGonagle, K. A., Zhao, S., Nelson, C. B., Hughes, M., Eshleman, S., Wittchen, H. U., & Kendler, K. S. (1994). Lifetime and 12-month prevalence of DSM-III-R psychiatric disorders in the United States: Results from the National Comorbidity Survey. *Archives of General Psychiatry, 51*, 8–19.

Kleinman, A., Eisenberg, L., & Good, B. (1978). Culture, illness, and care. *Annals of Internal Medicine, 88*, 251–258.

Klerman, G. L. (1989). Comment to Mirowsky and Ross. *Journal of Health and Social Behavior, 30*, 26–32.

Mechanic, D. (1978). *Medical sociology* (2nd ed.). New York: The Free Press.

Mechanic, D. (1995). Sociological dimensions of illness behavior. *Social Science and Medicine, 41*, 1207–1216.

Millon, T. (1983). The DSM-III: An insiders' perspective. *American Psychologist, 38*, 804–814.

Mirowsky, J., & Ross, C. E. (1989). Psychiatric diagnosis as reified measurement. *Journal of Health and Social Behavior, 30*, 11–25.

NIH Consensus Development Panel on Depression in Late Life. (1992). Diagnosis and treatment of depression in late life. *Journal of the American Medical Association, 192*(268), 1018–1024.

Rogler, L. H. (1996). Framing research on culture in psychiatric diagnosis: The case of the DSM-IV. *Psychiatry, 59*, 145–155.

Rogler, L. H. (1997). Making sense of historical changes in the *Diagnostic and Statistical Manual of Mental Disorders*: Five propositions. *Journal of Health and Social Behavior, 38*, 9–20.

World Health Organization. (1990). *International classification of diseases and related health problems* (10th ed.). Geneva: Author.

DISCUSSION QUESTIONS

1. Bruce takes a more conciliatory approach to the psychiatric conceptualization of mental illness than do Conrad and Schneider. After reading both articles, which approach do you find most convincing? Why?

2. The author points to "the kinds of lives lived by people with schizophrenia" as evidence of society's intolerance towards people with diminished capacities. What have you learned or observed about the lives of people with schizophrenia that is consistent with the author's statement?

3. Bruce asserts that the medical model of disease does not negate the role of social factors in the study of mental illness. What does she mean by that? What place do social factors have in the medical model of disease?

What Is Mental Illness? Sociological Perspectives

Peter Conrad

The Discovery of Hyperkinesis[†]

This article, first published over 30 years ago, is considered a classic in the field. Although the specific information it presents about "hyperkinesis" (now known as attention deficit hyperactivity disorder) is out of date, its arguments regarding the processes through which deviant behaviors are medicalized and the implications of medicalization for individuals and society still ring true. As you read Conrad's article, consider whether his arguments apply to any other conditions with which you are familiar.

INTRODUCTION

The increasing medicalization of deviant behavior and the medical institution's role as an agent of social control has gained considerable notice (Freidson, 1970; Pitts, 1968; Kitterie, 1971; Zola, 1972). By medicalization we mean defining behavior as a medical problem or illness and mandating or licensing the medical profession to provide some type of treatment for it. Examples include alcoholism, drug addiction, and treating violence as a genetic or brain disorder.

THE MEDICAL DIAGNOSIS OF HYPERKINESIS

Hyperkinesis is a relatively recent phenomenon as a medical diagnostic category. Only in the past two decades has it been available as a recognized diagnostic category and only in the last decade has it received widespread notice and medical popularity. However, the roots of the diagnosis and treatment of this clinical entity are found earlier.

Conrad, Peter. 1975. "The discovery of hyperkinesis." *Social Problems* 23:12–21.

Hyperkinesis is also known as Minimal Brain Dysfunction, Hyperkinetic Syndrome, Hyperkinetic Disorder of Childhood, and by several other diagnostic categories. Although the symptoms and the presumed etiology vary, in general the behaviors are quite similar and greatly overlap.[1] Typical symptom patterns for diagnosing the disorder include: extreme excess of motor activity (hyperactivity); very short attention span (the child flits from activity to activity); restlessness; fidgetiness; often wildly oscillating mood swings (he's fine one day, a terror the next); clumsiness; aggressive-like behavior; impulsivity; in school he cannot sit still, cannot comply with rules, has low frustration level; frequently there may be sleeping problems and acquisition of speech may be delayed (Stewart, Ferris, Pitts, & Craig, 1966; Stewart, 1970; Wender, 1971). Most of the symptoms for the disorder are deviant behaviors.[2] It is six times as prevalent among boys as among girls. We use the term hyperkinesis to represent all the diagnostic categories of this disorder.

THE DISCOVERY OF HYPERKINESIS

It is useful to divide the analysis into what might be considered *clinical factors* directly related to the diagnosis and treatment of hyperkinesis and *social factors* that set the context for the emergence of the new diagnostic category.

Clinical Factors

Bradley (1937) observed that amphetamine drugs had a spectacular effect in altering the behavior of school children who exhibited behavior disorders or learning disabilities. Fifteen of the 30 children he treated actually became more subdued in their behavior. Bradley termed the effect of this medication paradoxical, since he expected that amphetamines would stimulate children as they stimulated adults. After the medication was discontinued the children's behavior returned to premedication level.

A scattering of reports in the medical literature on the utility of stimulant medications for "childhood behavior disorders" appeared in the next two decades. The next significant contribution was the work of Strauss and his associates (Strauss & Lehtinen, 1947) who found certain behavior (including hyperkinesis behaviors) in postencephaletic children suffering from what they called minimal brain injury (damage). This was the first time these behaviors were attributed to the new organic distinction of minimal brain damage.

---

[1] The U.S.P.H.S. report (Clements, 1966) included 38 terms that were used to describe or distinguish the conditions that it labeled Minimal Brain Dysfunction. Although the literature attempts to differentiate M.B.D., hyperkinesis, hyperactive syndrome, and several other diagnostic labels, it is our belief that in practice they are almost interchangeable.

[2] For a fuller discussion of the construction of the diagnosis of hyperkinesis, see Conrad (forthcoming), especially chapter 6.

This disorder did not appear as a specific diagnostic category until Laufer, Denhoff, and Solomons (1957) described it as the "hyperkinetic impulse disorder" in 1957. Upon finding "the salient characteristics of the behavior pattern... are strikingly similar to those with clear cut organic causation" these researchers described a disorder with no clear-cut history or evidence for organicity (Laufer, Denhoff, & Solomons, 1957).

In 1966 a task force sponsored by the U.S. Public Health Service and the National Association for Crippled Children and Adults attempted to clarify the ambiguity and confusion in terminology and symptomology in diagnosing children's behavior and learning disorders. From over three dozen diagnoses, they agreed on the term "minimal brain dysfunction" as an overriding diagnosis that would include hyperkinesis and other disorders (Clements, 1966). Since this time MBD has been the primary formal diagnosis or label.

In the middle 1950s a new drug, Ritalin, was synthesized, that has many qualities of amphetamines without some of their more undesirable side effects. In 1961 this drug was approved by the FDA for use with children. Since this time there has been much research published on the use of Ritalin in the treatment of childhood behavior disorders. This medication became the "treatment of choice" for treating children with hyperkinesis.

Since the early sixties, more research appeared on the etiology, diagnosis, and treatment of hyperkinesis (cf. DeLong, 1972; Grinspoon & Singer, 1973; Cole, 1975)—as much as three-quarters concerned with drug treatment of the disorder. There had been increasing publicity of the disorder in the mass media as well. The *Reader's Guide to Periodical Literature* had no articles on hyperkinesis before 1967, one each in 1968 and 1969 and a total of 40 for 1970 through 1974 (a mean of 8 per year).

Now hyperkinesis has become the most common child psychiatric problem (Gross & Wilson, 1974, 142); special pediatric clinics have been established to treat hyperkinetic children, and substantial federal funds have been invested in etiological and treatment research. Outside the medical profession, teachers have developed a working clinical knowledge of hyperkinesis' symptoms and treatment (cf. Robin & Bosco, 1973); articles appear regularly in mass circulation magazines and newspapers so that parents often come to clinics with knowledge of this diagnosis. Hyperkinesis is no longer the relatively esoteric diagnostic category it may have been 20 years ago, it is now a well-known clinical disorder.

Social Factors

The social factors affecting the discovery of hyperkinesis can be divided into two areas: (1) The Pharmaceutical Revolution and (2) Government Action.

(1) *The Pharmaceutical Revolution.* Since the 1930s the pharmaceutical industry has been synthesizing and manufacturing a large number of psychoactive drugs, contributing to a virtual revolution in drug making and drug taking in America (Silverman & Lee, 1974).

Psychoactive drugs are agents that affect the central nervous system. Benzedrine, Ritalin, and Dexedrine are all synthesized psychoactive stimulants which were indicated for narcolepsy, appetite control (as "diet pills"), mild depression, fatigue, and more recently hyperkinetic children.

Until the early sixties there was little or no promotion and advertisement of any of these medications for use with childhood disorders.[3] Then two major pharmaceutical firms (Smith, Kline and French, manufacturer of Dexedrine and CIBA, manufacturer of Ritalin) began to advertise in medical journals and through direct mailing and efforts of the "detail men." Most of this advertising of the pharmaceutical treatment of hyperkinesis was directed to the medical sphere; but some of the promotion was targeted for the educational sector also (Hentoff, 1972). This promotion was probably significant in disseminating information concerning the diagnosis and treatment of this newly discovered disorder.[4] Since 1955 the use of psychoactive medications (especially phenothiazines) for the treatment of persons who are mentally ill, along with the concurrent dramatic decline in inpatient populations, has made psychopharmacology an integral part of treatment for mental disorders. It has also undoubtedly increased the confidence in the medical profession for the pharmaceutical approach to mental and behavioral problems.

(2) *Government Action.* Since the publication of the USPHS report on MBD there have been at least two significant governmental reports on treating school children with stimulant medications for behavior disorders. Both of these came as a response to the national publicity created by the *Washington Post* report (1970) that 5 to 10 percent of the 62,000 grammar school children in Omaha, Nebraska were being treated with "behavior modification drugs to improve deportment and increase learning potential" (quoted in Grinspoon & Singer, 1973). Although the figures were later found to be a little exaggerated, it nevertheless spurred a Congressional investigation (U.S. Government Printing Office, 1970) and a conference sponsored by the Office of Child Development (1971) on the use of stimulant drugs in the treatment of behaviorally disturbed school children.

The Congressional Subcommittee on Privacy chaired by Congressman Cornelius E. Gallagher held hearings on the issue of prescribing drugs for hyperactive school children. In general, the committee showed great concern over the facility in which the medication was prescribed; more specifically that some children at least were receiving drugs from general practitioners whose primary diagnosis was based on teachers' and parents' reports that

---

[3] The American Medical Association's change in policy in accepting more pharmaceutical advertising in the late fifties may have been important. Probably the FDA approval of the use of Ritalin for children in 1961 was more significant. Until 1970, Ritalin was advertised for treatment of "functional behavior problems in children." Since then, because of an FDA order, it has only been promoted for treatment of MBD.

[4] The drug industry spends fully 25 percent of its budget on promotion and advertising. See Coleman et al. (1966) for the role of the detail men and how physicians rely upon them for information.

the child was doing poorly in school. There was also a concern with the absence of follow-up studies on the long-term effects of treatment.

The HEW committee was a rather hastily convened group of professionals (a majority were MD's) many of whom already had commitments to drug treatment for childrens' behavior problems. They recommended that only MD's make the diagnosis and prescribe treatment, that the pharmaceutical companies promote the treatment of the disorder only through medical channels, that parents should not be coerced to accept any particular treatment, and that long-term follow-up research should be done. This report served as blue ribbon approval for treating hyperkinesis with psychoactive medications.

DISCUSSION

How does deviant behavior become conceptualized as a medical problem? We assume that before the discovery of hyperkinesis this type of deviance was seen as disruptive, disobedient, rebellious, anti-social, or deviant behavior. Perhaps the label "emotionally disturbed" was sometimes used, when it was in vogue in the early sixties, and the child was usually managed in the context of the family or the school or in extreme cases, the child guidance clinic. How then did this constellation of deviant behaviors become a medical disorder?

The treatment was available long before the disorder treated was clearly conceptualized. It was 20 years after Bradley's discovery of the "paradoxical effect" of stimulants on certain deviant children that Laufer named the disorder and described its characteristic symptoms. Only in the late fifties were both the diagnostic label and the pharmaceutical treatment available. The pharmaceutical revolution in mental health and the increased interest in child psychiatry provided a favorable background for the dissemination of knowledge about this new disorder. The latter probably made the medical profession more likely to consider behavior problems in children as within their clinical jurisdiction.

There were agents outside the medical profession itself that were significant in "promoting" hyperkinesis as a disorder within the medical framework. These agents might be conceptualized in Becker's terms as "moral entrepreneurs," those who crusade for creation and enforcement of the rules (Becker, 1963).[5] In this case the moral entrepreneurs were the pharmaceutical companies and the Association for Children with Learning Disabilities.

The pharmaceutical companies spent considerable time and money promoting stimulant medications for this new disorder. From the middle 1960s on, medical journals and the free "throw-away" magazines contained elaborate advertising for Ritalin and Dexedrine. These ads explained the utility of treating hyperkinesis and urged the physician to diagnose and treat hyperkinetic children.

The pharmaceutical firms also supplied sophisticated packets of "diagnostic and treatment" information on hyperkinesis to physicians, paid for professional conferences on the subject, and supported research in the identification and treatment of the disorder. Clearly these corporations had a vested interest in the labeling and treatment of hyperkinesis; CIBA had

$13 million profit from Ritalin alone in 1971, which was 15 percent of the total gross profits (Charles, 1971; Hentoff, 1972).

The other moral entrepreneur, less powerful than the pharmaceutical companies, but nevertheless influential, is the Association for Children with Learning Disabilities. Although their focus is not specifically on hyperkinetic children, they do include it in their conception of Learning Disabilities along with aphasia, reading problems like dyslexia and perceptual motor problems. Founded in the early 1950s by parents and professionals, it has functioned much as the National Association for Mental Health does for mental illness: promoting conferences, sponsoring legislation, providing social support. One of the main functions has been to disseminate information concerning this relatively new area in education, Learning Disabilities. While the organization does have a more educational than medical perspective, most of the literature indicates that for hyperkinesis members have adopted the medical model and the medical approach to the problem. They have sensitized teachers and schools to the conception of hyperkinesis as a medical problem.

The medical model of hyperactive behavior has become very well accepted in our society. Physicians find treatment relatively simple and the results sometimes spectacular. Hyperkinesis minimizes parents' guilt by emphasizing "it's not their fault, it's an organic problem" and allows for nonpunitive management or control of deviance. Medication often makes a child less disruptive in the classroom and sometimes aids a child in learning. Children often like their "magic pills," which make their behavior more socially acceptable and they probably benefit from a reduced stigma also. There are, however, some other, perhaps more subtle ramifications of the medicalization of deviant behavior.

EXTENDING THE ANALYSIS

In a 2000 follow-up article, Conrad and his co-author Debra Potter analyze the expansion of ADHD to adults. They note that medicalization is not simply the result of "medical imperialism" but, rather, that laypersons actively collaborate in the process of medicalization in order to gain legitimacy. According to Conrad and Potter, both professionals and laypersons were involved in the construction of adult ADHD. Scientific studies which suggested that some children do not outgrow ADHD coupled with lay accounts written by adults who first became aware of their ADHD symptoms at later ages set the stage for professional and public acceptance of the diagnostic expansion. The largest ADHD support group, CHADD (Children and Adults with Attention Deficit Disorder), sponsored a national conference on adult ADHD, prepared publications promoting the diagnosis, and advocated for workplace legislation to protect the rights of adults with ADHD, thereby bringing lay and professional advocates together. The expansion in the diagnosis gained further support from pharmaceutical companies, and was solidified by the decision to incorporate impairment at work (rather than just at school and at home) into the Diagnostic and Statistical Manual of Mental Disorders (DSM) diagnostic criteria in 1994. As Conrad did in his earlier research on ADHD, he and Potter identify features of the broad social context that support the expansion of ADHD to adults (e.g., the increasing acceptance of Prozac and other pharmaceutical solutions, the rise of managed care and its emphasis on pharmaceutical treatments) and discuss possible implications for society, including the medicalization of underperformance and the creation of a new disability category. Conrad and Potter's article reminds us that the social construction of mental illness is an ongoing process that both reflects and reinforces societal attitudes and preferences.

Conrad, P., & Potter, D. (2000). From hyperactive children to ADHD adults: Observations on the expansion of medical categories. *Social Problems, 47,* 559–582.

1. The problem of expert control.   The medical profession is a profession of experts; they have a monopoly on anything that can be conceptualized as illness. Because of the way the medical profession is organized and the mandate it has from society, decisions related to medical diagnoses and treatment are virtually controlled by medical professionals.

Some conditions that enter the medical domain are not ipso facto medical problems, especially deviant behavior, whether alcoholism, hyperactivity, or drug addiction. By defining a problem as medical it is removed from the public realm where there can be discussion by ordinary people and put on a plane where only medical people can discuss it. The public may have their own conceptions of deviant behavior but that of the experts is usually dominant.

2. Medical social control.   Defining deviant behavior as a medical problem allows certain things to be done that could not otherwise be considered; for example, the body may be cut open or psychoactive medications may be given. This treatment can be a form of social control.

These relatively new and increasingly popular forms of social control could not be utilized without the medicalization of deviant behavior. As is suggested from the discovery of hyperkinesis, if a mechanism of medical social control seems useful, then the deviant behavior it modifies will develop a medical label or diagnosis. No overt malevolence on the part of the medical profession is implied: rather it is part of a complex process, of which the medical profession is only a part. The larger process might be called the individualization of social problems.

3. The individualization of social problems.   The medicalization of deviant behavior is part of a larger phenomenon that is prevalent in our society, the individualization of social problems. We tend to look for causes and solutions to complex social problems in the individual rather than in the social system. This view resembles Ryan's (1971) notion of "blaming the victim;"

seeing the causes of the problem in individuals rather than in the society where they live. We then seek to change the "victim" rather than the society. The medical perspective of diagnosing an illness in an individual lends itself to the individualization of social problems. Rather than seeing certain deviant behaviors as symptomatic of problems in the social system, the medical perspective focuses on the individual diagnosing and treating the illness, generally ignoring the social situation.

4. *The depoliticization of deviant behavior.* Depoliticization of deviant behavior is a result of both the process of medicalization and individualization of social problems. To our Western world, probably one of the clearest examples of such a depoliticization of deviant behavior occurred when political dissenters in the Soviet Union were declared mentally ill and confined in mental hospitals (cf. Conrad, 1972). This strategy served to neutralize the meaning of political protest and dissent, rendering it the ravings of mad persons.

The medicalization of deviant behavior depoliticizes deviance in the same manner. By defining the overactive, restless, and disruptive child as hyperkinetic we ignore the meaning of behavior in the context of the social system. If we focused our analysis on the school system we might see the child's behavior as symptomatic of some "disorder" in the school or classroom situation, rather than symptomatic of an individual neurological disorder.

References

Becker, H. S. (1963). *The Outsiders.* New York: Free Press.

Bradley, C. (1937, March). The behavior of children receiving Benzedrine. *American Journal of Psychiatry, 94,* 577–585.

Charles, A. (1971, October). The case of Ritalin. *New Republic, 23,* 17–19.

Clements, S. D. (1966). *Task Force I: Minimal Brain Dysfunction in Children.* National Institute of Neurological Diseases and Blindness, Monograph no. 3. Washington, DC: U.S. Department of Health, Education, and Welfare.

Cole, S. (1975, January). Hyperactive children: The use of stimulant drugs evaluated. *American Journal of Orthopsychiatry, 45,* 28–37.

Coleman, J., Katz, E., & Menzel, J. 1966). *Medical Innovation.* Indianapolis, IN: Bob Merrill.

Conrad, P. (1972). *Ideological Deviance: An Analysis of the Soviet Use of Mental Hospitals for Political Dissenters.* Unpublished manuscript.

DeLong, A. R. (1972, February). What have we learned from psychoactive drugs research with hyperactives? *American Journal of Diseases in Children, 123,* 177–180.

Freidson, E. (1970). *Profession of Medicine.* New York: Harper & Row.

Grinspoon, L., & Singer, S. (1973, November). Amphetamines in the treatment of hyperactive children. *Harvard Educational Review, 43,* 515–555.

Gross, M. B., & Wilson, W. B. (1974). *Minimal Brain Dysfunction.* New York: Brunner Mazel.

Hentoff, N. (1972, May). Drug pushing in the schools: The professionals. *The Village Voice, 22,* 21–23.

Kitterie, N. (1971). *The Right to be Different.* Baltimore: Johns Hopkins Press.

Laufer, M. W., Denhoff, E., & Solomons, G. (1957, January). Hyperkinetic impulse disorder in children's behavior problems. *Psychosomatic Medicine, 19,* 38–49.

Office of Child Development. (1971, January 11–12). *Report of the Conference on the Use of Stimulant Drugs in Treatment of Behaviorally Disturbed Children*. Washington, DC: Office of Child Development, Department of Health, Education and Welfare.

Pitts, J. (1968). Social control: The concept. In David Sills (Ed.), *International Encyclopedia of the Social Sciences* (Vol. 14). New York: Macmillan.

Robin, S. S., & Bosco, J. J. (1973, December). Ritalin for school children: The teachers perspective. *Journal of School Health, 47*, 624–628.

Ryan, W. (1970). *Blaming the Victim*. New York: Vintage.

Silverman, M. & Lee, P. R. (1974). *Pills, Profits and Politics*. Berkeley: University of California Press.

Stewart, M. A., Ferris, A., Pitts, N. P., & Craig, A. G. (1966, October). The hyperactive child syndrome. *American Journal of Orthopsychiatry, 36*, 861–867.

Strauss, A. A., & Lehtinen, L. E. (1947). *Psychopathology and Education and the Brain-injured Child*. (Vol. 1). New York: Grune and Strattan.

U.S. Government Printing Office. (1970). *Federal Involvement in the Use of Behavior Modification Drugs on Grammar School Children of the Right to Privacy Inquiry: Hearing Before a Subcommittee of the Committee on Government Operations*. Washington, D.C.: 91st Congress, 2nd session (September 29).

Wender, P. (1971). *Minimal Brain Dysfunction in Children*. New York: John Wiley and Sons.

Zola, I. (1972, November). Medicine as an institution of social control. *Sociological Review, 20*, 487–504.

DISCUSSION QUESTIONS

1. Conrad's use of the word "discovery" in the title of his article is intentionally ironic. In what sense was hyperkinesis "discovered"? Who was involved in the "discovery"?

2. What does Conrad mean by "moral entrepreneurs"? According to his analysis, who are the moral entrepreneurs who promoted hyperkinesis as a medical disorder? What might their motivations have been?

3. What are the costs and benefits of medicalizing deviant conditions? Have you observed any of these costs and benefits in the lives of people you know who are affected by ADHD?

4. Can you think of other conditions that have been medicalized but which could be understood using other frameworks? What individuals and groups would have a stake in how that condition is defined?

Anne E. Figert

The Three Faces of PMS: The Professional, Gendered, and Scientific Structuring of a Psychiatric Disorder

Figert analyzes the controversy over the inclusion of late luteal phase dysphoric disorder (LLPDD; now called premenstrual dysphoric disorder) in the Diagnostic and Statistical Manual of Mental Disorders, Third Edition, Revised (DSM-III-R) through a social problems perspective. Specifically, she considers three domains of conflict over "ownership" of the disorder: between psychiatrists and other medical professionals, between women affected by the symptoms of LLPDD and professionals, and among scientific communities. Her analysis offers insight into the process through which the American Psychiatric Association establishes definitions of mental disorders, and demonstrates that those definitions are often the products of negotiations among competing interests.

THE RESEARCH SITE

This paper is about a rare psychiatric condition known "officially" since 1986 as Late Luteal Phase Dysphoric Disorder (LLPDD). LLPDD is related to, yet distinct from, the more popular diagnosis of Premenstrual Syndrome (PMS). The LLPDD diagnosis was developed in recognition that a small percentage of menstruating women (approximately 5 percent) experience severe psychological and emotional symptoms in the premenstrual phase of their menstrual cycle (Spitzer, Severino, Williams, & Parry, 1989; Gitlin & Pasnau, 1989). The controversy and decision to place LLPDD in a research appendix of the *Diagnostic and Statistical Manual of Mental Disorders, Third Edition, Revised (DSM-III-R)* is notable because the *DSM* is seen as a basic reference book for mental health professionals (Kirk & Kutchins, 1992; Brown, 1990; Amchin, 1991). It provides standardized diagnostic criteria used by most insurance carriers and is recognized as the psychiatric profession's consensus over the diagnoses of mental disorders (Spitzer, Severino, Williams, & Parry, 1989; Fisher, 1986; Holden, 1986). Controversies over the inclusion or exclusion of psychiatric diagnoses provide valuable insight into the highly contested nature of psychiatric knowledge and the ways that important social and policy decisions are made in powerful organizations like the American Psychiatric Association (APA) (Bayer, 1987; Scott, 1990).

Figert, Anne E. 1995. "The Three Faces of PMS: The Professional, Gendered, and Scientific Structuring of a Psychiatric Disorder." *Social Problems* 42:56–73.

The American Psychiatric Association began the revision process to its *Diagnostic and Statistical Manual of Mental Disorders,* the *DSM-III,* in the early 1980s (American Psychiatric Association, 1980). Premenstrual Dysphoric Disorder was first proposed for inclusion in the *DSM-III-R* in June 1985 by an advisory committee to the American Psychiatric Association. The advisory committee was composed of scientific and medical experts and specialists on premenstrual syndrome (PMS) and was chaired by the head of the revision process, Robert Spitzer. This advisory panel, the LLPDD Advisory Committee, defined and established the parameters of the diagnosis using research criteria first established at a 1983 National Institute of Mental Health conference, and the panel voted to recommend inclusion of Premenstrual Dysphoric Disorder (PDD) in the *DSM-III-R* by a vote of 11 to 1 with one abstention (later polled as a no vote against the recommendation for inclusion).

The proposed diagnosis quickly met with more sustained opposition outside of the LLPDD Advisory Committee. A letter writing campaign against the inclusion of the diagnosis was initiated by a coalition of feminist health professionals within and outside of the APA. A special committee was appointed within the APA to settle the controversy; meetings were held, and a public protest at the APA's annual meeting was held in May 1986 (see Goleman, 1985; Boxer, 1987; DePaul, 1986; Holden, 1986; and Mickelson, 1986 for journalistic accounts of the controversy). On June 23, 1986, after a year of bitter dispute, the Board of Trustees of the American Psychiatric Association voted to place a diagnosis that was ultimately called Late Luteal Phase Dysphoric Disorder (LLPDD) in the soon to be published edition of the *DSM-III-R.* By this time, the diagnostic criteria of the diagnosis had undergone many revisions. The APA Board of Trustees also voted to place the proposed diagnosis in a research appendix under the heading "diagnosis in need of further study," which meant that it was neither granted official status as a coded primary diagnosis nor to receive third party insurance reimbursement. It was official enough however to continue studying it for research and diagnostic efforts. The *DSM-III-R* appeared in May 1987—two years past its projected completion date, due in part to objections over the inclusion of the PMS diagnosis.

AVAILABLE EXPLANATIONS

The decision to make PMS an official psychiatric disorder can be explained using a variety of social problems perspectives. I draw upon the social worlds and arenas perspective.

In the "social worlds" perspective, controversies occur when people from different *social worlds* (collective actors who share similar outlooks, concerns, and commitments) hold different perspectives about the way something should be defined, pursued, or created (Strauss, 1978; Becker, 1982; Fujimura, 1988; Clarke, 1990a). Scientific controversies take place in *arenas* of interaction, "a conceptual location where all of the groups that care about a given phenomena meet" (Clarke, 1990b, p. 19). The arena of PMS would include all groups interested in the debate over the inclusion of LLPDD in *DSM-III-R*. The actors and groups involved in the controversy "are not only those individually and collectively 'present,' articulate, and committed to action in that arena but also those implicated by actions in that arena. That is, the actions taken in that arena will be consequential for them, regardless of their current presence, organization, or action" (Clarke & Montini, 1993, p. 45). If different actors have different meanings of the artifact under construction or contestation, then there has to be a way to distinguish and locate the social worlds in relationship to one another.

In order to locate and distinguish the multiple social worlds involved in the contested arena of PMS, I employ the term "domain." This term allows for spatial understanding of the location of the actors, and it distinguishes the multiple meanings of the controversial fact or artifact. Domains constitute a social and analytical construct that is created by: the actors in the controversy, and the sociological analyst (myself in this case) who is making the connections between what the actors say, do, or are implicated in the struggle. Thus, a domain is simultaneously: (1) a place of social interaction where people and their shared interests in the fact or object interact—that is a social world; and (2) a theoretical and analytic construct that is fashioned by the analyst of the controversy and guided by work and theory in sociology.

DATA AND METHODS

In this study, I utilize primary data from the following sources. I conducted semi-structured personal interviews with four of the key participants in the controversy. The four psychiatrists equally represented pro-inclusion (Robert Spitzer and Sally Severino) and anti-inclusion (Jean Hamilton and Teresa Bernardez) stances and took a leadership role during the controversy. I also examined the APA archival records and materials deposited at the American Psychiatric Association headquarters in Washington, DC. These records consist of internal memos concerning the *DSM-III-R* and LLPDD, letters of protest written about LLPDD, and minutes of meetings of committees involved in the *DSM* revision and the LLPDD decision. In order to balance the official records and documents of the APA, I also gained access to the bulk of the anti-inclusion materials that are deposited at the Institute for Research on Women's Health in Washington, DC. These records consist of briefing and press booklets, petitions, and strategic correspondence about fighting the inclusion of LLPDD. Finally, I collected and examined published accounts of the controversy in the popular, medical, and scientific presses. Any reference or mention of the *DSM-III-R* or LLPDD was counted as data for this study.

The first text that I examined was the diagnostic criteria for LLPDD. These criteria are found in Table 1. LLPDD and its criteria appear here as a finished product or human made artifact. When examined as this finished product

Table 1 Research Criteria for Late Luteal Phase Dysphoric Disorder as found in Appendix A of *DSM-III-R* (copyright, American Psychiatric Association, 1987)

A. In most menstrual cycles during the past year, symptoms in B occurred during the last week of the luteal phase and remitted within a few days after onset of the follicular phase. In menstruating females, these phases correspond to the week before, and a few days after, the onset of menses. (In nonmenstruating females who have had a hysterectomy, the timing of luteal and follicular phases may require measurement of circulating reproductive hormones.)

B. At least five of the following symptoms have been present for most of the time during which symptomatic late luteal phase, at least one of the symptoms being either (1), (2), (3), or (4);

   (1) marked affective lability, e.g., feeling suddenly sad, tearful, irritable, or angry
   (2) persistent and marked anger or irritability
   (3) marked anxiety, tension, feelings of being "keyed up," or "on edge"
   (4) markedly depressed mood, feelings of hopelessness, or self-deprecating thoughts
   (5) decreased interest in usual activities, e.g., work, friends, hobbies
   (6) easy fatigability or marked lack of energy
   (7) subjective sense of difficulty in concentrating
   (8) marked change in appetite, overeating, or specific food cravings
   (9) hypersomnia or insomnia
   (10) other physical symptoms, such as breast tenderness or swelling, headaches, joint or muscle pain, a sensation of "bloating," weight gain

C. The disturbance seriously interferes with work or with usual social activities or relationships with others.

D. The disturbance is not merely an exacerbation of the symptoms of another disorder, such as Major Depression, Panic Disorder, Dysthymia, or a Personality Disorder (although it may be superimposed on any of these disorders).

E. Criteria A, B, C, and D are confirmed by prospective daily self-ratings during at least two symptomatic cycles. (The diagnosis may be made provisionally prior to this confirmation.)

and taken out of the context of the people, events, and actions that compose the controversy, LLPDD is just another psychiatric disorder with set criteria. In this form, the diagnosis does not appear so controversial, nor does it seem interesting sociologically. It exists, psychiatrists use it, women have it or they don't. How and why was this diagnosis so politically charged and complicated?

According to many who observed the controversy, making sense of LLPDD was simple. An analysis employed by journalists and some psychiatrists was that the LLPDD issue was a simple matter of opposition forces lumped under the heading "feminist" (DePaul, 1986; Keyser, 1986). Who opposed the diagnosis? Feminists. Why did they oppose it? They were feminists. The often employed account implies that "feminists" opposed it for only political reasons and not for scientific reasons (Fink, 1987; Goodwin & Guze, 1989). Explanation for the controversy is reduced to a simplistic political accounting of the events.

In the same way that a political account reduces LLPDD to an "inevitable" and "uncomplicated" political struggle between feminists and the APA, another popular account suggests the eventual outcome unfolded rationally and bureaucratically. This type of explanation was employed by several APA officers and pro-inclusion psychiatrists (Gitlin & Pasnau, 1989; Blumenthal & Nadelson, 1988; Spitzer & Williams, 1987). This account suggests that various bodies within the APA successively collected new information and made sequenced decisions according to a rational bureaucratic procedure. The outcome, that is the decision to place LLPDD in a research appendix, could be seen as the most reasonable, judicious, and even inevitable one (Frances, 1989; Gitlin & Pasnau, 1989). In addition, a chronological portrayal of the controversy suggests that the resulting diagnosis produced well-defined criteria for the psychiatric manifestation of PMS and thus a scientific "linear" improvement over previously established 1983 NIMH guidelines.

Identifying and constructing the public (newspaper, official explanations in journals and books, and press releases) versus the private (personal interviews and documents) accounts of the controversy are important steps in employing a social worlds approach to analyzing the LLPDD controversy. One of the most important hidden pieces of information about LLPDD is that the first and primary opposition to the diagnosis came not from outside "feminist groups" (as the press accounts portrayed) but rather from the APA's own Committee on Women. Most of these women would describe themselves as feminists; they are also eminent psychiatrists and scientists. This suggests that they would have a variety of sometimes conflicting interests in PMS. By focusing initially on this committee and talking to the two psychiatrists (Hamilton and Bernardez) who spearheaded opposition forces, the shape of my analysis of the controversy began to change.

Intensive focus upon the actions and strategies of the Committee on Women (i.e., the Committee on Women served as an analytical "wedge"), enabled me to "fashion" three distinct but overlapping domains of the controversy. Figure 1 summarizes graphically the three domains in which the battle over PMS and LLPDD was fought. The shaded area in the center points to the arena of PMS—which is what the three domains have in common. In each, actors struggled for what Gusfield has called "the ownership" of a social problem, in this case PMS. Gusfield writes:

> To "own" a social problem Is to possess the authority to name a condition a "problem" and to suggest what might be done about it. It is the power to influence the marshalling of public facilities—laws, enforcement abilities, opinion, goods and services—to help resolve the problem (Gusfield, 1989, p.6).

In linking Gusfield's term of ownership with domain analysis, I show that PMS and LLPDD were not just an issue for the two opposing groups, but for a constellation of often overlapping actors and social groups. All were trying to claim ownership of PMS and its psychiatric manifestation in LLPDD.

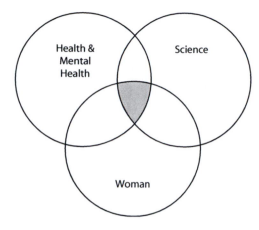

Figure 1 The Three Domains of PMS/LLPDD

There were three arenas of conflict that initially produced three differ-ent LLPDDs. First, the Committee on Women chose to go outside the APA and enlist other health, mental health, and legal professionals in creating an alliance to fight the inclusion of the diagnosis. I have called this the "health and mental health" domain. In doing this, the Committee linked LLPDD to larger professional concerns in the definition and treatment of mental ill-ness. It actively solicited support from organizations such as the American Psychological Association, the National Association of Social Workers, and the American Orthopsychiatric Association. Through strategies chosen by the APA's Committee on Women, LLPDD became the occasion for contests of professional dominance, raising questions about the hierarchy of authority in the health and mental health fields.

The Committee on Women also linked themselves to a variety of femi-nist and women's groups, for whom the diagnosis was not a "contest among professionals" but a struggle between experts and laity for the control over women's bodies and minds: a struggle over the definition of a normal and healthy woman. This "woman" domain included expert and professional women who made claims to speak on behalf of all women but also individ-ual women with PMS who claimed their own authority to speak for them-selves. The APA Committee on Women took LLPDD into this domain as it pursued certain strategies to advance its initial interest in getting this "anti-woman" diagnosis completely removed from *DSM-III-R*. When situated in feminist theories and critiques of science, gender studies, and historical and anthropological studies of women, and menstruation, LLPDD was a gen-dered artifact related to issues of stigmatization and control of women's bod-ies. Feminist health, mental health, and political groups/individuals pitted themselves in a gendered struggle against the effect of labeling all menstru-ating women as potentially "crazy."

Finally, the Committee on Women also chose to ground its opposition to the inclusion of a PMS-related diagnosis on the argument that there were insufficient scientific data to warrant such a move. This strategy moved LLPDD into yet a third domain: science. Here, LLPDD was neither a contest among professions nor a struggle between women and experts, but rather an example of "nature" (the reality of PMS and LLPDD) that was still being negotiated. PMS and LLPDD became part of a larger struggle for control over the construction of scientific truth in the midst of a public controversy.

HEALTH AND MENTAL HEALTH DOMAIN

The basic sociological issue in the Health and Mental Health Domain focuses on LLPDD as the battleground for professional dominance and control among various health and mental health professions and semi-professionals.

A major dispute over the ownership of PMS and LLPDD appeared between gynecologists and psychiatrists. Gynecologists made significant claims that they were better suited as a medical specialty not only to diagnose but to treat PMS because it was a physiological or biological disorder. For example, one physician wrote to the APA:

> How stupid can you get?! There is no wonder at all that the label, head shrinker (Shrink), is used. There is no significant justification (theoretical or practical) for any effort to classify the condition as a mental or emotional disorder (from Los Angeles, CA, June 26, 1986).

On the other hand, Robert Spitzer, the Head of the Work Group to revise *DSM-III* stated in the *Detroit Free Press* that:

> Gynecologists are totally irrelevant. This is purely a mental disorder. It is not a physical or neurological disease (in Mickelson, 1986).

How was this conflict among the two medical specialties negotiated and settled? The status of LLPDD as a diagnosis was changed by the APA Board of Trustees from a gynecologic to a psychiatric disorder by virtue of changing the code number of the diagnosis (from an International Classification of Diseases (ICD) gynecological code (307.90) to a psychiatric code (300.90) Unspecified Mental Disorder). Psychiatrists changed the code number of LLPDD in order to claim the psychological elements of PMS as part of their professional province and to avoid any further conflict with gynecologists. PMS as LLPDD could be diagnosed by a psychiatrist but PMS as a gynecological condition could still be diagnosed by a gynecologist. In spite of what gynecologists might have thought about the creation of this disorder and its separate code number, the power to create and classify psychiatric disorders ultimately rests with the APA. The APA chose to reinforce the division of labor within the medical profession by claiming jurisdictional control over the right to diagnose and treat the emotional and psychological disturbances of PMS.

The second dispute involved groups external to the psychiatric profession who have often engaged the APA in boundary disputes concerning the treatment and definition of mental illness. These groups included psychologists, social workers, and psychiatric nurses. They charged that psychiatrists have too much of an individually centered focus upon the psychoanalytic, physiological, chemical, or biological natures of mental illness, and failed to recognize the social and environmental influences upon human behavior. Why were these interprofessional disputes concerning LLPDD important? The *DSM-III-R* is the property and official statement of the APA and it is formally recognized as the means to code and reimburse mental health care. Other mental health workers are, in a sense, forced to recognize and use it, and this puts the APA in an organizational and structural position of power in the mental health hierarchy. If the more medical model of PMS and other psychiatric disorders was legitimated and emphasized in *DSM-III-R*, it would follow then that psychiatrists and not psychologists or other mental health practitioners should define and treat PMS as a mental illness. In constructing LLPDD as a psychiatric disorder, psychiatrists were seen as asserting their professional dominance among mental health professionals in claiming the ability to recognize the difference between PMS as a biological and psychiatric phenomenon, and treat the latter.

The opposition to the inclusion of LLPDD by the non-psychiatric professions was defeated with the inclusion of the diagnosis in the manual—even with its placement in the appendix. The argument that PMS has social, economic, and interpersonal bases in reality was not upheld in the settlement. The construction of the psychiatric diagnosis of LLPDD signified the addition of more mental health "professional turf" for psychiatrists. However, psychologists and social workers were successful in one aspect as a result of their opposition to the *DSM-III-R* revisions. Formal liaison positions to the committee that is revising *DSM-III-R* were extended to the American Psychological Association and the National Association of Social Workers. This gives these professions recognition and input in the future construction of psychiatric diagnosis in the DSM.

The final issue in this domain concerned the role of semiprofessional, self-help and nontraditional healers in treating and diagnosing PMS. This boundary was marked early in the debate. Robert Spitzer was very concerned about "a large number of semiprofessional groups treating this condition," which "need a psychiatrist's skill" (*Psychiatric News*, October 18, 1985, 6). Over the counter PMS tablets, self-help books, and PMS advice articles that focus on diet, stress, and exercise have all become a big business since the 1980s. At issue in this third conflict was whether or not PMS is something to be diagnosed and treated by a doctor or a psychiatrist or by alternative healers, including the patient herself. There were significant challenges to the professional expertise of psychiatry, such that Spitzer explicitly stated:

> When psychiatry is under attack, you must not equivocate. There is no doubt that what we call periluteal phase dysphoric disorder (the newly adopted name for what had been called premenstrual dysphoric disorder) exists as a clinically significant syndrome in some women, even though the causes and optimal therapy are unknown. We must call this a mental disorder!" (*The Psychiatric Times*, Vol. III, No. 8, August 1986)

The addition of LLPDD to the *DSM-III-R* signified that professional psychiatric expertise was needed to differentiate this "mental disorder." Over-the-counter medications or self-help books are not enough to treat PMS any longer. Neither are gynecologists, psychologists, or social workers necessarily the most qualified health or mental health professionals to recognize and treat LLPDD. In constructing PMS as a psychiatric disorder, the APA was successful in extending its professional boundaries on three fronts.

THE WOMAN DOMAIN

Two major issues structure the struggles around PMS in the Woman Domain. The first is the claim that the psychiatric labeling of PMS and LLPDD might incriminate all women as subject to their "raging hormones." The effects of labeling a severe form of PMS as a psychiatric disorder could have negative consequences for all women in this society. Feminist critics of LLPDD stated concerns about employment loss and discrimination and the possibility of women losing custody of their children due to having their PMS classified as a mental illness. These claims were usually made by women experts claiming the scientific or professional expertise (lawyers, psychiatrists, and psychologists) to speak on behalf of women. The second issue defining LLPDD as a gendered artifact is the assertions by individual women that the APA should listen to them and their individually grounded expertise and experiences with their bodies and PMS.

How PMS is defined—and who controls or owns the diagnoses related to it—is a matter of grave concern. Women's menstrually-related issues have historically either been ignored by physicians and scientists or women were told that any feelings or problems "are all in their heads." The degree to which PMS has become a major issue in modern society is best understood in light of studies indicating that anywhere between 20 to 90 percent of all menstruating women could qualify as having some of the more than 200 recognized symptoms of PMS (Olesen & Woods, 1986; Adler, 1990; Mitchell, Lentz, Woods, Lee, & Taylor, 1992). These changes include physical symptoms such as weight gain and bloating as well as emotional symptoms such as irritability, mood changes, and vivid dream cycles (Delaney, Lupton, & Toth, 1988). If this is indeed true, and if almost all menstruating women do have at least some of these symptoms, then the "stability" of women's moods and behaviors can be called into question by scientists, doctors, politicians, bosses, and lawyers.

Two events in particular generated publicity with substantial political and legal implications for women. In 1970, Dr. Edgar Berman (physician to Hubert Humphrey) stated publicly that women were unfit for certain jobs (e.g., President and surgeon) because of raging hormonal imbalances (see Fausto-Sterling, 1985; and Corea, 1985). In the early 1980s, two murder trials in Great Britain—in which two women received reduced sentences due to the successful claims of diminished capacity due to their PMS—created even greater public interest in the effect of PMS on women's emotions and actions (Rittenhouse, 1991; Laws, Hey, & Eagan, 1985). For some women, the publicity and legitimization of PMS and its symptoms has lead to a positive sense about themselves and this phenomenon (e.g., Taylor, 1988). However, a more negative image of PMS as something that controls women once a month, that makes them "crazy" and subject to their hormones is much more pervasive in our culture. This negative image is evident in the jokes, greeting cards, television shows, and advertisements for over-the-counter medications (Chrisler & Levy, 1990; Parlee, 1987, 1993; Heneson, 1984).

Issues of stigmatization were important in the debate as extensive arguments used by both sides over the negative social effect of LLPDD show. Members of the LLPDD Advisory Committee suggested that the diagnosis was really a good thing for women. The head of a PMS laboratory at NIMH stated that in spite of feminists' concerns "this is a gain for feminists" and that the inclusion of the diagnosis "will make it clear that the great majority of women do not suffer from 'raging hormones'" (Holden, 1986, p. 231). Sally Severino, a leading proponent of the diagnosis stated that the classification of PMS in the *DSM-III-R* "confers a legitimacy on a syndrome historically neglected by doctors and scientists" (DePaul, 1986, p. 20). Spitzer claimed that if a disorder isn't recognized formally by the psychiatric profession "it cannot be treated effectively" (Boxer, 1987, p. 82; Carey, 1986, p. 60).

Remarks such as these raise one of the major dilemmas in the feminist community about PMS. For centuries women have been told that PMS is all in their heads, that it isn't real. Yet, to actually call PMS a psychiatric disorder takes the diagnosis out of the hands of most women and into the control of a predominantly male profession. Throughout the debate opponents of LLPDD remained firm in their stance that the diagnosis was ultimately harmful for women. "They are trying to make something pathological out of a normal female function," stated the head of the APA's Office for Women's Programs (in Holden, 1986). Of major concern was the connection of a psychiatric diagnosis with women's menstrual cycles and the potential applicability to all women. The most basic question that epitomizes feminist opposition was addressed by the president of the Association of Women Psychiatrists: "Are women going to be labeled as having psychiatric illness every month?" (Keyser, 1986).

The Committee on Women of the APA (especially Bernardez and Hamilton) engaged in a coalition-building and tactical campaign that resulted in the placement of the diagnosis in a research appendix of *DSM-III-R*, rather than in the main text. Committee members were in a structural position of power and authority to fight on the behalf of all women and especially those immediately at risk from an LLPDD diagnosis. From the first meeting of the LLPDD

Advisory Committee in May 1985 until the publication of the *DSM-III-R* in 1987, the Committee on Women worked within the existing organizational structure of the APA to fight inclusion of the diagnosis. However, the political effectiveness of the Committee on Women's opposition was diminished so long as it remained focused only on an internal problem to the APA. In spite of exhortations to work within the APA, the Committee on Women went outside the organizational machinery of the APA and enlisted external allies to help fight the inclusion of LLPDD. It was through these tactics that opposition forces were effective in drawing public attention to women's health and mental health issues. The chair of the APA's Committee on Women commented:

> The Work Group didn't know how to handle the fact that psychiatrists and psychologists and social workers had formed a coalition...this said something about these groups who are usually competitors that banded together (personal interview with Teresa Bernardez, East Lansing, April 20, 1990).

According to one commentator, "[w]omen have seldom been as united as they were on this issue" (Braude, 1987, p. 30).

The Institute for Research on Women's Health in Washington, DC became a center of activity for the LLPDD opposition movement. As professional advocates for the health and mental health of all women, the strategy involved linking the diagnosis of LLPDD (and the other proposed controversial diagnoses) to wider scientific, economic, and political issues. In this domain, this meant going beyond professional interests as psychiatrists or psychologists and focusing on LLPDD as a feminist issue. Co-founder Hamilton stated:

> Because of that organization [the Institute for Research on Women's Health], I also had a mailing list and ties to other organizations and advocacy groups— interdisciplinary ties. So we put out the word. Also because I'm located in Washington and because I'm feminist and have connections to other nonprofit organizations in D.C., we know lobbyists and we knew press people....And those people put out the word in their newsletters or in their organizations so we had this sort of feminist networking process. So we had people writing letters and creating havoc and we had all these radio spots. And that really pissed them off—I mean it really pissed them off. I mean how dare we (personal interview, June 4, 1990, Washington, DC).

With the help of a mailing list from the National Coalition for Women's Mental Health, Hamilton states that women associated with the Institute for Research on Women's Health spent

> several months on putting together how best to present our position and then doing, you know, whatever mailings. We'd have group meetings, three or four people would come and we'd stuff envelopes...we must've mailed out to five or six hundred people" (personal interview, June 4, 1990, Washington, DC).

It was through these mailings and networking efforts that individual women were notified about the movement to make PMS a psychiatric disorder.

In particular, women who have PMS attempted to make their voices heard in the debate. In all the rhetoric and political maneuvering about LLPDD by the professional advocates, these women were not usually the focus of the controversy. Yet they did find ways to claim "ownership" of PMS. Many women wrote to the APA describing their experiences with PMS and protesting the inclusion of LLPDD. In their letters to the APA, these women had a strong sense of their own authoritative voice in defining PMS as *not* a psychiatric disorder. For example, a woman from Topeka, Kansas, wrote the following in claiming her own history with PMS:

> I believe that treating women with PMS syndrome in a standard psychiatric way—disregarding the biological effects this condition has upon women—is very dangerous. It is dangerous because this condition effects many aspects of the female personality as well as her biological character. I believe that my own case history might add some insight into this problem.

Another woman wrote:

> As a longtime sufferer of PMS I object vehemently to being labeled "mentally ill." Or did I all at once cease to be mentally ill upon my menopause? I admit my PMS gave me some mental anguish, but so do some of my physical ails today.

The significance of the placement of LLPDD in the appendix of *DSM-III-R* for these women with PMS is simply that they lost and their voices were rarely heard. Although "professional advocates" such as the Committee on Women continue to fight on their behalf, the women with PMS who protested the inclusion of the diagnosis of LLPDD appear to be silenced in the resulting settlement of the controversy. The inclusion of the diagnosis in the *DSM-III-R* even in the appendix and especially with a psychiatric coding signaled a defeat for these women who could be subject to the label of having a "mental illness."

THE SCIENCE DOMAIN

In the "Science Domain," LLPDD can be seen as a contest for the control and ownership of the "scientific truth" about PMS. The debate about the scientific validity of LLPDD and the research implications of creating such a diagnosis focused the debate on the nature and settlement of controversy in science and medicine.

What does the science of PMS tell us? Scientific research on the menstrual cycle has provided inconsistent and often contradictory findings. The 1983 NIMH-sponsored conference played a pivotal role in highlighting the lack of concrete scientific findings about PMS and was an impetus for the creation of the LLPDD label. Conference findings led to the conclusion that the current data on PMS are "seriously flawed" (Blume, 1983, p. 2866). Although some guidelines for conducting PMS research were agreed upon at this conference, many eminent PMS researchers supported the inclusion of LLPDD in the *DSM-III-R*. First, it provided *specific diagnostic criteria* for the 10 percent of women who suffer from severe and adverse forms of PMS. Second, it provided specific research criteria; LLPDD made PMS research more definable, specific, and fundable.

Proponents argued that the diagnosis's construction was consistent with the way science works. Sally Severino stated that:

> If we had waited until all the evidence was in, we would never have come up with the staging of heart disease or cancer. We have to begin by labeling, classifying, and defining. This is the way science progresses. (in Staver, 1986, p. 26)

Another one of the more consistent charges raised in the scientific domain was that the diagnosis was created only to secure more external funding grants from agencies such as NIMH. According to Hamilton, who was one of two dissenters on the LLPDD Advisory Committee and also a member of the Committee on Women:

> The concern was basically, look, NIMH isn't currently funding anything and they are not going to do it unless it's a diagnosis. Drug companies are not going to fund research on this unless we have a diagnosis because they are not going to give you money to test drugs for something that doesn't exist. We have to make an entity exist so we can study it. (personal interview, June 4, 1990, Washington, DC)

Scientific authority and data played an important role in the decision making about LLPDD. On the one hand, the expert knowledge of psychiatry and science was "at risk" because the social and political implications of the diagnostic process were well documented and exposed. Explicit connections to political and professional implications of the diagnosis and the process of *DSM-III* revisions were consistently made. For example, following the June 1986 decision to place the diagnosis in an appendix, the chair of the Committee on Women stated that:

> While I would have preferred to see the diagnoses dropped, I believe it is far better to have them in the appendix than in the text. Now while the proponents try to come up with scientific evidence to support inclusion in the text of *DSM-IV*, we will have the opportunity to educate our colleagues and the public. (Teresa Bernardez, as reported in Staver, 1986b, p. 41)

But what is interesting about this statement by Bernardez and by other psychiatrists is the basic belief that although the diagnostic *process* was political, somehow in the end, science will arrive at the truth about PMS and LLPDD. It was this basic belief in science and its role as the great arbitrator of the world that settled the question about LLPDD. In claiming the ultimate ownership of LLPDD, the APA Board of Trustees used the established cultural notions attached to the authority of science and effectively settled the controversy by postponing a final decision.

By including it in Appendix A of the *DSM-III-R* as a category in need of "further systematic clinical study and research" the Board of Trustees appealed to lack of scientific data about PMS. Statements made by the Board of Trustees about their decision to place the diagnosis in the appendix support this notion. Speaking for the Board, APA President Robert Pasnau stated:

> we are not yet convinced that the scientific evidence, while impressive, is sufficiently strong to warrant inclusion in the text of the manual at this time. But...[is] of sufficient clinical importance to justify publishing [it] in the appendix to the manual for research and educational purposes. (APA press release, July 1, 1986)

For those scientists who study PMS, the controversy and its settlement was a positive outcome. Even though the "scientific evidence" about the existence of LLPDD was called into question, its placement in an appendix under the heading of proposed diagnoses in need of further study made the scientists who study PMS big winners. Who benefits by further study of LLPDD? Scientists who conduct the study of PMS and who will receive grants in which to conduct their research.

CONCLUSIONS

The decision to place LLPDD in an appendix temporarily stabilized the controversy. However, disagreement still exists over this controversial diagnosis. Scientific and medical "consensus" about the psychological manifestations of PMS may never be achieved. A newly reformed LLPDD will once again be called "Premenstrual Dysphoric Disorder" and is scheduled to be included in the *DSM-IV.* It will appear as an example in the main text of a mood disorder (not otherwise specified), but the diagnosis itself will remain in the research appendix (Cotton, 1993).

In the end, controversies are not settled by "facts" or "science" alone. Latour reminds us that science is politics by other means (1987). The domain analysis offered here invites attention to significant and enduring sociological questions about the controversy and construction of scientific and medical artifacts: (1) "Who is making these claims and why?" (2) "On what grounds does a certain claim to truth exist?" (3) "How is this truth determined and settled?" The settlement of controversy certainly reflects the ability of some actors and groups to determine what becomes the accepted view of reality. It also reflects the social, political, and organizational processes through which this occurs. That these same processes can occur in *different* domains of interaction is a measure of the strength of this antireductionistic position.

References

Adler, T. (1990, January), Treatments for PMS are promising, but untested. *APA Monitor*, 11.

American Psychiatric Association. (1980). *Diagnostic and Statistical Manual of Mental Disorders* (3rd ed.). Washington, DC: Author.

American Psychiatric Association. (1987). *Diagnostic and Statistical Manual of Mental Disorders* (3rd ed., rev. ed.). Washington, DC: Author.

Amchin, J. (1991). *Psychiatric Diagnosis: A Biopsychosocial Approach Using DSM-III-R*. Washington, DC: American Psychiatric Association Press.

Bayer, R. (1987). *Homosexuality and American Psychiatry: The Politics of Diagnosis*. Princeton, NJ: Princeton University Press.

Becker, H. (1982). *Art Worlds*. Chicago: University of Chicago Press.

Blume, E. (1983). Methodological difficulties plague PMS research. *Journal of the American Medical Association, 249*, 2866.

Blumenthal, S., & Nadelson, C., (1988). Late Luteal Phase Dysphoric Disorder (premenstrual syndromes): Clinical implications. *Journal of Clinical Psychiatry, 49*, 469–474.

Boxer, S. (1987, August). The parable of the cheek-turners and the cheek-smiters. *Discover*, 80–83.

Braude, M. (1987). Further thoughts on DSM. *News for Women in Psychiatry 5*, 7.

Brown, P. (1990). The name game: Toward a sociology of diagnosis. *Journal of Mind and Behavior, 11*, 385–406.

Carey, J. (1986, May 26). Is PMS mental illness? Debate grows. *U.S. News & World Report, 100*, 60.

Chrisler, J., & Levy, K. (1990). The media construct a menstrual monster: A content analysis of PMS articles in the popular press. *Women & Health, 16*, 89–104.

Clarke, A. (1990a). Controversy and the development of reproductive science. *Social Problems, 37*, 18–37.

Clarke, A. (1990b). A social worlds research adventure: The case of reproductive science. In S. Cozzens and T. Gleryn (Eds.), *Theories of Science in Society* (pp. 15–42). Bloomington, IN.: Indiana University Press.

Clarke, A., & Montini, T. (1993). The many faces of RU486: Tales of situated knowledges and technological contestations. *Science, Technology & Human Values, 18*, 42–78.

Corea, G. (1985). *The Hidden Malpractice: How American Medicine Mistreats Women* (Updated version). New York: Harper Colophon Books.

Cotton, P. (1993). Psychiatrists set to approve DSM-IV. *Journal of the American Medical Association, 270*, 13–15.

DePaul, A. (1986, March 5). Defining new diseases of the mind: Feminist groups complain that a diagnosis of PMS will cause discrimination. *The Washington Post*, p. 20.

Delaney, J., Lupton, M., & Toth, E. (1988). *The Curse: A Cultural History of Menstruation*. Chicago: University of Illinois Press.

Fausto-Sterling, A. (1985). *Myths of Gender: Biological Theories About Women and Men*. New York: Basic Books.

Fink, P. (1987). Forward. In B. Ginsburg and B. F. Carter (Eds.), *Premenstrual Syndrome: Ethical and Legal Implications in a Biomedical Perspective*. New York: Plenum Press.

Fisher, K. (1986, July). DSM-III-R protest: Critics say psychiatry has been stonewalling. *APA Monitor*, 4–5.

Frances, A. (1989). Forward. In S. Severino and M. Moline (Eds.), *Premenstrual Syndrome: A Clinician's Guide*. New York: The Guilford Press.

Fujimura, J. (1988). Constructing doable problems in cancer research: Where social worlds meet. *Social Problems, 35,* 261–283.

Gitlin, M., & Pasnau, R. (1989). Psychiatric syndromes linked to reproductive function in women: A review of current knowledge. *American Journal of Psychiatry, 146,* 1413–1422.

Goleman, D. (1985, November 19). New psychiatric syndromes spur protest. *The New York Times,* pp. C1, C16.

Goodwin, D., & Guze, S. (1989). Preface. In D. Goodwin and S. Guz (Eds.), *Psychiatric Diagnosis* (4th ed.). New York: Oxford University Press.

Gusfield, J. (1989). Constructing the ownership of social problems: Fun and profit in the welfare state. *Social Problems, 36,* 431–441.

Heneson, N. (with Strain, C). (1984). The selling of P.M.S. *Science, 84 5,* 6671.

Holden, C. (1986). Proposed new psychiatric diagnoses raise charges of gender bias. *Science, 231,* 327–328.

Keyser, L. (1986, July 4). APA cuts manual to please feminists. *The Washington (D.C.) Times,* p. 80.

Kirk, S., & Kutchins, H. (1992). *The Selling of DSM: The Rhetoric of Science in Psychiatry.* Hawthorne, NY: Aldine de Gruyter.

Latour, B. (1987). *Science in Action.* Cambridge, MA: Harvard University Press.

Laws, S., Hey, V., & Eagan, A. (1985). *Seeing Red: The Politics of Premenstrual Tension.* London: Hutchinson.

Mickelsen, L. (1986, June 4). Battle of the couch: Who's ill? *The Detroit Free Press,* pp. 1B–3B.

Mitchell, E., Lentz, M., Woods, N., Lee, K., & Taylor, D. (1992). Methodological issues in the definition of premenstrual syndrome. In A. Dan and L. Lewis (Eds.), *Menstrual Health in Women's Lives* (pp. 7–14). Chicago: University of Illinois Press.

Olesen, V., & Woods, N. F. (1986). *Culture, Society and Menstruation.* Washington, DC: Hemisphere Publishing.

Parlee, M. B. (1987). Media treatment of premenstrual syndrome. In B. E. Ginsburg and B. F. Carter (Eds.), *Premenstrual Syndrome: Ethical and Legal Implications in a Biomedical Perspective* (pp. 189–205). New York: Plenum.

Parlee, M. B. (1993, November 21). Research on "premenstrual syndrome": Controversies and consolidation, 1968–1993. Paper presented at the Society for Social Studies of Science, Annual Meeting. West Lafayette, IN.

Psychiatric News. (1983–1987). The newspaper of the American Psychiatric Association. Articles are cited by date in the text.

The Psychiatric Times. (1986). Science or politics? DSM-III-R controversy grows. *III,* 17.

Rittenhouse, A. (1991). The emergence of Premenstrual Syndrome as a social problem. *Social Problems, 38,* 412–425.

Scott, W. (1990). PTSD in DSM-III: A case in the politics of diagnosis and disease. *Social Problems, 37,* 294–310.

Spitzer, R., & Williams, J. (1987). Introduction. In *Diagnostic and Statistical Manual of Mental Disorders* (3rd ed., Rev.). Washington, DC: American Psychiatric Association.

Spitzer, R., Severino, S., Williams, J., & Parry, B. (1989). Late luteal phase dysphoric disorder and DSM-III-R. *American Journal of Psychiatry, 146,* 892–897.

Staver, S. (1986, June 6). Diagnostic disputes: Proposed changes in diagnosis manual spark heated controversies. *American Medical News, 3,* 25–28.

Strauss, A. (1978). A social worlds perspective. In *Studies in Symbolic Interaction*, ed. Norman Denzin 1: 119–128. Greenwich: JAI Press.

Taylor, Dena. (1988). *Red Flower: Rethinking Menstruation*. Freedom, CA.: Crossing Press.

DISCUSSION QUESTIONS

1. What were the primary issues in each of the domains of conflict identified by Figert? How were those issues resolved?

2. How does Figert's analysis of PMS differ from Conrad's analysis of hyper-kinesis? What perspective does she use to guide her analysis? How might her analysis have differed if she had used a traditional medicalization perspective?

3. What does Figert's analysis suggest about the ability of science to resolve definitional controversies in psychiatry and other medical sciences? What scientific evidence would convince you that PMS should be defined as a mental disorder? What scientific evidence would convince you otherwise?

Culture and the Definition
of Mental Illness

Arthur Kleinman

What is a Psychiatric Diagnosis?[†]

Arthur Kleinman is a psychiatrist and medical anthropologist who has written extensively on the role of culture in illness experience. In this chapter from his book,
Rethinking Psychiatry: From Cultural Category to Personal Experience, *he asserts that psychiatric diagnoses are culturally-based interpretations of psychological, social, and biological experiences rather than objective classifications of naturally-occurring phenomena. Because interpretational systems vary from one culture to the next, diagnoses that are meaningful in one cultural context (e.g., neurasthenia in China) may not be meaningful in another. Kleinman's analysis raises important questions about the ability of psychiatric diagnoses to represent individual people's experiences faithfully, and about the challenges of studying mental disorders cross-culturally.*

I am sitting in a small interview room at the Hunan Medical College in south central China. It is August 1980 and the temperature is over 100 degrees. I am sweating profusely and so is the patient I am interviewing, a thin, pallid, 28-year-old teacher at a local primary school in Changsha whose name is Lin Xiling. Mrs. Lin, who has suffered from chronic headaches for the past six years, is telling me about her other symptoms: dizziness, tiredness, easy fatigue, weakness, and a ringing sound in her ears. She has been under the treatment of doctors in the internal medicine clinic of the Second Affiliated Hospital of the Hunan Medical College for more than half a year with increasing symptoms. They have referred her to the psychiatric clinic though against her objections, with the diagnosis of neurasthenia. Gently, sensing a deep disquiet behind the tight lips and mask-like squint, I ask Mrs. Lin if she feels depressed. "Yes, I am unhappy,," she replies. "My life has been difficult," she quickly adds as a justification. At this point Mrs. Lin looks away. Her thin

Kleinman, Arthur. 1988 "What is a psychiatric diagnosis?" Pp. 5–17 in *Rethinking Psychiatry: From Cultural Category to Personal Experience.* New York: Free Press.

lips tremble. The brave mask dissolves into tears. For several minutes she continues sobbing; the deep inhalations reverberate as a low wail.

After regaining her composure (literally reforming her "face"), Mrs. Lin explains that she is the daughter of intellectuals who died during the Cultural Revolution while being abused by the Red Guards. She and her four brothers and sisters were dispersed to different rural areas. Mrs. Lin, then a teenager, was treated harshly by both the cadres and peasants in the impoverished commune in the far north to which she was sent. She could not adapt to the very cold weather and the inadequate diet. After a year she felt that she was starving, and indeed had decreased in weight from 110 to 90 pounds. She felt terribly lonely: in five miserable years her *only* friend was a fellow middle school student with a similar background from her native city, who shared her complaints. Finally, in the mid-seventies she returned to Changsha. She then learned that one of her sisters had committed suicide while being "struggled" by the Red Guards and a brother had become paralyzed in a tractor accident. Three times Mrs. Lin took the highly competitive entrance examinations for university education, and each time, to her great shame, she failed to achieve a mark high enough to gain admission. Two years before our interview, she married an electrician in her work unit. The marriage was arranged by the unit leaders. Mrs. Lin did not know her husband well before their marriage, and afterward she discovered that both he and his mother had difficult, demanding, irascible personalities. Their marriage has been characterized by frequent arguments which end at times with her husband beating her, and her mother-in-law, with whom they live, attacking her for being an ungrateful daughter-in-law and incompetent wife. Both husband and mother-in-law hold her responsible for the stillbirth of a nearly full-term male fetus one year before.

Over the past two years, Mrs. Lin's physical symptoms have worsened and she has frequently sought help from physicians of both biomedicine and traditional Chinese medicine. When questioned by me, she admits to more symptoms—difficulty with sleep, appetite, and energy, as well as joylessness, anxiety, and feelings that it would be better to be dead. She has an intense feeling of guilt about the stillbirth and also about not being able to be practically helpful to her paraplegic brother. During the past six months she has developed feelings of hopelessness and helplessness, as well as self-abnegating thoughts. Mrs. Lin regards her life as a failure. She has fleeting feelings that it would be better for all if she took her life, but she has put these suicidal ideas to the side and has made no plans to kill herself.

From Mrs. Lin's perspective, her chief problem is her "neurasthenia." She remarks that if only she could he cured of this "physical" problem and the constant headache, dizziness, and fatigue it creates, she would feel more hopeful and would be better able to adapt to her family situation.

For a North American psychiatrist, Mrs. Lin meets the official diagnostic criteria for a major depressive disorder. The Chinese psychiatrists who interviewed her with me did not agree with this diagnosis. They did not deny that she was depressed, but they regarded the depression as a manifestation of neurasthenia, and Mrs. Lin shared this viewpoint. Neurasthenia—a syndrome of exhaustion, weakness, and diffuse bodily complaints believed to be caused by inadequate physical energy in the central nervous system—is an official diagnosis in China; but it is not a diagnosis in the American Psychiatric Association's latest nosology.

For the anthropologist, the problem seems more that of demoralization as a serious life distress due to obvious social sources than depression as a psychiatric disease. From the anthropological vantage point, demoralization might also be conceived as part of the illness experience associated with the disease, neurasthenia or depression. Here *illness* refers to the patient's perception, experience, expression, and pattern of coping with symptoms, while *disease* refers to the way practitioners recast illness in terms of their theoretical models of pathology.

Thus, a psychiatric diagnosis is an *interpretation* of a person's experience. That interpretation differs systematically for those professionals whose orientation is different. And other social factors—such as clinical specialty, institutional setting, and, most notably in Mrs. Lin's case, the distinctive cultural backgrounds of the psychiatrists—powerfully influence the interpretation. The interpretation is also, of course, constrained by Mrs. Lin's actual experience. Psychiatric diagnosis as interpretation must meet some resistance in lived experience, whose roots are deeply personal and physiological. The diagnosis does not create experience; mental disorder is part of life itself.

But that experience is perceived and expressed by Mrs. Lin through her own interpretation of bodily symptoms and problems of the self, so that the experience itself is always mediated. Because language, illness beliefs, personal significance of pain and suffering, and socially learned ways of behaving when ill are part of that process of mediation, the experience of illness (or distress) is always a culturally shaped phenomenon (like style of dress, table etiquette, idioms for expressing emotion, and aesthetic judgments). The interpretations of patient and family become part of the experience. Furthermore, professional and lay interpretations of experience are communicated and negotiated in particular relationships of power (political, economic, bureaucratic, and so forth). As a result, illness experiences are enmeshed in and inseparable from social relationships.

THE MEANING OF PSYCHIATRIC DIAGNOSIS TO THE PSYCHIATRIST

In a brilliant volume, McHugh and Slavney (1986), senior psychiatrists at Johns Hopkins Medical School, describe psychiatric diagnosis in a phenomenological idiom that I suspect most psychiatrists would find compelling. They refer to psychiatric disorders as naturally occurring forms of mental experience that can be observed in much the same way that the natural scientist observes the stratigraphy of mountains, the structures of the cell, or the forms of diseased arteries, rashes, and cancers. The problem of psychiatric diagnosis then becomes a question of verification. Are the forms present or not? McHugh and Slavney describe the two kinds of verification that psychiatric researchers struggle to establish in studies of the prevalence, manifestations, course, and treatment response of particular psychiatric disorders—namely, reliability and validity. Reliability they define as "verification of observations"; it is "the consistency with which one can make an observation...[it] is demonstrated by the correlation between the results of observers using the same technique to make that observation" (p. 4). Reliability is documented by the inter-rater correlation coefficient for congruence of diagnosis by psychiatrists trained in the same diagnostic methodology and using the same criteria.

Validity, on the other hand, is the "verification of presumptions," i.e., the verification of the psychiatric categories themselves. McHugh and Slavney correctly note that the "reliability of some psychiatric observations is high." That is to say, psychiatrists can he trained so as to make the same observations. But reliability reveals only that the measurement of the observations is consistent. It does not tell us if the observations are valid, i.e., whether a patient does or does not have an abnormal mental state such as delusions or hallucinations. After all, diagnosticians can be trained so that they are consistent but wrong.

For example, suppose ten North American psychiatrists are trained in the same diagnostic assessment technique and employ exactly the same diagnostic criteria. They are each asked to interview ten American Indians who are in the first weeks of bereavement following the death of a spouse. They may determine with 90 percent consistency (that is 9 out of 10 times) that the same seven subjects report hearing the voice of the dead spouse calling to them as the spirit travels to the afterworld. That is a high degree of reliability of observation. But the determination of whether such reports are a sign of an abnormal mental state is an interpretation based on knowledge of this group's behavioral norms and range of normal experiences of bereavement. Now it just so happens that in many American Indian tribes auditory experiences of the voices of the spirits of the dead calling to the living to join them in the afterworld are an expected and commonly experienced part of the sadness and loss that constitute the process of bereavement. This experience does not portend any dire consequences such as psychosis, protracted depression, or other complications of bereavement. Thus, to systematically interpret these normal auditory experiences in this cultural group as "hallucinations," with all that term connotes of abnormality, is an example of reliability without validity. Yet this is often done. I myself have been asked on four occasions to diagnose American Indian bereaved who were undergoing this culturally normative experience as psychotic, and thereby certifiable, by physicians who had made this invalid inference of hallucinations from normal sensory experience.

The problem lies in the positivist bias of most psychiatrists. For McHugh and Slavney, and most of us who have undergone the empiricist training in medical school, observations are direct representations of reality. A word, e.g., "hallucinations" or "delusions" points to an empirical entity, e.g.,

CULTURE-BOUND SYNDROMES

The *DSM-IV* defines a culture-bound syndrome as follows:

"The term *culture-bound syndrome* denotes recurrent, locality-specific patterns of aberrant behavior and troubling experience that may or may not be linked to a particular *DSM-IV* diagnostic category. Many of these patterns are indigenously considered to be 'illnesses,' or at least afflictions, and most have local names. Although presentations conforming to major *DSM-IV* categories can be found throughout the world, the particular symptoms, course, and social response are very often influenced by local cultural factors. In contrast, culture-bound syndromes are generally limited to specific societies or culture areas and are localized, folk, diagnostic categories that frame coherent meanings for certain repetitive, patterned, and troubling sets of experiences and observations" (American Psychiatric Association, 2000, p. 898).

Peter J. Guarnaccia and Lloyd Rogler (1999) note that we know very little about culture-bound syndromes. The little research that has been done typically applies the language and categories of dominant, Western psychiatric classification systems to culture-bound syndromes—for example, reinterpreting their symptoms as evidence of anxiety or depression—an approach that ignores their unique character. Guarnaccia and Rogler advocate a research agenda based on four key questions: (1) "How do we characterize the culture-bound syndrome within its cultural context? What are the defining features of the phenomenon?" (2) "Who are the people who experience culture-bound syndromes, and what is their social structural location? What situational factors provoke these symptoms?" (3) "How is the culture-bound syndrome empirically related to psychiatric disorder?" and (4) "When the culture-bound syndrome and psychiatric disorders coexist, what is the sequence of onset? How does the life history of the sufferer, particularly the experience of traumatic events, affect the sequence?"

Guarnaccia and Rogler illustrate the potential of their proposed agenda with reference to Ataques de nervios, an idiom of distress most common among Latinos from the Caribbean. Research shows that Ataques de nervios are very common among Puerto Rican adults (reported by 16 percent) and even more common in a sample of Puerto Rican and Dominican clients of mental health services in the United States (75 percent). Although psychiatric research has identified seizures and suicidal gestures as the prominent features of the syndrome, studies that ask sufferers to describe their experiences report that loss of emotional and physical control (e.g., screaming or crying uncontrollably) is the most common problem associated with the syndrome. With respect to the social distribution of the syndrome, it appears to be most common among women over the age of 45 with less than a high school education who are out of the labor force, and who recently experienced a marital separation or divorce. Ataques de nervios is highly comorbid with anxiety disorders and mood disorders although not all sufferers of one experience the other. Thus, Ataques de nervios appears to be a unique form of distress, related to but distinct from *DSM-IV* disorders and worthy of sustained research attention. A comparable research approach could prove equally illuminating if applied to other culture-bound syndromes.

American Psychiatric Association. 2000. *Diagnostic and Statistical Manual of Mental Disorders, Fourth Edition*, Text Revision. Washington, DC: American Psychiatric Association.
Guarnaccia, Peter J. and Lloyd H. Rogler. 1999. "Research on Culture-Bound Syndromes: New Directions." *American Journal of Psychiatry* 156:1322–1327.

an "abnormal mental state in the world." Advances in effective psychiatric treatment of specific disorders and recognition that clusters of symptoms and signs have the same prognosis not surprisingly encourage the view that depression, schizophrenia, and phobias are "things" in the real world. The picture is more complex. A word, after all, is a sign that signifies a meaningful phenomenon. That phenomenon, as noted above, exists in a world mediated by a cultural apparatus of language, values, taxonomies, notions of relevance, and rules for interpretation. Thus, observations of phenomena are judgments whose reliability can be determined by consistency of measurements but whose validity needs to be established by understanding the cultural context. Perception is theory-driven. The voice of a dead spouse is a hallucination (meaning abnormal sensory process) among most North Americans, for whose reference group the experience is not normative (though perhaps this is not true for some bereaved children (Egdell & Kolvin, 1972; Balk, 1983). But it is a normal experience of bereavement among members of many American Indian tribes. The term "hallucination," when used in its clinical sense to mean an abnormal percept, is an invalid interpretation for these individuals.

Validation of psychiatric diagnoses is not simply verification of the concepts used to explain observations. It is also verification of the meaning of the observations in a given social system (a village, an urban clinic, a research laboratory). That is to say, observation is inseparable from interpretation. Psychiatric diagnoses are not things, though they give name and shape to processes involving neurotransmitters, endocrine hormones, activity in the autonomic nervous system, and thoughts, feelings, and behaviors that show considerable stability. Rather, psychiatric diagnoses derive from categories. They underwrite the interpretation of phenomena, which themselves are congeries of psychological, social, and biological processes. Categories are the outcomes of historical development, cultural influence, and political negotiation. Psychiatric categories—though mental illness will not allow us to make of it whatever we like—are no exception.

If the cross-cultural perspective sharply raises the issue of validity, it surely does not resolve how it is to be decided. Clearly, validity cannot be a matter of pure subjectivity or complete relativity: the disease and its experience also constrain what diagnosis is valid. What are the criteria we can pose, then, for validity of diagnostic categories applied cross-culturally, i.e., how will we recognize a valid interpretation when we see it? What techniques can be specified that are likely to produce cross-culturally valid diagnoses? Anthropology poses the question, but offers only a tentative and quite modest answer: assuring the validity of psychiatric diagnoses should involve a conceptual tacking back and forth between the psychiatrist's diagnostic system and its rules of classification, alternative taxonomies, his clinical experience, and that of the patient, which includes the patient's interpretation. Validity is the negotiated outcome of this transforming interaction between concept and experience in a particular context. Thus, validity can be regarded as a type of ethnographic understanding of the meaning of an observation in a local cultural field.

Let us return to the diagnosis of Mrs. Lin's disorder. For her Chinese internists and psychiatrists, the disorder is neurasthenia—a putative "chronic malfunction" of the cerebral cortex associated with nervousness, weakness, headaches, and dizziness, thought to be common among "brain workers" and to have psychosocial as well as biological causes. But it is held to be a physical illness and therefore neither conveys the marked stigma Chinese attribute to mental illness nor implies personal accountability for the associated physical impairment or emotional distress. The way in which Mrs. Lin presents her symptoms is also influenced by the category neurasthenia, which is not only a technical psychiatric taxonomic entity in China but one widely understood in the popular culture. Mrs. Lin's perception of her symptoms selects out and lumps together those symptoms that are familiar and salient to her, namely the ones that fit the popular blueprint of neurasthenia. This practice is reinforced by the relatives, friends, and practitioners to whom she tells the story of her illness, who attend to and emphasize precisely those symptoms that they expect to be present in the neurasthenic syndrome. Thus, Mrs. Lin's symptom report is already an interpretation and therefore a diagnosis.

For myself, the North American psychiatrist who interviewed Mrs. Lin, neurasthenia was not a diagnostic possibility. Ironically "neurasthenia," a term coined by the New York neurologist George Beard in 1869 to describe a disorder he called the "American Disease" because of its presumed prevalence in the United States, was formally expunged from the American Psychiatric Association's *Diagnostic and Statistical Manual of Mental Disorders, Third Edition (DSM-III),* in 1980. It had ceased being an acceptable professional term several decades before. In the same year *DSM-III*'s rejection of the term meant neurasthenia was no longer a disease in the United States, I conducted a study of 100 neurasthenic patients in the outpatient psychiatry clinic at the Hunan Medical College. I showed that most of these patients could be rediagnosed, using a standard North American psychiatric protocol translated into Chinese together with *DSM-III* diagnostic criteria, as cases of major depressive disorder (Kleinman, 1986). But there was a rub. Unlike the great majority of chronically, depressed patients, these depressed patients responded only partially to antidepressant medication. Although many of the symptoms associated with depression improved, their chief somatic complaints and medical help seeking ended only when they were able to resolve major work and family problems (Kleinman & Kleinman, 1985; Kleinman, 1986).

I concluded that there were several ways to explain these findings. Neurasthenia might represent culturally shaped illness experience underwritten by the disease depression. The biologically based disease responded to the "therapeutic trial" of drugs; the illness experience ended only when powerful social contingencies "conditioning" the sick role behavior were removed. Chronic pain and other chronic conditions associated with depression have been shown to have a similar treatment response. Once the illness behavior becomes chronic, treatment of the depression may or may not remove the symptoms of depression, but the illness behavior persists (Katon, Kleinman, & Rose, 1982). Alternatively, both neurasthenia and depression might be regarded as the products of distinctive Chinese and American professional psychiatric taxonomies. In that sense, the experience that both psychiatric systems mapped might be thought of as a case solely of the psychobiology of chronic demoralization, and the mapping itself as a medicalized turning away from the social sources of human misery. In this alternative formulation, the psychiatric diagnosis does not point toward the solution. Rather it disguises the problem.

Other schools of psychiatrists might interpret Mrs. Lin's case and the 100 cases in the Hunan sample drawing on the diagnostic systems of psychoanalytic, behavioral, or other approaches to psychiatry. The World Health Organization (WH0) sponsors a diagnostic system, the International Classification of Disease, Ninth Revision (ICD-9), which does include neurasthenia as an official diagnosis. Although ICD-9 is not used in the United States, it is used in much of the world. Neurasthenia is no longer widely diagnosed in North America, South America, or Western Europe, but it is still a popular diagnosis in Eastern Europe, China, and several Southeast Asian societies. Furthermore, the symptoms and behaviors neurasthenia labels in those societies, which are much like those described in Beard's classic definition, are still common in the United States, despite the fact that the term "neurasthenia" lacks coherence in the North American popular culture. In the West now, new diagnostic labels are employed, which emphasize distinctive aspects of this syndrome: depressive disorder, anxiety disorder, somatization disorder, chronic pain syndrome, and in the North American popular culture, stress syndrome. A characteristic of these newer terms is that sometimes they describe syndromes that are predominantly bodily, like neurasthenia in China and in nineteenth-century New York, and other times clusters that are predominantly psychological. The presumption is that psychopathology creates both varieties of symptoms. (In this sense, unlike neurasthenia, these disorders, which imply psychosomatic factors, are not regarded as legitimate physical disorders. For that reason chronic viral disorders, like hypoglycemia and other putative physical disorders a decade ago, are the currently fashionable exemplars of "real" disease used to legitimate psychosomatic conditions. Both forms of symptoms are common in the West, but the overtly psychological variety is decidedly uncommon in most nonWestern societies.

THE CATEGORY FALLACY

If psychiatrists in the United States were to diagnose North American patients similar to Mrs. Lin as cases of neurasthenia, their decision would be seen by their peers as an invalid anachronism. The reification of one culture's diagnostic categories and their projection onto patients in another culture, where those categories lack coherence and their validity has not been established, is a category fallacy (Kleinman, 1977). Obeyesekere (1985) offers a telling example. Suppose, he suggests, a psychiatrist in South Asia, where semen loss syndromes are common, traveled to the United States, where these syndromes have neither professional nor popular coherence. Let us imagine that this South Asian psychiatrist has first operationalized the symptoms of semen loss in a psychiatric diagnostic schedule, translated this interview protocol into English, had other bilingual persons translate it back into the original language to check the accuracy of the translation, adjusted those items that were mistranslated, and then trained a group of American psychiatrists in its use and established a high level of consistency in their diagnoses. Using this schedule, he could derive prevalence data for "semen loss syndrome" in the United States. But would these findings have any validity in a society in which there are neither folk nor professional categories of semen loss and in which semen loss is not reported as a disturbing symptom?

This egregious example of the category fallacy is amusing but deplorable. Regrettably, much of cross-cultural psychiatry has been conducted in a rather similar manner, though with one important difference. By and large, cross-cultural studies in psychiatry are carried out by Western psychiatrists (or by members of the indigenous culture who arc trained either in departments of psychiatry dominated by Western paradigms or in the West itself) working in the non-Western world.

Dysthymic disorder in *DSM-III*, or neurotic depression in 1CD-9, may be an example of a category fallacy. Chronic states of depression associated with feelings of demoralization and despair have been prominent in the West since the time of Hippocrates (Jackson, 1986). Yet in Chinese and other non-Western societies they have not received a great deal of attention. They are influential in the West, especially for the more affluent members of society.

However, dysthymia would seem to be an instance of the medicalization of social problems in much of the rest of the world (and perhaps often in the West as well), where severe economic, political, and health problems create endemic feelings of hopelessness and helplessness, where demoralization and despair are responses to actual conditions of chronic deprivation and persistent loss, where powerlessness is not a cognitive distortion but an accurate mapping of one's place in an oppressive social system, and where moral, religious, and political configurations of such problems have coherence for the local population but psychiatric categories do not. This state of chronic demoralization, moreover, is not infrequently associated with anemia and other physiological concomitants of malnutrition and chronic tropical disorders that mirror the *DSM-III* symptoms of dysthymic disorder (e.g., sleep, appetite, and energy disturbances). In such a setting, is the psychiatrist who is armed with a local translation of the major North American diagnostic instruments and who applies these to study the prevalence of dysthymic disorder any different than his hypothetical Bangladeshi colleague studying semen loss in midtown Manhattan? Clearly, great care must be taken before applying this diagnostic category to assure that its use is valid.

For the psychiatric epidemiologist, it is crucial to distinguish a case of a disorder from a person with distress but no disorder. Depression, after all, could be a disease, a symptom, or a normal feeling. Operational definitions that specify inclusion and exclusion criteria are what enable the epidemiologist to proceed. In making the distinction between distress and disorder, taxonomy can become entangled in its own decision rules. For patients with loss of energy due to malaria, appetite disturbance, and psychomotor retardation owing to the anemia of hookworm infestation, sleeplessness associated with chronic diarrheal disease, and dysphoria owing to poverty and powerlessness, labeling these four somatic symptoms and one emotion the diagnostic criteria of major depressive disorder is the difference between becoming a case of the disease depression and an instance where depression is a symptom of distress due to a socially caused form of human misery and its biological consequences. Neither *DSM-III* nor ICD-9 was created with such problems in mind. But they are applied in such settings. The upshot is both a distorted view of pathology and an inappropriate use of diagnostic categories.

There is overwhelming evidence that certain psychiatric diagnoses are valid worldwide—e.g., organic brain disorders, schizophrenia, manic-depressive psychosis, certain anxiety disorders, and perhaps major depressive disorder. But we have substantial reason to doubt whether other psychiatric diagnoses currently popular in the West—e.g., dysthymic disorder, anorexia nervosa, agoraphobia, and personality disorders—are valid categories for other societies.

There is, however, good justification to apply psychiatric diagnoses with rigor and precision. Certain psychiatric conditions are treatable; and without effective treatment, they lead to pain, suffering, disability, considerable expense and even death. Effective treatment and prevention require a usable diagnostic system. Attempts to create airtight systems of diagnoses are ineffective, costly, and dangerous. Diagnostic systems do have unintended consequences, one of which is to serve bureaucratic interests of social control that may not be healthy for patients. There are also intended consequences of diagnostic systems, such as providing official listings for third-party reimbursement, legal procedures, and disability determinations that go beyond the technical needs of the diagnostician but are essential for the patient and the broader society. Both intended and unintended consequences shape the diagnostic system. For example, *DSM-III* is so organized that every conceivable psychiatric condition is listed as a disease to legitimate remuneration to practitioners from private medical insurance and government programs.

Perhaps the most useful contribution of cultural analysis to psychiatry is to continually remind us of these dilemmas. Cross-cultural comparison, appropriately applied, can challenge the hubris in bureaucratically motivated attempts to medicalize the human condition. It can make us sensitive to the potential abuses of psychiatric labels. It encourages humility in the face of alternative cultural formulations of the same problems, which are viewed not as evidence of the ignorance of laymen, but as distinctive modes of thinking about life's troubles. And it can create in the psychiatrist a sense of being uncomfortable with mechanical application of all too often taken-for-granted professional categories and the tacit "interests" they represent. There is, thank goodness, an obdurate grain of humanness in all patients that resist diagnostic pigeonholing. Most experienced psychiatrists learn to struggle to translate diagnostic categories into human terms so that they do not dehumanize their patients or themselves. Yet, the potential for failure in this core clinical skill is built into the very structure of diagnostic systems. An anthropological sensibility regarding the cultural assumptions and social uses of the diagnostic process can be an effective check on its potential misuses and abuses. Irony, paradox, ambiguity, drama, tragedy, humor—these are the elemental conditions of humanity that should humble even master diagnosticians.

References

Balk, David. 1983. "Adolescents' Grief Reactions and Self-Concept Perceptions Following Sibling Death." *Journal of Youth and Adolescence* 12:137–161.

Egdell, H. G., and Israel Kolvin. 1972. "Child Hallucinations." *Journal of Child Psychology and Psychiatry* 13:279–287.

Katon, Wayne J., Arthur Kleinman, and G. Rosen. 1982. "Depression and Somatization. Parts 1 and 2." *American Journal of Medicine* 72:127–135, 241–247.

Kleinman, Arthur. 1986. *Social Origins of Distress and Disease: Depression, Neurasthenia, and Pain in Modern China.* New Haven: Yale University Press.

Kleinman, Arthur, and Joan Kleinman. 1985. "Somatization." Pp. 429–490 in *Culture and Depression*, A. Kleinman and B. Good, eds. Berkeley: University of California Press.

Kleinman, Arthur. 1977. "Depression, Somatization, and the New Cross-Cultural Psychiatry." *Social Science and Medicine* 11:3–10.

McHugh, Paul H., and Philip R. Slavney. 1986. *The Perspectives of Psychiatry*. Baltimore: Johns Hopkins University Press.

Obeyesekere, G. 1985. Depression, Buddhism, and the Work of Culture in Sri Lanka. Pp. 134–142 in *Culture and Depression*, A. Kleinman and B. Good, eds. Berkeley: University of California Press.

DISCUSSION QUESTIONS

1. According to Kleinman, what is the distinction between illness and disease? How are illness and disease shaped by culture?

2. What does Kleinman mean when he says, "(p)sychiatric diagnosis as interpretation must meet some resistance in lived experience, whose roots are deeply personal and physiological. The diagnosis does not create experience; mental disorder is part of life itself"?

3. *Ataques de nervios* is a syndrome reported primarily among Latinos from the Caribbean but also known among other Latin American and Latin Mediterranean groups (see sidebar). It is characterized by a sense of being out of control, uncontrollable shouting, attacks of crying, trembling, heat in the chest that rises into the head, and verbal or physical aggression; some people also experience seizures or fainting episodes. Ataques de nervios frequently occur as a result of stressful events relating to the family. This psychiatric diagnosis is not recognized in the *Diagnostic and Statistical Manual of Mental Disorders*. If a patient presented to a U.S. psychiatrist with these symptoms, on what basis should the psychiatrist assign a diagnosis? How useful is the *DSM* as a guide in that instance? Would your answer be different depending on whether or not the patient was Latino? Why or why not?

Kathryn Schulz

Did Antidepressants Depress Japan?

This selection comes from the New York Times, one of the most highly-respected news publications in the United States. The author, Kathryn Schulz, describes the introduction of antidepressant medications into Japan and the attendant changes in the culture. Use the concepts from this section to analyze what happened. How was depression interpreted in Japan prior to the introduction of antidepressant medications? Who was involved in promoting medicalized interpretations of depression in Japan? What challenges to that interpretation have been made? How might the medicalization of depression change Japanese culture?

Schulz, Kathryn. 2004. "Did Antidepressants Depress Japan?" *New York Times*, August 24.

If you had lived in Japan for the last five years, you would know by now that your *kokoro* is at risk of coming down with a cold. Your kokoro is not part of your respiratory system. It is not a member of your family. Its treatment lies well beyond the bailiwick of your average ear, nose, and throat doctor. Your kokoro is your soul, and the notion that it can catch cold (*kokoro no kaze*) was introduced to Japan by the pharmaceutical industry to explain mild depression to a country that almost never discussed it.

Talking about depression in Japanese has always been a fundamentally different undertaking than talking about it in English. In our language, the word for depression is remarkably versatile. It can describe dips in landscapes, economies, or moods. It can refer to a devastating psychiatric condition or a fleeting response to the Cubs losing the pennant. It can be subdivided almost endlessly: major, minor, agitated, anxious, bipolar, unipolar, postpartum, premenstrual.

But in Japanese, the word for depression (*utsubyo*) traditionally referred only to major or manic depressive disorders and was seldom heard outside psychiatric circles. To talk about feelings, people relied on the word *ki* or "vital energy." A literal translation of Japanese synonyms for sorrow reads, to Westerners, like the kind of emotional troubles that might befall a kitchen sink: *ki ga fusagu*, sadness because your ki is blocked; *ki ga omoi*, sadness because your ki is sluggish; *ki ga meiru*, sadness because your ki is leaking.

Inside every neologism lies a compact history of cultural change—think McJobs, metrosexuals, the blogosphere. In Japan, the coining of kokoro no kaze marked a sea change in people's thinking about depression. That transformation was triggered by the pharmaceutical industry's other contribution to Japan in 1999: along with providing a catchy slogan for mild depression, the industry provided a cure: modern antidepressants. More than a decade ago, Peter Kramer chronicled the capacity of those drugs to reshape the cultural landscape in *Listening to Prozac*. But back then the culture they reshaped was the culture that had shaped them. Now, a huge campaign by the pharmaceutical industry is publicizing mild depression, which most Japanese didn't realize existed until recently. Japan has become a proving ground for what we stand to gain and lose by the global expansion of Western psychopharmacology.

Certainly, Japan is a compelling candidate for a mental health makeover. Serious mental illness has long been inadequately addressed there. The suicide rate is more than twice that of the United States. The average hospitalization for mental illness lasts 390 days, compared with the American average of less than 10. Until recently, depression was regarded in much the same light as schizophrenia, and treatment was available almost exclusively in institutions. There was no such thing as "mild" depression. Talk therapy was rare (and remains so), and quasi-official policy dissuaded open discussion. "The Ministry of Health considered 'depression' a bad word," Yukio Saito, who helped found Japan's national mental health hotline in 1971, said. For decades, Saito's requests to post hotline ads in public places were routinely denied.

Last year, in a volte-face that reflects the shifting cultural tides of the last five years, the Ministry of Health launched a committee to help educate the public about depression. The actress Nana Kinomi talked publicly about her postmenopausal depression in 2000. Other celebrities followed suit. And last month, the Imperial Household Agency acknowledged that Crown Princess Masako is on antidepressants and in counseling for depression and an "adjustment disorder."

Over the past five years, according to the Japanese Bookstore Association, 177 books about depression have been published, compared with a mere 27 from 1990 to 1995. Earlier this month, the country's most popular online bulletin board, Channel 2, carried 713 conversation threads about depression—more than music (582), or food (691), and almost as many as romance (716).

Depression has gone from bad word to buzzword. "The media mention depression almost every week," said Yutaka Ono, a psychiatrist and professor at Keio University and one of Japan's leading depression experts. People have even come to his office with newspaper in hand, he said, and asked if what they have is depression. Ono has been practicing for 25 years, but, he said, the number of patients who have consulted him about mild depression has surged in the last 4 or 5. Most Japanese epidemiological data doesn't differentiate between degrees of depression, but the Ministry of Mental Health and the leading psychiatrists with whom I spoke agree that mild depression accounts for the vast majority of new cases—of which there are a staggering number. According to IMS Health, a company that tracks global health care and pharmaceutical information, depression-related doctor vists in Japan increased 46 percent from 1999 to 2003.

Disease rates typically increase because more people get sick or because diagnosis and reporting improve. But neither explanation fully accounts for the rise in mild depression in Japan. "There's no question in my mind that severe clinical depression is a real disease," said Arthur Kleinman, a psychiatry professor, chairman of Harvard's anthropology department and coeditor of the definitive work "Culture and Depression." "I could take you all over the world, and you would have no difficulty recognizing severely depressed people in completely different settings. But mild depression is a totally different kettle of fish. It allows us to relabel as depression an enormous number of things."

As the idea of mild depression has gained traction in Japan, it may be that more people haven't gotten sick; they have simply come to define what's ailing them as a disease. Mild depression is not contagious but it can be considered, in the root sense of the word, communicable—and for the last five years, the pharmaceutical industry and the media have communicated one consistent message: your suffering might be a sickness. Your leaky vital energy, like your runny nose, might respond to drugs.

Looking back, Naoya Mitake thinks he might have first experienced depression while in college. "I was about to graduate, and my friends had all been hired by Japanese companies," he recalled. "I couldn't imagine doing that, but I didn't know what else to do." He felt incompetent and worthless, unable to make decisions about his future. He might have been depressed back then, but, he said, "the word never came to mind."

Mitake, now 39, steered clear of corporate Japan and instead became an associate professor of comparative politics at Komazawa University. In 2001, he consulted a doctor about his longstanding battles with insomnia and fatigue. The doctor prescribed antidepressants—a common treatment for insomnia—but Mitake's sleep didn't improve. (People on antidepressants frequently have to try different pills and dosages before finding an effective treatment.) Meanwhile, Mitake became increasingly anxious, frightened, and sad. He stopped taking the first set of antidepressants, and his problems persisted. This time, he said, he knew he was "extremely depressed."

Mitake is handsome, warm, and articulate. He talked about his experiences with an appealing blend of curiosity and tranquillity, although the emotions he described were far from tranquil. "I'd wake up in the middle of the night with this strange, strong anxiety," he remembered. "I couldn't be alone. I felt too afraid. I couldn't teach my classes anymore."

Three months after his mood plummeted, he turned to antidepressants again and felt considerably better but not perfect. For almost two years, he cycled through various pills, with his melancholy waxing and waning. It wasn't until the summer of 2003, when he accidentally discovered a nonmedical treatment of his own, that his depression lifted.

In the *Diagnostic and Statistical Manual of Mental Disorders*—the American Psychiatric Association's compendium of mental disorders—depression is divided into discrete categories. In reality, though, there is no discernible line where moodiness crosses over into mild depression, or mild depression into severe. Moreover, mild depression does not feel mild to those who experience it. When I asked Mitake if his soul had a cold, he laughed, then paused and said he shouldn't have laughed. "The phrase did some good. It changed people's perception and made depression easier to talk about."

In a country famous for its reticence, that is no small achievement—especially since talking about depression is one effective way to treat it. But counseling is still rare in Japan; in books and speeches, Yutaka Ono has tried to encourage people to discuss their depression with a professional, but, he said, psychotherapy has been far slower to catch on than medication. The current idiom also has its limits: Mitake, for one, said he never uses the expression kokoro no kaze. "Maybe for some people depression is like a cold," he said. "If so, their colds are a lot worse than mine. Or my depression is a lot worse than theirs."

For 1,500 years of Japanese history, Buddhism has encouraged the acceptance of sadness and discouraged the pursuit of happiness—a fundamental distinction between Western and Eastern attitudes. The first of Buddhism's four central precepts is: suffering exists. Because sickness and death are inevitable, resisting them brings more misery, not less. "Nature shows us that life is sadness, that everything dies or ends," Hayao Kawai, a clinical psychologist who is now Japan's commissioner of cultural affairs, said. "Our mythology repeats that; we do not have stories where anyone lives happily ever after." Happiness is nearly always fleeting in Japanese art and literature. That bittersweet aesthetic, known as aware, prizes melancholy as a sign of sensitivity.

This traditional way of thinking about suffering helps to explain why mild depression was never considered a disease. "Melancholia, sensitivity, fragility—these are not negative things in a Japanese context," Tooru Takahashi, a psychiatrist who worked for Japan's National Institute of Mental Health for 30 years, explained. "It never occurred to us that we should try to remove them, because it never occurred to us that they were bad."

The medical model of depression, by contrast, sees suffering as pathological and prescribes a pill in response. That outlook is partly pragmatic: call depression a disease and health insurance covers its treatment.

Patient advocates also argue that reclassifying depression as a disease helps to diminish its stigma. But probably most important, the pharmaceutical industry has the financial incentive to recast moods as medical problems, creating what Kleinman calls "a pharmacology of remorse and regret." It is, Kleinman said, "one of the most powerful aspects of globalization, and Japan is at its leading edge."

In the late 1980s, Eli Lilly decided against selling Prozac in Japan after market research there revealed virtually no demand for antidepressants. Throughout the 90s, when Prozac and other selective serotonin reuptake inhibitors, or SSRI's, were traveling the strange road from chemical compound to cultural phenomenon in the West, the drugs and the disease alike remained virtually unknown in Japan.

Then, in 1999, a Japanese company, Meiji Seika Kaisha, began selling the SSRI Depromel. Meiji was among the first users of the phrase kokoro no kaze. The next year, GlaxoSmithKline—maker of the antidepressant Paxil—followed Meiji into the market. Koji Nakagawa, GlaxoSmithKline's product manager for Paxil, explained: "When other pharmaceutical companies were giving up on developing antidepressants in Japan, we went ahead for a very simple reason: the successful marketing in the United States and Europe."

Direct-to-consumer drug advertising is illegal in Japan, so the company relied on educational campaigns targeting mild depression. As Nakagawa put it: "People didn't know they were suffering from a disease. We felt it was important to reach out to them." So the company formulated a tripartite message: "Depression is a disease that anyone can get. It can be cured by medicine. Early detection is important."

Like the Bush administration, GlaxoSmithKline has spent the last four years staying relentlessly on-message. Its 1,350 Paxil-promoting medical representatives visit selected doctors an average of twice a week. Awareness campaigns teach general practitioners and the public to recognize the following symptoms of depression (the translation is the company's): "head feels heavy, cannot sleep, stiff shoulders, backache, tired and lazy, no appetite, not intrigued, feel depressed."

The psychiatrist Yutaka Ono advocates raising awareness about depression, but GlaxoSmithKline's marketing made him uncomfortable. "They ran a very intense campaign about mild depression where a beautiful young lady comes out all smiles and says, 'I went to a doctor and now I'm happy.' You know, depression is not that easy. And if it is that easy, it might not be depression."

Whatever misgivings Ono and other doctors may have about the medicalization of mild depression, it has been a resounding financial success. As one psychiatrist, Kenji Kitanishi, noted wryly, "Japanese psychiatry is in the bubble economy now." Between 1998 and 2003, sales of antidepressants in Japan quintupled, according to IMS Health. GlaxoSmithKline alone saw its sales of Paxil increase from $108 million in 2001 to $298 million in 2003. According to the company, during one seven-month ad campaign it ran last year, 110,000 people in a population of 127 million consulted their doctors about depression.

In late 2001, one of those people was Mitake. "From the things I'd read, I knew about these chemicals in the brain, serotonin and so forth," Mitake said. "And I thought, O.K., this is a chemical phenomenon, so it needs to be cured by a chemical substance." In fact, no one understands the etiology of depression, and the role serotonin plays is ambiguous. Ask people with mild depression to explain its origins, and most will offer autobiography, not biochemistry: difficult families, dissolved relationships, demanding jobs. Japanese mental health specialists consistently cite the collapse of the bubble economy and disintegrating social structures as major factors in the nation's soaring depression rates.

The idea that depression is a neurochemical malfunction dodges a fundamental chicken-and-egg problem. Screwy neurochemistry can cause depression, but depression can also wreak havoc on your neurochemistry. Likewise, research has shown brain chemistry can change in response to any number of interventions: medication, talk therapy, exercise, prayer. The question, then, isn't whether depression is biochemical phenomenon; it is. So is the act of formulating a thought. So, in a sense, is sorrow. The question is, What do we gain, and what do we lose, by understanding the darker acts of our brains as diseases?

One side effect of the antidepressants Mitake was taking was weight gain, so in August 2003 he went on a fasting retreat in the mountains. He thought he'd do some reading, but after the fourth day, he recounted: "You can't even think. You just kind of lie there." Toward the end of his fast, Mitake went to a hot spring. "There I was, totally naked with this breeze blowing and the sun shining, and suddenly I started to feel better," he recalled. Mitake credits the fast with ending his depression. "It's like because I couldn't think for a while, the cycle just broke. All those negative feelings were gone." His depression hasn't returned, although on his doctor's advice, he continued to take antidepressants until last month.

Mitake was quick to sound a cautionary note: "I don't dare tell my friends with depression, 'Oh, you should go fast.' I tell them to find a good doctor and take medication as prescribed. I really believe the fast is what worked in my case, but I'd never recommend it as a cure."

Andrew Solomon, author of *The Noonday Demon* (Simon & Schuster, 2002), champions antidepressants, but even he ultimately concludes that the best cure is the one you believe in. "If you have cancer and try an exotic treatment and then think you are better, you may well be wrong," he writes. "If you have depression and try an exotic treatment and think you are better, you are better." Yet the medicalization of depression makes it difficult to believe in any treatment but medicine. Rather than expanding options for care for those who suffer, the globalization of psychopharmacology may ultimately sow a monocrop of ideas about health and sickness.

Writing about changing understandings of depression in other countries risks romanticizing suffering and other cultures. But not writing about them contributes to a kind of silence already evident in Japan. "There is this almost invisible pressure that makes it difficult to freely raise questions," Saito, one of the founders of Japan's mental health hotline, noted. "I find myself doubting whether medicalization is a good trend. But being in the position I'm in, needing some support from the medical system, I don't usually make comments like this."

Thomas Hardy once noted, "What we gain by science is, after all, sadness." He meant the more we learn about nature, the crueler it seems and the less individual experience matters. The century since he wrote has seen stunning technological advances, but we haven't made much progress figuring out how to integrate science with other ways of understanding what it means to be human. These days, we may lose even sadness.

PREVALENCE AND PATTERNS OF MENTAL ILLNESS

P sychiatric epidemiology is a field of research concerned with the distribution of psychological distress and mental disorders in the population: the overall prevalence (percentage of people who experience symptoms or have a disorder) as well as which subgroups of the population are at greatest risk. Research in psychiatric epidemiology relies on community surveys in which large samples of people respond to questions about symptoms they are currently experiencing or have experienced in the past. How psychological distress and mental disorders are measured importantly determines what we learn from those surveys. We begin this section with three selections that describe common approaches to measurement in psychiatric epidemiological studies. In the first selection, Switzer and colleagues present a brief history of measurement and introduce important controversies that have shaped the field. In the second and third selections, Kessler, followed by Mirowsky and Ross, elaborate on those controversies. While the controversies could be conceived as narrowly technical, they raise more fundamental questions about the existence of mental disorders and the nature of human distress.

The final three selections present results from recent studies of the prevalence of mental disorders in the United States and worldwide. These selections introduce the methods of psychiatric epidemiological research and the major patterns in the distribution of mental disorders.

The Measurement of Mental Health and Mental Illness

Galen E. Switzer, Mary Amanda Dew, and Evelyn J. Bromet

Issues in Mental Health Assessment[†]

The first selection in this section begins with a brief history of how mental illness has been measured in psychiatric epidemiological studies. Historical changes in measurement reflect more general methodological developments as well as changes in the Diagnostic and Statistical Manual of Mental Disorders itself. The authors define two important dimensions of measurement quality—reliability and validity—and discuss how categorical and dimensional measures of mental health compare on those dimensions. Although somewhat technical, this selection presents information that will be important to your understanding of the results of psychiatric epidemiological studies.

Deviations from "normal" emotional functioning have been recognized and documented for as long as written accounts of history have existed. Parables concerning mental disorder appear in the written works of all major religions, and statutes concerning the mentally ill were a part of early Roman law (Eaton, 1980). Depending on the particular historical period in which they lived, those whose behavior did not conform to accepted norms were labeled variously as possessed, holy, mad, or insane. In the late 19th and early 20th centuries, as mental disorders increasingly came under the purview of medical science, the previous broad categories of mental disorder (e.g., raving, melancholic, lunatic, idiot; Jarvis, 1971) began to be subdivided into more specific "diagnostic" categories. This categorization process, or nosology, has continued to the present day and is currently embodied in its most specific form as the American Psychiatric

Switzer, Galen E., Mary Amanda Dew, and Evelyn J. Bromet. 1999. "Issues in Mental Health Assessment." Pp. 81–104 in *Handbook of the Sociology of Mental* Health, edited by C. S. Aneshensel and J. C. Phelan. New York: Kluwer Academic-Plenum Publishers.

Association's *Diagnostic and Statistical Manual of Mental Disorders* (*DSM-IV*; American Psychiatric Association, 1994), and the International Classification of Diseases (ICD-10; World Health Organization, 1992), which describe the symptoms and diagnostic criteria of more than 250 psychiatric disorders.

Brief History of Community Mental Health Assessment

Dohrenwend and Dohrenwend (1982) identified several distinct periods or eras of instrumentation and methodological developments that have culminated in what they refer to as "third generation" studies. Each of the three generations of studies and instrument types has distinctive characteristics, which are summarized in Table 1.

Conducted prior to World War II, the first set of community mental health studies attempted to assess broad patterns of mental disorder in the community by gathering information from informants, medical records, and, occasionally, from direct interviews (e.g., Jarvis, 1971). One of the first systematic efforts to assess treated prevalence of mental disorder in the community was conducted by Faris and Dunham (1939). These sociologists reviewed all medical records of Illinois state mental hospitals from 1922 through 1931 and drew inferences about the rates of diagnosed general mental disorder, and of schizophrenia specifically, in the adult population living in and around Chicago. Their expectation was supported that a variety of sociological factors would result in higher rates of general disorder and schizophrenia in more densely populated, less affluent, inner-city areas. This application of sociological and epidemiological methodology to the assessment of mental disorder in the community was a significant departure from the traditional individualized methods used in clinic settings. The clinical setting tends to emphasize the unique aspects of each individual's personal history as distinct from the commonalities that exist across groups of similar persons, or among those exposed to similar environmental conditions.

Table 1 Characteristics of Three Generations of Epidemiological Research

	Timespan	Method	Assessor	Primary goal	Limitations
First generation	1850–1950	Key informant Agency records Direct interview	Clinician	General disorder type	Validity Reliability
Second generation	1950–1980	Direct interview	Clinician or lay interviewer	Impairment	Validity
Third generation	1980– present	Direct interview Self-report survey Computer assisted	Clinician, lay interviewer, or self	Diagnosis or impairment	Validity

Source: Based on Dohrenwend & Dohrenwend (1982).

The primary limitation of such first-generation community mental health studies was the fact that prevalence estimates were based on treated (rather than general population) samples; rates of individuals seeking mental health treatment were used directly to estimate rates of disorder in the population. It is now well established that only a fraction of those with mental disorders ever seek treatment, meaning that these initial community studies almost certainly underestimated "true" prevalence rates (Dohrenwend & Dohrenwend, 1982). In addition, the lack of standardized guidelines for diagnosing disorders at that time led to problems with comparability among these studies (Faris & Dunham, 1939).

The involvement of the United States in World War II ushered in the second generation of assessment studies. In the 1940s, the Neuropsychiatric Screen Adjunct (NSA) was developed by the U.S. Army to eliminate from the armed forces those individuals who could not serve effectively as soldiers (Star, 1950; Stouffer et al., 1950). The NSA, designed to assess general psychiatric status, found much higher prevalence rates of psychiatric impairment than expected based on pre–World War II studies. The necessity of evaluating large numbers of individuals for military service, coupled with the strikingly high observed rates of impairment, provided the impetus for the further development and refinement of instruments for use in community settings in the postwar period.

Two classic studies from this second generation—the Midtown Manhattan Study in New York (Srole et al., 1962), and the Stirling County Study in Nova Scotia (Leighton, Harding, Macklin, Macmillan, & Leighton, 1963)—were designed and conducted by sociologist Leo Srole and psychiatrist Alexander Leighton, respectively. Both studies drew on, and expanded, the Selective Service NSA items as a basis for rating individuals along five- or six-point continuums of psychiatric impairment ranging from completely well to completely or severely impaired. Both studies used relatively sophisticated techniques—including solicitation of a diverse set of expert opinions, pilot testing items, and assessment agreement between interview items and psychiatric ratings—to improve their instruments. In addition, these studies used state-of-the-art probabilistic sampling methods to select several hundred respondents who were representative of their respective communities. Advantages of these second-generation studies over previous efforts to assess population-based mental health included the use of community samples and direct interviewing, methods that had not previously been feasible. These new methods were made possible by the fact that these new instruments could be administered by nonclinician lay interviewers rather than psychiatrists, making them substantially less costly. Finally, there was growing evidence that instruments developed during this second phase of epidemiological investigation were considerably more reliable than their predecessors (Dohrenwend, 1995).

However, second-generation efforts did evoke some of the same validity concerns as first-generation studies. First, instruments used in these studies did not adequately assess the full range of clinical diagnostic categories, including impairment resulting from behavioral disorders or substance abuse. Second, and perhaps more important, there was ample evidence that psychiatric impairment, as defined by instruments used in the community, was not comparable to disorder as defined by psychiatrist clinicians; impairment was measured on a continuous scale quite different from discrete diagnostic categories (Srole et al., 1962; Leighton et al., 1963). Given that diagnosis of disorder was not the central purpose, however, it is important to acknowledge that many of these instruments did provide relatively stable dimensional assessments of areas such as general distress and depression (Link & Dohrenwend, 1980). Finally, additional validity concerns arose during this period as researchers and psychiatrists noticed large differences in the rates of psychiatric disorders between countries. The most striking example involved reported rates of manic–depressive psychosis in Britain that were 20 times those found in the United States (Kramer, 1961), which led to a large multisite study in the two nations (Cooper et al., 1972). This collaborative study—in which the Present State Examination (PSE) was chosen as the standard instrument—revealed that the cross-national differences had been produced by disparities in instrumentation and methods of diagnosis, findings that led to further refinement and standardization of community diagnostic instruments.

In a reflexive process, the demand for reliable instruments for epidemiological and clinical-based research spurred the psychiatric community to undertake several major revisions in its core diagnostic manual. Increasing detail and specificity of the *DSM*, in turn, led to the development of a third generation of instruments based on the more specific diagnostic categories found in the *DSM*. In response to the high cost of having clinicians administer these instruments in the community, the National Institute of Mental Health (NIMH) developed a fully structured interview that could be administered by lay interviewers. The Diagnostic Interview Schedule (DIS; Robins et al., 1988), based on the *DSM-III*, was designed for use in the Epidemiologic Catchment Area (ECA) studies conducted at five sites in major U.S. cities and has now been translated into several other languages (Regier & Robins, 1991). In the past two decades, the number and variety of psychiatric assessment instruments designed specifically for use in the community has proliferated. Currently, a variety of fully structured and semistructured diagnostic instruments are available for community-based research.

REVIEW AND SUMMARY OF MAJOR
ASSESSMENT TECHNIQUES

In general, mental health measures used in community settings currently fall into two categories, referred to here as dimensional and diagnostic. Dimensional instruments—also called screening instruments or symptom inventories (depending on how they are used and the type of data they gather) and designed for use by lay interviewers in research contexts—were designed to provide information about an individual's relative symptom level rather than a discrete diagnosis. These instruments can be fully structured (no deviations in how questions are asked) for lay interviews, semi-structured (with probes as needed to gather maximum information) for clinician interviews, or self-administered questionnaires.

In contrast, diagnostic instruments—also called schedules or examinations—are based very closely on the specific symptoms described by the *DSM-IV*, or, more recently, the ICD-10, used to make diagnostic judgments in the clinic. One of the central goals in the development of diagnostic instruments was to allow nonclinicians to conduct fully or semistructured interviews that provide the equivalent of psychiatric diagnoses. Although there are many differences between diagnostic and dimensional instruments, perhaps the central distinction is that diagnostic instruments categorize individuals into dichotomous outcomes (e.g., meets criteria for major depression or not), whereas dimensional instruments place individuals along a continuum of symptom severity (e.g., more or less depressed).

The debate over the relative advantages and disadvantages of diagnostic versus dimensional approaches continues both at academic and policy levels. Proponents of the diagnostic approach argue that discrete categorization of mental illness is necessary from the practical standpoint of determining who is eligible for insurance and/or social service assistance. In addition, they assert that diagnostic typology, founded on consistent decision rules, will produce more precise assessment of mental status than will dimensional systems (Regier et al., 1984; Weissman, 1987). Moreover, they argue that mental illness is more than a matter of degree of severity along a continuous dimension; conditions such as schizophrenia and major depression are qualitatively distinct from normal human functioning. In contrast, proponents of a dimensional approach suggest that diagnostic approaches rely too heavily on microbiological models that view individuals as either diseased or not diseased. Mirowsky and Ross (1989a) argue that the discipline of psychiatry is inherently motivated to adhere to this medical model in order to retain its traditional preeminence over other disciplines concerned with mental health issues. They contend that discrete measurement of nondiscrete psychological phenomena (1) disregards useful information about the degree and characteristics of psychological distress; (2) confounds information on symptoms, causes, and consequences of distress; and (3) provides assessments that are relatively insensitive to changes in mental status (see Mirowsky & Ross, 1989a, 1989b). Clearly, the controversy over techniques for community mental health assessment will continue, and we suggest that prior to selecting an instrument, researchers become familiar with the major arguments on both sides of the issue.

Diagnostic Instruments

As noted earlier, proponents of categorical instruments argue that each mental disorder is qualitatively distinct from other disorders and from normality

(Clementz & Iacono, 1993). These instruments generally assign only one primary diagnosis using a hierarchical system. One of the drawbacks of using these instruments (e.g., Structured Clinical Interview for *DSM-IV* [SCID] and PSE) in a hierarchical format is that, although assigning a single primary diagnosis may be useful for guiding treatment decisions in clinic settings, the high degree of comorbidity in psychiatric disorders may make it less desirable for assessing prevalence of psychiatric disorders in the population. Additionally, diagnostic instruments can be fairly lengthy, because they cover a broad range of areas and may lead to respondent fatigue.

Traditionally, diagnostic instruments used in the community have demonstrated only moderate reliability and relatively low validity (Ustun & Tien, 1995). For example, researchers using a variety of diagnostic instruments, including the DIS (Robins, Helzer, Ratcliff, & Seyfried, 1982), the SCID (Williams, 1992), and the Schedule for Affective Disorders and Schizophrenia (SADS; Bromet, Dunn, Connell, Dew, & Schulberg, 1986) have typically found fewer reported symptoms when the instrument is administered a second time to the same individuals (Robins, 1985). One of the difficulties in establishing reliability for diagnostic instruments is that the criteria for verifying reliability are relatively strict. To be deemed reliable, a diagnostic instrument must identify the same individuals as cases and as noncases in a second administration of the schedule as in the initial administration (Robins, 1985; Dohrenwend, 1989). This dichotomous, or "hard," approach to reliability is generally more stringent than the correlation coefficient used to establish reliability of a dimensional scale.

Validity concerns about diagnostic instruments are currently even more pressing than reliability concerns. Although category definitions have become much more specific and well defined—improving the face validity of included items—diagnostic instruments may still lack criterion validity. For example, DIS diagnoses obtained during the ECA studies (Anthony et al., 1985; Helzer et al., 1985) differed significantly from the number and type of diagnoses assigned to the same samples through clinical interviews (Anthony et al., 1985; Shrout, 1994). As Murphy (1995) notes, however, there is some controversy over whether clinical interviews should serve as the gold standard by which to assess the validity of community-based instruments. In the ECA studies, prevalence rates assigned by psychiatrists, as well as those assigned by the DIS, varied significantly across the metropolitan administration sites (Robins, 1985), suggesting that neither assessment technique provides completely reliable and valid estimates of prevalence.

Similarly, concerns have been raised about the construct validity of diagnostic instruments. The primary technique for validating diagnostic measures has been to assess the degree of correspondence of diagnoses obtained in the community with psychiatrists', clinical psychologists', or psychiatric social workers' diagnoses of the same individuals through clinical interviews. Thus, experienced clinicians' diagnoses—rather than a latent condition particular to the individual—become the construct represented in diagnostic instruments (Mirowsky & Ross, 1989a). Given the considerable variance in clinician-assigned diagnoses for individuals exhibiting similar symptoms and mental health histories, it has been argued that validating instruments against such diagnoses is tenuous at best (Mirowsky & Ross, 1989a).

COMPOSITE INTERNATIONAL DIAGNOSTIC INTERVIEW (CIDI) DEPRESSION SECTION

The following questions come from the depression section of the CIDI, a categorical assessment based on the *DSM-IV*. The first few questions give respondents an opportunity to describe their depressed feelings using a number of different terms—"sad, empty, or depressed," discouraged," or as having "lost interest." Respondents who have had any of those experiences meet the most basic criterion for the diagnosis of major depressive episode. The subsequent questions evaluate the degree of impairment associated with the episode, and the extent to which respondents experienced other symptoms of depression at the same time, things like feeling hopeless or having a smaller appetite than usual. The answers to these questions are used to determine whether each respondent satisfies the diagnostic criteria for major depression according to the *DSM-IV*. We have simplified the instrument for purposes of presentation but have retained its general format and content to give you a flavor for how categorical assessments work.

Have you ever in your life had a period lasting several days or longer when most of the day you felt sad, empty, or depressed?

Have you ever had a period lasting several days or longer when most of the day you were very discouraged about how things were going in your life?

Have you ever had a period lasting several days or longer when you lost interest in most things you usually enjoy like work, hobbies, and personal relationships?

Did you ever have an episode of being (sad, discouraged, or uninterested in things) that lasted most of the day, nearly every day, for two weeks or longer?

How severe was your emotional distress during those times—mild, moderate, severe, or very severe?

How often was your emotional distress so severe that nothing could cheer you up – often, sometimes, rarely, or never?

How often was your emotional distress so severe that you could not carry out your daily activities—often, sometimes, rarely, or never?

In answering the next questions, think about the period during that episode when your (sadness, discouragement, or loss of interest) and other problems were most *severe and frequent*. During that period, which of the following problems did you have *most of the day* nearly *every day:*

Did you feel sad, empty, or depressed most of the day nearly every day during that period of (several days/two weeks)?

Did you feel so sad that nothing could cheer you up nearly every day?

During that period of (several days/two weeks), did you feel discouraged about how things were going in your life most of the day nearly every day?

Did you feel hopeless about the future nearly every day?

During that period of (several days/two weeks), did you lose interest in almost all things like work and hobbies and things you like to do for fun?

Did you feel like nothing was fun even when good things were happening?

Did you have a much smaller appetite than usual nearly every day during that period of (several days/two weeks)?

Did you have a much *larger* appetite than usual nearly every day?

Did you gain weight without trying to during that period of (several days/two weeks)?

Did you *lose* weight without trying to?

Did you have a lot more trouble than usual either falling asleep, staying asleep, or waking too early nearly every morning during that period of (several days/two weeks)?

Did you sleep a lot more than usual nearly every night during that period of (several days/two weeks)?

Did you sleep much less than usual and still not feel tired or sleepy?

Did you feel tired or low in energy nearly every day during that period of (several days/two weeks) even when you had not been working very hard?

Did you have a lot more energy than usual nearly every day during that period of (several days/two weeks)?

Did you talk or move more slowly than is normal for you nearly every day?

Were you so restless or jittery nearly every day that you paced up and down or couldn't sit still?

Did your thoughts come much more slowly than usual or seem mixed up nearly every day during that period of (several days/two weeks)?

Did your thoughts seem to jump from one thing to another or race through your head so fast you couldn't keep track of them?

Did you have a lot more trouble concentrating than is normal for you nearly every day?

Were you unable to make up your mind about things you ordinarily have no trouble deciding about?

Did you lose your self-confidence?

Did you feel that you were not as good as other people nearly every day?

Did you feel totally worthless nearly every day?

Did you feel guilty nearly every day?

Did you feel irritable, grouchy, or in a bad mood nearly every day?

Did you feel nervous or anxious most days?

During that time, did you have any sudden attacks of intense fear or panic?

Did you often think a lot about death, either your own, someone else's, or death in general?

During that period, did you ever think that it would be better if you were dead?

Did you think about committing suicide?

Did you make a suicide plan?

Did you make a suicide attempt?

http://www.hcp.med.harvard.edu/ncs/replication.php

Dimensional Instruments

Although dimensional instruments have been developed to assess a wide variety of impairment types, we focus here on five categories of impairment that are most frequently assessed: anxiety, depression, personality, social adjustment, and multiple distress domains. Anxiety, depression, and social adjustment (the ability to function effectively in social contexts) are generally considered to be state-like, or episodic in nature. Anxiety and depression are embodied in several of the primary Axis I disorders recognized by the *DSM-IV* and also are the most frequently assessed subcomponents on multiple distress instruments. In contrast, personality is typically regarded as an enduring trait, and is the central component of *DSM-IV* Axis II disorders. Measures in these five domains typically contain a series of items asking respondents to rate the presence–absence, frequency, and/or intensity of psychiatric symptoms during a timeframe of the past 1–2 weeks. Dimensional instruments differ from diagnostic instruments in several important ways. First, many of these instruments assess only one or two areas of symptomatology rather than a broad range of disorders, as found in most diagnostic instruments. Second, rather than defining caseness as a dichotomy, these instruments provide an overall score for the area of distress, based on a sum or average of the individual items in the instrument. Subscale scores for particular types of symptoms may also be computed. Symptoms are presumed to reflect quantitative departures from normal functioning (Clementz & Iacono, 1993). Most published dimensional instruments do, however, provide cutpoints or threshold levels that differentiate between "cases" and "noncases," where caseness is typically defined as a high, clinically significant level of symptomatology, or as showing a high likelihood of meeting psychiatric diagnostic criteria in a formal clinical assessment. These cutpoints may, however, have very low convergence with diagnoses based on clinical interviews and ratings (Dohrenwend, 1995). Finally, most dimensional instruments measure only current distress—as opposed to past episodes or lifetime rates—limiting the amount and type of information they provide.

Like diagnostic instruments, dimensional instruments have suffered from criticisms concerning reliability and validity. Although the internal consistency of established scales is relatively high—in the range of .80 to .85—test-retest reliability has been less consistent (Murphy, 1985). Variability in test–retest reliability may in part reflect the fact that some instruments (e.g., General Health Questionnaire [GHQ]) conceptualize and assess symptomatology or distress as acute (atypical, time-discrete symptoms), whereas others (e.g., Hopkins Symptom Checklist [HSCL]) focus on more chronic aspects of the symptomatology (may be typical and enduring symptoms). As might be expected, instruments assessing chronic symptomatology tend to have higher test–retest coefficients than those assessing episodic or acute symptoms (Murphy, 1995) in part because the phenomenon being assessed is inherently more stable over time.

Link and Dohrenwend (1980) found that early versions of dimensional instruments demonstrated very low correspondence with diagnosable disorder, thus raising serious questions about the validity of such instruments as measures of psychiatric disorders. Even more recently developed instruments (e.g., Center for Epidermiologic Studies-Depression Scale [CES-D]) may exhibit this weakness (Breslau, 1985). However, positive evidence concerning validity has been found for some dimensional scales (e.g., Hopkins Symptom Check List [HSCL], Symptom Check List [SCL-90]), which have relatively stable underlying factor structures that seem to correspond to specific clinical syndromes (Derogatis & Cleary, 1977). However, as noted by Dohrenwend and Dohrenwend (1965, 1982), the high correlations among virtually all dimensional instruments (even when they were designed to assess different domains of psychiatric impairment) raise serious questions about the legitimacy of interpreting the measures as assessing different constructs. Instead, these instruments all may be measuring a more general factor such as nonspecific distress or demoralization (Dohrenwend & Dohrenwend, 1965, 1982).

In general, although diagnostic and dimensional instruments were developed with divergent goals, their application in community assessment studies may be quite similar. Dimensional instruments assess symptomatology on a continuous scale but are frequently published with a threshold or cut-point above which individuals are defined as "cases," or as experiencing "significant distress." Conversely, in addition to reporting caseness, studies using diagnostic instruments often report continuous variables such as the number of symptoms endorsed or average level of symptom severity. This merging of diagnosis and dimensionality and intensity may be the ultimate future of community mental health assessment.

THE CENTER FOR EPIDEMIOLOGIC STUDIES-DEPRESSION SCALE

The Center for Epidemiologic Studies Depression Scale is one of the most frequently used dimensional assessments in sociological research. The questions in the scale inquire about a range of thoughts, feelings, and behaviors that characterize depression. Scores on the scale are calculated by adding up the responses to the individual questions according to the following metric: 0 = rarely or none of the time (less than 1 day), 1 = some or a little of the time (1–2 days), 2 = occasionally or a moderate amount of time (3–4 days), most or all of the time (5–7 days). As there are 20 items, the total score can range from 0 to 60. Some research suggests that scores over 16 indicate a clinically-relevant level of depression.

Select the statement that best describes how often you felt this way during the past week.

1. I was bothered by things that usually don't bother me
2. I did not feel like eating; my appetite was poor
3. I felt that I could not shake off the blues even with help from my family and friends
4. I felt that I was just as good as other people
5. I had trouble keeping my mind on what I was doing
6. I felt depressed
7. I felt like everything I did was an effort
8. I felt hopeful about the future
9. I thought my life had been a failure
10. I felt fearful
11. My sleep was restless

12. I was happy
13. I talked less than usual
14. I felt lonely
15. People were unfriendly
16. I enjoyed life
17. I had crying spells
18. I felt sad
19. I felt that people disliked me
20. I could not "get going"

Radloff, L. S. (1977). The CES-D Scale: A Self-report Depression Scale for Research in the General Population. *Applied Psychological Measurement*, 1:385–401.

CONTROVERSIES IN MENTAL HEALTH ASSESSMENT: RELIABILITY AND VALIDITY ISSUES

Maximizing Reliability at the Expense of Validity?

Most individuals interested in research understand that a measure's ability to perform consistently (reliability), and to measure the targeted underlying construct (validity), are both highly desirable and necessary elements of the assessment process. The relationship between reliability and validity concerns is sometimes less explicitly stated. First, reliability is a necessary but not sufficient condition for establishing validity (i.e., an unreliable measure can never be valid). Second, validity is neither a necessary nor a sufficient condition for establishing reliability (i.e., a measure's reliability is independent of its validity). Finally, because it is a precondition for, and generally much easier to achieve than validity, reliability tends to be the focus of psychometric analysis of instrumentation.

The history of the *DSM*, and of community-based instruments founded on *DSM* definitions (e.g., CIDI and DIS), is one of increasing specificity in nomenclature, in diagnostic criteria, and in the number of different disorders identified. The increasing specificity and detail of these measures and continued refinement of items and assessment techniques has led to great improvements in the reliability of clinical research and community mental health assessment. However, this improvement should not be interpreted as an indication that the measures are simultaneously becoming increasingly valid (see Kirk & Kutchins, 1992). Although it is true that community assessment techniques must produce consistent results if they are to be claimed as valid, it is also true that a measure may be 100 percent reliable and 0 percent valid. Thus, while community-based measures have become increasingly reliable, there are enduring questions about their validity (Dohrenwend,

1995; Murphy, 1995). These questions stem in part from the lack of correspondence between diagnoses assigned to patients by community assessments and those assigned by expert clinicians; the severity of this problem varies according to the type of disorder being diagnosed. Although it is not clear if either assessment technique should be used as the "gold standard," the lack of agreement between the two assessment modalities raises serious validity concerns. Because the *DSM*, and community-based diagnostic instruments based on it, rely on conservative criteria for diagnosis—typically, observable behavioral criteria—community-based measures may tend to underestimate the prevalence of some disorders.

Assessment Context

We close the body of this chapter by coming full circle to the issue of the broader context within which beliefs about, descriptions of, and attempts to assess mental health and disorder take place. Assessment techniques are tools created in a particular social context to gather information about the empirical world. As such, these instruments are not "objective" and can be no better or worse than the assumptions on which they are founded. A society's beliefs about the causes of mental disorders and their likely solutions will ultimately be reflected in the instruments used to assess mental health by that society. More broadly, the particular social arrangements—including the distributions of power, status, and resources—will all influence the creation, selection, and administration of instruments.

Numerous examples of the influence of social and political context on the definition and assessment of mental disorders can be found simply by charting the flow of diagnostic categories into and out of the *DSM*. The recent creation and addition of posttraumatic stress disorder (PTSD) to the *DSM* was a direct result of concerted post-Vietnam War lobbying efforts by American military veterans. The elimination of homosexuality as a diagnostic category was a result of lobbying by gay and lesbian organizations, changes in prevailing societal attitudes, and the greater willingness on the part of the medical community to acknowledge the lack of empirical evidence that homosexuality reflects psychopathology. The fact that posttraumatic symptoms and homosexuality have been a consistent part of human experience while their status as mental disorders has changed dramatically in the last 15 years is evidence of the subjective and transmutable nature of psychiatric categorization. These same societal forces have, at various times, defined broad population groups (e.g., women, ethnic minorities) as being "by nature" more vulnerable to psychiatric disorders. The emphasis on genetic or organic factors as a source of mental disorders has demonstrated the power of such explanations for some disorders (e.g., Alzheimer's disease), and their failure for others (e.g., major depression). The increased specificity of organic and genetic explanations—by helping to define both what biology can and cannot explain—has actually fostered the growth of sociological and epidemiological explanations for and investigations of mental health issues. The disciplines of mental health currently find themselves in a social context that encourages interdisciplinary efforts to assess and weigh the importance of physical, psychological, social, and environmental factors as precursors of mental disorder.

In summary, there has been dramatic progress in our ability to assess community mental health and disorder during the past 150 years. Technical advances, such as the development of improved sampling methods, more reliable instruments, and more powerful analytical tools have been accompanied by the emergence of an increasingly complex interdisciplinary paradigm to explain mental disorder. Sociologists and epidemiologists, as relative newcomers to the field of mental health assessment, have provided valuable insights not only about how to conduct broad-based community studies but also about the critical effects of environmental and social forces on mental health. The future seems to hold continued interdisciplinary collaboration, further development of instruments combining the strengths of diagnostic and dimensional instruments and/or use of multimethod techniques, and increasing application of computer technology to mental health assessment.

References

American Psychiatric Association. (1994). *Diagnostic and statistical manual of mental disorders* (4th ed, rev.). Washington, DC: Author.

Anthony, J. C., Folstein, M., Romanoski, A. J., Von Korff, M. R., Nestadt, G. R., Chahal, R., Merchant, A., Hendricks Brown, C., Shapiro, S., Kramer, M., & Gruenberg, E. (1985). Comparison of the lay diagnostic interview schedule and a standardized psychiatric diagnosis: Experience in Eastern Baltimore. *Archives of General Psychiatry, 42,* 667–675.

Breslau, N. (1985). Depressive symptoms, major depression and generalized anxiety: A comparison of self-reports on CES-D and results from diagnostic interviews. *Psychiatry Research, 15,* 219–229.

Bromet, E. J., Dunn, L. O., Connell, M. M., Dew, M. A., & Schulberg, H. C. (1986). Long-term reliability of diagnosing lifetime major depression in a community sample. *Archives of General Psychiatry, 43,* 435.

Clementz, B. A., & Iacono, W. G. (1993). Nosology and diagnosis. In A. S. Bellack & M. Hersen (Eds.), *Psychopathology in adulthood* (pp. 3–20. Needham Heights, MA: Allyn & Bacon.

Cooper, J. E., Kendell, R. E., Gurland, B. J., Sharpe, L., Copeland, J. R. M., & Simon, R. (1972). *Psychiatric diagnosis in New York and London.* London: Oxford University Press.

Derogatis, L. R., & Cleary, P. A. (1977). Confirmation of the dimensional structure of the SCL-90: A study in construct validation. *Journal of Clinical Psychology, 33,* 981–989.

Dohrenwend, B. P. (1995). The problem of validity in field studies of psychological disorders. In M. T. Tsuang, M. Tohen, & G. E. P. Zahner (Eds.), *Textbook in psychiatric epidemiology* (pp. 3–20). New York: Wiley.

Dohrenwend, B. P. (1989). The problem of validity in field studies of psychological disorders revisited. *Psychological Medicine, 20,* 195–208.

Dohrenwend, B. P., & Dohrenwend, B. S. (1982). Perspectives on the past and future of psychiatric epidemiology. *American Journal of Public Health, 72*, 1271–1279.

Dohrenwend, B. P., & Dohrenwend, B. S. (1965). The problem of validity in field studies of psychological disorder. *Journal of Abnormal Psychology. 70, 52–69.*

Eaton, W. W. (1980). *The sociology of mental disorders.* New York: Praeger Publishers.

Faris, R. L., & Dunham, H. W. (1939). *Mental disorders in urban areas.* Chicago: University of Chicago Press.

Helzer, J. E., Robins, L. N., McEnvoy, L. T., Spitznagel, E. L., Stoltzman, R. K., Farmer, A., & Brockington, I. F. (1985). A comparison of clinical and diagnostic interview schedule diagnoses: Physician reexamination of lay-interviewed cases in the general population. *Archives of General Psychiatry, 42*, 657–666.

Jarvis, E. (1971). *Insanity and idiocy in Massachusetts.* Cambridge, MA: Harvard University Press.

Kirk, S. A., & Kutchins, H. (1992). *The selling of DSM: The rhetoric of science in psychiatry.* New York: Aldine de Gruyter.

Kramer, M. (1961). Some problems for international research suggested by observations on differences in first admission rates to the mental hospitals of England and Wales of the United States. *Proceedings of the Third World Congress of Psychiatry, 3*, 153–160.

Leighton, D. C., Harding, J. S., Macklin, D. B., Macmillan, A. M., & Leighton, A. H. (1963). *The character of danger.* New York: Basic Books.

Link, B., & Dohrenwend, B. P. (1980). Formulation of hypotheses about the true prevalence of demoralization in the United States. In B. P. Dohrenwend, B. S. Dohrenwend, M. S. Gould, B. Link, R. Neugebauer, & R. Wunsch-Hitzig (Eds.), *Mental illness in the United States: Epidemiological estimates* (pp. 114–132). New York: Praeger.

Mirowsky, J., & Ross, C. E. (1989a). *Social causes of psychological distress.* New York: Aldine de Gruyter.

Mirowsky, J., & Ross, C. E. (1989b). Psychiatric diagnosis as reified measurement. *Journal of Health and Social Behavior, 30*, 114–125.

Murphy, J. M. (1995). Diagnostic schedules and rating scales in adult psychiatry. In M. T. Tsuang, M. Tohen, & G. E. P. Zahner (Eds.), *Textbook in Psychiatric Epidemiology* (pp. 253–271). New York: Wiley.

Murphy, J. M., Neff, R. K., Sobol, A. M., Rice, J. X., & Olivier, D. C. (1985). Computer diagnosis of depression and anxiety: The Stirling County Study. *Psychological Medicine, 15*, 99–112.

Regier, D. A., Myers, J. E., Kramer, M., Robins, L. N., Blazer, D. G., Hough, R. L., Eaton, W. W., & Lock, B. Z. (1984). The NIMH Epidemiologic Catchment Area program: Historical context, major objectives, and study population characteristics. *Archives of General Psychiatry, 41*, 934–941.

Regier D. A., & Robins, L. N. (1991). Introduction. In L. N. Robins & D. A. Regier (Eds.), *Psychiatric disorders in America* (pp. 1–10). New York: Free Press.

Robins, L. N. (1985). Epidemiology: Reflections on testing the validity of psychiatric interviews. *Archives of General Psychiatry, 42*, 918–924.

Robins, L. N., Helzer, J., Ratcliff, K. S., & Seyfried, W. (1982). Validity of the Diagnostic Interview Schedule, Version II: DSM-III diagnoses. *Psychological Medicine, 12*, 855–870.

Robins, L. N., Wing, J. K., Wittchen, H. U., Helzer, J. E., Babor, T. F., Burke, J., Farmer, A., Jablenski, A., Pickens, R., Regier, D. A., Sartorius, N., & Towle, L. H. (1988). The Composite International Diagnostic Interview: An epidemiologic instrument suitable for use in conjunction with different diagnostic systems and in different cultures. *Archives of General Psychiatry, 45*, 1069–1077.

Shrout, P. (1994). The NIMH Epidemiologic Catchment Area program: Broken promises and dashed hopes? *International Journal of Methods and Psychiatric Research, 4*, 113–122.

Srole, L., Langner, T. S., Michael, S. T., Opler, M. K., & Rennie, T. A. C. (1962). *Mental health in the metropolis*. New York: McGraw-Hill.

Star, S. A. (1950). The screening of psychoneurotics in the army: Technical developments of tests. In S. A. Stouffer, L. Guttman, E. A. Suchman, P. F. Lazarsfeld, S. A. Star, & J. A. Clausen (Eds.), *Measurement and prediction* (pp. 486–547). Princeton, NJ: Princeton University Press.

Stouffer, S. A., Guttman, L., Suchman, E. A., Lazarsfeld, P. F., Star, S.,A., & Clausen, J. A. (1950). *The American soldier: Measurement and prediction* (Vol. IV). Princeton, NJ: Princeton University Press.

Ustun, T. B., & Tien, A. Y. (1995). Recent developments for diagnostic measures in psychiatry. *Epidemiologic Reviews, 17*(1), 210–220.

Weissman, M. M. (1987). Advances in psychiatric epidemiology: Rates and risks for major depression. *American Journal of Public Health, 77*, 445–451.

Williams, J. B. W. (1992). The structured clinical interview for DSM-III-R (SCID): II. Multisite test–retest reliability. *Archives of General Psychiatry, 49*, 630–636.

World Health Organization. (1992). *International statistical classification of diseases and related health problems: ICD-10* (Vol I, 10th ed. rev.). Geneva: Author.

DISCUSSION

1. What are the main differences between dimensional and diagnostic assessments?

2. Based on the authors' review, develop a list of the relative advantages and disadvantages of dimensional and diagnostic assessments. Which type of assessment would sociologists likely favor and why?

3. Can you think of other sociological concepts that could be measured using either a dimensional or categorical assessment procedure? What considerations would inform the choice?

Ronald C. Kessler

The categorical versus dimensional controversy in the sociology of mental illness[†]

Sociologists wrestle with the question of whether or not to adopt psychiatric concep-tualizations and measures of mental disorders in their research. On the one hand, social constructionist research reveals that definitions of mental disorders are social products rather than objective realities, which calls into question their validity as representations of human experience. Official definitions of mental disorders also assume that it is possible to cleanly distinguish persons who have a disorder from those who do not and, in the process, ignore substantial variation in the number and severity of symptoms that people experience. On the other hand, psychiatry speaks the "language" of official definitions of mental disorders and, as a result, those defi-nitions are more influential in clinical practice and in program and policy develop-ment. The two selections that follow present a much-abbreviated account of a debate on these issues that was held at a meeting of the American Sociological Association in 2000.

The controversy surrounding the use of categorical assessments (yes/no decisions regarding whether a person does or does not have a mental illness) versus dimensional assessments (each person receiving a score on a continu-ous scale of psychological distress with no cut-point to designate a threshold between those with and without a presumed illness) to create outcomes in sociological studies of mental illness can be traced back nearly half a cen-tury to the early community psychiatric studies of mental illness that were carried out shortly after World War II (Leighton et al., 1963; Srole et al., 1962). Many sociologists came down on the side of dimensional assessment at that time, and many sociologists have continued to use dimensional measures of distress as the main outcomes in their community surveys of mental illness ever since. The two main reasons advanced for preferring dimensional to categorical measures are that (1) the relationships between predictors and syndromes of psychological distress are more accurately captured in statisti-cal models that specify dimensional rather than categorical representations of distress and that (2) there is no evidence for the existence of true discrete mental illnesses that account for the patterns observed among symptoms in dimensional assessments. Mainstream psychiatric epidemiologists (some of whom were trained as sociologists), in comparison, moved away from an ini-tial use of dimensional assessments to categorical assessments, and then to a more recent use of both types of assessments in tandem. I argue in this paper that the tandem approach makes more sense than an exclusive use of either

Kessler, Ronald C. 2002. "The categorical versus dimensional controversy in the sociol-ogy of mental illness." *Journal of Health and Social Behavior* 43:171–188.

dimensional or categorical assessments. I also argue that the decision to use either categorical, dimensional, or both types of assessment should be made independent of whether the researcher believes that there is a true discrete illness that accounts for the symptoms under investigation.

BACKGROUND

The earliest dimensional scales of nonspecific psychological distress used in community epidemiological surveys were the 22-item Langner (1962) Scale used in the Midtown Manhattan Study (Srole et al., 1962) and the 20-item Health Opinion Survey (Macmillan 1957) used in the Stirling County Study (Leighton et al., 1963). Both the Langner and Health Opinion Survey scales were based on a more detailed screening scale, the Neuropsychiatric Screening Adjunct (Star, 1950), developed for Selective Service screening during World War II. These early scales were all designed to be first-stage screening tools used to target respondents with broadly defined emotional problems for more in-depth clinical assessment. This comparison between screening scores and clinical evaluations of mental illness led to the establishment of optimal cut-points on the screening scales for differentiating "cases" and "noncases." These validated cut-points were then used in later surveys to report prevalence rates (i.e., percentages of respondents with mental illness), without clinical follow-up to transform dimensional screening scale scores into dichotomous case definitions. However, controversies arose regarding the appropriate cut-points on these scales for case thresholds in community surveys (Seiler 1973). These controversies were fueled by the absence of a consistent way of defining clinical cases in the validation phase of the research, which led to inconsistencies in prevalence estimates across surveys (Dohrenwend & Dohrenwend, 1974). In addition, differences in prevalence across community samples and clinical samples led to differences in the positive predictive values of screening scale scores (the proportion of respondents with a given screening scale score who would be confirmed as a "case" by a clinical reinterviewer) across samples. Failure to account for differences in positive predictive values introduced further imprecision into community survey prevalence estimates. In the face of the confusion caused by these problems, and in the presence of evidence that the symptoms included in these screening scales have a strong unidimensional component (Dohrenwend et al., 1980), these screening scales came to be reported only in dimensional form (e.g., means, plots of distributions) in later surveys (e.g., Myers, Lindenthal, & Pepper, 1975).

The cut-point debate focused initially on a narrow clinical question: "What is the correct cut-point to define clinical significance of psychiatric symptoms?" However, the labeling theory debate in sociology (Gove & Howell, 1974; Scheff, 1974), which was going on at roughly the same time as the cut-point debate, raised a deeper question: "Does it make sense to believe that there is any true illness that provides a principled basis for deciding on a cut-point?" The recognition that the diagnostic criteria for mental disorders stipulated in the American Psychiatric Association's *Diagnostic and Statistical Manual of Mental Disorders* (*DSM*) often had as much to do with votes by committees as scientific evidence (Kirk & Kutchins, 1992) added a conceptual rationale to the predisposition of sociologists to favor the use of dimensional rather than categorical assessments. The situation has not changed much in the intervening three decades. Despite a dramatic expansion in our knowledge of the neurobiology of psychiatric syndromes (Charney, 1999), psychiatry continues to be unable to develop definitive biological tests for any mental disorder. As a result, the preference for dimensional over categorical assessments of these syndromes among sociologists continues to this day. There is also a strong movement within psychiatry for favoring dimensional measures over arbitrary categories based on similar reasoning in addition to an emphasis on clinical usefulness (Goldberg, 2000).

Link and Dohrenwend (1980), in a detailed review of the content and interpretation of dimensional screening scales of nonspecific psychological distress, showed that these scales typically include questions about a heterogeneous set of cognitive, behavioral, emotional, and psychophysiological symptoms that are elevated among people with a wide range of different mental disorders. These authors also demonstrated that, despite this heterogeneous content, the vast majority of the symptoms in these scales tap a single broad underlying dimension of nonspecific psychological distress. It is not surprising, based on these findings, that studies of correlations among categorical measures of psychiatric diagnoses in psychiatric epidemiological surveys find high rates of comorbidity (Kessler, 1995; Robins, Locke, & Regier, 1991).

Despite this evidence of a strong unidimensional core to psychological distress, psychiatric epidemiological surveys find that a sizeable number of people have pure categorical mental disorders (i.e., one and only one disorder). Based on this kind of evidence, researchers who favor dimensional assessment have moved beyond an exclusive interest in measures of psychological distress to study distinct dimensional measures of anxiety, depression, and several of the other syndromes that have been differentiated in research on the structure of psychological distress (Derogatis 1983; Dohrenwend et al. 1980).

The situation is quite different in mainstream psychiatric epidemiology, which moved away from the use of screening scales of nonspecific psychological distress in community surveys beginning in the early 1980s. This move occurred as a result of the influential Epidemiologic Catchment Area (ECA) Study (Robins & Regier, 1991). It is noteworthy that a number of sociologists played key roles in the ECA Study. The cut-point problem was resolved in the ECA study by taking advantage of the fact that the newly created *DSM-III* diagnostic system (American Psychiatric Association, 1980) provided rules for operationalizing diagnostic criteria that were much clearer than in previous versions of the *DSM*. These rules were used to develop a fully structured interview schedule (i.e., an interview schedule that could be used by trained interviewers who are not clinicians), the Diagnostic Interview Schedule (Robins et al., 1981), to generate diagnoses according to the definitions and criteria of *DSM-III*. It was only due to the fact that the Diagnostic Interview Schedule was easy to administer and did not require clinical interviewers that the massive ECA study (over 20,000 respondents selected across five different sites interviewed at multiple points in time) was logistically and financially feasible. Importantly, the Diagnostic Interview Schedule was argued to have acceptable concordance with independent *DSM-III* clinical diagnoses based on subsequent blind ECA reinterviews carried out by psychiatrists (Helzer et al., 1985), although the empirical data comparing Diagnostic Interview Schedule and independent clinical diagnoses actually showed concordance to be rather poor (Anthony et al., 1985).

The ECA was an enormously influential study in psychiatry. A number of Diagnostic Interview Schedule surveys based on the ECA were subsequently carried out in countries throughout the world (e.g., Bland, Orn, & Newman, 1988; Canino et al., 1987; Hwu, Yeh, & Chang, 1989; Lee et al., 1990; Lépine et al., 1989; Wells et al., 1989; and Wittchen et al., 1992). Cross-national comparative studies of these surveys showed impressive consistencies in patterns and correlates of disorders (Cross-National Collaborative Group, 1992). However, as most countries around the world use the World Health Organization's (WHO) International Classification of Diseases rather than the *DSM* system to diagnose mental disorders, there was a need for a fully structured interview to generate diagnoses based on the definitions and criteria of the International Classification of Diseases. Recognizing this need, collaboration was established between the WHO and the developers of the Diagnostic Interview Schedule to create a broader interview that would generate both International Classification of Diseases and *DSM* diagnoses. The resulting instrument, the World Health Organization Composite International Diagnostic Interview (Robins et al., 1988), was subsequently used in a number of community epidemiological surveys around the world (World Health Organization International Consortium of Psychiatric Epidemiology, 2000). Composite International Diagnostic Interview diagnoses have generally been shown in these surveys to have acceptable concordance with clinical diagnoses based on blind clinician reinterviews (Wittchen, 1994).

It is important to realize that the impressive body of work that has occurred since the early 1980s in community epidemiological studies of categorical diagnoses depended fundamentally on the existence of a fully structured diagnostic interview like the Diagnostic Interview Schedule and that the creation of the Diagnostic Interview Schedule would not have been possible without the existence of the clear diagnostic classification rules that were first introduced in 1980 in the *DSM-III*. Agreement among clinicians and clinical researchers to adopt these rules led to a resolution of the question raised by psychiatric epidemiologists in the early post-World War II categorical-dimensional assessment debate regarding the appropriate place to make clinical cut-points. However, it did not address the deeper question asked by sociologists regarding whether categorical distinctions make sense at all. The *DSM-III* categorical distinctions were made based on practical considerations having to do with presumed magnitudes of clinically significant distress and impairment combined with evidence regarding treatment response, rather than based on biological evidence justifying the diagnostic distinctions. The developers of the *DSM-III* were also sensitive to the fact that the system would be used for insurance billing purposes. This explains why so many "not otherwise specified" categories are included in the classification scheme. This creation of a document that met many needs led Jablensky (1999), a psychiatrist intimately involved in the classification process, to say that the *DSM-III* and later modification of the *DSM* and International Classification of Diseases systems created an agreement on nomenclature but not a logical system for classifying mental disorders.

Interestingly, even though the *DSM-III* system set the stage for the dominance of categorical classification in psychiatric epidemiological research over the next two decades, clinicians have continued to make use of dimensional scales, both to screen for mental illness in primary care (Goldberg, 1972) and to assess symptom severity and treatment effectiveness in clinical studies (Rush et al., 1996). Similar to the screening scales developed shortly after World War II, the screening scales used in primary care are designed to be short, nonspecific measures that provide broad-gauged assessment of the presence of any mental disorder. More detailed clinical assessment is required among patients who screen positive to determine which disorders they have. The screening scales used to study symptom severity and treatment effectiveness, in comparison, are designed for use only among people known to have a specific disorder, rather than in the general population. This means that the questions in these clinical scales are much more specific to particular disorders than the questions included in scales designed for use in the general population. In addition, the thresholds of the questions in these clinical scales are a good deal higher than those found in the scales designed for use in the general population.

Many clinical decisions are based on the results of dimensional rather than categorical assessment, albeit in patient samples defined on the basis of prior categorical evaluations (Andrews, forthcoming). For example, clinical experience shows that the usefulness of drug therapy in conjunction with behavioral therapy, rather than behavioral therapy alone, to treat phobias is related to the severity of phobic reactions assessed on dimensional scales such as the Marks Fear Questionnaire (Marks & Mathews, 1979) and the Liebowitz Social Anxiety Scale (Liebowitz, 1987). These scales are only administered after first determining, on the basis of an initial categorical clinical interview, that the patient does meet criteria for a phobia. Although it is possible, at least in principle, to carry out both types of assessment with a single dimensional scale that evaluates a clinical threshold and also evaluates symptom severity above that threshold, this is not done in practice because the types of information obtained in the two phases of assessment do not lend themselves to a consistent response format. In the categorical assessment, for example, it is usually quite important to ask about age of onset, course, family history, and range of trigger stimuli that lead to phobic fear and avoidance. In the symptom severity assessment, in comparison, the interviewer begins with the recognition that a phobia exists and asks the respondent to focus on the severity of their fear during exposure and the persistence of their efforts to avoid exposure to the feared stimuli. It is much more convenient to carry out these categorical and dimensional assessments separately rather than to devise a single dimensional assessment that can be administered to an unrestricted general population sample.

THE CASE FOR CATEGORICAL ASSESSMENT

There are three important attractions of categorical assessment. The first is that from the perspective of the clinician, treatment decisions are often categorical. Blood pressure is measured dimensionally and has a monotonic relationship with risk of subsequent stroke. However, clinicians have to decide when to intervene in this continuous distribution and this is usually a categorical decision. As a result, the National Heart, Lung, and Blood Institute has provided a categorical definition of hypertension (systolic blood pressure $\geq$ 140 mmHg or diastolic blood pressure $\geq$ 90 mmHg) in order to guide clinical categorical treatment decisions (NHLBI, 1998). This cut-point was selected based on external considerations concerning epidemiological data on risks of heart attack and stroke associated with specific combinations of systolic and diastolic blood pressure. In cases of this sort, where external criteria are used to define rational cut-points, it is reasonable to assume that the cut-points will change over time. Changes of this sort can occur based on considerations of cost-effectiveness (e.g., average treatment cost per year of life saved due to the treatment), or can be based on considerations of competing risks that compare the decrease in risk of morbidity and increase in estimated longevity created by treatment to the increase in risk of morbidity and decrease in estimated longevity created by other illnesses that might occur as an indirect result of the treatment (Gold et al., 1996). Political and financial considerations also come into play in making these changes.

The second attraction of categorical assessment is that it allows researchers to estimate prevalence of dimensional scores above the cut-points that are recognized as clinically significant. This is of considerable importance for needs assessment research, where some sort of threshold is required to determine how many people in the population are defined as in need of treatment. The definition of need can have dimensional characteristics, as when we discriminate among people classified as having severe disorders, serious but not severe disorders, and non-severe disorders. The definition can be influenced by moral as well as by scientific consideration and can consequently be made in different ways by different societies. However, this decision takes on a practical reality once it is made.

The third attraction of categorical assessment is that it makes it possible to obtain (usually retrospectively) information about lifetime occurrence. Dimensional measures, in comparison, limit assessment to recent time intervals such as the past week (e.g., Radloff, 1977) or the past month (e.g., Derogotis, 1983). The fact that categorical assessment makes it possible to speak about a discrete syndrome means that we can ask respondents about such things as how old they were when this syndrome first occurred and whether the syndrome has been episodic or chronic since that time. It is also possible to ask about such aspects as number of episodes, length of episodes, time between the end of one episode and the beginning of the next, and whether the length or time between episodes has become systematically shorter or longer over time. Information of this sort enriches our understanding of the natural history of these syndromes in a single survey much more than does the information obtained in dimensional measures on current symptom distributions.

THE CASE FOR DIMENSIONAL ASSESSMENT

Although treatment decisions are categorical, the evidence on which a treatment decision is based is almost always dimensional. How severe is the asthma? What are the scores on the dimensional liver function tests? In cases where the relevant dimensional measures are of borderline clinical significance, watchful waiting might be the appropriate initial clinical reaction even if the patient has the full set of symptoms. Treatment might be suggested if the dimensional scores are more elevated, while hospitalization might be the recommended course of action in even more extreme cases. Dimensional information is commonly used in this way in psychiatry. For example, cutpoints for mild, moderate, and severe depression based on the dimensional Hamilton Rating Scale for Depression (Hamilton, 1960) are routinely used to help guide clinical decisions regarding the use of medications and whether inpatient treatment might be needed.

A different attraction of dimensional assessment exists for the risk factor researcher, where studies of the predictors of scores on dimensional symptom scales are much easier to carry out and offer much greater statistical power than analyses of the predictors of categorical transformations of these dimensional scales. However, the usefulness of dimensional analysis hinges centrally on whether or not the risk factors are linearly related to scores on the dimensional scale. If the researcher wants his or her results to be relevant to the policy audience or to the clinical research audience, then the decision to focus on dimensional outcomes needs to be justified by demonstrating relevance at the clinical or policy threshold. In the absence of such a demonstration, potential users of the results have no way of excluding the possibility that significant predictors of the dimensional score are due to nonlinear effects of the predictors outside the clinical range.

THE INTEGRATION OF CATEGORICAL AND DIMENSIONAL ASSESSMENT IN EPIDEMIOLOGICAL RESEARCH

These observations should make it clear that there are benefits of integrating categorical and dimensional assessments. One can see this kind of integration in clinical trials, where it is conventional to present results in terms of mean differences between treatment and control arms on a dimensional symptom severity scale and also in terms of proportions of treatment and control respondents with various categorically defined outcomes. The two most commonly reported categorical outcomes are treatment response, defined as some specified magnitude of reduction (usually 50 percent) in the symptom severity score, and recovery, defined as a reduction in the symptom severity score to some specified low point that is considered no longer clinically significant. It is not uncommon for these various outcomes to yield different results, such as showing that the treatment leads to a significant reduction in average symptom severity and to widespread improvement, but to little recovery.

One can easily imagine a similar mix of outcomes being useful in community surveys both to describe the distribution of mental health problems in the population and to study predictors and social consequences. Indeed, work along these lines is already beginning to appear in the literature. For example, there has been a great deal of interest over the past few years in the distribution and correlates of social phobia (Davidson, 2000; Lecrubier et al., 2000; Lépine & Pelissolo, 2000; Montgomery, 1999; Stein & Gorman, 2001; Wittchen, 2000) based on the finding in recent community surveys that a surprisingly high proportion of the population meets criteria for this disorder and the low proportion of these people who ever seek treatment (Chartier, Hazen, & Stein, 1998; Davidson et al., 1993; Kessler, Stein, & Berglund, 1998). This work has shown, though, that the mean of these community cases on standard dimensional scales of clinical severity is quite low and that only a minority of community cases can be classified categorically as having the subtype of social phobia that has been found in clinical studies to be associated with serious impairment (Stein, Walker, & Forde, 1994). In addition, the predictors and social consequences of categorically defined social phobia and dimensionally defined social anxiety symptoms have been shown to differ in ways that shed light on the determinants of initial onset of the syndrome and determinants of increases in symptom severity (Kessler, forthcoming).

SUMMARY

The decision by sociological researchers to use dimensional rather than categorical outcomes in studies of mental illness has traditionally rested on the twin assumptions that the associations of predictors with psychological distress syndromes are most accurately operationalized by using dimensional measures rather than categorical measures of these syndromes and that no true underlying discrete mental illnesses can reasonably be inferred to exist that would justify the creation of dichotomous transformations of dimensional measures. These assumptions have been asserted rather than tested. Methods now exist to test these assumptions. Such tests should be required to justify the use of dimensional assessments in future empirical studies. The critical test should be whether the predictors are consistently related to differences in symptom severity across the full relevant range of the dimensional distribution. If they are, then analysis of the dimensional version of the symptom scale makes most sense. If the predictors are not consistently related to differences in symptom severity, analysis of either a categorical, a truncated dimensional, or a nested set of categorical and dimensional transformations of the original dimensional scale make the most sense.

References

American Psychiatric Association. 1980. *Diagnostic and Statistical Manual of Mental Disorders (Third Edition): DSM-III.* Washington, DC: American Psychiatric Association.

Anthony, James C., Marshal F. Folstein, Alan J. Romanoski, Michael R. Von Korff, Gerald R. Nestadt, Raman Chahal, Altaf Merchant, C. Hendricks Brown, Sam Shapiro, Morton Kramer, and Ernest M. Gruenberg. 1985. "Comparison of the Lay Diagnostic Interview Schedule and Standardized Psychiatric Diagnosis: Experience in eastern Baltimore." *Archives of General Psychiatry* 42:667–75.

Bland, Roger C., Helene Orn, and Stephen C. Newman. 1988. "Lifetime Prevalence of Psychiatric Disorders in Edmonton." *Acta Psychiatrica Scandinavica Supplementum* 338:24–32.

Canino, Glorisa J., Hector R. Bird, Patrick E. Shrout, Maritza Rubio-Stipec, Milagros Bravo, Ruth Martinez, M. Sesman, and Luz M. Guevara. 1987. "The Prevalence of Specific Psychiatric Disorders in Puerto Rico." *Archives of General Psychiatry* 44:727–35.

Charney, Dennis S. 1999. *Neurobiology of Mental Illness.* New York, NY: Oxford University Press.

Chartier, Mariette J., Andrea L. Hazen, and Murray B. Stein. 1998. "Lifetime Patterns of Social Phobia: A Retrospective Study of the Course of Social Phobia in a Nonclinical Population." *Depression and Anxiety* 7:113–21.

Cross-National Collaborative Group. 1992. "The Changing Rate of Major Depression: Cross-national Comparisons." *Journal of the American Medical Association* 268:3098–105.

Davidson, Jonathan R.T. 2000 "Social Anxiety Disorder under Scrutiny." *Depression and Anxiety* 11:93–98.

Davidson, Jonathan R.T., Dana C. Hughes, Linda K. George, and Dan G. Blazer. 1993. "Epidemiology of Social Phobia: Findings from the Duke Epidemiological Catchment Area Study." *Psychological Medicine* 23:709–18.

Derogatis, Leonard R. 1983. *SCL-90-R Revised Manual.* Baltimore, MD: Johns Hopkins School of Medicine.

Dohrenwend, Bruce P. and Barbara S. Dohrenwend. 1974. "Social and Cultural Influences on Psychopathology." *Annual Review of Psychology* 25:417–52.

Dohrenwend, Bruce P., Patrick E. Shrout, Gladys Ergi, and Frederick S. Mendelsohn. 1980. "Measures of Non-specific Psychological Distress and Other Dimensions of Psychopathology in the General Population." *Archives of General Psychiatry* 37:1229–36.

Gold, Marthe R., Joanna E. Siegel, Louise B. Russell, and Milton C. Weinstein. 1996. *Cost-Effectiveness in Health and Medicine.* Oxford, UK: Oxford University Press.

Goldberg, David P. 1972. *The Detection of Psychiatric Illness by Questionnaire: A Technique for the Identification and Assessment of Non-Psychotic Psychiatric Illness.* London, UK: Oxford University Press.

Goldberg, David. 2000. "Plato versus Aristotle: Categorical and Dimensional Models for Common Mental Disorders." *Comprehensive Psychiatry* 41(suppl. 1):8–13.

Gove, Walter R. and Petter Howell. 1974. "Individual Resources and Mental Hospitalization: A Comparison and Evaluation of the Societal Reaction and Psychiatric Perspectives." *American Sociological Review* 39(1):86–100.

Hamilton, Max. 1960. "A Rating Scale for Depression." *Journal of Neurology, Neurosurgery, and Psychiatry* 23:56–62.

Harris, Grant T., Marnie E. Rice, and Vernon L. Quinsey. 1994. "Psychopathy as a Taxon: Evidence that Psychopaths Are a Discrete Class." *Journal of Counseling and Clinical Psychology* 62:387–97.

Helzer, John E., Lee N. Robins, Larry T. McEvoy, and Edward Spitznagel. 1985. "A Comparison of Clinical and Diagnostic Interview Schedule Diagnoses: Physician Re-examination of Lay-interviewed Cases in the General Population." *Archives of General Psychiatry* 42:657–66.

Hwu Hai-Gwo, Eng Kung Yeh, and L. Y. Chang. 1989. "Prevalence of Psychiatric Disorders in Taiwan Defined by the Chinese Diagnostic Interview Schedule." *Acta Psychiatrica Scandinavica* 79:136–47.

Jablensky, Assen. 1999. "The Nature of Psychiatric Classification: Issues Beyond ICD-10 and DSM-IV" *Australian & New Zealand Journal of Psychiatry* 33(2):137–44.

Kendall, Robert E. 1989. "Clinical Validity." *Psychological Medicine* 19:1–55.

Kessler, Ronald C. 1995. "Epidemiology of Psychiatric Comorbidity." Pp. 179–97 in *Textbook in Psychiatric Epidemiology*, edited by Ming T. Tsuang, Mauricio Tohen, and Gwendolyn E. P. Zahner. New York: John Wiley and Sons.

Kessler, Ronald C., Murray B. Stein, and Patricia A. Berglund. 1998. "Social Phobia Subtypes in the National Comorbidity Survey." *The American Journal of Psychiatry* 155:613–19.

Kirk, Stewart A. and Herb Kutchins. 1992. *The Selling of the DSM: The Rhetoric of Science in Psychiatry.* New York: Aldine De Gruyter.

Langner, Thomas S. 1962. "A Twenty-two Item Screening Score of Psychiatric Symptoms Indicating Impairment." *Journal of Health and Human Behavior* 3:269.

Lecrubier, Yves, Hans-Ulrich Wittchen, Carlo Favavelli, Julio Bobes, Anita Patel, and Martin Knapp. 2000. "A European Perspective on Social Anxiety Disorder." *European Psychiatry* 15:5–16.

Lee, Chung Kyoon, Young Sook Kwak, Joe Yamamoto, Hee Rhee, Y. S. Kim, J-H Han, J. O. Choi, and Y. H. Lee. 1990. "Psychiatric Epidemiology in Korea. Part I: Gender and Age Differences in Seoul. *Journal of Nervous and Mental Disease* 178:242–6.

Leighton, Dorothea C., John H. Harding, David B. Macklin, Allister M. MacMillan, and Alexander H. Leighton. 1963. *The Character of Danger: Psychiatric Symptoms in Selected Communities.* Vol 3, *The Sirling County Study.* New York: Basic Books.

Lépine, Jean Pierre, and Antoine Pelissolo. 2000. "Why take Social Anxiety Disorder Seriously?" *Depression and Anxiety* 11:87–92.

Lépine, Jean Pierre, Joseph Lellouch, A. Lovell, M. Teherani, C. Ha, M. H. Verdier-Taillefer, N. Rambourg, and T. Lemperiere. 1989. "Anxiety and Depressive Disorders in a French Population: Methodology and Preliminary Results." *Psychiatric Psychobiology* 4:267–74.

Liebowitz, Michael R. 1987. "Social Phobia." *Modern Problems of Pharmacopsychiatry* 22:141–73.

Link, Bruce G. and Bruce P. Dohrenwend. 1980. "Formulation of Hypotheses about the True Relevance of Demoralization in the United States." Pp. 114–32 in *Mental*

Illness in the United States: Epidemiological Estimates, edited by Bruce P. Dohrenwend, Barbara S. Dohrenwend, Madelyn S. Gould, Bruce Link, Richard Neugebauer, and Robin Wunsch-Hitzig. New York, NY: Praeger.

MacMillan, Allister M. 1957. "The Health Opinion Survey: Techniques for Estimating Prevalence of Psychoneurotic and Related Types of Disorder in Communities." *Psychological Reports* 3:325.

Marks, Isaac M. and Andrew M. Mathews. 1979. "Brief Standard Self-rating Scale for Phobic Patients." *Behavior Research and Therapy* 17:263–7.

Montgomery, Stuart A. 1999. "Social Phobia: Diagnosis, Severity, and Implications for Treatment." *European Archives of Psychiatry and Clinical Neuroscience* 249:1–6.

Myers, Jerome K., Jacob J. Lindenthal, and Max P. Pepper. 1975. "Life Events, Social Integration and Psychiatric Symptomatology." *Journal of Health & Social Behavior* 16:421–7.

National Heart, Lung, and Blood Institute (NHLBI) Obesity Education Initiative Expert Panel on the Identification, Evaluation, and Treatment of Overweight and Obesity in Adults. 1998. "Clinical Guidelines on the Identification, Evaluation, and Treatment of Overweight and Obesity in Adults." Washington, DC: National Heart, Lung, and Blood Institute, June.

Radloff, Lori S. 1977. "The CES-D Scale: A Self-report Depression Scale for Research in the General Population." *Applied Psychological Measurement* 1:385–401.

Robins, Lee N., John E. Helzer, Jack L. Croughan, and Kathryn S. Ratcliff. 1981. "National Institute of Mental Health Diagnostic Interview Schedule: Its History, Characteristics and Validity." *Archives of General Psychiatry* 38:381–9.

Robins, Lee N., Ben Z. Locke, and Darrel A. Regier. 1991. "An Overview of Psychiatric Disorders in America." Pp. 328–66 in *Psychiatric Disorders in America: The Epidemiologic Catchment Area Study,* edited by Lee N. Robins and Darrel A. Regier. New York: Free Press.

Robins, Lee N. and Darrel A. Regier. 1991. *Psychiatric Disorders in America: The Epidemiologic Catchment Area Study.* New York, NY: The Free Press.

Robins, Lee N., John K. Wing, Hans-Ulrich Wittchen, John E. Helzer, Thomas F. Babor, Jack D. Burke, A. Farmer, A. Jablenski, R. Pickens, Darrel A. Regier, Norman Sartorius, and L. H. Towle. 1988. "The Composite International Diagnostic Interview: An Epidemiologic Instrument Suitable for Use in Conjunction with Different Diagnostic Systems and in Different Cultures." *Archives of General Psychiatry* 45:1069–77.

Rush, John A., Christina M. Gullion, Monica R. Basco, Robin B. Jarrett, and Madhukar H. Trivedi. 1996. "The Inventory of Depressive Symptomatology (IDS): Psychometric Properties." *Psychological Medicine* 3:477–86.

Scheff, Thomas J. 1974. "The Labeling Theory of Mental Illness." *American Sociological Review* 39(3):444–52.

Seiler, Lauren H. 1973. "The 22-Item Scale Used in Field Studies of Mental Illness: A Question of Method, a Question of Substance, and a Question of Theory." *Journal of Health and Social Behavior* 14(3):252–64.

Srole, Leo, Thomas S. Langner, Stanley T. Michael, Marvin K. Opler, and Thomas A. C. Rennie. 1962. *Mental Health in the Metropolis: The Midtown Manhattan Study.* New York, New York: McGraw-Hill.

Star, Shirley A. 1950. "The Screening of Psychoneurotics in the Army: Technical Development of Tests." Pp. 486–547 in *The American Soldier: Measurement and Prediction,* edited by S. Stouffer, L. Guttman, and E. Suchman. Princeton, NJ: Princeton University Press.

Stein, Murray B., and Jack M. Gorman. 2001. "Unmasking Social Anxiety Disorder."
    Journal of Psychiatry and Neuroscience 26:185–9.
Stein, Murray B., John R. Walker, and David R. Forde. 1994. "Setting Diagnostic
    Thresholds for Social Phobia: Considerations from a Community Survey of Social
    Anxiety." *The American Journal of Psychiatry* 151:408–12.
Wells, J. E., John A. Bushnell, Andrew R. Hornblow, Peter R. Joyce, and Mark A.
    Oakley-Browne. 1989. "Christchurch Psychiatric Epidemiology Study. Part
    I. Methodology and Lifetime Prevalence for Specific Psychiatric Disorders."
    Australian and New Zealand Journal of Psychiatry 23:315–26.
Wittchen, Hans-Ulrich. 1994. "Reliability and Validity Studies of the WHO
    —Composite International Diagnostic Interview (CIDI): A Critical Review."
    Journal of Psychiatric Research 28:57–84.
———. 2000. "The Many Faces of Social Anxiety Disorder." *International Clinical
    Psychopharmacology* 15:S7–12.
Wittchen, Hans-Ulrich, Cecilia A. Esau, Detlev von Zerssen, Jrgen-Christianson
    Krieg, and Michael Zaydig. 1992. "Lifetime and Six-Month Prevalence of Mental
    Disorders in the Munich Follow-up Study." *European Archives of Psychiatry and
    Clinical Neuroscience* 241:247–58.

John Mirowsky and Catherine E. Ross

Measurement for a Human Science[†]

Measures of mental health should represent and assess elements of human
experience clarified and refined from that experience but not removed from
it. Research in mental health speaks most true when it takes measure of life
as people feel it, sense it, and experience it.

THE ADVANTAGES OF INDEXES OVER DIAGNOSTIC CATEGORIES

Real but Not Dichotomous

Psychological problems are real, but they are not discrete. They are not something that is entirely present or entirely absent, without shades in between.
Psychological problems are not entities. They are not alien things that get
into a person and wreak havoc. Nevertheless, psychiatrists speak of depression and other psychological problems as if discrete entities enter the bodies
and minds of hapless victims. The psychiatrist detects the presence of an
entity and determines its species (makes a diagnosis), then selects an appropriate weapon against it (usually drug treatment). The imagery of detection

---

Mirowsky, John and Catherine E. Ross. 2002. "Measurement for a Human Science."
    Journal of Health and Social Behavior 43:152–170.

follows from the language of discrete entities. This categorical language is the legacy of 19th- century epidemiology and microbiology. A person is diseased or not. The disease is malaria or not, cholera or not, schistosomiasis or not. A language of categories fits some realities better than others. It fits the reality of psychological problems poorly (Mirowsky & Ross 1989a, 1989b).

Assessing the Type and Severity of Problems

Instead of diagnosing people, we can assess the type and severity of symptoms using indexes or scales. The fact is that we do not have to place people in diagnostic categories in order to know which subpopulations suffer more than others. Counting the number of persons in a diagnostic category is easily replaced by counting the number of symptoms of a particular type that various people have. The later strategy avoids the proliferation of diseases, each with its own name and mythical status as a unique, discrete entity. We need to remember, though, that a category of symptoms is a mental pigeon hole too. People are the real entities. The symptoms are merely things that some people feel or think or do more than others, for reasons we would like to know. Some of those things appear together more frequently than others, and those are the ones we treat as a single type of symptom.

It is useful to think in terms of the *type* and *severity* of psychological problems (Mirowsky & Ross 1989a, 1989b). Depression is a type of psychological problem. So is anxiety. Each type of problem ranges on a continuum from not at all severe to very severe. People score at all points on the continuum—from very few symptoms to many symptoms. People can get a severity score for each type of psychological problem. Contrast this with the diagnostic approach. Imagine two people on either side of some arbitrary cutoff that defines depression. One has just enough symptoms to get a diagnosis, and the other is just short of enough. Although the type and severity of their problems are very similar, one is diagnosed as depressed and the other is not. The diagnostic imposition ignores their similarity. Imagine another two people. One is happy, fulfilled, and productive. The other is demoralized, hopeless, and miserable, but just short of meeting the criteria for a diagnosis of depression. The diagnostic imposition ignores their differences. Diagnosis throws away information on the similarity of some cases and on the dissimilarity of others (Mirowsky & Ross 1989a, 1989b).

Unreliability of Dichotomous Measures

Throwing away information doesn't help us understand problems, it hinders us. Imagine being asked, "Are you depressed—yes or no?" You think about how to answer. You feel depressed at times and are not enjoying life very much, you don't feel too hopeful that things will get better, and sometimes you lie awake at night, troubled; on the other hand, you get out of bed every day, go to work and care for your children, you don't feel unable to concentrate at all, and you don't feel totally alone or think about death. Are you depressed? The crude dichotomy does not allow you to give a meaningful answer about how you feel. A more accurate assessment would allow you to tell the interviewer about the frequency of each symptom more exactly. Only people in perfect mental health, on the one hand, or extremely depressed to the point of considering suicide, on the other, could easily answer yes or no. For the large majority, the dichotomy is too insensitive to describe their subjective experience. Yet diagnostic instruments often force people to answer yes or no to questions about how they feel.

Insensitivity of Diagnoses

A diagnosis of depression is a profoundly insensitive measure. As a consequence, it can be difficult to find meaningful changes or differences in diagnosed depression. For example, a community study finds education and family income do not predict whether a person gets a diagnosis of depression or not (Weissman, 1987). One of the researchers concludes that "depression equally affects the educated and uneducated, the rich and poor, white and black Americans, blue and white collar workers" (Weissman, 1987, 448). Nothing could be further from the truth. No theory, whether social, psychological, genetic, or environmental, predicts that the poor, the uneducated, the blacks, and the blue collar workers have the same exposure to the causes of depression as the rich, the educated, the whites, and the white collar workers. With a sufficiently insensitive measure, we cannot hear the suffering of millions, and cannot see the causes.

Using diagnosis ignores almost all information about people, treating everyone within the category (depressed) as the same, and everyone outside the category (not depressed) as the same. In reality, people who qualify for a diagnosis of depression differ in their depression levels, as do people who do not qualify for a diagnosis. This loss of information weakens correlations (Cohen, 1983).

People Do Not Need to Be Diagnosed to Be Helped

Often the argument for categorizing people as ill versus well is that those categorized as ill can be treated. A diagnosis may or may not be handy, but it is not necessary. Anyone who feels very depressed and seeks treatment or is referred for treatment can be treated for depression. We do not need to label people as depressives, schizophrenics, or alcoholics in order to recognize that they feel bad, or their thoughts are disorganized and bizarre, or they have problems with alcohol. Certainly, we need to assess the type and extent of a person's problems, but the assessment does not need to be categorical. A person does not have to be diagnosed to be helped. Just the opposite may be true. Once a person receives a label, such as "schizophrenic," the diagnosis is treated as if it were the person's preeminent trait. Often the rest of the person's life and their other psychological problems are ignored. Clinical social workers use official psychiatric diagnoses primarily for insurance purposes, but they find the diagnoses of little or no value for understanding clients' psychological problems or the origins of these problems in family or work life, for understanding or predicting clients' behavior, or for planning treatment (Kirk & Kutchins, 1992; Kutchins & Kirk, 1988).

The Proliferation of Diagnostic Categories

Even when types of symptoms are empirically distinct, it does not mean that we can neatly assign individuals to a set of mutually exclusive diagnostic categories, saying some are depressed, others are anxious, and others are schizophrenic. Attempts to produce a set of exhaustive and mutually exclusive diagnostic categories lead to a proliferation of diagnoses that describe people who happen to have symptoms from more than one cluster. Thus, we get diagnostic categories like "schizo-affective," which is given when the clinician can't decide whether to diagnose schizophrenia (disorganized and bizarre thoughts and perceptions) or affective disorder (severe depression and anxiety). Worse than the introduction of unnecessary complexity, such a practice may obscure the fact that the causes of some symptoms on which a diagnosis is based are different than the causes of other symptoms on which the diagnosis is based.

Even with a profusion of diagnoses for people who are between categories (schizoaffective disorder), or just outside a category (schizophreniform disorder), or have an atypical disorder (atypical depression), or a mild disorder (dysthemia), a large minority of patients cannot be classified (Srole & Fischer, 1980), and many problems occur together. In the National Comorbidity Survey, atypical major depression was also associated with conduct disorder, social phobia, interpersonal dependence, and alcohol/drug use disorder (Sullivan, Kessler, & Kendler, 1998). Even with the profusion of diagnoses, the odds of qualifying for a diagnosis of schizophrenia are 28.5 times greater for those who also qualify for a diagnosis of major depression than for those who do not (Boyd et al., 1984).

Psychological problems are not discrete. Diagnostic categories do not reflect the reality of psychological problems. Indexes are superior scientifically to diagnostic categories, but continuums are not as useful in convincing the public, other physicians, insurance companies, or government agencies that psychiatric problems are real, serious problems that deserve insurance coverage and funding (Wilson, 1993). American psychiatry had an interest in developing diagnostic measures (Horwitz, 2002).

CONCLUSION

For researchers who decide to create knowledge that gives power to those who suffer or risk suffering, certain things follow. In one way or another they all come down to one thing: respect for the autonomy and self-determination of the people we study. Logically, then, the science we create should be designed to educate rather than to manipulate. It should use common language as much as possible. It should take measure of life as people feel it, sense it, and experience it. We connect our science to the lives of those we study by measuring the shades and grades of misery, anguish, distress, and alarm common to human beings—the human burden of tension, worry, mistrust, apprehension, fear, dejection, despair, sadness, loneliness, shame, frustration, humiliation, resentment, indignation, hostility, scorn, and anger. Although most measures have focused on the negative end of human experience, we hope to likewise connect by measuring the qualities of existence humans enjoy and seek: happiness, delight, serenity, fervor, gratification, hope, joy, purpose, accomplishment, affection, and acceptance. Let the sociology of mental health observe, think, and speak in such terms. Let us create a human science.

References

Boyd, Jeffrey H., J.D. Burke, E. Gruenberg, C.E. Holzer, D.S. Rae, L.K. George, M. Karno, R. Stolzman, L. McEnvoy, and G. Nestadt. 1984. "Exclusion Criteria of DSM-III: A Study of Co-occurrence of Hierarchy-free Syndromes." *Archives of General Psychiatry* 41:9 83–9.

Cohen, Jacob. 1983. "The Cost of Dichotomization." *Applied Psychological Measurement* 7:249–53.

Horwitz, Allan V. 2002. *Creating Mental Illness.* Chicago: University of Chicago Press.

Kirk, Stuart A. and Herb Kutchins. 1992. *The Selling of DSM: The Rhetoric of Science in Psychiatry.* New York: Aldine de Gruyter.

Kutchins, Herb and Stuart A. Kirk. 1988. "The Business of Diagnosis: DSM-III and Clinical Social Work." *Social Work* 33: 215–20.

Mirowsky, John, and Catherine E. Ross. 1989a. "Psychiatric Diagnosis as Reified Measurement." *Journal of Health and Social Behavior* 30(1):11–25.

Mirowsky, John and Catherine E. Ross. 1989b. *Social Causes of Psychological Distress.* New York: Aldine de Gruyter.

Srole, Leo and Anita Kassen Fischer. 1980. "To the Editor." *Archives of General Psychiatry* 37: 1424–6.

Sullivan, P.F., Ronald C. Kessler, and K.S. Kendler. 1998. "Latent Class Analysis of Lifetime Depressive Symptoms in the National Comorbidity Survey." *American Journal of Psychiatry* 155:1398–406.

Weissman, Myrna M. 1987. "Advances in Psychiatric Epidemiology: Rates and Risks for Major Depression." *American Journal of Public Health* 77:445–51.

Wilson, Mitchell. 1993. "DSM-III and the Transformation of American Psychiatry." *American Journal of Psychiatry* 150:399–410.

DISCUSSION QUESTIONS

1. How do the authors' arguments relate to the earlier selections you read about mental illness definitions? What do you see as the major points of disagreement in this debate?

2. Do you find Kessler's arguments about the advantages of categorical assessments persuasive? Why or why not? How would Mirowsky and Ross respond to his points?

3. What different insights do categorical and dimensional assessments of mental illness offer? Which do you think provides the most useful information for program and policy development? For analyses of the distribution of human joy and misery in the population?

Current Prevalence Estimates in the United States

Ronald C. Kessler, Olga Demler, Richard G. Frank, Mark Olfson,
Harold Alan Pincus, Ellen E. Walters, Philip Wang, Kenneth B. Wells,
Alan M. Zaslavsky

Prevalence and Treatment of Mental Disorders, 1990 to 2003

What proportion of people in the United States experience a major mental disorder in their lifetimes, has the proportion changed over time, and how many of those people receive treatment? Mental health researchers rely on surveys of the general population to find answers to questions such as these. Interviewers ask respondents a series of questions designed to determine whether respondents meet diagnostic criteria for specific mental disorders and whether and where they received treatment. Based on that information, they develop estimates of the prevalence of disorder and treatment. The article that follows presents summary results from the original National Comorbidity Survey and the National Comorbidity Survey-Replication, the most comprehensive studies of the prevalence of mental disorders in the United States. The authors find that the prevalence of mental disorders did not change in the ten years between the surveys but that the prevalence of treatment did.

Kessler, Ronald C., Olga Demler, Richard G. Frank, Mark Olfson, Harold Alan Pincus, Ellen E. Walters, Philip Wang, Kenneth B. Wells, and Alan M. Zaslavsky. 2005. "Prevalence and Treatment of Mental Disorders, 1990–2003." *New England Journal of Medicine* 352:2515–2523.

ABSTRACT

Background

Although the 1990s saw enormous change in the mental health care system in the United States, little is known about changes in the prevalence or rate of treatment of mental disorders.

Methods

We examined trends in the prevalence and rate of treatment of mental disorders among people 18 to 54 years of age during roughly the past decade. Data from the National Comorbidity Survey (NCS) were obtained in 5388 face-to-face household interviews conducted between 1990 and 1992, and data from the NCS Replication were obtained in 4319 interviews conducted between 2001 and 2003. Anxiety disorders, mood disorders, and substance-abuse disorders that were present during the 12 months before the interview were diagnosed with the use of the American Psychiatric Association's *Diagnostic and Statistical Manual of Mental Disorders*, fourth edition (DSM-IV). Treatment for emotional disorders was categorized according to the sector of mental health services: psychiatry services, other mental health services, general medical services, human services, and complementary–alternative medical services.

Results

The prevalence of mental disorders did not change during the decade (29.4 percent between 1990 and 1992 and 30.5 percent between 2001 and 2003, P = 0.52), but the rate of treatment increased. Among patients with a disorder, 20.3 percent received treatment between 1990 and 1992 and 32.9 percent received treatment between 2001 and 2003 (P < 0.001). Overall, 12.2 percent of the population 18 to 54 years of age received treatment for emotional disorders between 1990 and 1992 and 20.1 percent between 2001 and 2003 (P < 0.001). Only about half those who received treatment had disorders that met diagnostic criteria for a mental disorder. Significant increases in the rate of treatment (49.0 percent between 1990 and 1992 and 49.9 percent between 2001 and 2003) were limited to the sectors of general medical services (2.59 times as high in 2001 to 2003 as in 1990 to 1992), psychiatry services (2.17 times as high), and other mental health services (1.59 times as high) and were independent of the severity of the disorder and of the sociodemographic characteristics of the respondents.

Conclusions

Despite an increase in the rate of treatment, most patients with a mental disorder did not receive treatment. Continued efforts are needed to obtain data on the effectiveness of treatment in order to increase the use of effective treatments.

The U.S. Surgeon General's report on mental health[1] and the President's New Freedom Commission on Mental Health[2] have both called for expanding treatment for mental disorders. Planning this expansion requires accurate data on the prevalence and rate of treatment of mental disorders. In the 1980s, the Epidemiologic Catchment Area (ECA) Study found that 29.4 percent of the adults interviewed had had a mental disorder at some time in the 12 months before the interview (referred to as a "12-month mental disorder"), according to the criteria of the American Psychiatric Association's *Diagnostic and Statistical Manual of Mental Disorders*, third edition (DSM-III).[3] A fifth of those with a 12-month disorder received treatment. Half of those who received treatment did not meet the criteria for a 12-month disorder according to the ECA Study or the DSM-III. A decade later, the National Comorbidity Survey (NCS) found that 30.5 percent of people 15 to 54 years of age had conditions that met the criteria for a 12-month mental disorder according to the criteria of the DSM-III, revised (DSM-III-R).[4] A fourth of these patients received treatment. Roughly half those who received treatment did not meet the criteria for a 12-month mental disorder according to the NCS or the *DSM-III-R*.

The results of the ECA study and the NCS are no longer valid owing to changes in the delivery of mental health care. The Substance Abuse and Mental Health Services Administration found that annual visits to mental health specialists (i.e., psychiatrists and psychologists) increased by 50 percent between 1992 and 2000.[5] The National Ambulatory Medical Care Survey found that the number of people receiving treatment for depression tripled between 1987 and 1997.[6] The Robert Wood Johnson Foundation Community Tracking Survey found that the number of people with a serious mental illness who were treated by a specialist increased by 20 percent between 1997 and 2001.[7]

The aim of our study was to present more comprehensive data on national trends with regard to the prevalence and rate of treatment of 12-month mental disorders based on the NCS, conducted from 1990 to 1992,[4] and the NCS Replication (NCS-R), conducted from 2001 to 2003.[8] In our study, unlike the study by the Substance Abuse and Mental Health Services Administration and the National Ambulatory Medical Care Survey, we examined data on the rate of treatment inside and outside the health care system. Unlike the Community Tracking Survey, which contained only rough data based on screening measures of prevalence, our study analyzed detailed diagnostic assessments.

METHODS

Samples

The NCS and NCS-R are nationally representative, face-to-face household surveys of respondents 15 to 54 years of age (NCS) or 18 years of age and older (NCS-R). In the NCS, the response rate was 82.4 percent, and the total number of completed interviews was 8098; in the NCS-R, the response rate was 70.9 percent, and the total number of completed interviews was 9282.[4,8] All respondents had a diagnostic interview that focused on mental disorders. Respondents who had received a diagnosis of a mental disorder and a randomly selected subgroup of those who did not were interviewed to assess risk factors, treatment, and consequences of having a mental disorder. Weights were used to adjust for bias due to differences in responses and within-household differences in the probability of selection. Residual discrepancies between data from the U.S. Census and data on our sample with regard to demographic and geographic distributions were corrected with a final weight. A detailed discussion of samples and weights has been presented elsewhere.[4,8] The data presented in this report are from the part II assessment of respondents in the overlapping age range of the two samples (among respondents 18 to 54 years old, 5388 completed interviews in the NCS, and 4319 in the NCS-R).

Recruitment and Consent

Introductory explanatory materials that were mailed to households included the NCS and NCS-R survey samples before an interviewer visited to answer any remaining questions respondents might have and to obtain informed consent and schedule interviews. As an incentive to respond, respondents included in the NCS received $25 and those included in the NCS-R received $50. A subgroup of those who did not initially agree to be interviewed received higher incentives ($50 in the NCS, and $100 in the NCS-R) to encourage them to complete a screening interview. The human-subjects committees of the University of Michigan and Harvard Medical School approved these procedures.

Diagnostic Assessment

Diagnosis was based on the World Health Organization's Composite International Diagnostic Interview (CIDI) in conjunction with the DSM-III-R in the NCS[9] and CIDI in conjunction with the fourth edition of DSM (DSM-IV) in the NCS-R.[10] Diagnoses included anxiety disorders (e.g., panic disorder, generalized anxiety disorder, phobias, and posttraumatic stress disorder), mood disorders (e.g., major depression, dysthymia, and bipolar disorder), and substance-abuse disorders (e.g., alcohol and drug abuse and dependence). Interviews conducted for clinical reappraisal documented good concordance and conservative estimates of prevalence, as compared with diagnoses made by clinicians who were unaware of the responses given in the diagnostic interview.[11,12] Twelve-month disorders were considered to be present if they had occurred at any time during the 12 months before the interview, even if the disorders had subsequently remitted with treatment.

Because the criteria of the DSM-III-R and of the DSM-IV differ too greatly to justify direct comparisons of prevalence in the data from the NCS and NCS-R, the trend analysis was based on a recalibration of both surveys according to a summary rating of severity that was developed for the NCS-R and then applied (imputed) to the data from the NCS. This rating has been described in detail elsewhere.[13] In brief, a serious disorder was defined as either one that met the 12-month criteria for schizophrenia, any other non-affective psychosis, bipolar I disorder or bipolar II disorder, or substance dependence with a syndrome of physiological dependence, a suicide attempt or having a suicide plan in conjunction with a diagnosis of a disorder according to the criteria of the NCS-R and DSM-IV, a self-report of "severe" impairment in role functioning in two or more areas owing to a mental disorder, or a self-reported functional impairment associated with a mental disorder consistent with a score of 50 or less according to the Global Assessment of Functioning Scale (scores range from 0 to 100, with higher scores indicating better functioning).[14] A mental disorder that did not meet the criteria for a serious disorder was classified as a moderate or mild disorder on the basis of the subject's responses to disorder-specific questions on the Sheehan Disability Scales for the assessment of clinical severity.[15]

The imputation of scores for severity of disorder to cases included in the NCS was based on estimates calculated with the use of logistic-regression equations in the NCS-R in which symptom measures available in both surveys were used to predict the presence of a serious disorder in one respondent as compared with all other respondents, a serious-to-moderate disorder as compared with mild disorders in all other respondents, and the presence of any disorder as compared with no disorder. The accuracy of prediction was good with all three equations (area under the curve, 0.7 for a serious disorder, 0.8 for a serious-to-moderate disorder, and 0.8 for any disorder). The coefficients in these equations were used to generate predicted probabilities for each respondent included in both surveys for each nested outcome, and these probabilities, in turn, were used to impute discrete scores on the scale for severity (with a range from none to serious).

Treatment

All respondents who were interviewed to assess risk factors in both surveys were asked whether they had sought treatment for an emotional disorder within the 12 months before the interview from a list of providers and settings. Responses were classified according to the providers in the sector of mental health services — psychiatrist, other mental health specialist, general medical provider (e.g., a general medical doctor or a nurse practitioner), or complementary–alternative medical provider.

Analysis

Trends were assessed with the use of risk ratios, defined as the proportional increase in the prevalence in the NCS-R as compared with the NCS. Variation in trends among subgroups in the sample, which were defined according to sociodemographic characteristics, was assessed with the use of pooled logistic-regression analysis. Predictors included time, sociodemographic characteristics, and interactions between time and the sociodemographic characteristics. Trends in treatment were also assessed, as a function of the severity of the disorder. Standard errors were obtained with the use of the Taylor series linearization method.[16] Adjustment for imprecision in the imputed scores for severity was made with the use of the multiple-imputation method.[17] Ten independent pseudosamples were drawn from the original NCS-R sample for this purpose, with the use of predicted probabilities of severity that were converted into dichotomous case classifications on the basis of probability distributions. The pseudosamples were used to build uncertainty with regard to classification into the standard error of the estimate; this was done by defining the square of the standard error as the sum of the average design-adjusted coefficient-variance estimates within the 10 pseudosamples and the variance of the coefficients across these pseudo-samples. Logistic-regression coefficients and standard errors were exponentiated to create odds ratios with 95 percent confidence intervals. The significance of sets of multiple predictors was evaluated with the Wald χ^2 tests with the use of design-adjusted, multiply-imputed coefficient variance–covariance matrixes.

RESULTS

Trends in Prevalence

The estimated prevalence of a 12-month mental disorder that met the criteria of the DSM-IV did not differ significantly between the surveys (29.4 percent between 1990 and 1992 and 30.5 percent between 2001 and 2003, P = 0.52). There was no significant change in the prevalence of serious disorders (5.3 percent vs. 6.3 percent, P = 0.27), moderate disorders (12.3 percent vs. 13.5 percent, P = 0.30), or mild disorders (11.8 percent vs. 10.8 percent, P = 0.37), and no statistically significant interactions between time and sociodemographic characteristics in the prediction of prevalence (data not shown).

Trends in Treatment

The prevalence of treatment for an emotional disorder within the 12 months before the interview was 12.2 percent between 1990 and 1992 and 20.1 percent between 2001 and 2003 (risk ratio, 1.65, P < 0.001) (Table 1). The association between greater severity and receipt of treatment was positive, significant (P < 0.001), and did not differ over time. It was substantively moderate in the pooled data, however, calculated with the use of a Pearson's contingency coefficient (a polychotomous extension of the phi coefficeint of 0.14). Only a minority of respondents with a serious mental disorder received treatment (24.3 percent between 1990 and 1992 and 40.5 percent between 2001 and 2003). Approximately half those who received treatment (49.0 percent between 1990 and 1992 and 49.9 percent between 2001 and 2003) had none of the disorders considered here (Table 1).

Table 1. Treatment of 12-Month Disorders According to Severity and Sector of Mental Health Services among 5388 Respondents to the National Comorbidity Survey (NCS), 1990–1992, and 4319 Respondents to the National Comorbidity Survey Replication (NCS-R), 2001–2003.[*]

Variable	Any	PSY	OMH	GM	HS	CAM
			percentage ± SE[†]			
NCS						
Serious	24.3 ± 3.8	7.3 ± 2.2	11.4 ± 2.5	8.2 ± 3.0	4.5 ± 1.9	8.4 ± 1.9
Moderate	25.4 ± 2.4	5.8 ± 1.2	13.6 ± 1.6	8.6 ± 1.4	5.5 ± 1.1	7.1 ± 1.2
Mild	13.3 ± 2.4	2.5 ± 1.2	4.9 ± 1.3	4.3 ± 1.4	3.0 ± 1.2	3.0 ± 0.8
Any	20.3 ± 1.5	4.8 ± 0.8	9.7 ± 1.0	6.8 ± 1.0	4.3 ± 0.7	5.7 ± 0.7
None	8.8 ± 0.7	1.4 ± 0.3	3.5 ± 0.4	2.6 ± 0.4	1.9 ± 0.3	2.3 ± 0.3
Total	12.2 ± 0.6	2.4 ± 0.3	5.3 ± 0.3	3.9 ± 0.4	2.6 ± 0.3	3.3 ± 0.3
NCS-R						
Serious	40.5 ± 4.7	14.4 ± 3.3	19.4 ± 3.5	22.1 ± 3.5	6.5 ± 1.6	6.2 ± 1.5
Moderate	37.2 ± 3.0	13.0 ± 1.6	15.8 ± 1.8	19.5 ± 2.4	5.5 ± 1.2	4.6 ± 1.0
Mild	23.0 ± 3.8	5.1 ± 1.3	9.0 ± 2.2	11.8 ± 2.9	3.9 ± 1.5	2.9 ± 0.9
Any	32.9 ± 2.0	10.5 ± 1.0	14.1 ± 1.3	17.3 ± 1.3	5.1 ± 0.8	4.3 ± 0.6
None	14.5 ± 0.9	2.9 ± 0.4	5.9 ± 0.6	6.8 ± 0.6	2.7 ± 0.4	1.9 ± 0.3
Total	20.1 ± 0.8	5.2 ± 0.3	8.4 ± 0.5	10.0 ± 0.5	3.5 ± 0.3	2.7 ± 0.3
			risk ratio ± SE[‡]			
Ratio of NCS-R to NCS						
Serious	1.68 ± 0.35	2.01 ± 0.84	1.72 ± 0.49	2.91 ± 1.33	1.53 ± 0.70	0.74 ± 0.25
Moderate	1.47 ± 0.19[§]	2.27 ± 0.57[§]	1.17 ± 0.19	2.29 ± 0.46[§]	1.01 ± 0.29	0.65 ± 0.17
Mild	1.74 ± 0.35[§]	2.17 ± 1.14	1.85 ± 0.57	2.82 ± 1.04	1.34 ± 0.64	0.97 ± 0.38
Any	1.62 ± 0.15[§]	2.21 ± 0.40[§]	1.46 ± 0.18[§]	2.58 ± 0.41[§]	1.19 ± 0.25	0.76 ± 0.14
None	1.65 ± 0.16[§]	2.05 ± 0.50[§]	1.71 ± 0.26[§]	2.57 ± 0.46[§]	1.42 ± 0.32	0.86 ± 0.16
Total	1.65 ± 0.10[§]	2.17 ± 0.27[§]	1.59 ± 0.15[§]	2.59 ± 0.29[§]	1.32 ± 0.19	0.81 ± 0.10

	χ^2	P Value	χ^2	P Value	χ^2	P Value	χ^2	P Value	χ^2	P Value	χ^2	P Value
Statistical significance[¶]												
Severity	194.6	<0.001	112.2	<0.001	118.1	<0.001	105.3	<0.001	23.0	<0.001	82.9	<0.001
Time	56.8	<0.001	34.5	<0.001	22.7	<0.001	72.4	<0.001	3.3	0.07	3.3	0.07
Time-by-severity	0.5	0.93	0.2	0.98	3.0	0.40	0.3	0.96	0.9	0.82	1.2	0.76

[*] Mental disorders were diagnosed according to the criteria of the DSM-IV. Respondents in both surveys were 18 through 54 years of age. Any denotes any sector of mental health services, PSY the sector of psychiatry services, OMH other mental health services, GM general medical services, HS human services, CAM complementary-alternative medical services, and χ^2 the Wald χ^2 test. Standard errors (SEs) are the design-based multiply-imputed standard errors of the estimated values.

[†] Percentages are the proportions of respondents in the total sample who received any treatment or treatment within the indicated sector of mental health services.

[‡] The risk ratio is not always equal to the ratio of the estimated percentages, because of the use of the multiple-imputation method.

[§] P values of less than 0.05 (in a two-sided test) indicate statistical significance.

[¶] Each χ^2 test for severity has 3 degrees of freedom. Each χ^2 test for time has 1 degree of freedom. Significance tests for interactions between time and severity evaluate the significance of changes between the two surveys. Each time-by-severity χ^2 test has 3 degrees of freedom.

The trends in the rate of treatment according to the sectors of mental health services were similar to the overall trends in two respects (Table 1). First, the severity of a disorder was significantly related to the rate of treatment (P < 0.001), and second, this association did not change significantly over time. A significant difference in these trends was found among sectors (P < 0.001). In the sector of general medical services, the rate of treatment increased from 3.9 percent to 10.0 percent (risk ratio, 2.59), in that of psychiatry services it increased from 2.4 percent to 5.2 percent (risk ratio, 2.17), and in the sector of other mental health services it increased from 5.3 percent to 8.4 percent (risk ratio, 1.59). In the sector of human services, it increased from 2.6 percent to 3.5 percent (risk ratio, 1.32; P = 0.07), the rate in the sector of complementary–alternative medical services decreased from 3.3 percent to 2.7 percent (risk ratio, 0.81; P = 0.07).

A shift in the distribution of treatment among the sectors occurred because of differences within the sectors. The distribution of treatment in the sector of general medical services increased from 31.5 percent to 49.6 percent (P < 0.001), in that of psychiatry services from 19.6 percent to 25.8 percent (P = 0.007), in that of other mental health services from 43.5 percent to 41.9 percent (P = 0.59), in that of human services from 21.5 percent to 17.2 percent (P = 0.11), and in that of complementary–alternative medical services from 26.8 percent to 13.2 percent (P < 0.001). The changes in distribution did not vary significantly according to severity of disorder.

Sociodemographic Variables and Treatment

We examined associations between seven sociodemographic variables and the measures of the six sectors in which treatment was provided (Table 2). Of the 42 associations, 10 were found to be significant with the use of a threshold of 0.001 as an approximate control for type 1 error. Predictors of the receipt of treatment within any sector of mental health services included age greater than 24 years, female sex, non-Hispanic white race, and marital status (separated, widowed, divorced, or never married). Race was self-reported. Predictors of treatment specific to the sector of services included age (older age correlated positively with treatment in the sector of general medical services and negatively with that of other mental health services), sex (female sex correlated positively with treatment in the sector of general medical services and negatively with that of complementary–alternative medical services), marital status (respondents who had never married were more likely than those who were currently married to receive treatment in the sector of other mental health services), education (more years of education correlated negatively with treatment in the sector of general medical services), and urban as compared with rural area (rural areas related negatively to sector of services). These associations are all moderate in magnitude (Pearson's contingency coefficient, 0.04 to 0.07). Income was the only sociodemographic variable that was not significantly related to treatment in any sector of mental health services. Interactions with time and severity of mental disorder were shown to be nonsignificant with the use of a threshold of 0.001 (Table 2).

Table 2. Sociodemographic Characteristics That Were Predictors of the Receipt of Treatment for Any 12-Month Mental Disorder in the Total Sample of 9707 Respondents and as a Proportion of Treatment Provided in All Sectors of Services.[*]

Characteristic	Any	PSY	OMH	GM	HS	CAM
	odds ratio (95 percent confidence interval)					
Age group						
18–24 yr	0.6 (0.5–0.8)[†]	0.6 (0.4–1.0)	2.6 (1.7–3.9)[†]	0.4 (0.3–0.6)[†]	2.1 (1.2–3.8)[†]	0.9 (0.6–1.5)
25–34 yr	0.9 (0.7–1.1)	0.6 (0.4–0.8)[†]	1.9 (1.3–2.6)[†]	0.6 (0.4–0.8)[†]	1.5 (0.9–2.6)	1.2 (0.8–1.7)
35–44 yr	1.1 (0.9–1.4)	0.7 (0.5–0.9)[†]	1.7 (1.3–2.3)[†]	0.8 (0.6–1.1)	1.3 (0.8–2.2)	1.1 (0.8–1.5)
45–54 yr[‡]	1.0	1.0	1.0	1.0	1.0	1.0
P value	<0.001	0.007	<0.001	<0.001	0.07	0.70
Sex						
Female	1.7 (1.4–1.9)[†]	0.7 (0.6–0.9)[†]	1.0 (0.8–1.2)	1.8 (1.4–2.3)[†]	1.1 (0.8–1.5)	0.7 (0.5–0.8)
Male[‡]	1.0	1.0	1.0	1.0	1.0	1.0
P value	<0.001	0.01	0.71	0.001	0.69	<0.001
Race or ethnic group[§]						
Hispanic	0.6 (0.5–0.9)[†]	0.5 (0.3–0.8)[†]	1.0 (0.6–1.6)	0.8 (0.5–1.2)	1.5 (0.8–2.7)	0.8 (0.4–1.4)
Non-Hispanic black	0.5 (0.4–0.7)[†]	0.9 (0.6–1.5)	0.7 (0.5–1.1)	0.5 (0.5–1.4)	1.9 (1.2–3.0)[†]	0.6 (0.4–1.0)
Other	0.5 (0.4–0.7)[†]	0.9 (0.5–1.7)	1.0 (0.4–2.5)	0.8 (0.2–2.6)	0.7 (0.3–1.9)	0.7 (0.3–1.5)
Non-Hispanic white[‡]	1.0	1.0	1.0	1.0	1.0	1.0
P value	<0.001	0.02	0.47	0.68	0.01	0.22
Marital status						
Separated, widowed, or divorced	1.8 (1.5–2.2)[†]	1.0 (0.7–1.3)	1.8 (1.4–2.5)[†]	0.6 (0.4–0.8)†	1.3 (0.8–2.1)	1.5 (1.0–2.3)
Never married	1.3 (1.1–1.6)[†]	1.2 (0.8–1.6)	1.3 (1.0–1.8)†	0.8 (0.5–1.1)	1.0 (0.6–1.6)	0.9 (0.6–1.4)
Married[‡]	1.0	1.0	1.0	1.0	1.0	1.0
P value	<0.001	0.59	<0.001	0.003	0.39	0.05
Education						
0–11 yr	1.1 (0.8–1.5)	0.9 (0.6–1.3)	0.6 (0.4–0.9)†	2.6 (1.7–4.1)[†]	0.4 (0.2–0.8)[†]	1.1 (0.7–1.8)
12 yr	1.0 (0.8–1.3)	0.8 (0.6–1.2)	0.6 (0.4–0.9)†	2.2 (1.5–3.2)[†]	0.8 (0.5–1.2)	1.0 (0.7–1.5)
13–15 yr	1.2 (0.9–1.4)	0.7 (0.5–0.9)[†]	0.8 (0.6–1.0)	2.1 (1.4–3.1)[†]	0.8 (0.5–1.2)	0.8 (0.6–1.2)
≥16 yr[‡]	1.0	1.0	1.0	1.0	1.0	1.0
P value	0.32	0.04	0.02	<0.001	0.03	0.48
Income[¶]						
Low	1.1 (0.8–1.4)	1.2 (0.8–1.9)	1.0 (0.7–1.6)	0.9 (0.5–1.4)	2.1 (1.1–3.8)[†]	1.4 (0.9–2.2)
Low-average	0.9 (0.7–1.1)	0.9 (0.6–1.4)	1.0 (0.7–1.4)	1.2 (0.8–1.8)	1.9 (1.1–3.2)[†]	1.6 (1.1–2.5)[†]
High-average	0.9 (0.7–1.1)	0.8 (0.5–1.2)	0.9 (0.7–1.3)	1.1 (0.8–1.6)	1.6 (1.0–2.1)[†]	1.5 (1.0–2.1)
High[‡]	1.0	1.0	1.0	1.0	1.0	1.0
P value	0.25	0.07	0.94	0.21	0.10	0.08

(continued)

Table 2 continued

Characteristic	Any	PSY	OMH	GM	HS	CAM
Urban vs. rural area‖						
Large MSA–central city	1.6 (0.9–2.6)	0.8 (0.3–2.1)	3.2 (1.3–7.6)	0.7 (0.3–1.4)	0.3 (0.1–0.7)	2.9 (1.0–8.4)†
Large MSA–suburb	1.5 (0.9–2.4)	0.7 (0.2–2.0)	3.0 (1.3–7.2)	0.7 (0.4–1.4)	0.5 (0.2–1.1)	2.6 (0.9–7.3)
Small MSA–central city	1.5 (0.9–2.4)	0.5 (0.2–1.4)	4.0 (1.7–9.4)	1.0 (0.5–1.9)	0.4 (0.2–0.9)†	1.9 (0.7–5.6)
Small MSA–suburb	1.4 (0.8–2.4)	0.5 (0.2–1.4)	3.2 (1.4–7.4)	1.1 (0.6–2.0)	0.5 (0.2–1.1)	1.6 (0.6–4.4)
Adjacent area	1.2 (0.8–1.9)	0.6 (0.2–1.6)	3.6 (1.5–8.6)	1.1 (0.5–1.7)	0.5 (0.2–1.1)	2.0 (0.8–5.2)
Rural area‡	1.0	1.0	1.0	1.0	1.0	1.0
P value	0.35	0.23	0.06	0.36	0.10	0.006

* Odds ratios have been adjusted for the severity of the disorder and for the time period. Any denotes any sector of mental health services, PSY psychiatry services, OMH other mental health services, GM general medical services, HS human services, and CAM complementary–alternative medical services.

† P values of less than 0.05 (in a two-sided test) indicate statistical significance.

‡ Respondents in this category served as the reference group.

§ Race was self-reported.

¶ Income was defined as a multiple of the federal poverty line (for 1990 in the NCS and for 2001 in the NCS-R) for a family with the same composition as that of the respondent: low denotes a ratio of income to poverty (I:P) of less than 1.5:1, low-average an I:P between 1.5:1 and < 3:1, high-average an I:P between 3:1 and < 6:1, and high an I:P of ≥6:1.

‖ Urban vs. rural area was coded according to the definitions of the U.S. Census Bureau for 1990 (NCS) and 2000 (NCS-R) to distinguish between large metropolitan statistical areas (MSAs) (at least 2 million residents) and smaller MSAs (< 2 million) and between central cities and the suburbs of such cities.

DISCUSSION

Although there are limitations to our study, there were five important results. First, no notable change occurred in the prevalence or severity of mental disorders in the United States between 1990 and 1992 or between 2001 and 2003. There are two possible explanations for this result: that the prevalence of mental disorders would have been higher in the early 2000s than in the early 1990s were it not for the increase in the rate of treatment, and that this increase did not result in a decrease in the number and type of disorders. Consistent with the first possibility is the fact that an economic recession began shortly before and deepened throughout the field-study period of the NCS-R, even though the attacks on September 11, 2001, occurred in the middle of the field-study period. The prevalence of mental disorders might have increased in the absence of an increase in the rate of treatment. However, there is more evidence that is consistent with the second explanation. Studies show that most treatment for mental disorders falls below the minimal standards of quality.[18] In addition, such treatment is typically brief, which means that treatment would influence the duration of an episode of mental disorder more than it would the prevalence of mental disorders in the 12 months before the interview.

Finally, the increase in the rate of treatment was largely in the sector of general medical services, and treatment was provided to patients without disorders that were classified according to criteria of the NCS-R and DSM-IV. Controlled treatment trials have provided no evidence that pharmacotherapy significantly improves mild disorders, making it unlikely that pharmacotherapy could prevent a significant increase over time in the prevalence of such disorders.

ESTIMATING THE PREVALENCE OF MENTAL DISORDERS AMONG U.S. RACIAL AND ETHNIC MINORITIES

National surveys of mental illness, such as the National Comorbidity Survey Replication, do not include sufficiently large samples of racial/ethnic minority groups to permit meaningful estimates of the prevalence of mental disorders in those groups. Some surveys have been conducted within specific racial or ethnic groups, but they often cover only certain specific regions of the country or include only English-speaking respondents; as a result, they leave out large segments of the population and cannot be used to generate national estimates of prevalence. The National Latino and Asian American study (NLAAS) was conducted to address these limitations. The study provides the first national estimates of the prevalence of mental disorders in subgroups of the U.S. Latino and Asian American populations. The study investigators pay special attention to differences in the prevalence of mental disorders based on ethnic origin and immigrant status—two important sources of variation in minority group members' experiences. For example, Margarita Alegría and her colleagues observed that, among U.S. Latino populations, Puerto Ricans had the highest prevalence rates of mental disorders, that rates of disorder were higher among Latinos with high as compared to low English language proficiency, higher among U.S.-born Latinos than among immigrants, and that, among immigrants, rates of disorder increased with the length of time they had lived in the U.S. In contrast, David Takeuchi and colleagues found that, among Asian Americans, there were few differences in rates of disorder by country of origin and that the associations of immigration-related factors with rates of mental disorder differed markedly for men and women. U.S. born women had higher rates of disorder than immigrant women but there were few differences in rates of disorders based on country of birth for men. Men with high levels of English proficiency had lower rates of disorders than men with low levels of English proficiency; English proficiency was not associated with rates of disorder for women. Length of residence in the U.S. was not associated with rates of disorder for men or women in Asian American populations, in contrast to the results for Latinos. These results suggest that there is dramatic variation in the mental health of members of racial and ethnic minority groups depending on group and individual immigration histories and depending on the experiences they encounter in the United States. For example, because Puerto Ricans are U.S. citizens, they may feel a greater sense of disappointment when their expectations for life in the U.S. are not met. As scholars give greater attention to the complexity of minority group members' lives, we will learn more about their specific experiences as well as about the general processes through which the social environment affects well-being.

Alegría, Margarita, Norah Mulvaney-Day, Maria Torres, Antonio Polo, Zhun Cao, and Glorisa Canino. 2007. "Prevalence of Psychiatric Disorders Across Latino Subgroups in the United States." *American Journal of Public Health* 97:68–75.

Takeuchi, David T., Nolan Zane, Seunghye Hong, David H. Chae, Fang Gong, Gilbert C. Gee, Emily Walton, Stanley Sue, and Margarita Alegría. 2007. "Immigration-Related Factors and Mental Disorders among Asian Americans." *American Journal of Public Health* 97:84–90.

Second, a substantial increase in the rate of treatment occurred between 1990 to 1992 and 2001 to 2003 in the proportion of the population treated for emotional disorders, even though the majority of those with such disorders still received no treatment. The increased rate of treatment may have been due to aggressive, direct-to-consumer marketing of new psychotropic medications[19]; the development of new community programs to promote the awareness of mental disorders and provide screening and help in seeking care[20]; the expansion of primary care, managed care, and behavioral "carveout" programs of mental health services[21]; and new legislation and policies to promote access to these services.[22] Presumably, increased access played an independent role in the increase in the proportion of the population treated for emotional disorders.[23] Insurance coverage expanded throughout the decade, whereas cost sharing by consumers declined.

Third, the increase in the rate of treatment varied among the sectors of mental health services, leading to a shift in the type of treatment, most notably an increase of more than 150 percent in the rate of treatment in the sector of general medical services. Despite the hope that mental disorders might be treated more efficiently owing to this shift, the data show that many patients receiving treatment in this sector of services did not complete the clinical assessment or receive treatment or the appropriate ongoing monitoring in accordance with accepted standards of care.[18] In addition, a high proportion of patients continued to receive treatment provided in the sectors of human services and complementary–alternative medical services for which rigorous evidence of effectiveness is lacking.

Fourth, the increase in the rate of treatment was unrelated to sociodemographic variables. As a result, the increase did not reduce the sociodemographic differences shown in the baseline NCS.[24] Indeed, in absolute terms, these inequalities increased. For example, in both the NCS and the NCS-R, among non-Hispanic blacks and whites, blacks were only 50 percent as likely to receive psychiatric treatment as whites when both received a diagnosis of a disorder of the same severity, but the fact that the rate of psychiatric treatment increased by more than 100 percent suggests that this difference resulted in an absolute gap in the receipt of treatment between non-Hispanic blacks and whites that increased by more than 100 percent.

Fifth, although a small positive association was found in both surveys between the severity of the disorder and the receipt of treatment, severity did not interact with time in predicting receipt of treatment. Thus, the proportional increase in the rate of treatment was essentially the same for all levels of severity. The positive association between severity and treatment has been interpreted as evidence of rationality in the distribution of treatment resources.[24] However, the fact that in roughly half the respondents who received treatment, the mental disorder did not meet the criteria of the *DSM* for any disorder assessed in the NCS and NCS-R has led to controversy with regard to the relationship between severity and the need for treatment.[25,26] Some commentators have argued that treatment resources should be focused on serious disorders.[27] Others have argued that the treatment of mild disorders[28] and subthreshold syndromes[29] might be cost-effective and might prevent the onset of serious disorders in the future. No comparative data on cost-effectiveness are available to use in considering these contending views.

Two limitations of the study need to be noted. First, severity was assessed indirectly between 1990 and 1992 with the use of imputation, and second, the adequacy of treatment was not assessed. Both the strong relationship of imputed values to direct measures of severity in the NCS-R and the use of the multiple-imputation method to adjust for the increase in error variance when testing for significance tend to minimize concern with regard to the first limitation. The second limitation is of more concern, because research has shown that many patients with a mental disorder receive inadequate treatment.[18] We were unable to study the adequacy of treatment, however, because the information on processes of care in the NCS was insufficient for such an analysis.

Our data suggest two directions for future research and policy analysis. First, because most people with a mental disorder do not receive treatment, efforts are needed to increase access to and demand for treatment. The persistence of low rates of treatment among traditionally underserved groups calls for special initiatives.[30] The Surgeon General's report on undertreatment among racial and ethnic groups[1] and the National Institute of Mental Health initiative with regard to undertreatment among men[31] may provide useful models that should be evaluated. Programs to expand resources for treatment in targeted locations might also be of value,[32] as might initiatives such as legislation to encourage the use of mental health services by vulnerable elderly patients.[22] Efforts are also needed to evaluate widely used treatments for which there are as yet no data on effectiveness and to increase the use of evidence-based treatments. The expansion of disease-management programs, quality-assurance programs for treatment, and the use of "report cards" are important steps in this direction. Substantial barriers continue to exist, however, including competing clinical demands and distorted treatment incentives.[33,34] Initiatives aimed at overcoming these barriers are under way.[35,36] Future surveys of trends in the prevalence and treatment of mental disorders need to include data on treatment processes, such as those in the NCS-R, to permit changes in the quality of treatment to be tracked.

Supported by grants from the John D. and Catherine T. Mac-Arthur Foundation, the Pfizer Foundation, the U.S. Public Health Service (R13-MH066849, R01-MH069864, and R01 DA016558), the Fogarty International Center (FIRCA R01-TW006481), the Pan American Health Organization, Eli Lilly, Ortho-McNeil Pharmaceutical, GlaxoSmithKline, and Bristol-Myers Squibb. The National Comorbidity Survey was supported by grants from the National Institute of Mental Health (NIMH) (R01 MH46376, R01 MH49098, and R01 MH52861), with supplemental support from grants from the National Institute of Drug Abuse (NIDA) (MH46376) and the William T. Grant Foundation (90135190), and the National Comorbidity Survey Replication is supported by a grant from the NIMH (U01-MH60220), with supplemental support from grants from the NIDA, the Substance Abuse and Mental Health Services Administration, the Robert Wood Johnson Foundation (044708), and the John W. Alden Trust.

The views expressed in this article are those of the authors and do not necessarily represent the views of the sponsoring organizations, agencies, or the U.S. government.

We are indebted to the staff of the World Mental Health Data Collection and Data Analysis Coordination Centers for assistance with instrumentation, fieldwork, and consultation on the data analysis; and to Bedirhan Ustun for helpful comments on the manuscript.

APPENDIX

In addition to the authors, the following were collaborating investigators: K. Merikangas (co-principal investigator, NIMH), J. Anthony (Michigan State University), W. Eaton (Johns Hopkins University), M. Glantz (NIDA),

D. Koretz (Harvard University), J. McLeod (Indiana University), G. Simon (Group Health Cooperative Health Care System), M. Von Korff (Group Health Cooperative Health Care System), E. Wethington (Cornell University), and H.-U. Wittchen (Max Planck Institute of Psychiatry).

References

1. Department of Health and Human Services. Mental health: a report of the Surgeon General. Bethesda, Md.: National Institute of Mental Health, 1999. (Accessed May 20, 2005, at http://www.surgeongeneral.gov/library/mental-health/home.html.)
2. President's New Freedom Commission on Mental Health. Achieving the promise: transforming mental health care in America. (Accessed May 20, 2005, at http://www.mentalhealthcommission.gov/reports/ finalreport/fullreport.htm.)
3. Robins LN, Regier DA, eds. Psychiatric disorders in America: The Epidemiologic Catchment Area Study. New York: Free Press, 1991.
4. Kessler RC, McGonagle KA, Zhao S, et al. Lifetime and 12-month prevalence of DSM-III-R psychiatric disorders in the United States: results from the National Comorbidity Survey. Arch Gen Psychiatry 1994;51: 8-19.
5. Manderscheid RW, Atay JE, Hernandez-Cartagana MR, et al. Highlights of organized mental health services in 1998 and major national and state trends. In: Manderscheid RW, Henderson MJ, eds. Mental health, United States, 2000. Washington, D.C.: Government Printing Office, 2001:135-71.
6. Olfson M, Marcus SC, Druss B, Elinson L, Tanielian T, Pincus HA. National trends in the outpatient treatment of depression. JAMA 2002;287:203-9.
7. Mechanic D, Bilder S. Treatment of people with mental illness: a decade-long perspective. Health Aff (Millwood) 2004;23(4):84-95.
8. Kessler RC, Berglund P, Chiu WT, et al. The US National Comorbidity Survey Replication (NCS-R): design and field procedures. Int J Methods Psychiatr Res 2004;13:69-92.
9. Robins LN, Wing J, Wittchen HU, et al. The Composite International Diagnostic Interview: an epidemiologic instrument suitable for use in conjunction with different diagnostic systems and in different cultures. Arch Gen Psychiatry 1988;45:1069-77.
10. Kessler RC, Ustun TB. The World Mental Health (WMH) Survey Initiative version of the World Health Organization (WHO) Composite International Diagnostic Interview (CIDI). Int J Methods Psychiatr Res 2004;13:93-121.
11. Kessler RC, Berglund PA, Demler O, Jin R. Walters EE. Lifetime prevalence and age-of-onset distributions of DSM-IV disorders in the National Comorbidity Survey Replication (NCS-R). Arch Gen Psychiatry 2005;62:593-602.
12. Kessler RC, Wittchen H-U, Abelson JM, et al. Methodological studies of the Composite International Diagnostic Interview (CIDI) in the US National Comorbidity Survey. Int J Methods Psychiatr Res 1998;7:33-55.
13. Kessler RC, Chiu W-T, Demler O, Walters EE. Prevalence, severity, and comorbidity of twelve-month DSM-IV disorders in the National Comorbidity Survey Replication (NCS-R). Arch Gen Psychiatry 2005;62:617-27.
14. Endicott J, Spitzer RL, Fleiss JL, Cohen J. The Global Assessment Scale: a procedure for measuring overall severity of psychiatric disorders. Arch Gen Psychiatry 1976;33:766-71.

15. Leon AC, Olfson M, Portera L, Farber L, Sheehan DV. Assessing psychiatric impairment in primary care with the Sheehan Disability Scale. Int J Psychiatry Med 1997;27:93-105.
16. Wolter KM. Introduction to variance estimation. New York: Springer-Verlag, 1985.
17. Rubin DB. Multiple imputation for non-response in surveys. New York: John Wiley, 1987.
18. Wang PS, Berglund P, Kessler RC. Recent care of common mental disorders in the United States: prevalence and conformance with evidence-based recommendations. J Gen Intern Med 2000;15:284-92.
19. Rosenthal MB, Berndt ER, Donohue JM, Frank RG, Epstein AM. Promotion of prescription drugs to consumers. N Engl J Med 2002;346:498-505.
20. Jacobs DG. National Depression Screening Day: educating the public, reaching those in need of treatment, and broadening professional understanding. Harv Rev Psychiatry 1995;3:156-9.
21. Sturm R. Tracking changes in behavioral health services: how have carve-outs changed care? J Behav Health Serv Res 1999:26:360-71.
22. Bender E. Better access to geriatric mental health care goal of new house bill. Psychiatric News. August 16, 2002:2.
23. Frank RG, Glied S. Better but not well: US mental health policy 1950-2000. Baltimore: Johns Hopkins University Press (in press).
24. Kessler RC, Zhao S, Katz SJ, et al. Past-year use of outpatient services for psychiatric problems in the National Comorbidity Survey. Am J Psychiatry 1999:156:115-23.
25. Regier DA, Kaelber CT, Rae DS, et al. Limitations of diagnostic criteria and assessment instruments for mental disorders: implications for research and policy. Arch Gen Psychiatry 1998;55:109-15.
26. Mechanic D. Is the prevalence of mental disorders a good measure of the need for services? Health Aff (Millwood) 2003;22(5): 8-20.
27. Narrow WE, Rae DS, Robins LN, Regier DA. Revised prevalence estimates of mental disorders in the United States: using a clinical significance criterion to reconcile 2 surveys' estimates. Arch Gen Psychiatry 2002; 59:115-23.
28. Wakefield JC, Spitzer RL. Lowered estimates — but of what? Arch Gen Psychiatry 2002;59:129-30. [Erratum, Arch Gen Psychiatry 2002;59:416.]
29. Kessler RC, Merikangas KR, Berglund P, Eaton WW, Koretz DS, Walters EE. Mild disorders should not be eliminated from the DSM-V. Arch Gen Psychiatry 2003;60:1117-22.
30. Smedley BD, Stith AY, Nelson AR, eds. Unequal treatment: confronting racial and ethnic disparities in health care. Washington, D.C.: National Academy Press, 2003.
31. Real Men, Real Depression program. Bethesda, Md.: National Institute of Mental Health, 2003. (Accessed May 20, 2005, at http://menanddepression.nimh.nih.gov.)
32. Rost K, Fortney J, Fischer E, Smith J. Use, quality, and outcomes of care for mental health: the rural perspective. Med Care Res Rev 2002;59:231-65.
33. Williams JW Jr. Competing demands: does care for depression fit in primary care? J Gen Intern Med 1998:13:137-9.
34. Klinkman MS. Competing demands in psychosocial care: a model for the identification and treatment of depressive disorders in primary care. Gen Hosp Psychiatry 1997;19:98-111.

35. Pincus HA, Hough L, Houtsinger JK, Rollman BL, Frank RG. Emerging models of depression care: multi-level ('6 P') strategies. Int J Methods Psychiatr Res 2003;12:54-63.
36. Wang PS, Simon G, Kessler RC. The economic burden of depression and the cost-effectiveness of treatment. Int J Methods Psychiatr Res 2003;12:22-33.

DISCUSSION QUESTIONS

1. What might account for the high prevalence of mental disorders in the United States? Should we be concerned that over one-quarter of the population meets criteria for a mental disorder sometime in their lifetimes? Why or why not?

2. What might account for the low rates of treatment receipt among people with mental disorders? How do those rates vary over time and across sociodemographic groups? What do those variations suggest about possible explanations?

Allan V. Horwitz and Jerome C. Wakefield

The Epidemic in Mental Illness: Clinical Fact or Survey Artifact?

Detailed reports from the National Comorbidity Survey and the National Comorbidity-Survey Replication suggest that about half of the American population experiences a major mental disorder at some point in their lives. The authors of this selection, Allan V. Horwitz and Jerome C. Wakefield, challenge the validity of that claim. Their challenge relies on a detailed critique of the kinds of questions that are used to assess mental disorders in community surveys. We encourage you to read this selection together with two surrounding articles by Ronald C. Kessler and colleagues. Taken together, what do these three selections suggest about the strengths and limitations of psychiatric epidemiological studies?

Do half of all Americans suffer from mental disorders at some point in their lives? Or do surveys misdiagnose the distress that is a normal part of every life?

According to large, community-based research studies that the media report with great fanfare, alarming numbers of Americans suffer from mental disorders. The most frequently cited study, the National Comorbidity Survey, claims that half the population suffers from a mental illness at some point. Moreover, these same studies show that few people diagnosed as mentally ill seek professional treatment.

Policy discussions, scientific studies, media reports, advocacy documents, and pharmaceutical advertisements routinely cite such figures to show that mental disorder is a public health problem of vast proportions, that few sufferers receive appropriate professional treatment, that untreated disorders incur huge economic costs, and that more people need to take medication or seek psychotherapy to overcome their suffering. Awareness of large numbers of untreated, mentally ill people in the community has reshaped mental health policy, justifying efforts to address this "unmet need for treatment"— for example, by training general practitioners or public school personnel to screen for and treat mental disorders.

Despite their rhetorical value, the high rates are a fiction; the studies establish no such thing. In fact, the extraordinarily high rates of untreated mental disorder reported by community studies are largely a product of survey methodologies that inherently overstate the number of people with a mental disorder. The inflated rates stem from standard questions about symptoms with no context provided that might distinguish the normal distress experienced in life from genuinely pathological conditions that

Horwitz, Allan V. and Jerome C. Wakefield. 2006. "The Epidemic in Mental Illness: Clinical Fact or Survey Artifact?" *Contexts* 5:19–23.

indicate an underlying mental illness. Both get classified as signs of disorders. Moreover, because people experiencing normal reactions to stressful events are less likely than the truly disordered to seek medical attention, such questions are bound to inflate estimates of the rate of untreated disorders.

We use depression to illustrate such exaggeration. However, our argument applies equally well to estimates of other presumed mental illness such as sexual dysfunctions, anxiety disorders, or drug and alcohol abuse. Some history will help to frame the problem.

Origins of Symptom-based Diagnosis

All major surveys in psychiatric epidemiology, the field that assesses the patterns of mental illness in a population, attempt to translate as exactly as possible into survey questions the diagnostic criteria published in various editions of the American Psychiatric Association's *Diagnostic and Statistical Manual of Mental Disorders (DSM)*. Often called the "Bible of psychiatry" because of its authoritative status and almost universal use by clinicians, researchers, and medical insurers, the *DSM* provides official diagnostic definitions for all mental disorders.

Since its third edition, published in 1980, the *DSM* has attempted to provide precise, reliable, easily applied criteria for diagnosing each mental disorder. This approach was a response to a variety of criticisms of psychiatry common at the time, many of which hinged on the unreliability of psychiatric diagnosis. That is, different clinicians were likely to diagnose the same individual in different ways. Two problems led to this embarrassing result. First, members of different theoretical schools often conceived of and defined disorders differently, on the basis of their own theoretical concepts, whether psychodynamic, biological, or behavioral. Second, earlier definitions were generally vague and referred to fuzzily defined internal processes. To increase reliability, the third edition of the *DSM (DSM-III)* addressed both problems by stating diagnostic criteria strictly in terms of observable or reportable symptoms. Theoretical concepts were left out of diagnosis, which became "theory neutral." The new definitions used only symptoms that clinicians could precisely describe and reliably ascertain.

The *DSM-III* approach of defining disorders by presenting lists of symptoms is still used in the current edition published in 2000. For example, the definition of depressive disorder requires that five of the following nine symptoms be present during a two-week period: depressed mood, lack of pleasure or interest in usual activities, change in appetite or weight, insomnia or excessive sleep, psychomotor agitation or retardation (slowing down), fatigue or loss of energy, feeling worthless or inappropriately guilty, lack of concentration or indecisiveness, and recurrent thoughts of death, suicide, or a suicide attempt. Cases of normal bereavement after the death of a loved one are exempted from diagnosis, but only if the grief involves no severe symptoms and lasts no more than two months.

Using Standardized Questions in Community Surveys

Epidemiologists study rates and patterns of disease in order to find clues about causes and determine possible treatments. They eagerly embraced the *DSM's* symptom-based approach to diagnosis. Because researchers generally accepted the *DSM* criteria as authoritative, psychiatric epidemiologists could use them without having to do elaborate studies of their own to establish their validity. Moreover, the approach seemed to resolve a series of problems that plagued contemporary community studies of mental disorder.

Early studies in psychiatric epidemiology had simply surveyed various treatment settings and relied on the diagnoses contained in medical charts to determine rates of mental disorder. But it soon became apparent that the number of treated patients did not reliably indicate the degree of mental disorder in a community for a variety of reasons, such as lack of access to appropriate treatment, people's reluctance to seek professional help because of stigma or cost, and variations in diagnostic practices. Community studies of mental disorders try to get around these problems by attempting to determine directly how many people in the community have various mental disorders, regardless of whether they have undergone treatment. This requires interviewing many normal as well as disordered people.

In contrast to respondents in treatment studies, most of the people in community studies have never been diagnosed with mental disorders. Thus, to establish rates of disorders in the overall population, community surveys must collect thousands of cases. This poses formidable challenges. For one thing, psychiatric or other professional interviewers are expensive. For another, unless questions are carefully standardized, there is a danger of unreliability in the way the interviews are conducted. Additionally, valid analysis of qualitative data such as psychiatric interviews is extremely difficult.

The *DSM's* symptom-based diagnostic criteria offered a solution to these problems. Epidemiologists conducting community studies simply translated the *DSM's* symptoms into closed-format questions about symptoms experienced by respondents. This yielded a questionnaire that nonprofessionals could be trained to administer, allowing cost-effective collection of data from large numbers of people. Computer programs using the *DSM* criteria could determine if a disorder was present.

Accurate estimates of prevalence require that different interviewers ask these questions in exactly the same way. As one study notes, "The interviewer reads specific questions and follows positive responses with additional prescribed questions. Each step in the sequence of identifying a psychiatric symptom is fully specified and does not depend upon the judgment of the interviewers." Without such standardization, even minor variations in wording or in the interviewer's probes or instructions can lead to different results. The resulting standardized interview format excluded any discussion of the reported symptoms and their context. The rigid approach of structured interviews improves the consistency of symptom assessment across interviewers and research sites and thus the reliability of diagnostic decisions. Note, however, that the decision to use decontextualized, symptom-based measures in community studies assumes an uncritical acceptance of the *DSM's* symptom-based criteria and is based largely on considerations of practicality and cost, not on independent tests that prove the accuracy of such methods in identifying disorders in the community.

Are Survey-based Diagnoses Equivalent to Clinical Diagnoses?

The diagnoses of particular disorders in surveys, however reliable they may be, provide poor measures of mental illness in community populations. The core assumption in community studies is that tightly structured questions allow researchers to obtain diagnoses that are comparable to those of a psychiatrist, since the questions match the *DSM's* symptom criteria. This assumption rests in turn on the assumption that those criteria are valid for identifying disorders. However, those diagnosed as having mental disorders in community populations differ in two fundamental ways from those who seek mental health treatment.

First, people seeking help are highly self-selected and use all sorts of contextual information to decide for themselves if their feelings exceed ordinary and temporary responses to stressful events. David Karp, for example, found that depressed people sought help from psychiatrists only after they attributed their symptoms to internal psychological problems and not to stressful situations:

> [O]nce it becomes undeniable that something is really wrong, that one's difficulties are too extreme to be pushed aside as either temporary or reasonable, efforts begin in earnest to solve the problem. Now choices to relieve pain are made with a conscious and urgent deliberation. The shift in thinking often occurs when the presumed cause of pain is removed, but the difficulty persists. Tenure is received, you finally get out of an oppressive home environment, a destructive relationship is finally ended, and so on, but the depression persists. Such events destroy theories about the immediate situational sources of depression and force the unwelcome interpretation that the problem might be permanent and have an internallocus. One has to consider that it might be a problem of the self rather than the situation.

People who enter treatment thus have already decided that their problems go beyond normal reactions.

Second, clinicians as well as patients make contextual judgments of symptoms when they diagnose mental illness in treated populations. Psychiatrists have long recognized that symptoms such as depressed mood, loss of interest in usual activities, insomnia, loss of appetite, inability to concentrate, and so on might naturally occur in response to major losses, humiliations, or threats to one's meaning system, such as having a marriage unravel, losing one's job or pension, or failing a test that has serious implications for one's career.

Such reactions, even when quite intense, are part of normal human nature. Applying the *DSM's* symptom-based criteria literally, with no professional judgment, would result in classifying such normal reactions as disordered. Clinical diagnosis has a built-in backup system for catching such potential misdiagnoses: the clinician takes a psychiatric history in an interview that includes questions about context. The clinician is free to deviate from the literal *DSM* criteria in arriving at a diagnostic judgment and is responsible for doing so when the criteria erroneously classify a normal reaction as disordered. How often clinicians actually use this corrective option is unknown, but at least it exists in principle.

Thus, in treated populations, contextual judgments by both patients and clinicians precede clinical diagnosis. In contrast, the diagnostic process in community studies, which involves neither self-evaluation by respondents nor clinical judgment, ignores the context in which symptoms develop. Survey interviewers are forbidden to judge the validity of responses or to discuss the intent of questions, and they neither exercise clinical discretion nor use flexible probes about responses. Even if the respondent seems to misunderstand a question, the interviewer is instructed to repeat the question verbatim. The absence of interviewer probes can produce seriously misleading results for example, when asked, "Have you ever had a period of two weeks or more when you had trouble sleeping," a person might recall a time when ongoing construction across the street interrupted her sleep. In such a case, she can disregard the literal meaning of the question, self-censor her response, and not report the "symptom." Or she can give an answer that is literally true, with the result that her troubled sleep will be counted as a potential symptom of a mental illness. The lack of clinical judgment based on exploring context can easily inflate reported rates of pathological conditions.

The Prevalence of Depression

The most widely cited estimates of the prevalence of depression in the United States in the scientific, policy, and popular literatures stem from the National Comorbidity Survey (NCS) conducted in the early 1990s, with a ten-year follow-up, and from a similar study, the Epidemiologic Catchment Area (ECA) study undertaken in the early 1980s. The NCS uses two steps to obtain diagnoses of depression based on *DSM* criteria. First, respondents must answer yes to at least one of the following stem questions at the beginning of the interview: (1) "In your lifetime, have you ever had two weeks or more when nearly every day you felt sad, blue, or depressed?"; (2) "Have you ever had two weeks or more when nearly every day you felt down in the dumps, low, or gloomy?"; (3) "Have there ever been two weeks or more when you lost interest in most things like work, hobbies, or things you usually liked to do?" and (4) "Have you ever had two weeks or more during which you felt sad, blue, depressed or where you lost all interest and pleasure in things that you usually cared about or enjoyed?" Since these questions are so broad and do not allow for reference to the circumstances in which the moods arose, it is no surprise that 56 percent of the population replies yes to at least one of them. Later in the interview, these respondents are asked questions about symptoms derived from the *DSM* criteria for Major Depressive Disorder. To be diagnosed with depression, community members must report having depressed mood or inability to feel pleasure along with four additional symptoms, such as loss of appetite, difficulty sleeping, fatigue, or inability to concentrate on ordinary activities.

The NCS estimates that about 5 percent of subjects have a current (30-day) episode of major depression, about 10 percent had this condition in the past year, about 17 percent at some point in their lives, and about 24 percent report enough symptoms for a lifetime diagnosis of either depression or dysthymia, a related disorder. It also finds that relatively few people diagnosed with these conditions have sought professional help: only about a third of those with survey-identified Major Depressive Disorders had sought professional treatment, and far fewer sought any kind of help from mental health professionals.

Are the many cases of Major Depressive Disorder uncovered in such community studies equivalent to treated clinical cases? In contrast to clinical settings, where the judgments of both lay persons and clinicians distinguish ordinary sadness from depressive disorders, symptom-based diagnoses in community studies consider everyone who reports enough symptoms as having the mental disorder of depression. A respondent might recall symptoms such as depressed mood or insomnia that lasted longer than two weeks after the breakup of a romantic relationship, during a loved one's serious illness, or the unexpected loss of a job. Although these symptoms might have dissipated as soon as a new relationship developed, the loved one recovered, or another job was found, this person would be counted among the many millions who suffer from the presumed disorder of depression each year. For example, in the ECA study the most commonly reported symptoms are "trouble falling asleep, staying asleep, or waking up early" (33.7 percent); being "tired out all the time" (22.8 percent); and "thought a lot about death" (22.6 percent). College students during exam periods, people who must work overtime, who are worried about an important upcoming event, or who take the survey soon after the death of a famous person would all naturally experience such symptoms.

Symptoms that neither respondents nor clinicians would see as requiring treatment may nevertheless qualify as signs of disorder in community surveys. Moreover, the duration criteria only require that the symptom last for a two-week period, so that many transient and self-correcting symptoms are counted as disordered. In other cases, reported symptoms could be normal responses to long-standing conditions of poverty, oppression, or injustice. Diagnostically oriented community studies, rather than uncovering high rates of depressive disorders, simply show that the natural results of acute or chronic stressful experiences could be distressing enough to fit the *DSM* definition of a disorder.

Why Are the High Rates Perpetuated?

The exaggerated rates of mental disorder in community surveys do not mean that untreated psychiatric disorders are not a significant problem. Nor do they mean that people who experience normal distress may not sometimes benefit from drugs or psychological treatments. It does, however, contribute to a pervasive medicalization of many problems that we might view more constructively as expectable results of social circumstances.

Community surveys could more adequately separate normal responses to stressful situations from mental disorders by including questions about the context in which symptoms develop and persist. Interviewers could ask, for example, if symptoms of depression emerged during periods of intense stress and disappeared as soon as these crises were over. Clinical interviews often include such probes, which are also compatible with basic principles of survey methodology; psychiatrists have always recognized the need for such considerations. The decision not to include contextual criteria in community surveys may involve not only the efficiency and practicality of decontextualized, standardized methods but also resistance to change by groups that benefit from the reported high rates of mental illnesses.

During the 1960s the National Institute of Mental Health (NIMH) promoted an expansive agenda of community mental health and sponsored projects that attempted to alleviate poverty, combat juvenile delinquency, and promote social change, but political changes in the 1970s forced the NIMH to change its focus from social and economic problems to specific diseases. This was more politically palatable than addressing controversial social problems. In addition, the rise of the biological paradigm in psychiatry naturally shifted emphasis from the social circumstances that can produce mental illness toward internal sources. The NIMH funded the epidemiological studies in the 1980s and 1990s in an effort to show that presumed disease conditions were widespread yet untreated. The resulting belief in high prevalence rates, which became the focus of well-known and widely disseminated documents such as the Surgeon General's Report on Mental Health, insulated the agency from political pressures, expanded its mandate, enhanced the importance of the problem it addressed, and protected its budget. Political support is more likely for an agency devoted to preventing and curing widespread disease than for one that confronts controversial social problems.

Pharmaceutical companies have also capitalized on these survey findings, which create a broader market for their products. Their ads focus on symptoms such as sadness, loneliness, exhaustion, and anxiety that are common among normal people. These ads also routinely feature the alleged numbers of people who suffer from particular mental disorders, sending the message that potential consumers are not unique but share their problems with millions of others. The explosive growth in sales of antidepressants shows the effectiveness of this appeal.

Family advocacy groups such as the National Alliance for the Mentally Ill embrace claims about the prevalence of mental disorders, which allow them to equate the millions of people that community surveys identify with the far smaller number of people with truly serious mental disorders. This presumably reduces the social distance between the mentally disordered and others, and lowers the stigma of mental illness, potentially aiding efforts to obtain more funding for treatment.

These groups promote high prevalence rates in the belief that if they can convince politicians that mental illnesses are widespread, they can gain more funding for mental health services. But their efforts to get more treatment for currently untreated cases are just as likely to shift resources from people who truly need professional mental health services to those who might be distressed but are not disordered. Moreover, such high rates may make the problem of mental illness seem so overwhelming and potentially costly that it will not be addressed. Erasing the distinction between normal and disordered conditions and calling both mental disorders may harm the truly disabled.

DISCUSSION QUESTIONS

1. According to Horwitz and Wakefield, why do community surveys overestimate rates of mental disorders? What changes do they suggest to how those surveys are conducted?
2. What problems do Horwitz and Wakefield identify with overestimates of rates of mental disorders? Who stands to gain and lose from high reported rates?

Current Cross-National Prevalence Estimates

Ronald C. Kessler, Matthias Angermeyer, James C. Anthony, Ron de Graaf, Koen Demyttenaere, Isabelle Gasquet, Giovanni de Girolamo, Semyon Gluzman, Oye Gureje, Josep Maria Haro, Norito Kawakami, Aimee Karam, Daphna Levinson, Maria Elena Medina Mora, Mark A. Oakley Browne, José Posada-Villa, Dan J. Stein, Cheuk Him Adley Tsang, Sergio Aguilar-Gaxiola, Jordi Alonso, Sing Lee, Steven Heeringa, Beth-Ellen Pennell, Patricia Berglund, Michael J. Gruber, Maria Petukhova, Somnath Chatterji, T. Bedirhan Üstün for the WHO World Mental Health Survey Consortium

Lifetime Prevalence and Age-of-Onset Distributions of Mental Disorders in the World Health Organization's World Mental Health Survey Initiative

The selection that follows describes the most comprehensive, worldwide assessment of mental disorders to date. The authors present estimates of the lifetime prevalence and the lifetime risk of mental disorders in many different countries. This research

Kessler, Ronald C., Matthias Angermeyer, James C. Anthony, Ron De Graaf, Koen Demyttenaere, Isabelle Gasquet, Giovanni De Girolamo, Semyon Gluzman, Oye Gureje, Josep Maria Haro, Norito Kawakami, Aimee Karam, Daphna Levinson, Maria Elena Medina Mora, Mark A. Oakley Browne, José Posada-Villa, Dan J. Stein, Cheuk Him Adley Tsang, Sergio Aguilar-Gaxiola, Jordi Alonso, Sing Lee, Steven Heeringa, Beth-Ellen Pennell, Patricia Berglund, Michael J. Gruber, Maria Petukhova, Somnath Chatterji, T. Bedirhan Üstün, for the WHO World Mental Health Survey Consortium. 2007. "Lifetime Prevalence and Age-of-Onset Distributions of Mental Disorders in the World Health Organizations' World Mental Health Survey Initiative." *World Psychiatry* 6:168–176.

builds on the previous selections you have read while also raising questions about the comparability of psychiatric diagnoses and mental health assessments in different cultures.

Although psychiatric epidemiological surveys have been carried out since after World War II (1), absence of a common format for diagnosis hampered cross-national syntheses. This situation changed in the early 1980s, with the development of fully structured research diagnostic interviews (2) and the implementation of large-scale psychiatric epidemiological surveys in many countries (3–5). The World Health Organization (WHO) developed a diagnostic instrument, the WHO Composite International Diagnostic Interview (CIDI) (6,7), based on extensive cross-national field trials, for use in cross-national epidemiological surveys (8–14). In 1998, the WHO created the WHO International Consortium in Psychiatric Epidemiology (ICPE) to coordinate comparative analyses of these surveys. The ICPE launched the WHO World Mental Health (WMH) Survey Initiative shortly thereafter to conduct coordinated CIDI surveys in all parts of the world. The current report presents the first cross-national results regarding age of onset, lifetime prevalence, and projected lifetime risk of mental disorders from the 17 WMH surveys so far completed.

Data of this sort are sorely needed by policy planners to assess the societal burden of mental disorders, unmet need for treatment, and barriers to treatment. These data are especially important given evidence from the WHO Global Burden of Disease Study that mental disorders impose enormous burdens worldwide, due to their combination of high prevalence and high disability (15), and evidence that, despite efficacious treatments, substantial unmet need for treatment exists throughout the world (16). While earlier studies found high lifetime prevalence and generally early age-of-onset distributions of mental disorders, they did not make systematic disorder-specific age-of-onset comparisons. The latter are important for targeting early interventions, which are coming to be seen as critical for an effective public health response to mental disorders (17–19). Previous studies also focused on lifetime prevalence (the proportion of the population with a lifetime disorder up to age at interview) rather than projected lifetime risk (the estimated proportion of the population who will have the disorder by the end of their life), even though the latter is more important for policy planning purposes. We consider both prevalence and risk in this report.

METHODS

Samples

WMH surveys were administered in Africa (Nigeria, South Africa); the Americas (Colombia, Mexico, United States), Asia and the Pacific (Japan, New Zealand, Beijing and Shanghai in the People's Republic of China, henceforth referred to as Metropolitan PRC), Europe (Belgium, France, Germany, Italy, the Netherlands, Spain, Ukraine) (20); and the Middle East (Israel, Lebanon). Seven of these countries are classified by the World Bank as less developed (China, Colombia, Lebanon, Mexico, Nigeria, South Africa, Ukraine), while the others are classified as developed (21).

Most WMH surveys were based on stratified multistage clustered area probability household samples. Samples of areas equivalent to counties or municipalities in the United States were selected in the first stage, followed by one or more subsequent stages of geographic sampling (e.g., towns within counties, blocks within towns, households within blocks) to arrive at a sample of households. In each of them, a listing of household members was created and one or two people were selected to be interviewed. No substitution was allowed when the originally sampled household resident could not be interviewed. The household samples were selected from census area data in all countries other than France (where telephone directories were used) and the Netherlands (where postal registries were used). Several WMH surveys (Belgium, Germany, Italy) used municipal resident registries to select respondents without listing households. The Japanese sample is the only totally unclustered sample, with households randomly selected in each of the four sample areas and one random respondent selected in each sample household. Nine of the 17 surveys were based on nationally representative household samples, while 2 others were based on nationally representative household samples in urbanized areas (Colombia, Mexico).

All surveys were conducted face-to-face by trained lay interviewers in multi-stage household probability samples, with 85,052 respondents. Country-level samples ranged from 2,372 (Netherlands) to 12,992 (New Zealand). The weighted average cross-national response rate was 71.1 percent, with a 45.9–87.7 percent range (Table 1).

The Part I interview schedule, completed by all respondents, assessed core diagnoses. All respondents who met criteria for any diagnosis plus a probability sub-sample of other Part I respondents were administered Part II, which assessed disorders of secondary interest and a wide range of correlates. Part I data were weighted to adjust for differential probabilities of selection and to match population distributions on socio-demographic and geographic data. The Part II sample was additionally weighted for the oversampling of Part I respondents with core disorders. The interview schedule and other study materials were translated using standardized WHO translation and back-translation protocols. Consistent interviewer training procedures and quality control monitoring were used in all surveys (22,23). Informed consent was obtained in all countries using procedures approved by local Institutional Review Boards.

Measures

Diagnoses were based on CIDI Version 3.0 (24), which generates both ICD-10 (25) and *DSM-IV* (26) diagnoses. *DSM-IV* criteria are used here to facilitate comparison with previous epidemiological surveys. Core diagnoses included anxiety disorders (panic disorder, agoraphobia without panic disorder, specific phobia, social phobia, generalized anxiety disorder, post-traumatic stress disorder, and separation anxiety disorder), mood disorders (major depressive disorder, dysthymic disorder, bipolar disorder I or II or subthreshold bipolar disorder), impulse control disorders (intermittent explosive disorder, oppositional-defiant disorder, conduct disorder, attention-deficit/hyperactivity disorder), and substance use disorders (alcohol and drug abuse with or without dependence). Not all disorders were assessed in all countries. The Western European countries did not assess bipolar disorders and drug dependence. Only three countries (Colombia, Mexico, United States) assessed all impulse control disorders.

The disorders that require childhood onset (oppositional defiant disorder, conduct disorder, and attention-deficit/hyperactivity disorder) were included in Part II and limited to respondents in the age range 18–39/44, because of concerns about recall bias among older respondents. All other disorders were assessed for the full sample age range. Organic exclusion rules and hierarchy rules were used to make all diagnoses other than substance use disorders, which were diagnosed without hierarchy, because abuse often is a stage in the progression to dependence. Clinical calibration studies (27) found CIDI to assess these disorders with generally good validity in comparison to blinded clinical reappraisal interviews using the Structured Clinical Interview for *DSM-IV* (SCID) (28). CIDI prevalence estimates were not higher than SCID prevalence estimates. Retrospective age-of-onset reports were based on a question series designed to avoid the implausible response patterns obtained in using the standard CIDI age-of-onset question (29). Experimental research has shown that this question sequence yields responses with a much more plausible age-of-onset distribution than the standard CIDI age-of-onset question (30). Predictor variables included cohort (defined by ages at interview 18–34, 35–49, 50–64, 65+), sex, and education (students versus non-students with low, low-average, average-high, and high education categories based on country-specific distributions). Education was coded as a time-varying predictor by assuming an orderly educational history.

Analysis Procedures

Age of onset and projected lifetime risk as of age 75 were estimated using the two-part actuarial method implemented in SAS 8.2 (31). Predictors were examined using discrete-time survival analysis with person-year as the unit of analysis (32). Standard errors were estimated using the Taylor series linearization method (33) implemented in the SUDAAN software system (34). Multivariate significance tests were made with Wald χ^2 tests, using Taylor series design-based coefficient variance-covariance matrices. Standard errors of lifetime risk were estimated using the jackknife repeated replication method (35) implemented in a SAS macro (31). Significance tests were all evaluated at the .05 level with two-sided tests.

Table 1 Sample Characteristics of the World Mental Health Surveys

Country	Survey	Field dates	Age range	Sample size Part I	Sample size Part II	Sample size Part II and age ≤44[a]	Response rate
Belgium	ESEMeD	2001–2	18+	2419	1043	486	50.6
Colombia	NSMH	2003	18–65	4426	2381	1731	87.7
France	ESEMeD	2001–2	18+	2894	1436	727	45.9
Germany	ESEMeD	2002–3	18+	3555	1323	621	57.8
Israel	NHS	2002–4	21+	4859	—	—	72.6
Italy	ESEMeD	2001–2	18+	4712	1779	853	71.3
Japan	WMHJ 2002–2003	2002–3	20+	2436	887	282	56.4
Lebanon	LEBANON	2002–3	18+	2857	1031	595	70.0
Mexico	M-NCS	2001–2	18–65	5782	2362	1736	76.6
Netherlands	ESEMeD	2002–3	18+	2372	1094	516	56.4
New Zealand	NZMHS	2004–5	16+	12992	7435	4242	73.3
Nigeria	NSMHW	2002–3	18+	6752	2143	1203	79.3
People's Republic of China	B-WMH S-WMH	2002–3	18+	5201	1628	570	74.7
South Africa	SASH	2003–4	18+	4315	—	—	87.1
Spain	ESEMeD	2001–2	18+	5473	2121	960	78.6
Ukraine	CMDPSD	2002	18+	4725	1720	541	78.3
United States	NCS-R	2002–3	18+	9282	5692	3197	70.9

ESEMeD—European Study of the Epidemiology of Mental Disorders; NSMH—Colombian National Study of Mental Health; NHS—Israel National Health Survey; WMHJ 2002–2003—World Mental Health Japan Survey; LEBANON—Lebanese Evaluation of the Burden of Ailments and Needs of the Nation; M-NCS—Mexico National Comorbidity Survey; NZMHS—New Zealand Mental Health Survey; NSMHW—Nigerian Survey of Mental Health and Wellbeing; B-WMH—Beijing World Mental Health Survey; S-WMH—Shanghai World Mental Health Survey; SASH—South Africa Health Survey; CMDPSD—Comorbid Mental Disorders during Periods of Social Disruption; NCS-R—U.S. National Comorbidity Survey Replication.

The response rate is calculated as the ratio of the number of households in which an interview was completed to the number of households originally sampled, excluding from the denominator households known not to be eligible either because of being vacant at the time of initial contact or because the residents were unable to speak the designated languages of the survey

[a]All countries were age restricted to ≤44, with the exception of Nigeria, People's Republic of China, and Ukraine, which were age restricted to ≤39

RESULTS

Lifetime Prevalence

The estimated lifetime prevalence of having one or more of the disorders considered here varies widely across the WMH surveys, from 47.4 percent in the United States to 12.0 percent in Nigeria. The inter-quartile range (IQR; 25th–75th percentiles across countries) is 18.1–36.1 percent. Symptoms consistent with the existence of one or more lifetime mental disorders were reported by more than one-third of respondents in five countries (Colombia, France, New Zealand, Ukraine, United States), more than one-fourth in six (Belgium, Germany, Lebanon, Mexico, The Netherlands, South Africa), and more than one-sixth in four (Israel, Italy, Japan, Spain). The remaining two countries, Metropolitan PRC (13.2 percent) and Nigeria (12.0 percent), had considerably lower prevalence estimates, which are likely to be downwardly biased (36,37). Prevalence estimates for other developing countries were all above the lower bound of the inter-quartile range (Table 2).

All four classes of disorder were important components of overall prevalence. Anxiety disorders were the most prevalent in ten countries (4.8–31.0 percent, IQR 9.9–16.7 percent) and mood disorders in all but one other country (3.3–21.4 percent, IQR 9.8–15.8 percent). Impulse control disorders were the least prevalent in most countries that included a relatively full assessment of these disorders (0.3–25.0 percent, IQR 3.1–5.7 percent). Substance use disorders were generally the least prevalent elsewhere (1.3–15.0 percent, IQR 4.8–9.6 percent). The Western European countries did not assess illicit drug abuse-dependence, though, leading to artificially low prevalence estimates (1.3–8.9 percent) compared to other countries (2.2–15.0 percent). Substance dependence was also assessed only in the presence of abuse, possibly further reducing estimated prevalence (38). Lifetime disorder co-occurrence was quite common, as seen by noting that the sum of prevalence across the four disorder types was generally between 30 percent and 50 percent higher than the prevalence of any disorder. Within-class co-occurrence cannot be seen in the reported results, but is even stronger than between-class co-occurrence (results available on request).

Age-of-onset Distributions

Despite the wide cross-national variation in estimated lifetime prevalence, considerable cross-national consistency exists in standardized age-of-onset distributions (detailed results are not reported here, but are available on request).

Impulse control disorders have the earliest age-of-onset distributions, both in terms of early median ages of onset (7–9 years of age for attention deficit hyperactivity disorder, 7–15 for oppositional-defiant disorder, 9–14 for conduct disorder, and 13–21 for intermittent explosive disorder) and an extremely narrow age range of onset risk, with 80 percent of all lifetime attention-deficit/hyperactivity disorder beginning in the age range 4–11 and the vast majority of oppositional-defiant disorder and conduct disorder beginning between ages 5 and 15. Although the age-of-onset distribution is less concentrated for intermittent explosive disorder, fully half of all lifetime cases have onsets in childhood and adolescence.

The situation is more complex with anxiety disorders, as the age-of-onset distributions fall into two distinct sets. The phobias and separation anxiety disorder all have very early ages of onset (medians in the range 7–14, IQR 8–11). Generalized anxiety disorder, panic disorder, and posttraumatic

Table 2 Lifetime Prevalence and Projected Lifetime Risk as of Age 75 of *DSM-IV* Disorders

| | Any Anxiety Disorder | | | | | Any Mood isorder | | | | |
| | Prevalence | | | Projected lifetime risk | | Prevalence | | | Projected lifetime risk | |
Country	%	N[a]	SE	%	SE	%	N[a]	SE	%	SE
Belgium	13.1	219	1.9	15.7	2.5	14.1	367	1.0	22.8	1.7
Colombia	25.3	948	1.4	30.9	2.5	14.6	666	0.7	27.2	2.0
France	22.3	445	1.4	26.0	1.6	21.0	648	1.1	30.5	1.4
Germany	14.6	314	1.5	16.9	1.7	9.9	372	0.6	16.2	1.3
Israel	5.2	252	0.3	10.1	0.9	10.7	524	0.5	21.2	1.6
Italy	11.0	328	0.9	13.7	1.2	9.9	452	0.5	17.3	1.2
Japan	6.9	155	0.6	9.2	1.2	7.6	183	0.5	14.1	1.7
Lebanon	16.7	282	1.6	20.2	1.8	12.6	352	0.9	20.1	1.2
Mexico	14.3	684	0.9	17.8	1.6	9.2	598	0.5	20.4	1.7
Netherlands	15.9	320	1.1	21.4	1.8	17.9	476	1.0	28.9	1.9
New Zealand	24.6	3171	0.7	30.3	1.5	20.4	2755	0.5	29.8	0.7
Nigeria	6.5	169	0.9	7.1	0.9	3.3	236	0.3	8.9	1.2
PR China	4.8	159	0.7	6.0	0.8	3.6	185	0.4	7.3	0.9
South Africa	15.8	695	0.8	30.1	4.4	9.8	439	0.7	20.0	2.4
Spain	9.9	375	1.1	13.3	1.4	10.6	672	0.5	20.8	1.2
Ukraine	10.9	371	0.8	17.3	2.0	15.8	814	0.8	25.9	1.5
United States	31.0	2692	1.0	36.0	1.4	21.4	2024	0.6	31.4	0.9

[a]The numbers reported here are the numbers of respondents with the disorders indicated in the column heading. The denominators used to calculate prevalence estimates based on these numbers of cases are reported in Table 1. In the case of anxiety disorders and substance use disorders, the denominators are the numbers of respondents in the Part II sample. In the case of mood disorders, the denominators are the numbers of respondents in the Part I sample. In the case of impulse control disorders and any disorders, the denominators are the numbers of respondents aged ≤44 in the Part II sample

stress disorder, in comparison, have much later age-of-onset distributions (median 24–50, IQR 31–41), with much wider cross-national variation than for the impulse control disorders or the phobias or separation anxiety disorder.

The age-of-onset distributions for mood disorders are similar to those for generalized anxiety disorder, panic disorder, and posttraumatic stress disorder. Prevalence is consistently low until the early teens, at which time a roughly linear increase begins that continues through late middle age, with a more gradual increase thereafter. The median age of onset of mood disorders ranges between the late 20s and the early 40s (29–43, IQR 35–40).

The age-of-onset distribution of substance use disorders is consistent across countries, in that few onsets occur prior to the mid-teens and cumulative increase in onset is rapid in adolescence and early adulthood. Considerable cross-national variation exists, though, in the sharpness of the change in the slope as well as in the age range of this change. This cross-national variation leads to wider cross-national variation in both the median and the inter-

Any impulse control disorder					Any substance use disorder					Any disorder				
Prevalence			Projected lifetime risk		Prevalence			Projected lifetime risk		Prevalence			Projected lifetime risk	
%	Nᵃ	SE	%	SE	%	Nᵃ	SE	%	SE	%	Nᵃ	SE	%	SE
5.2	31	1.4	5.2	1.4	8.3	195	0.9	10.5	1.1	29.1	519	2.3	37.1	3.0
9.6	273	0.8	10.3	0.9	9.6	345	0.6	12.8	1.0	39.1	1432	1.3	55.2	6.0
7.6	71	1.3	7.6	1.3	7.1	202	0.5	8.8	0.6	37.9	847	1.7	47.2	1.6
3.1	31	0.8	3.1	0.8	6.5	228	0.6	8.7	0.9	25.2	573	1.9	33.0	2.5
_b	—	—	—	—	5.3	261	0.3	6.3	0.4	17.6	860	0.6	29.7	1.5
1.7	27	0.4	_c	—	1.3	56	0.2	1.6	0.3	18.1	612	1.1	26.0	1.9
2.8	11	1.0	_c	—	4.8	69	0.5	6.2	0.7	18.0	343	1.1	24.4	1.8
4.4	53	0.9	4.6	1.0	2.2	27	0.8	—	_c	25.8	491	1.9	32.9	2.1
5.7	152	0.6	5.7	0.6	7.8	378	0.5	11.9	1.0	26.1	1148	1.4	36.4	2.1
4.7	37	1.1	4.8	1.1	8.9	210	0.9	11.4	1.2	31.7	633	2.0	42.9	2.5
_b	—	—	—	—	12.4	1767	0.4	14.6	0.5	39.3	4815	0.9	48.6	1.5
0.3	9	0.1	_c	—	3.7	119	0.4	6.4	1.0	12.0	440	1.0	19.5	1.9
4.3	37	0.9	4.9	0.9	4.9	128	0.7	6.1	0.8	13.2	419	1.3	18.0	1.5
_b	—	—	—	—	13.3	505	0.9	17.5	1.2	30.3	1290	1.1	47.5	3.7
2.3	40	0.8	2.3	0.8	3.6	180	0.4	4.6	0.5	19.4	842	1.4	29.0	1.8
8.7	91	1.1	9.7	1.3	15.0	293	1.3	18.8	1.7	36.1	1074	1.5	48.9	2.5
25.0	1051	1.1	25.6	1.1	14.6	1144	0.6	17.4	0.6	47.4	3929	1.1	55.3	1.2

ᵇImpulse control disorders not assessed
ᶜCell size was too small to be included in analysis
ᵈProjected lifetime risk to age 65 due to the sample including only respondents up to age 65

quartile range of the age-of-onset distributions than for impulse control disorders or phobias or separation anxiety disorder, but lower variation than for mood disorders or other anxiety disorders.

Projected Lifetime Risk

Projected lifetime risk of any disorder as of age 75 is between 17 percent (United States) and 69 percent (Israel) higher than estimated lifetime prevalence (IQR 28–44 percent) (Table 2). The highest risk-to-prevalence ratios (57–69 percent) are in countries exposed to sectarian violence (Israel, Nigeria, and South Africa). Excluding these three, there is no strong difference in ratios of less developed (28–41 percent) versus developed (17–49 percent) countries. The highest class-specific proportional increase in projected risk is for mood disorders (45–170 percent, IQR 61–98 percent) and the lowest for impulse control disorders (0–14 percent, IQR 0–2 percent), consistent with the former having the latest and the latter having the earliest age-of-onset distribution. The projected lifetime risk estimates suggest that approximately half the population (47–55 percent) will eventually have a mental disorder in six countries (Colombia, France, New Zealand, South Africa, Ukraine, United States), approximately one-third (30–43 percent) in six other countries (Belgium, Germany, Israel, Lebanon, Mexico, the Netherlands), approximately one-fourth (24–29 percent) in three others (Italy, Japan, Spain), and approximately one-fifth (18–19 percent) in the remaining countries (Metropolitan PRC, Nigeria).

Cohort Effects

Previous research has suggested that projected lifetime risk might be increasing in recent cohorts (39). Prospective tracking studies are required to monitor cohort effects directly. However, indirect approximations can be obtained in cross-sectional data using retrospective age-of-onset reports. This was done in the WMH data using discrete-time survival analysis to predict onset of disorders across age groups 18–34, 35–49, 50–64, and 65+. As these surveys were completed between 2002 and 2005, the most recent cohorts (aged 18–34 at interview) roughly correspond to those born in the years from 1968+. Respondents aged 35–49 at interview correspond roughly to cohorts born in 1953–1970, while those aged 50–64 were born in 1938–1955, and those aged 65+ were born before 1938. Survival analysis finds that the odds ratios for anxiety, mood, and substance use disorders are generally higher in recent compared to older cohorts, while not for impulse control disorders (Tables 3–5). No meaningful difference exists between less developed and developed countries, although cross-national variation exceeds chance expectations.

DISCUSSION

Three possible biases could have led to under-estimating prevalence. First, people with mental illness have been found to be less likely than others to participate in surveys, because of sample frame exclusions (e.g., excluding homeless people), differential mortality, or greater reluctance to participate (40). Variation in the magnitude of such under-representation across countries could help account for the wide between-country variation in prevalence-risk estimates. Second, previous research suggests that lifetime prevalence is sometimes under-reported because of respondent reluctance to admit mental illness (41). This bias might be especially strong in less developed countries with no strong tradition of independent public opinion research, which could help account for the especially low prevalence-risk estimates in Nigeria and Metropolitan PRC. Third, interviewer error might have led to under-reporting, especially in countries where there was an indirect incentive to rush through interviews, because interviewers were paid by the interview rather than by the hour. The most plausible bias that could have led to over-estimating prevalence, in comparison, is that the interview thresholds for defining disorders might have been too liberal. However, as noted in the section on measures, clinical reappraisal studies carried out in some of the countries with the highest prevalence estimates found no evidence of such bias (27).

Two possible biases of other sorts are also noteworthy. First, the method used to estimate lifetime risk was based on the assumption of constant conditional risk of first onset in a given year of life across cohorts. The existence of an apparent cohort effect means that this assumption is incorrect, probably causing an under-estimation of lifetime risk in younger cohorts. Second, age of onset might have been recalled with error related to age at interview, which could produce the data pattern found here as indirect evidence for a cohort effect (42). Evidence for age-related bias has been documented in previous epidemiological research (29), although the novel probing strategy used in the WMH surveys has been shown to minimize this problem (30).

Based on these considerations, the wide cross-national variation in WMH prevalence and risk estimates should be interpreted with caution, because it is likely over-estimated due to between-country differences in some of the biases enumerated above. The overall prevalence-risk estimates, which are consistent with previous cross-national research (8–14, 39), are likely to be conservative, as the most plausible biases lead to underestimation. The evidence for cohort effects is more difficult to judge, as both substantive and methodological interpretations are plausible. The options are either that the prevalence of mental disorders is on the rise or that prevalence is stable but under-estimated among older respondents.

Given the high prevalence-risk estimates even with the possibility of conservative bias, a question can be raised about the meaningfulness of these estimates. Our clinical reappraisal studies, consistent with comparable studies carried out in conjunction with previous community psychiatric epidemiological surveys (43), show that the high prevalence estimates are genuine (i.e., consistent with expert clinician judgments) rather than due to CIDI errors. It is important to recognize, though, that not all mental disorders are severe. WMH measures of disorder severity were applied only to 12-month cases, so we have no way to estimate severity of lifetime cases. Analysis of 12-month cases, though, finds the majority rated mild on a clinical rating scale with categories mild, moderate, and severe (22). These cases are nonetheless meaningful, because even mild cases can be impairing and often evolve into more serious disorders over time (44).

The age-of-onset distributions reported here are consistent with those in previous epidemiological surveys (39,45). Given the enormous personal and societal burdens of mental disorders, the finding that many cases have early ages of onset suggests that public health interventions might profitably begin in childhood. Importantly, studies of initial contact with the treatment system (46–48) show that people with these early-onset disorders often wait more than a decade before seeking treatment, and present with seriously impairing disorders that might have been easier to treat if they had sought treatment earlier in the course of illness. Interventions aimed at

Table 3 Inter-Cohort Differences in Lifetime Risk of Any *DSM-IV* Anxiety Disorder[a]

Country	18–34			35–49			50–64			65+[b]			χ^2	df	N
	OR	95% CI	N	OR	95% CI	N	OR	95% CI	N	OR	95% CI	N			
Belgium	2.6*	1.3–5.0	254	1.6	0.8–3.2	331	1.3	0.6–2.6	278	1.0	—	180	14.2*	3	1043
Colombia	1.6*	1.2–2.1	1125	1.3	0.9–1.8	818	1.0	—	438	—	—	—	10.0*	2	2381
France	3.1*	1.5–6.4	388	3.2*	1.5–6.7	472	1.6	0.8–3.3	362	1.0	—	214	21.3*	3	1436
Germany	3.1*	1.9–5.1	316	2.3*	1.4–3.9	436	2.3*	1.3–4.1	345	1.0	—	226	21.8*	3	1323
Israel	4.7*	2.6–8.3	1627	2.7	1.6–4.4	1302	2.1*	1.4–3.3	1069	1.0	—	861	27.3*	3	4859
Italy	1.5	0.7–3.0	496	1.6	0.9–2.8	516	1.3	0.8–2.2	454	1.0	—	313	3.3	3	1779
Japan	5.6*	2.2–13.8	155	2.8*	1.3–6.1	219	2.6*	1.2–5.6	295	1.0	—	218	14.9*	3	887
Lebanon	3.2*	1.6–6.2	349	2.5*	1.2–5.1	348	1.0	0.5–2.1	199	1.0	—	135	24.1*	3	1031
Mexico	2.4*	1.6–3.4	1183	1.6*	1.1–2.4	750	1.0	—	429	—	—	—	25.3*	2	2362
Netherlands	3.6*	2.1–6.1	264	4.5*	3.0–6.8	358	3.0*	2.0–4.6	302	1.0	—	170	60.6*	3	1094
New Zealand	3.4*	2.7–4.2	2394	2.6*	2.1–3.1	2474	2.1*	1.7–2.7	1517	1.0	—	927	126.3*	3	7312
Nigeria	3.1*	1.4–6.9	971	2.3*	1.1–4.9	549	2.8*	1.5–5.4	369	1.0	—	254	11.1*	3	2143
PR China	1.7	0.6–4.4	379	1.1	0.5–2.5	726	1.6	0.7–3.9	357	1.0	—	166	3.3	3	1628
South Africa	2.3*	1.3–4.0	2172	1.8*	1.1–3.1	1264	1.3	0.8–2.1	638	1.0	—	241	16.5*	3	4315
Spain	3.8*	2.2–6.5	545	2.8*	1.5–5.2	556	1.3	0.8–2.2	456	1.0	—	564	28.7	3	2121
Ukraine	1.7*	1.1–2.6	420	1.0	0.6–1.6	434	1.0	0.7–1.6	412	1.0	—	454	6.5	3	1720
United States	3.5*	2.8–4.4	1939	3.4*	2.7–4.1	1831	2.5*	2.0–3.0	1213	1.0	—	709	159.2*	3	5692

[a]Based on discrete-time survival models with person-year as the unit of analysis, controls are time intervals.
[b]Referent category.
*Significant at the .05 level, two-sided test.

Table 4 Inter-Cohort Differences in Lifetime Risk of Any *DSM-IV* Mood Disorder[a]

Country	18–34			35–49			50–64			65+[b]			χ^2	df	N
	OR	95% CI	N	OR	95% CI	N	OR	95% CI	N	OR	95% CI	N			
Belgium	11.3*	6.1–20.9	573	4.9*	3.2–7.5	775	3.6*	2.0–6.4	570	1.0	—	501	87.3*	3	2419
Colombia	6.3*	4.2–9.3	2000	2.3*	1.6–3.1	1577	1.0	—	849	—	—	530	92.7	2	4426
France	9.0*	6.0–13.5	743	3.0*	2.2–4.2	942	1.8*	1.2–2.6	719	1.0	—	490	146.4*	3	2894
Germany	12.2*	7.1–21.0	815	5.2*	3.5–7.7	1180	2.4*	1.6–3.4	893	1.0	—	667	94.4*	3	3555
Israel	6.5*	4.5–9.4	1627	2.8*	2.0–4.0	1302	1.8*	1.3–2.5	1069	1.0	—	861	118.4*	3	4859
Italy	5.7	3.8–8.4	1326	3.6*	2.6–5.0	1393	2.3*	1.6–3.3	1153	1.0	—	840	91.3*	3	4712
Japan	23.7*	13.4–42.0	410	7.7*	4.5–13.2	571	3.8*	2.4–5.8	764	1.0	—	691	146.2*	3	2436
Lebanon	6.2*	3.0–12.8	965	3.1*	1.4–6.7	931	1.7	0.8–3.2	553	1.0	—	408	60.5*	3	2857
Mexico	4.0*	2.6–6.1	2871	1.6*	1.1–2.3	1888	1.0	—	1023	—	—	646	65.0*	2	5782
Netherlands	11.7	6.6–20.8	564	6.4*	4.0–10.2	729	2.9*	1.7–4.8	627	1.0	—	452	115.7	3	2372
New Zealand	10.0*	8.2–12.2	3747	5.0*	4.1–6.0	4102	2.9*	2.4–3.6	2697	1.0	—	2244	653.9*	3	12790
Nigeria	3.7	1.8–7.6	3175	1.8	0.9–3.6	1631	1.2	0.7–2.1	1104	1.0	—	842	19.4*	3	6752
PR China	20.8*	9.4–45.8	1209	4.4*	2.3–8.4	2261	2.5*	1.4–4.4	1184	1.0	—	547	76.5*	3	5201
South Africa	9.6*	5.5–16.7	2172	5.5*	3.1–9.9	1264	2.5*	1.4–4.4	638	1.0	—	241	95.6	3	4315
Spain	9.6*	6.6–13.9	1567	4.2*	3.0–5.9	1431	2.2*	1.6–3.0	1024	1.0	—	1451	176.3*	3	5473
Ukraine	1.9*	1.4–2.4	1194	1.0	0.8–1.3	1225	0.9	0.8–1.1	1180	1.0	—	1126	38.2*	3	4725
United States	9.5*	7.3–12.4	3034	5.0*	3.7–6.6	2865	3.0*	2.3–3.9	1922	1.0	—	1461	383.6*	3	9282

[a]Based on discrete-time survival models with person-year as the unit of analysis, controls are time intervals.
[b]Referent category.
*Significant at the .05 level, two-sided test.

Table 5 Inter-Cohort Differences in Lifetime Risk of Any *DSM-IV* Substance Use Disorder[a]

Country	18–34 OR	18–34 95% CI	18–34 N	35–49 OR	35–49 95% CI	35–49 N	50–64 OR	50–64 95% CI	50–64 N	65+[b] OR	65+[b] 95% CI	65+[b] N	χ^2	df	N
Belgium	5.0*	2.6–9.8	254	3.6*	1.7–7.3	331	2.6*	1.2–5.4	278	1.0	—	180	26.7*	3	1043
Colombia	2.3*	1.6–3.3	2000	1.1	0.7–1.6	1577	1.0	—	849	—	—	530	39.3*	2	4426
France	5.8*	3.3–10.0	388	3.3*	2.0–5.7	472	2.5*	1.4–4.2	362	1.0	—	214	44.1*	3	1436
Germany	5.6*	2.9–10.7	316	3.7*	2.0–6.8	436	3.9*	2.1–7.1	345	1.0	—	226	35.0*	3	1323
Israel	11.3*	5.9–21.6	1627	4.6*	2.4–9.0	1302	2.5*	1.2–5.1	1069	1.0	—	861	119.9*	3	4859
Italy	2.6*	1.0–6.7	496	1.8	0.8–4.1	516	1.6	0.6–3.9	454	1.0	—	313	5.5	3	1779
Japan	1.9	0.6–6.0	155	2.3*	1.1–4.9	219	2.5*	1.1–5.7	295	1.0	—	218	6.7	3	887
Lebanon[c]	—	—	—	—	—	—	—	—	—	—	—	—	—	—	—
Mexico	1.7*	1.3–2.4	2871	1.2	0.9–1.7	1888	1.0	—	1023	—	—	646	12.8*	2	5782
Netherlands	12.4*	7.0–21.8	264	7.0*	3.8–13.1	358	6.8*	3.4–13.9	302	1.0	—	170	85.3*	3	1094
New Zealand	8.1*	6.1–10.7	3747	3.5*	2.7–4.7	4102	2.5*	1.9–3.3	2697	1.0	—	2244	283.7*	3	12790
Nigeria	3.4*	1.1–10.1	971	4.9*	1.8–13.3	549	2.9	1.0–8.7	369	1.0	—	254	11.8*	3	2143
PR China	8.2*	1.0–67.2	379	4.0	0.6–28.2	726	1.5	0.2–11.2	357	1.0	—	166	31.9*	3	1628
South Africa	2.6*	1.3–5.4	2172	1.5	0.8–2.9	1264	1.0	0.6–1.9	638	1.0	—	241	29.1	3	4315
Spain	9.3*	3.6–24.2	545	5.0*	1.8–13.7	556	1.5	0.6–4.2	456	1.0	—	564	38.1*	3	2121
Ukraine	10.8*	5.8–20.1	420	5.0*	2.4–10.4	434	2.8*	1.3–5.8	412	1.0	—	454	116.4*	3	1720
United States	6.7	4.6–10.0	1939	4.9*	3.5–7.0	1831	3.5*	2.4–5.3	1213	1.0	—	709	111.0*	3	5692

[a]Based on discrete-time survival models with person-year as the unit of analysis, controls are time intervals.
[b]Referent category.
[c]Cell size too small to be included in analysis.
*Significant at the .05 level, two-sided test.

early detection and treatment might help reduce the persistence or severity of these largely primary anxiety and impulse control disorders and prevent the onset of secondary disorders. More preclinical and clinical research is needed on treatments of early cases, though, to determine whether this is true. Epidemiological research is also needed on the long-term consequences of early interventions for long-term secondary prevention.

Acknowledgments

The surveys discussed in this article were carried out in conjunction with the World Health Organization's World Mental Health (WMH) Survey Initiative. We thank the WMH staff for assistance with instrumentation, fieldwork, and data analysis. These activities were supported by the U.S. National Institute of Mental Health (R01-MH070884), the John D. and Catherine T. MacArthur Foundation, the Pfizer Foundation, the U.S. Public Health Service (R13-MH066849, R01-MH069864, and R01-DA016 558), the Fogarty International Center (FIRCA R01-TW006481), the Pan American Health Organization, Eli Lilly and Company, Ortho-McNeil Pharmaceutical, Inc., GlaxoSmithKline, and Bristol-Myers Squibb. The Chinese World Mental Health Survey Initiative is supported by the Pfizer Foundation. The Colombian National Study of Mental Health (NSMH) is supported by the Ministry of Social Protection, with supplemental support from the Saldarriaga Concha Foundation. The ESEMeD project is funded by the European Commission (Contracts QLG5–1999-01042; SANCO 2004123), the Piedmont Region (Italy), Fondo de Investigación Sanitaria, Instituto de Salud Carlos III, Spain (FIS 00/0028), Ministerio de Ciencia y Tecnología, Spain (SAF 2000–158-CE), Departament de Salut, Generalitat de Catalunya, Spain, and other local agencies, and by an unrestricted educational grant from GlaxoSmithKline. The Israel National Health Survey is funded by the Ministry of Health, with support from the Israel National Institute for Health Policy and Health Services Research and the National Insurance Institute of Israel. The World Mental Health Japan (WMHJ) Survey is supported by the Grant for Research on Psychiatric and Neurological Diseases and Mental Health (H13-SHOGAI-023, H14-TOKUBETSU-026, H16-KOKORO-013) from the Japan Ministry of Health, Labour and Welfare. The Lebanese National Mental Health Survey (LEBANON) is supported by the Lebanese Ministry of Public Health, the WHO (Lebanon), anonymous private donations to IDRAAC, Lebanon, and unrestricted grants from Janssen Cilag, Eli Lilly, GlaxoSmithKline, Roche, and Novartis. The Mexican National Comorbidity Survey (MNCS) is supported by the National Institute of Psychiatry Ramon de la Fuente (INPRFMDIES 4280) and by the National Council on Science and Technology (CONACyT-G30544-H), with supplemental support from the Pan American Health Organization. Te Rau Hinengaro: The New Zealand Mental Health Survey (NZMHS) is supported by the New Zealand Ministry of Health, Alcohol Advisory Council, and the Health Research Council. The Nigerian Survey of Mental Health and Wellbeing (NSMHW) is supported by the World Health Organization (Geneva), the World Health Organization (Nigeria), and the Federal Ministry of Health, Abuja, Nigeria. The South Africa and Health Study (SASH) is supported by the U.S. National Institute of Mental Health (R01-MH059575) and National Institute of Drug Abuse, with supplemental funding from the South African Department of Health and the University of Michigan. The Ukraine Comorbid Mental Disorders during Periods of Social Disruption (CMDPSD) study is funded by the U.S. National Institute of Mental Health (R01-MH61905). The U.S. National Comorbidity Survey Replication (NCS-R) is supported by the National Institute of Mental Health (U01-MH60220), with supplemental support from the National Institute of Drug Abuse, the Substance Abuse and Mental Health Services Administration (SAMHSA), the Robert Wood Johnson Foundation (Grant 044780), and the John W. Alden Trust.

References

1. Cooper B. *Psychiatric Epidemiology*. London: Croom Helm; 1987.
2. Robins LN, Helzer JE, Croughan JL, et al. National Institute of Mental Health Diagnostic Interview Schedule: its history, characteristics and validity. *Arch Gen Psychiatry*. 1981;38:381–389.
3. Cross-National Collaborative Group. The changing rate of major depression: cross-national comparisons. *JAMA*. 1992;268:3098–3105.
4. Weissman MM, Bland RC, Canino GJ, et al. The cross-national epidemiology of panic disorder. *Arch Gen Psychiatry*. 1997;54:305–309.
5. Weissman MM, Bland RC, Canino GJ, et al. Cross-national epidemiology of major depression and bipolar disorder. *JAMA*. 1996;276:293–299.
6. Wittchen HU. Reliability and validity studies of the WHO Composite International Diagnostic Interview (CIDI): a critical review. *J Psychiatr Res*. 1994;28:57–84.
7. World Health Organization. *Composite International Diagnostic Interview (CIDI, Version 1.0)*. Geneva: World Health Organization; 1990.
8. Andrade L. Lifetime prevalence of mental disorders in a catchment area in São Paulo, Brazil. Presented at the 7th Congress of the International Federation of Psychiatric Epidemiology, Santiago, August 1996.
9. Bijl RV, van Zessen G, Ravelli A, et al. The Netherlands Mental Health Survey and Incidence Study (NEMESIS): objectives and design. *Soc Psychiatry Psychiatr Epidemiol*. 1998;33:581–586.
10. Caraveo J, Martinez J, Rivera B. A model for epidemiological studies on mental health and psychiatric morbidity. *Salud Mental*. 1998;21:48–57.
11. Kessler RC, McGonagle KA, Zhao S, et al. Lifetime and 12-month prevalence of DSM-III-R psychiatric disorders in the United States. Results from the National Comorbidity Survey. *Arch Gen Psychiatry*. 1994;51:8–19.
12. Kylyc C. *Mental Health Profile of Turkey: Main Report*. Ankara: Ministry of Health Publications; 1998.
13. Vega WA, Kolody B, Aguilar-Gaxiola S, et al. Lifetime prevalence of DSM-III-R psychiatric disorders among urban and rural Mexican Americans in California. *Arch Gen Psychiatry*. 1998;55:771–778.
14. Wittchen H-U, Perkonigg A, Lachner G, et al. Early Developmental Stages of Psychopathology study (EDSP): objectives and design. *Eur Addict Res*. 1998;4:18–27.

15. Murray CJL, Lopez AD. *The Global Burden of Disease: A Comprehensive Assessment of Mortality and Disability from Diseases, Injuries and Risk Factors in 1990 and Projected to 2020.* Cambridge: Harvard University Press; 1996.
16. Bijl RV, de Graaf R, Hiripi E, et al. The prevalence of treated and untreated mental disorders in five countries. *Health Aff.* 2003;22:122–133.
17. Amminger GP, Leicester S, Yung AR, et al. Early-onset of symptoms predicts conversion to non-affective psychosis in ultra-high risk individuals. *Schizophr Res.* 2006;84:67–76.
18. McGue M, Iacono WG. The association of early adolescent problem behavior with adult psychopathology. *Am J Psychiatry.* 2005;162:1118–1124.
19. Thompson KN, Conus PO, Ward JL, et al. The initial prodrome to bipolar affective disorder: prospective case studies. *J Affect Disord.* 2003;77:79–85.
20. Alonso J, Angermeyer MC, Bernert S, et al. Sampling and methods of the European Study of the Epidemiology of Mental Disorders (ESEMeD) project. *Acta Psychiatr Scand.* 2004;420(Suppl.):8–20.
21. World Bank. *World Development Indicators 2003.* Washington: World Bank; 2003.
22. Demyttenaere K, Bruffaerts R, Posada-Villa J, et al. Prevalence, severity, and unmet need for treatment of mental disorders in the World Health Organization World Mental Health Surveys. *JAMA.* 2004;291:2581–2590.
23. Kessler RC, Merikangas KR. The National Comorbidity Survey Replication (NCS-R): background and aims. *Int J Methods Psychiatr Res.* 2004;13:60–68.
24. Kessler RC, Ustun TB. The World Mental Health (WMH) Survey Initiative Version of the World Health Organization (WHO) Composite International Diagnostic Interview (CIDI). *Int J Methods Psychiatr Res.* 2004;13:93–121.
25. World Health Organization. *International Classification of Diseases (ICD-10).* Geneva: World Health Organization; 1991.
26. American Psychiatric Association. *Diagnostic and Statistical Manual of Mental Disorders*, 4th ed. Washington: American Psychiatric Association; 1994.
27. Haro JM, Arbabzadeh-Bouchez S, Brugha TS, et al. Concordance of the Composite International Diagnostic Interview Version 3.0 (CIDI 3.0) with standardized clinical assessments in the WHO World Mental Health Surveys. *Int J Methods Psychiatr Res.* 2006;15:167–180.
28. First MB, Spitzer RL, Gibbon M, et al. *Structured Clinical Interview for DSM-IV Axis I Disorders, Research Version, Non-patient Edition (SCID-I/NP).* New York: Biometrics Research, New York State Psychiatric Institute; 2002.
29. Simon GE, VonKorff M. Recall of psychiatric history in cross-sectional surveys: implications for epidemiologic research. *Epidemiol Rev.* 1995;17:221–227.
30. Knauper B, Cannell CF, Schwarz N, et al. Improving the accuracy of major depression age of onset reports in the US National Comorbidity Survey. *Int J Methods Psychiatr Res.* 1999;8:39–48.
31. SAS Institute. *SAS/STAT Software: Changes and Enhancements, Release 8.2.* Cary: SAS Publishing; 2001.
32. Efron B. Logistic regression, survival analysis, and the Kaplan-Meier curve. *J Am Stat Assoc.* 1988;83:414–425.
33. Wolter KM. *Introduction to Variance Estimation.* New York: Springer; 1985.
34. Research Triangle Institute. *SUDAAN: Professional Software for Survey Data Analysis.* Research Triangle Park: Research Triangle Institute; 2002.
35. Kish L, Frankel MR. Inferences from complex samples. *J Royal Stat Soc.* 1974;36:1–37.

36. Gureje O, Lasebikan VO, Kola L, et al. Lifetime and 12-month prevalence of mental disorders in the Nigerian Survey of Mental Health and Well-Being. *Br J Psychiatry*. 2006;188:465–471.
37. Shen YC, Zhang MY, Huang YQ, et al. Twelve-month prevalence, severity, and unmet need for treatment of mental disorders in metropolitan China. *Psychol Med*. 2006;36:257–267.
38. Hasin DS, Grant BF. The co-occurrence of DSM-IV alcohol abuse in DSM-IV alcohol dependence: results of the National Epidemiologic Survey on Alcohol and Related Conditions on heterogeneity that differ by population subgroup. *Arch Gen Psychiatry*. 2004;61:891–896.
39. WHO International Consortium in Psychiatric Epidemiology. Cross-national comparisons of the prevalences and correlates of mental disorders. *Bull World Health Organ*. 2000;78:413–426.
40. Allgulander C. Psychoactive drug use in a general population sample, Sweden: correlates with perceived health, psychiatric diagnoses, and mortality in an automated record-linkage study. *Am J Publ Health*. 1989;79:1006–1010.
41. Cannell CF, Marquis KH, Laurent A. A summary of studies of interviewing methodology: 1959–1970. *Vital Health Stat*. 1977;2:69.
42. Giuffra LA, Risch N. Diminished recall and the cohort effect of major depression: a simulation study. *Psychol Med*. 1994;24:375–383.
43. Kessler RC, Wittchen H-U, Abelson JM, et al. Methodological studies of the Composite International Diagnostic Interview (CIDI) in the US National Comorbidity Survey. *Int J Methods Psychiatr Res*. 1998;7:33–55.
44. Kessler RC, Merikangas KR, Berglund P, et al. Mild disorders should not be eliminated from the DSM-V. *Arch Gen Psychiatry*. 2003;60:1117–1122.
45. Christie KA, Burke JDJ, Regier DA, et al. Epidemiologic evidence for early onset of mental disorders and higher risk of drug-abuse in young-adults. *Am J Psychiatry*. 1988;145:971–975.
46. Christiana JM, Gilman SE, Guardino M, et al. Duration between onset and time of obtaining initial treatment among people with anxiety and mood disorders: an international survey of members of mental health patient advocate groups. *Psychol Med*. 2000;30:693–703.
47. Olfson M, Kessler RC, Berglund PA, et al. Psychiatric disorder onset and first treatment contact in the United States and Ontario. *Am J Psychiatry*. 1998;155:1415–1422.
48. Wang PS, Angermeyer M, Borges G, et al. Delay and failure in treatment seeking after first onset of mental disorders in the World Health Organization's World Mental Health Survey Initiative. *World Psychiatry*. 2007;6:177–185.

DISCUSSION QUESTIONS

1. Based on what you have learned about mental illness definitions and psychiatric epidemiological research, what challenges are there to conducting cross-national research on mental disorders?

2. Choose one meaningful pattern of results (i.e., a difference in prevalence across countries or across disorders) from Table 2, describe it, and develop

a plausible explanation for it. What kinds of data would you need to evaluate your explanation?

3. Rates of anxiety, mood, and substance use disorders are consistently higher in more recent cohorts than in older cohorts in almost every country. How well can the cohort difference be explained by genetic or biological factors? Cultural factors? Structural factors?

THE SOCIAL ORIGINS OF MENTAL HEALTH AND ILLNESS

Research on the social origins of mental illness highlights another of sociology's unique contributions to the study of mental illness: its analysis of the relevance of social statuses and conditions to the risk of mental health problems. In contrast to clinical researchers who emphasize the prediction of risk for specific disorders, sociologists emphasize the broad implications of socially-structured arrangements for psychological well-being. Sociological theories about the origins of mental illness begin with the identification of potentially consequential social conditions, such as an economic recession or conflicting role demands, and move from those arrangements to their effects on individuals. As a result, sociological theories are often nonspecific: they assert that social conditions manifest in a range of mental health problems rather than in any specific disorder. Sociological theories also assume that mental illness is not an unexpected outcome of a failed social order. Rather, mental illness is an expected outcome of a hierarchical social system built on inequality.

The first three selections in this section present orienting frameworks to guide your reading of the selections that follow. Aneshensel considers the general issue of how sociological analyses of the predictors of mental illness differ from analyses by researchers in clinical fields such as psychology and psychiatry. Pearlin introduces the stress process framework—a general framework for understanding how socially-structured inequalities affect mental health. In a selection that is both theoretical and empirical, Thoits, moves away from the analysis of inequalities per se to consider how the roles we occupy influence our well-being.

These three broad frameworks motivate the empirical selections that follow. From Turner and colleagues' analysis of the social distribution of stress to Schieman and colleagues' analysis of age differences in distress, each of the selections provides compelling evidence for the effects of social conditions, statuses, and roles on mental health.

Basic Concepts

Carol S. Aneshensel

Research in Mental Health: Social Etiology versus Social Consequences[†]

We open this section with a selection by Carol S. Aneshensel who presents a strong statement for the unique insights sociology brings to the study of mental health. She begins by comparing and contrasting two distinct approaches to identifying social risk factors for mental health problems: the social etiology model and the social consequences model. She then identifies the primary differences between the models and advocates for sociologists to adopt a social consequences orientation. By highlighting the distinctions between the models, Aneshensel encourages sociologists to be mindful of their broad disciplinary mission, and sets the stage for the empirical articles that follow.

S ociological research on mental health is typically focused on identifying how social organization and processes affect mental health. This orientation has tended to emphasize the impact of social structure, examining in particular the mental health consequences of socioeconomic stratification (McLeod & Nonnemaker, 1999). Other research in this tradition has emphasized gender stratification, especially differences in the occurrence of disorder between men and women, but also variation among women according to their social role occupancy (Bird, 1999; Simon, 2002). Other aspects of stratification studied within this tradition include race-ethnicity (Williams, Takeuchi, & Adair, 1992; Jackson, 1997), age (Mirowsky & Ross, 1992; Schieman, Van Gundy, & Taylor, 2001), and marital status (Barrett, 2000; Simon, 2002). The stress process (Pearlin, 1999) has figured prominently in attempts to connect social stratification to risk of mental disorder, along with the elaboration of mediating concepts such as mastery, social support, and

Aneshensel, Carol S. 2005. "Research in Mental Health: Social Etiology versus Social Consequences." *Journal of Health and Social Behavior* 46:221–228.

coping. The common element linking these specific undertakings is a shared focus on explaining how society influences the mental health of its members and this connection is the topic of this article, specifically its differentiation from seemingly similar endeavors. The key issue to be addressed is whether the task at hand concerns identifying the social antecedents of a specific disorder, or the overall mental health consequences of various social arrangements.

THE SOCIAL ETIOLOGY MODEL

The social etiology model is concerned with the occurrence of one particular disorder and the identification of social risk factors associated with its occurrence. It is etiological given that its motivation is to locate the causes or origins of the disorder. Primary goals of this type of inquiry pertain to the prevention and treatment of the disorder under investigation. This model is employed in not only sociology but also public health, but it derives from medicine insofar as it is concerned with etiology. Although sociological investigators have begun to examine multiple or alternative mental health outcomes (e.g., Simon, 2002), the disorder-specific etiologic model continues to predominate in sociological research.

The defining characteristic of this model is its focus on a single disorder, such as major depression. Persons with the disorder are treated as being positive on the outcome under investigation, that is, depressed. Other persons are treated as negative on the outcome, that is, not depressed. In very simplistic terms, people who have the disorder are compared to those who do not, that is, depressed versus not depressed. This classification strategy is internally consistent with the etiologic goals of this type of study. In other words, the intent of the research—to identify the causes of a particular disorder—and the measurement method match one another.

Within this disorder-specific model, people with different disorders are implicitly classified as "well" because they do not have the one particular disorder singled out for investigation. For example, a study of major depression will by default consider a nondepressed person who has a substance abuse disorder to be "well" (i.e., negative on the outcome) because the person does not have major depression. Indeed, the presence of other disorders may not be assessed, despite evidence that comorbidity for psychiatric disorders is extensive (Kessler et al., 1994). Again, this measurement strategy is consistent with the goal of identifying the causes of the one disorder singled out for investigation, major depression in our running example.

The disorder-specific etiological model is an extremely powerful model. It is used in most medical and epidemiological research. This model has generated a good deal of what we know about what makes people sick, including most of what we know about the social factors that make people sick. It is a good model—when used in the service of the etiologic goals of epidemiological and medical research.

THE SOCIAL CONSEQUENCES MODEL

The disorder-specific etiological model is a problem for sociologists, however, because the goals of sociological inquiry are usually not etiological, but rather emphasize the consequences of various social arrangements on people's lives. The subject of inquiry is the structural factor, such as concentrated poverty, racial segregation, or gender stratification. Disorder is of interest, by and large, because it is seen as an important outcome of these social factors; it is not the object of explanation in and of itself. In other words, the goal is to elucidate the ways in which society impacts mental health as distinct from isolating the causes of a particular mental health problem in order to prevent or treat it.

When sociological research limits itself to identifying the social anteced-ents of a particular disorder, the research is indistinguishable from the dis-order-specific etiological model; all that differs, perhaps, is the disciplinary background of the investigators and the journals in which the research is published. In other words, social etiological investigations implicitly adopt an inherently medical model as distinct from what I am labeling the social consequences model. Whereas the etiologic model is concerned with the social antecedents of a particular disorder, the social consequences model, I reiterate, is concerned with the mental health consequences of specific social arrangements.

Moreover, from the sociological perspective, the mental health conse-quences of social organization are typically assumed to be nonspecific, not limited to one particular disorder. Although a good deal of this litera-ture focuses on depression and nonspecific psychological distress, research into the mental health consequences of social organization has examined a diverse set of other disorders as well. This list includes anger, violence, anti-social behavior, alcohol and substance abuse, anxiety, antisocial personality disorder, and suicide.

By and large, examples such as those just cited examine single mental health outcomes in isolation from other potential outcomes of the same set of social conditions. Consequently, these studies implicitly adopt the disor-der-specific model. The point, however, is that findings from these studies *collectively* demonstrate that social organization is associated with a broad spectrum of potential mental health outcomes and is not linked to a sin-gle disorder to the exclusion of other disorders. Studies examining multiple mental health outcomes also support the conclusion that the mental health effects of social organization are nonspecific (e.g., Aneshensel, Rutter, & Lachenbruch, 1991; Barrett, 2000; Horwitz & White, 1987; Horwitz, White, & Howell-White, 1996; Pearlin, 1989; Simon, 1998, 2002). In other words, the assumption of nonspecific effects is a viable one.

The best evidence supporting the need for multiple outcomes studies comes from two epidemiologic studies that estimated the prevalence of a broad range of common psychiatric disorders, the Epidemiologic Catchment Area Study (Robins & Regier, 1991) and the National Comorbidity Survey (Kessler et al., 1994) and its replication (Kessler et al., 2003). These investigations examined the distribution of each of these disorders across a variety of social risk factors.

Two general patterns of findings can be distinguished. In the first, the social characteristic has a fairly consistent association with a broad range of psychiatric disorders. For example, socioeconomic status, operationalized as education and income, is inversely associated with the rates of almost all disorders (Kessler & Zhao, 1999). In the second pattern, the social characteristic is associated with some disorders, but not others, or in the extreme case bears a positive association with the occurrence of some disorders but a negative association with the occurrence of other disorders. Gender fits this pattern, for example, with females having higher rates than men of mood disorders (with the exception of mania for which there is no gender difference), anxiety disorders, and nonaffective psychoses, and men having higher rates than women of substance use disorders and antisocial personality disorder (Kessler & Zhao, 1999).

Findings from these studies demonstrate quite conclusively that empirical results concerning associations between social attributes and mental health outcomes are contingent on the specific type of disorder selected for investigation. If the goal is, as it so often is in sociological research, to address the general mental health impact of the social attribute, then the full range of relevant outcomes needs to be considered.

A second key element of the social consequences model is the assumption that the impact of social organization on mental health is causative in nature (Aneshensel, 1992; Wheaton, 2001). Empirical associations between indicators of social placement and mental health have also been studied for evidence of social selection (e.g., McLeod & Kaiser, 2004). For example, Miech and colleagues (1999) examine anxiety, depression, antisocial disorder, and attention deficit disorder and find that each disorder has a unique relationship in terms of causation versus social selection regarding educational attainment. However, most work in this area has been devoted to explicating models that assume a causal connection between social placement and risk of adverse mental health outcomes.

From this perspective, indicators of social placement, such as socioeconomic status, gender, race or ethnicity, and age, are often cast in the role of independent variable, indeed are often the focal point of the investigation. In this tradition, Link and Phelan (1995) treat social placement as a fundamental cause of disease, including mental disorder. In contrast, etiologic studies often treat this same set of variables as potential confounders, set to the side as control variables. This distinction, between causality and noise, is one of the key differences between sociological and etiological research, emphasizing explanation and prediction, respectively. The social consequences model treats indicators of social placement as signifying ongoing social processes that organize people's lives in ways that influence their mental health. For example, indicators of social placement are associated with mental health at least in part because these statuses and roles regulate exposure to social stress and access to psychosocial resources (Aneshensel, 1992; Pearlin, 1989; Turner & Lloyd, 1999; Turner, Wheaton, & Lloyd, 1995).

A final key element of the social consequences model is the idea that mental and emotional disorder is a normal byproduct of society (Aneshensel, 1992; Aneshensel & Phelan, 1999; Pearlin, 1989). In other words, the very structures and processes that make social life possible for most people create circumstances that are intolerable for some persons. For example, in a capitalist society, some people will always experience the stress of unemployment; the only question is who is most likely to encounter it. Unemployment-related disorder, then, is an inevitable occurrence given the organization of the occupational sphere.

This orientation distinctly differs from the disease model of medicine in which disorder is viewed as abnormal, the outcome of some dysfunction in social or other etiological factors. This pathological orientation leads inevitably to the individualization of risk. In contrast, the social consequences model examines regularities in social organization and processes that place populations, as distinct from individuals, at elevated risk. This means that sociological research tends to look for the sources of mental disorder in the usual, not the esoteric (Pearlin, 1989). For example, the emphasis is more likely to be on ongoing strains within marital and occupational roles than on the once-in-a-lifetime occurrence of a natural disaster. (However, sociologists may well be concerned with how social status shapes responses to such unusual occurrences.) Thus, the social consequences model is typically concerned with the ways in which location in society shapes everyday experiences in ways that are deleterious to the mental health of some.

IMPLICATIONS

Sociological research shortchanges itself by adopting the social etiological model.

First, the mental health consequences of various social arrangements are underestimated. The mental health "cost" of poverty among children is not limited to the impact of poverty on problematic behavior but includes as well its impact on emotional distress (McLeod & Edwards, 1995). In the disorder-specific model, only those children having the condition under investigation, for example, problem behavior, are counted, whereas those who adversely react to poverty in other ways are counted as "well," for example, those who are emotionally distressed. That is, these children are misclassified as "unaffected" by their exposure to poverty. Thus, the disorder-specific model undercounts the number of persons affected by adverse social conditions. This undercount occurs whenever the social condition affects more than one domain of functioning. Since many social conditions meet this criterion, the extent of this undercount is pervasive.

Second, we obtain a biased estimate of the mental health impact of social arrangements when we consider only one condition instead of the full range of relevant conditions (Aneshensel et al., 1991). In most empirical applications, impact is estimated either as an ordinary least squares or a logistic regression coefficient. For example, the logistic regression coefficient for condition A (relative to not A) is obviously not equivalent to one for conditions A, B, C, or D (relative to none of these conditions). The direction of this bias is unknown; it depends on the strength of the association for the various outcomes. When we estimate the social antecedents of disorder A, then, we get a biased estimate of the mental health consequences of that social condition whenever the condition also impacts any other mental health outcome, that is, B, C, or D.

Unfortunately, there is no easy solution, in large part because different types of disorder are not equivalent to one another precisely because they represent distinctly different domains of functioning. This is the proverbial problem of trying to add apples and oranges. Thus, attempts to create a composite of various domains of functioning seem to be fraught with more conceptual and empirical difficulties than warrant the effort. Instead, the optimal approach, in my opinion, is to examine a broad array of outcomes. This conclusion is based on the assumption, stated above, that the impact of social arrangements on mental health tends to be nonspecific.

The array of outcomes to be investigated should include at least a sample of the full spectrum of outcomes that are relevant to the social arrangements being examined. The identification of outcomes should begin with the nature of the social arrangements being studied. Existing research has emphasized, as noted earlier, aspects of social stratification and inequality, an emphasis that is relevant to depressive outcomes but also easily applies to other outcomes, such as substance use. This focus on stratification, however, should not divert attention from other aspects of society that impact mental health, such as family relationships, socialization practices, or stigmatization. The key point is that the nature of the outcomes to be investigated should be dictated by the aspect of social life that is being probed, not vice versa.

The question of selecting several outcomes ought to be fundamentally the same as selecting the outcome when only one disorder is being investigated. I suspect, however, that the selection of a specific disorder is more often driven by its own characteristics than by the aspect of society being probed. Prominent among these characteristics are considerations that make a disorder a public health concern, such as high prevalence, severity of disability, or chronic course. In this regard, sociological research has often fashioned itself on epidemiologic research and has, on more than one occasion, lost sight of its sociological objectives.

As a result, theory is generally underdeveloped with regard to why particular aspects of social life ought to be related to specific types of disorder. The processes and dynamics linking various aspects of social organization to particular outcomes warrant further development. This task is usually undertaken for the one disorder under investigation, showing its relevance to the aspect of society being studied. This step is necessary but not sufficient from the perspective of the social consequences model. Theory should also address what other outcomes are relevant and identify those that are not pertinent. These considerations are often overlooked insofar as the disorder-specific model by default treats all other disorders as nondisorders. In sum, theories need to specify not simply that a particular outcome is relevant but rather to identify the full range of relevant outcomes in order to operationalize the social consequences model.

It should be clear that the array of outcomes investigated need not include all possible outcomes. It is not necessary to assess, for example, all disorders identified in the *Diagnostic and Statistical Manual of Mental Disorders* (American Psychiatric Association, 2000). If one concludes that a large array of outcomes is necessary, one could sample disorders much in the way we sample populations or constructs. Indeed, this is often done already insofar as mental health surveys typically measure more than one outcome. The goal is to better articulate the reasons why these particular outcomes are most relevant to the social conditions under investigation. Moreover, once measured, these multiple outcomes need to be simultaneously analyzed.

CONCLUSIONS

The social etiology and social consequences models are not in opposition to one another, but they do serve different purposes and therefore require distinctive research approaches. I think sociologists are uniquely advantaged to articulate a research agenda that emphasizes the broad impact of social conditions on mental health. This viewpoint is underappreciated in a research environment that is organized around specific diseases, such as at the National Institutes of Health, and, as I have emphasized, is bound to underestimate the influence of social arrangements on people's mental health. The way in which society is organized is consequential to the ways in which people think, act, and feel. This impact is broad in scope, and the methods we use should reveal this impact, not conceal it. We as sociologists should take the lead, I submit, in developing a research agenda that speaks to the multitude of ways in which society affects the mental health of its members.

References

American Psychiatric Association. 2000. *Diagnostic and Statistical Manual of Mental Disorders.* 4th ed., text rev. Washington, DC: American Psychiatric Association.

Aneshensel, Carol S. 1992. "Social Stress: Theory and Research." *Annual Review of Sociology* 18:18–38.

Aneshensel, Carol S. and Jo C. Phelan. 1999. "The Sociology of Mental Health: Surveying the Field." Pp. 3–17 in *Handbook of the Sociology of Mental Health,* edited by Carol S. Aneshensel and Jo C. Phelan. New York: Kluwer.

Aneshensel, Carol S., Carolyn M. Rutter, and Peter A. Lachenbruch. 1991. "Social Structure, Stress, and Mental Health: Competing Conceptual and Analytic Models." *American Sociological Review* 56:166–78.

Barrett, Anne E. 2000. "Marital Trajectories and Mental Health." *Journal of Health and Social Behavior* 41:451–64.

Bird, Chloe E. 1999. "Gender, Household Labor, and Psychological Distress: The Impact of the Amount and Division of Housework." *Journal of Health and Social Behavior* 40:32–45.

Horwitz, Allan V. and Helene Raskin White. 1987. "Gender Role Orientations and Styles of Pathology among Adolescents." *Journal of Health and Social Behavior* 28:158–70.

Horwitz, Allan V., Helene R. White, and Sandra Howell-White. 1996. "The Use of Multiple Outcomes in Stress Research: A Case Study of Gender Differences in Responses to Marital Dissolution." *Journal of Health and Social Behavior* 37:278–91.

Jackson, Pamela Braboy. 1997. "Role Occupancy and Minority Mental Health." *Journal of Health and Social Behavior* 38:237–55.

Kessler, Ronald C., Patricia Berglund, Olga Demler, Robert Jin, Doreen Koretz, Kathleen R. Merikangas, A. John Rush, Ellen E. Walters, and Philip S. Want. 2003. "The Epidemiology of Major Depressive Disorder: Results from the National Comorbidity Survey Replication (NCRS-R)." *Journal of the American Medical Association* 289:3095–105.

Kessler, Ronald C., Katherine A. McGonagle, Shanyang Zhao, Christopher B. Nelson, Michael Hughes, Suzann Eshleman, Hans-Ulrich Wittchen, and Kenneth S. Kendler. 1994. "Lifetime and 12-Month Prevalence of DSM-III-R Psychiatric Disorders in the United States: Results from the National Comorbidity Survey." *Archives of General Psychiatry* 51:8–19.

Kessler, Ronald C. and Shanyang Zhao. 1999. "Overview of Descriptive Epidemiology of Mental Disorders." Pp. 127–50 in *Handbook of the Sociology of Mental Health*, edited by Carol S. Aneshensel and Jo C. Phelan. New York: Kluwer.

Link, Bruce G. and Jo C. Phelan. 1995. "Social Conditions as Fundamental Causes of Disease." *Journal of Health and Social Behavior* 36(extra issue):80–94.

McLeod, Jane D. and Kevan Edwards. 1995. "Contextual Determinants of Children's Responses to Poverty." *Social Forces* 73:1487–516.

McLeod, Jane D. and Karen Kaiser. 2004. "Childhood Emotional and Behavioral Problems and Educational Attainment." *American Sociological Review* 69:636–58.

McLeod, Jane D. and James M. Nonnemaker. 1999. "Social Stratification and Inequality." Pp. 321–44 in *Handbook of the Sociology of Mental Health*, edited by Carol S. Aneshensel and Jo C. Phelan. New York: Kluwer.

Miech, Robert A., Avshalom Caspi, Terrie E. Moffitt, Bradley R. Entner Wright, and Phil A. Silva. 1999. "Low Socioeconomic Status and Mental Disorders: A Longitudinal Study of Selection and Causation during Young Adulthood." *American Journal of Sociology* 104:1096–131.

Mirowsky, John and Catherine E. Ross. 1992. "Age and Depression." *Journal of Health and Social Behavior* 33:187–205.

Pearlin, Leonard I. 1989. "The Sociological Study of Stress." *Journal of Health and Social Behavior* 30:241–56.

———. 1999. "The Stress Process Revisited: Reflections on Concepts and Their Interrelationships." Pp. 395–415 in *Handbook of the Sociology of Mental Health*, edited by Carol S. Aneshensel and Jo C. Phelan. New York: Kluwer.

Robins, Lee N. and Darrel A. Regier. 1991. *Psychiatric Disorders in America: The Epidemiologic Catchment Area Study*. New York: Free Press.

Schieman, Scott, Karen Van Gundy, and John Taylor. 2001. "Status, Role, and Resource Explanations for Age Patterns in Psychological Distress." *Journal of Health and Social Behavior* 42:80–96.

Simon, Robin. 1998. "Assessing Sex Differences in Vulnerability among Employed Parents: The Importance of Marital Status." *Journal of Health and Social Behavior* 39:38–54.

———. 2002. "Revisiting the Relationships among Gender, Marital Status, and Mental Health." *American Journal of Sociology* 107:1065–96.

Turner, R. Jay and Donald A. Lloyd. 1999. "The Stress Process and the Social Distribution of Depression." *Journal of Health and Social Behavior* 40:374–404.

Turner, R. Jay, Blair Wheaton, and Donald A. Lloyd. 1995. "The Epidemiology of Social Stress." *American Sociological Review* 60:104–25.

Wheaton, Blair. 2001. "The Role of Sociology in the Study of Mental Health...and the Role of Mental Health in the Study of Sociology." *Journal of Health and Social Behavior* 42:221–34.

Williams, David R., David T. Takeuchi, and Russell K. Adair. 1992. "Socioeconomic Status and Psychiatric Disorder among Blacks and Whites." *Social Forces* 71:179–94.

DISCUSSION QUESTIONS

1. According to Aneshensel, what are the most important differences between the "social etiology" and "social consequences" model? Why does she see the latter as more consistent with the goals of sociology than the former?

2. At the end of the article, Aneshensel notes that the National Institutes of Health organize research funding in a way that encourages researchers to adopt the "social etiology" model. How might our knowledge about the social risk factors for mental health problems be biased by the organization of research funding? What could we gain by applying a "social consequences" model?

Leonard I. Pearlin

The Sociological Study of Stress[†]

Stress research is an interdisciplinary field with major contributions from psychology, social work, and medicine as well as from sociology. In this article, Leonard I. Pearlin introduces the stress process framework—one of the most important theoretical frameworks in contemporary sociological research on mental health and illness. His discussion emphasizes the unique insights of a sociological approach to stress research and, by so doing, makes a strong case for the centrality of sociology to the study of mental health.

Sociologists have an intellectual stake in the study of stress. It presents an excellent opportunity to observe how deeply well-being is affected by the structured arrangements of people's lives and by the repeated experiences that stem from these arrangements. Yet stress is not generally seen as part of a sociological mainstream, partly, I believe, because those of us who are engaged in stress research are not consistently attentive to the sociological character of the field. In this paper I attempt to identify what I regard as some of the conceptual and analytic issues that should be considered in bringing the study of stress closer to sociology.

THE STRUCTURAL CONTEXTS OF THE STRESS PROCESS

Most research into stress starts with an experience—an exigency that people confront and their perceptions of that exigency as threatening or burdensome. Many stressful experiences, it should be recognized, don't spring out of a vacuum but typically can be traced back to surrounding social structures and people's locations within them. The most encompassing of these structures are the various systems of stratification that cut across societies, such as those based on social and economic class, race and ethnicity, gender, and age. To the extent that these systems embody the unequal distribution of resources, opportunities, and self-regard, a low status within them may itself be a source of stressful life conditions.

Another important structural context is found in social institutions and their arrangements of statuses and roles. Incumbency in a major institutionalized role necessarily entails persistent encounters with a host of conditions and expectations that exert a structuring force on experience. Because the roles themselves persist in time, experiences within them tend to become a repeated feature of their incumbents' lives. When these experiences are

Pearlin, Leonard I. 1989. "The sociological study of stress." *Journal of Health and Social Behavior* 30:241–256.

threatening and problematic, they may result in stress. Relationships formed by role sets are relatively enduring and stable, and typically are of considerable importance to the parties involved. Consequently, when such relationships are problematic and filled with conflict, they can produce considerable stress.

"Interrelated" levels of social structure—social stratification, social institutions, interpersonal relationships—mold and structure the experiences of individuals; these experiences, in turn, may result in stress. Therefore the structural contexts of people's lives are not extraneous to the stress process but are fundamental to that process. They are the sources of hardship and privilege, threat and security, conflict and harmony. In searching for the origins of stress, we may begin fruitfully by scrutinizing the social arrangements of society and the structuring of experience within these arrangements. This search, I believe, will reveal how ordinary people can be caught up in the disjunctures and discontinuities of societies, how they can be motivated to adopt socially valued dreams and yet can find their dreams thwarted by socially erected barriers, and how as engaged members of society they come into conflict with others and with themselves.

The distinguishing mark of sociological inquiry is its effort to uncover patterns and regularities shared by people whose social characteristics and circumstances are similar. The essential element of the sociological study of stress is the presence of similar types and levels of stress among people who are exposed to similar social and economic conditions, who are incumbents in similar roles, and who come from similar situational contexts. There can be little, if any, sociological interest in randomly distributed problems or randomly distributed responses to the problems. Such random or idiosyncratic stress is of legitimate interest to clinicians or biologists, but not to sociologists. Therefore a salient feature of sociological stress research is its concern with the socially patterned distribution of components of the stress process: stressors, mediators, and outcomes. Such patterns provide a cue that individuals' potentially stressful experiences and the ways in which they are affected by these experiences may originate in the social orders of which they are a part.

SOCIAL STRESSORS

Historically, stress research has been guided by two modal concerns: one having a primary interest in naturalistic stressors and the other in the mediation and outcomes of stress. As the preceding discussion suggests, sociologists have been and should be interested in the former. For other scientists, who are more concerned with stress outcomes and their psychological and biological dimensions, the nature and origins of the stressors are less important. To those researchers it makes little difference whether stress is controlled experimentally in the laboratory, is unique to individuals, or is anchored in highly unusual circumstances. From their viewpoint, the response of the organism to stress is legitimately of greater interest than the cause of the stress (Pearlin, 1982). Sociological attention, by contrast, is more fixed on the stressors and their naturalistic sources.

Stressors, of course, refer to the experiential circumstances that give rise to stress. Although virtually all *social* scientists engaged in stress research are interested in stressors, they differ considerably as to how they conceptualize stressors and as to the importance they attach to different types of stressors. In recent years, attention generally has been divided between *life events*, on the one hand, and more enduring or recurrent life problems, sometimes referred to as *chronic strains*, on the other.

Life Events as Stressors

Life events have occupied by far the most research attention in the past 20 years. Indeed, in some circles life events inappropriately have become a metaphor for stress research. There are at least three reasons for the impressive surge of life events research in the past two decades. First, the pioneering work of Hans Selye (1982) provided an important theoretical foundation for events research. Second, in response to Selye's theoretical inspiration, a method was developed to assess in seemingly simple and objective fashion the magnitude of eventful change experienced by individuals. Third, interest in research into life events was spurred by its early success in showing relationships between the scope of eventful change and various indicators of health. All in all, stress researchers who attempted to identify and measure stressors found a theory to stimulate their work, a method by which to carry it out, and empirical results to reward their efforts.

Since the launching of life events research, however, its theory, its methods, and its findings have been called into question. With regard to underlying theory, it is now clear that a key assumption about life events as stressors is untenable. Following from the implications of Selye's observations of laboratory animals' responses to environmental changes, the theory held that *all* change is potentially harmful because all change requires readjustment. Sociologists should find this notion difficult to accept because change is a normal and inexorable feature of every level of social life and of aging. At any rate, the weight of current evidence shows that not change per se but the quality of change is potentially damaging to people. Specifically, changes that are undesired, unscheduled, nonnormative, and uncontrolled are most harmful (Fairbank & Hough, 1979; Gersten, Langner, Eisenberg, & Simcha-Hogan, 1977; Thoits, 1981; Vinokur & Seltzer, 1975). I believe that researchers no longer accept unquestioningly the assumption that change is categorically bad for people or that the magnitude of change is harmful independent of its quality.

Next, the instruments used to identify life events are misleading in crucial respects. Many events that typically appear on inventories such as the Holmes and Rahe Social Readjustment Rating Scale (1967) are simply

SOCIAL READJUSTMENT RATING SCALE

Holmes and Rahe's (1967) Social Readjustment Rating Scale was the most influential measure of life event exposure in early research on social stress. The authors of the scale identified events for inclusion by reviewing the medical records of U.S. Navy personnel for events that were commonly associated with injury or the onset of illness. A convenience sample of judges then rated the events for the amount of "readjustment" they required. Their ratings were averaged and converted into a standard scale on which "death of a spouse" was assigned a weight of 100. The scale has been criticized for including "injury and illness" (which may be outcomes of stress rather than life events), for failing to distinguish between positive events (such as getting married) and negative events (such as losing a job), and for failing to include events common to women and people of lower status. Despite its limitations, the scale still serves as an important example of "checklist" measures of acute stress. When you read the article by Turner and his colleagues, you can compare Holmes and Rahe's measure to theirs and see how far social stress research has progressed since the 1960s.

1. Death of a spouse	100
2. Divorce	73
3. Marital Separation	65
4. Jail term	63
5. Death of a close family member	63
6. Personal injury or illness	53
7. Marriage	50
8. Fired at work	47
9. Marital reconciliation	45
10. Retirement	45
11. Change in health of family member	44
12. Pregnancy	40
13. Sex difficulties	39
14. Gain of a new family member	39
15. Business readjustments	39
16. Change in financial state	38
17. Death of a close friend	37
18. Change to different line of work	36

19.	Change in no. of arguments with spouse	35
20.	Mortgage over $ 50,000	31
21.	Foreclosure of mortgage	30
22.	Change in responsibilities at work	29
23.	Son or daughter leaving home	29
24.	Trouble with in-laws	29
25.	Outstanding Personal achievements	28
26.	Wife begins or stops work	26
27.	Begin or end school	26
28.	Change in living conditions	25
29.	Revision of personal habits	24
30.	Trouble with boss	23
31.	Change in work hours or conditions	20
32.	Change in residence	20
33.	Change in school	20
34.	Change in recreation	19
35.	Change in religious activities	19
36.	Change in social activities	18
37.	Loan less than 50,000	17
38.	Change in sleeping habits	16
39.	Change in no. of family gettogether	15
40.	Change in eating habits	15
41.	Vacation	13
42.	Holidays	12
43.	Minor violation of laws	11

Holmes, Thomas H., & Richard H. Rahe. 1967. The Social Readjustment Rating Scale. *Journal of Psychosomatic Research* 11:213–218.

markers or surrogate indicators of ongoing conditions; they do not represent free-standing or discrete life change. The loss of a home through foreclosure or a jail sentence, for example, is not an event that erupts unexpectedly. More likely, the event is merely an episodic segment of continuing problems. Because the event inventory allows us to see only the segment and not its history, we ignore the more extended life circumstances of which the event may be a part. Thus questions that presumably are asked about events may in fact elicit information about nonevents. Therefore the tools used to assess eventful change tend to confuse events with more enduring stressors.

This confusion, in turn, brings into question the meaning of past research findings showing relationships between events and health, relationships that have provided much of the empirical support for the interest in life events as stressors. To the extent that events are surrogate indicators of noneventful, ongoing circumstances, empirical relationships between events and health may be explained more accurately by the continuing circumstances in which the event is embedded. Thus in interpreting events-health relationships we are susceptible to exaggerating the importance of eventful change and to minimizing—or overlooking altogether—the problematic continuities of people's lives. The confusion between an event and a more chronic life strain, I submit, impedes a clear understanding of the social etiology of ill health and emotional distress.

Chronic Strains as Stressors

The second major type of stressor involves the relatively enduring problems, conflicts, and threats that many people face in their daily lives. The very number and diversity of this type of stressor and the formidable measurement problems that they entail are among the reasons why life event inventories, by comparison, are so inviting a research tool. One way in which sociologists can gain some conceptual control over the extensive array of potential chronic stressors is to focus their attention on problems that arise within the boundaries of major social roles and role sets. As I argued above, problems rooted in institutionalized social roles are often enduring, for the activities and the interpersonal relationships they entail are enduring. Moreover, when problems—or strains, as I refer to them—occur within roles, they are likely to affect their incumbents, because typically we attach considerable importance to our major roles. Difficulties in job, marriage, or parenthood have important effects because the roles themselves are important. Furthermore, the focus on role strains can reinforce the links between the contexts that largely structure people's activities, relationships, and experiences, and their well-being.

Several types of role strain were assessed in our earlier work (Pearlin, 1983; Pearlin & Schooler, 1978); only a brief review of those types is presented here. One type is *role overload,* a condition that exists when demands on energy and stamina exceed the individual's capacities. Role overload is found most commonly in occupational and homemaker roles as well as in specialized roles, such as among informal caregivers to seriously impaired relatives. *Interpersonal conflicts within role sets* are the type of chronic strain reported most often. This type of strain assumes many forms, but they all entail problems and difficulties that arise among those who interact with each other in sets of complementary roles, such as wife-husband, parent-child, or worker-supervisor. Still another type of strain, *inter-role conflict,* is found at the juncture of different roles. It entails the incompatible demands of multiple roles, especially demands of work and family. Commonly individuals cannot satisfy the demands and expectations of one of these roles without forsaking those of the other. A different strain involves *role captivity,* which exists when one is an unwilling incumbent of a role. People experiencing this type of strain include housewives or retirees who would prefer outside employment or employed workers who would prefer to be at home with young children. The roles that these people occupy might not be onerous or filled with conflict; the people simply prefer to be and to do things outside the confines of the unwanted role.

Finally, *role restructuring* is an important but overlooked type of strain that certainly deserves more attention. It is virtually inevitable that relationships in role sets undergo change. Although the actors and the role sets remain the same, either the aging process or extraneous exigencies force alterations in long-established patterns of expectation and interaction. This phenomenon can be observed in a variety of situations, such as the rebellious adolescent who complains that he is treated as a baby, the apprentice who grows restless with his mentor as he masters his craft, or adult children who must assume increasing responsibility for the care of aged parents. Often the restructuring of entrenched relationships is not easy; it can result in a sense of betrayal, status loss, and the violation of expectations. These kinds of strains may develop insidiously and may persist until people readjust to the new expectations and norms governing the relationships.

Not all severe strains are found within major roles. Living in or close to poverty, residing in neighborhoods where there is reason to fear crime or violence, and having a serious chronic illness are among the *ambient strains* that cut across roles and envelop people. Still other strains may arise in more informal and elective roles, such as in voluntary activities and associations or in dealing with friends and acquaintances. Thus the strains that people experience in their institutionalized roles by no means represent all chronic stressors.

The Convergence of Events and Chronic Strains

Even if it were possible to overcome the difficulties in measuring and assessing both life events and chronic strains, our research still would be encumbered by conceptual blinders. A serious limitation of inquiry into stressors is the tendency toward "either-or" thinking. In searching for stressors, we usually focus either on life events or on chronic strains. As a result of this unwitting tendency we have missed opportunities to observe the ways in which events and strains converge in people's lives. There are at least three ways in which events and strains come together in stressful experience: (1) events lead to chronic strains; (2) chronic strains lead to events; and (3) strains and events provide meaning contexts for each other.

Consider first the capability of events to cause strains. Studies of events typically examine the events as direct causes of stress in individuals. Yet events also cause stress in an indirect manner by altering adversely the more enveloping and enduring life conditions. These conditions, in turn, become potent sources of stress in their own right—perhaps more potent than the precipitating event. This process, in which events adversely restructure social and economic conditions of life, has been demonstrated empirically for at least three events: involuntary job loss (Pearlin, Lieberman, Menagham, & Mullan, 1981), divorce (Pearlin & Johnson, 1977), and death of spouse (Pearlin & Lieberman, 1978). These events commonly result in such circumstances as increased economic hardship, heightened interpersonal conflict, or greater social isolation. These kinds of circumstances, in turn, may be stronger antecedents of stress than the events that helped to create the circumstances.

Just as stressful chronic problems may be created by events, stressful events can be triggered by persisting problems. As I argued earlier, research into events usually does not separate the events from the strains that might have preceded them. Consequently there has been little study examining how enduring strains give rise to events. Some scattered evidence, however, suggests that this situation occurs. We know, for example, that continued marital conflict can result in separation and divorce (Menaghan, 1982). Indeed, it is reasonable to speculate that in general, prolonged interpersonal conflict can precipitate events which mark the disruption of or withdrawal from the troubled relationships.

In the third way in which events and strains converge in stressful experience, each provides the meaning context for the other. Thus the nature of relevant conditions preceding the event may influence whether or not an event is experienced as stressful. It would be a mistake, for example, to assume that divorce is uniformly stressful without considering whether the couple's prior marital life was characterized solely by strife and frustration or whether it also contained fulfillment and satisfaction. Indeed, Wheaton (1988) shows that the intensity of the strains experienced in roles tends to govern the levels of stress that follow transitions out of the roles. Depending on prior circumstances, the same transitional events might be experienced either as liberating or as depriving. Moreover, just as *preceding* conditions color the meaning and the impact of the event, *consequent* conditions also may regulate the impact of the event. Retirement, for example, might have a negative effect on well-being if the retirement results in a loss of status or the atrophying of prized skills; it might have a positive effect if one finds in retirement the opportunity to pursue self-fulfilling passions that previously had been held in abeyance.

Events, then, typically do not stand as stressors separate from the durable stains that people experience, nor do the strains necessarily persist apart from the events they may precipitate. Events and strains often flow together in people's experiences, although researchers might see them as separate and unrelated. Events can create stressful strains; strains can precipitate stressful events; and events and strains each constitute the contexts that shape the meanings and the stressful effects of the other. Merely correlating events or strains with health outcomes fails to capture an accurate picture of an ante-cedent process that often involves a dynamic connection between events and relatively durable strains.

Primary and Secondary Stressors

Underlying the above discussion is the assumption that significant stressors rarely, if ever, occur singly. If people are exposed to one serious stressor, it is very likely that they will be exposed to others as well. One event leads to another event or triggers chronic strains; strains, for their part, beget other strains or events. Thus clusters of stressors may develop, each cluster made up of a variety of events and strains. Furthermore, the clustered stressors may be formed by problems that originated in different institutionalized roles (Wheaton, in press): job loss may engender economic strains, occu-pational strains may create marital strains, and so on. It is reasonable that stressors should proliferate and diffuse within and across institutional lines, because the multiple sectors of people's lives are interrelated such that dis-ruptions in one sector are likely to cause disruptions in others. Moreover, the stressors experienced by one individual often become problems for others who share the same role sets. Thus a married person who is in a difficult work situation probably has a spouse who is under stress as a consequence (Pearlin & McCall, in press).

For the sociological stress researcher, the multiplication and the contagion of stressors means that studies must cast a wide net to capture the full array of stressors that are present in an individual's life. If we fail to discern all the appreciable stressors that are contemporaneous, we also will fail to interpret correctly the outcomes that we observe. Suppose, for example, we wished to study the relationship between serious physical injury and depression. Our inquiry would be incomplete, if not misleading, if we assumed that the injury was the only stressor present; in such a case we would ignore possible concomitant economic, occupational, family, and social problems. Variations in depression thus reflect not only the seriousness of the injury itself but also variations in the clustering of stressors. It is not an event or a strain that mer-its the sociologist's attention, but how the *organization of people's lives* may be disrupted in the stress process.

One step toward bringing this organization into view is to distinguish *primary* and *secondary* stressors. Primary stressors are those that are likely to occur first in people's experience. The stressor may be an event, especially one that is undesired and eruptive, such as the untimely death of a loved one, involuntary job loss, or injury; or it could be a more enduring or repeated stressor, such as those experienced in marriage or occupation. Whereas pri-mary stressors can be conceptualized as occurring first in experience, sec-ondary stressors come about as a consequence of the primary stressors. I do not refer to them as secondary because they are less potent than the pri-mary stressors. On the contrary, once established, secondary stressors inde-pendently may become capable of producing even more intense stress than those we consider to be primary. They are secondary only on the basis of their presumed order in the stress process, not on the basis of their importance to the process.

Examples of secondary stressors resulting from more primary stressors may be drawn from our current studies of specialized caregiving roles, those involving the care of impaired relatives or friends (Pearlin, Semple, & Turner, 1988; Pearlin, Turner, & Semple, 1989). Informal caregiving to impaired people is an extreme instance of role restructuring: usually it occurs within established relationships, and when impairment is severe, prolonged, and progressive, the caregiving comes to dominate the interactions between actors whose previous relationships were organized in a very different way. A number of primary stressors, those involved directly in providing care to the impaired person, can be observed. They include the vigilance that may be required to monitor and control the patient, the psychological losses that accumulate with the patient's continued deterioration, and exhaustion and overload. Several secondary stressors stem from these primary problems. For example, increased conflict with others is quite common, as when the caregiver feels abandoned by family members. Caregivers holding outside jobs may find themselves unable to devote themselves fully to one activity without neglecting the requirements of the other. Economic strain arising from diminished income or increased expenditure is another frequently observed secondary stressors, as are the losses of desired social relationships and activities outside the caregiving situation. Once set in motion, these secondary stressors produce their own stressful outcomes.

These examples are intended to illuminate pivotal point: important life problems, whether in the form of events or of durable strains, do not exist in isolation from other problems. The very integration of individuals' activities and relationships means that disruptions in one area of their lives serve to create other disruptions. Therefore sociological stress researchers cannot confine their attention to a single event or to groups of events, nor can they examine only one role strain on the assumption that it is the only problem or the most important problem faced by the individual. Instead, the presence and the organization of constellations of stressors need to be discerned and measured independently. The discernment of this organization, in turn, may be enhanced by distinguishing primary and secondary stressors. This distinction will help to discriminate between people who may be similar with regard to their exposure to one stressor but who differ appreciably with regard to the array of stressors to which they are exposed. Such discrimination can go far in explaining why people who seem to be alike with regard to the problems that they face differ sharply with regard to the intensity and range of the stress outcomes that they manifest. People who are treated analytically as similar may, in fact, be different.

I would like to raise a final issue with regard to the identification and specification of stressors; this issue concerns values. As I have emphasized, a central task of research into stress is to explain why individuals exposed to stressor conditions that appear to be similar do not necessarily suffer the same outcomes. Part of this explanation lies in social values. By values I refer to what is defined socially as good, desirable, and prized or as something to be eschewed (Williams, 1960, pp. 397–470). Although the importance of values to stress research has been recognized (Lazarus & Folkman, 1984, pp. 77–81), their part in the stress process has not yet been examined systematically. Values, I believe, regulate the effects of experience by regulating the meaning and the importance of the experience (Pearlin, 1988).

To understand the role of values in regulating the impact of stressors, one must understand that conditions are stressful when they are threatening. I use "threat" in the broadest sense to include reactions to such disparate constructs as loss, unfulfilled needs, violation of self-image, and blocked aspirations. Some conditions may be intrinsically threatening, as when one's life is at stake. More often, however, the threat that people experience from the circumstances they face depends to some degree on the values they hold—that is, on what they define as important, desirable, or to be cherished. An example can be provided from a study that showed that marital partners from unequal status backgrounds also tended to have higher levels of marital stress (Pearlin, 1975). Further analytic probing revealed that these inequalities were related to stress primarily among people who held certain status values. Specifically, hypogamous people—those who "married down"—were particularly vulnerable to marital stress, but only when they valued status enhancement and upward mobility. Others who also had married down but who were not status strivers were unaffected by their hypogamous marriage. Thus the cause of stress was neither a structural arrangement alone nor a value alone but a particular combination of the two.

The careful study of stressors, then, should provide the researcher with an opportunity to learn something about social life as it bears on individual functioning. The sociological study of stressors can reveal the connections between social organization and the organization of lives. To find these connections, however, we cannot treat stress as stemming from unconnected happenings. Instead the antecedents of stress need to be understood in terms of process, whereby broad structured and institutional forces, constellations of primary and secondary stressors, and widely shared values converge over time to affect people's well-being. Most certainly, the sociological study of social stress does not rely on predictive models. We must guide our effort not simply by identifying and adding together all factors that might contribute to the variance of an outcome but also by asking how and why these contributions come about. Prediction alone does not make us wiser sociologists; for that purpose we need also to be good explainers and interpreters.

THE MEDIATORS AND THEIR INTERVENTIONS

I have already suggested two explanations for the fact that the same stressors do not necessarily lead to the same stressful outcomes: different configurations of unobserved stressors may surround the observed stressor, or different values may endow the same stressor with different meanings. Yet by far the largest responsibility for explaining outcome differences has been placed on constructs that I refer to collectively as mediators. They are mediators in the sense that they have been shown to govern (or mediate) the effects of stressors on stress outcomes. Coping and social support have received the most attention in the research literature; for this reason I shall confine my attention to these mediators. Other constructs, however, also have been cast analytically as mediators; in particular these include the self-concepts of self-esteem and mastery (Pearlin & Schooler, 1978). These aspects of self represent personal resources and appear to serve as appreciable barriers to the stressful effects of difficult life conditions.

Although coping and social support certainly intersect, they are quite distinct; each has its own conceptual problems. Briefly and selectively I shall point out some of these problems. Then I shall consider strategies for evaluating mediating effects within the stress process.

Coping

Coping refers to the actions that people take in their own behalf as they attempt to avoid or lessen the impact of life problems (Pearlin & Schooler, 1978). Although coping refers to individuals' actions and perceptions, it is of sociological interest because important elements of coping may be learned from one's membership and reference groups in the same ways as other behaviors are learned and internalized. Because interest in coping was rooted initially in clinical concerns, researchers tend to think of a person's coping repertoire as representing a clinical profile unique to the individual and to ignore the shared, normative basis of individual coping. Although aspects of one's coping indeed may be unique, it is likely that people who interact with each other and who share important life circumstances will also share coping behaviors. Consequently part of the sociologists' research agenda should be aimed at identifying the associations between people's social and economic circumstances and their coping repertoires.

Is coping a set of general dispositions activated when one is faced with threatening problems, or does it consist of more specific responses invoked selectively in dealing with specific kinds of problems? From a personality perspective, coping may be seen as a tendency to react in characteristic ways to threat, regardless of the nature of the threat or the context in which it arises. It is distinctly possible that there are general coping dispositions which cut across different situations. Perhaps, for example, people who engage in denial in one situation will do the same in a very different situation. Yet the sociologist finds it difficult to accept the notion that people cope with retirement from the job, for example, in the same way as with being fired from the job, or with conflict with one's boss in the same way as with conflict with one's child. There is simply no reason to assume that coping will be the same regardless of the nature of the impinging stressors, the institutional contexts in which they occur, or the relationships they might involve.

Individuals have personalities that retain their integrity from one situation to another. Yet the coping responses that mediate the stressful impact of one situation may be entirely inappropriate to another. Therefore the researcher who is sensitive to the social and contextual origins of stressors also must be sensitive to the situation-specific character of coping.

Even so, the *functions* of coping are essentially the same in all situations, although the *forms* of coping might vary from one situation to another. As we described in detail elsewhere (Pearlin & Schooler, 1978), all coping—regardless of the nature of the stressors—serves either to *change the situation* from which the stressors arise, to *manage the meaning* of the situation in a manner that reduces its threat, or to *keep the symptoms of stress within manageable bounds*. Therefore we possess a conceptual framework for the study of coping that has general application, even though the behavioral elements of coping are more specific to the particular stressor that is being experienced and vary with that stressor (Pearlin & Aneshenselm 1986).

Social Support

It would appear that among the major mediating constructs, social support should have the clearest and best established theoretical links to social theory. Somewhat surprisingly, however, this is not the case. Perhaps one reason is that sociologists who are interested in social networks tend not to be the same as those working in stress and social support. Networks refer more directly than supports to the structure of people's social attachments. These attachments, of course, differ in extensiveness and composition for different groups in the society. As Lin and his colleagues describe (Lin, Dean, & Ensel, 1986, pp. 17–30, 53–70), most people's attachments include some mix of formal and informal, primary and secondary, and strong and weak ties; some attachments exist with friends and others with relatives; some involve frequent face-to-face interaction and others do not. The organization of one's social network mirrors the organization of one's engagement with the larger society.

Whereas the social network can be regarded as the totality of the social resources on which one potentially may draw, social support represents the resources that one actually uses in dealing with life problems (Pearlin, 1985). In most instances, of course, one's sources of support in dealing with any given stressor will be much more restricted than one's total network. Consequently stress researchers tend to ignore network and its structure and to deal only with support as it is perceived by the individual. Certainly there is nothing wrong with data that bear on perceived support; studies indicate that perceived support indeed has a mediating function in the stress process (Turner, 1983). Yet, when the study of perceived support is separated from the study of networks, we are unable to see how individuals' support is associated with their integration into various social institutions and contexts. The identification of the connections between individuals' social life and their inner well-being could be enhanced, I submit, by joining the study of social support more closely to the study of social networks.

Aside from its separation from network, the study of support lacks sociological substance for still another reason: typically it considers only the recipient of support and ignores the donors of support and their interactions with the recipient (Pearlin, 1985; Pearlin & McCall, in press). A construct that is inherently interactional is treated instead as an individual attribute. When the social and interactional nature of social support is ignored, we are left with an incomplete, if not distorted, picture of how it functions. The forms of support, its reciprocity, the connections between seeking and receiving support, its stability, and even whether or not it is welcomed depend not on the recipient alone but on the donor-recipient relationship.

Supporting relationships are found in virtually all institutional and social contexts: religion, occupation, family, neighborhood, voluntary associations, the medical care system, and elsewhere. Just as the forms and functions of support may vary with the nature of the relationship from which support is drawn, there is some evidence (House, 1981) that the effect of support is constrained or enhanced by the context in which the relationships exist. Thus we need to learn more both about the interactional aspects of support and about the effects of social contexts on its forms, functions, and efficacy. Sociologists should be foremost among the contributors to this research.

How Do Mediators Mediate?

The very words "coping" and "social support" contain implicit consequences. Once a behavior is labeled as coping, we assume that it succeeds in relieving stress; if someone is labeled as the recipient of support, he is perforce supported. These assumed beneficial consequences, inherent in the very language we use to refer to stress mediators, inadvertently may have diverted us from asking whether in fact the mediators do mediate, and, if so, how. At any rate, insufficient effort has been devoted to evaluating the efficacy of the mediators, especially in the case of coping.

In raising this issue here, I am concerned less with the methodology of determining how much difference the mediators make than with where to look for these differences. In this regard it is useful to recall that stressful situations may contain constellations of primary and secondary stressors. Moreover, each type of stressor may contain multiple subtypes of stressors. This conceptualization of the stress process suggests ways to search for the effects of coping and social support that currently are not recognized. Specifically, we should expand our assessments of efficacy to include the ability of the mediators to inhibit the scope and severity both of the primary stressors and of the secondary stressors that follow. To whatever extent the mediators succeed in constraining the intensity, number, and diffusion of stressors, they also must succeed eventually in constraining the extent and intensity of stress outcomes. These *indirect* effects of the mediators may be every bit as instrumental in minimizing stress outcomes as the *direct* effects to which attention usually is limited.

The evaluation of indirect effects of mediators should help further to illuminate the question that now has been raised at several points of this paper:

What accounts for variations in the outcomes of stressful life conditions? Our understanding of the variability of stress outcomes will be enhanced by observing how coping and social support affect each step of the process that precedes the outcomes. If we confine our assessment of the mediators solely to their direct effects on outcomes, we will not be able to detect their important indirect effects, those which are exercised through their regulation of antecedent conditions.

OUTCOMES

Outcomes refer to the manifestations of organismic stress. Many manifestations exist, and they are found at multiple levels of organismic functioning. Indeed, the multiplicity of stress indicators has led some researchers to question whether the very notion of stress is useful (Elliott & Eisdorfer, 1982). A construct that subsumes such diverse (although presumably related) phenomena as the immunological and endocrine systems, the digestive and cardiovascular systems, anxiety, depression, and mental health—to name just a few—is bound to create confusion. The confusion is compounded understandably by the fact that several disciplines have developed their own distinctive approaches to the study of stress and its indicators. Yet despite its ambiguity, the notion of stress provides a framework sufficiently flexible to encompass the broad and diverse range of constructs found in sociological studies of stress and health. Thus for sociologists, an attractive feature of the stress concept is its ability to absorb the far-reaching notion of inseparability between the circumstances of social life and individual functioning.

What outcomes should be considered in sociological research into stress? Understandably, the answer to this query is based on the kinds of data to which sociologists have ready access as well as on their theoretical perspectives. For example, sociologists typically do not look at endocrine secretions or at the immunological system because they possess neither the skills nor the facilities to do so without the costly collaboration of others. Instead we usually examine outcomes that can be assessed through direct observation, medical records, or self-evaluations and reports. Examples of stress indicators found in sociological studies include health histories, symptoms of physical health, symptom scales measuring a variety of dimensions of mental health, the abuse of alcohol or of mindaltering drugs, inability to fulfill role obligations, and the disruption of social relationships. None of these outcomes has a compelling theoretical priority over the others, but there may be a theoretically compelling reason to avoid reliance on a single outcome in assessing the stressfulness of social conditions.

The observation of multiple outcomes is highly desirable because people having different social and economic characteristics also may have different modes of manifesting stress. As a result, we run the risk of seriously misjudging the effects of difficult life circumstances if we judge effect only on the basis of a single outcome. Gender differences again provide a telling illustration. It has been shown repeatedly that women more than men are host to depressive symptoms and emotional distress. In turn, this finding has led to speculation that women may be more vulnerable than men to certain stressful circumstances, such as network losses (e.g., Kessler & McLeod, 1984). Yet before we can accept the assumption of vulnerability, we must be sure that we have considered a full range of relevant outcomes. Perhaps men and women do not differ in their overall vulnerability to stressors, but differ instead with regard to the particular outcomes to which they are vulnerable. This warning emerges from the work of Aneshensel (1988), who showed that apparent gender differences in vulnerability to the impact of events disappear when excessive drinking and other outcomes are considered along with depression. That is, the stressful events are no less harmful for men than for women, a fact that was obscured when only depression was examined. We must keep in mind that structurally demarcated groups may manifest stress in different ways. Unless multiple outcomes are considered, we can mistakenly exaggerate the vulnerability of some groups while underestimating at the same time the general impact of the stressors under examination.

SUMMARY AND DISCUSSION

In this paper I have not sought to lay out steps to be followed; rather, I have attempted to raise issues to be considered in the sociological study of stress. The overarching strategy of social research into stress is the identification of the many links that join forms of social organization to individual stress. I have suggested a number of conceptual and analytic perspectives that I believe will enable us to advance this agenda. One crucial element is the examination of statuses and other background circumstances at each step of the stress process. We need to know how these social factors bear on the kinds of stressors to which people are exposed, the personal and social resources to which people have access, and the emotional, behavioral, and physical disorders through which stress is manifested. This proposal contains nothing new; it deserves emphasis only because researchers tend either to limit the analyses of social background factors or to relegate them to serving as controls through which the independent effects of other conditions are established. Yet the sociological stake in stress research requires the careful and comprehensive analysis of information about the structural contexts of people's lives.

Many important life experiences, some of them stressful, are rooted in these contexts. Stressful experiences may take on different forms and configurations and it is unlikely that they can be fully captured by examining either life events or life strains separately and apart from each other. Over time, stressors typically surface as groups or constellations of stressors, some primary and others secondary, that blend events with more durable strains. This is a useful way to look at the antecedent process, and is consistent with available empirical evidence. It seeks stressors in the organization of lives and in the structure of experience rather than among unrelated "risk factors."

One of the analytic tasks of the stress researcher is to explain variations in stress outcomes. First, some of the variation in outcomes is to be found in the constellations of stressors. When we observe events and strains singly while ignoring broader clusters of primary and secondary stressors, we may incorrectly assume more similarity in exposure to stressful experience than actually exists. In other words, part of the unexplained variations in outcomes may be due to relevant stressors that are not being observed and whose effects therefore cannot be assessed.

Second, even though we have probably relied too heavily on the explanatory power of coping and support, nevertheless we may systematically have underestimated their mediating effects. We cannot appreciate the full capacity of these mediators until we examine their effects in limiting the number and severity of primary and secondary stressors. These are the indirect effects which soften stress outcomes but which are not in view when we concern ourselves only with the direct effects of the mediators on outcomes.

Finally, some of the difficulty, encountered in analytically explaining variations in outcomes lies with the range of outcomes selected for study. Focusing exclusively on a single outcome, such as depression, may lead to the mistaken conclusion that some groups of people are affected adversely by stressors that leave others unaffected. These putative variations in vulnerability, however, may be an artifact of the ways in which different social and economic groups channel and manifest stress. Consequently the inclusion of a reasonable range of outcomes should prevent us from making inappropriate assumptions of differential vulnerability to common stressors.

However one thinks of the stress process, it obviously consists of multiple conceptual components; each component potentially has multiple aspects or dimensions. The richness and the complexity of the process invite us to phrase research questions in very different ways. One study, for example, may be concerned mainly with the epidemiological distribution of depression; another may have as its central question the buffering effects of social support on depression; a third might seek to evaluate the effects of a particular event or role strain on depression. Each question places a somewhat different set of issues at the center of its interests. Although the questions may generate overlapping data, the data essentially serve different research goals.

When studies start with questions about the parts played across the stress process by the social and economic arrangements in which people's lives are embedded, they produce knowledge that has a distinctive emphasis. Although studies of this type share with other approaches an interest in individuals' well-being, they also help to illuminate those aspects of social organization which pertain particularly to the differential exposure to and meaning of stressors, to differences in the various kinds of resources that people can mobilize in responding to stressful circumstances, and, finally, to differences in the manifestation of stress. The sociological study of stress, I believe, can contribute uniquely both to an understanding of social life and to an understanding of how the fates of individuals come to be bound to it.

References

Aneshensel, Carol S. 1988. "Disjunctures between Public Health and Medical Models." Paper presented at the meetings of the American Public Health Association, Boston.

Elliott, Glenn R. and Carl Eisdorfer. 1982. "Conceptual Issues in Stress Research." Pp. 11–45 in *Stress and Human Health*, edited by G.R. Elliott and C. Eisdorfer. New York: Springer.

Fairbank, Dianne T. and Richard L. Hough. 1979. "Life Events Classification and the Event-Illness Relationship." *Journal of Health and Social Behavior* 19:41–7.

Gersten, Joanne C., Thomas S. Langner, Jeanne G. Eisenberg, and Ora Simcha-Hogan. 1977. "An Evaluation of the Etiologic Role of Stressful Life-Change Events in Psychological Disorders." *Journal of Health and Social Behavior* 18:228–44.

Holmes, Thomas H. and Richard H. Rahe. 1967. "The Social Readjustment Rating Scale." *Journal of Psychosomatic Research* 11:213–18.

James S. House. 1981. *Work Stress and Social Support*. Reading, MA: Addision Wesley.

Kessler, Ronald C. and Jane D. McLeod. 1984. "Sex Differences in Vulnerability to Undesirable Life Events." *American Sociological Review* 49:620–31.

Lazarus, Richard S. and Susan Folkman. 1984. *Stress, Appraisal and Coping*. New York: Springer.

Lin, Nan, Alfred Dean, and Walter Ensel. 1986. *Social Support, Life Events, and Depression*. Orlando, FL: Orlando Academic Press.

Menaghan, Elizabeth G. 1982. "Assessing the Impact of Family Transition on Marital Experience." Pp. 90–108 in *Family Stress, Coping and Social Support*, edited by H.I. McCubbin, A.E. Cauble, and J.M. Patterson. Springfield, IL: Thomas.

Pearlin, Leonard I. 1975. "Status Inequality and Stress in Marriage." *American Sociological Review* 40: 344–57.

———. 1982. "The Social Contexts of Stress." Pp. 367–79 in *Handbook of Stress*, edited by L. Goldberger and S. Breznitz. New York: Free Press.

———. 1983. "Role Strains and Personal Stress." Pp. 3–32 in *Psychosocial Stress: Trends in Theory and Research*, edited by Howard B. Kaplan. New York: Academic Press.

———. 1985. "Social Process and Social Supports." Pp. 43–60 in *Social Support and Health*, edited by Sheldon Cohen and Leonard Syme. New York: Academic Press.

———. 1988. "Social Structure and Social Values; The Regulation of Structural Effects." Pp. 252–64 in *Surveying Social Life*, edited by Hubert O'Gorman. Middletown, CT: Wesleyan University Press.

Pearlin, Leonard I. and Carol Aneshensel. 1986. "Coping and Social Supports: Their Functions and Applications." Pp. 53–74, *Applications of Social Science to Clinical Medicine and Health*, edited by L.H. Aiken and D. Mechanic. New Brunswick, NJ: Rutgers University Press.

Pearlin, Leonard I. and Joyce S. Johnson. 1977. "Marital Status, Life Strains and Depression." *American Sociological Review* 42:704–15.

Pearlin, Leonard I. and Morton A. Lieberman. 1978. "Social Sources of Emotional Distress." Pp. 217–48 in *Research in Community and Mental Health*. Vol. 1. edited by R. Simmons. Greenwich, CT: JAI.

Pearlin, Leonard I. and Mary McCall. In press. "Occupational Problems and Marital Support." In *The Transmission of Stress Between Work and Family*, edited by J. Eckenrode and S. Gore. New York: Plenum.

Pearlin, Leonard I. and Carmi Schooler. 1978. "The Structure of Coping." *Journal of Health and Social Behavior* 19:2–21.

Pearlin, Leonard I., Shirley Semple, and Heather Turner. 1988. "Stress of AIDS Caregiving." *Death Studies* 12:501–17.

Pearlin, Leonard I., Heather Turner, and Shirley Semple. 1989. "Coping and the Mediation of Caregiver Stress." In *Alzheimer's Disease Treatment and Family Stress: Directions for Research,* edited by E. Light and B. Liebowitz. Washington, DC: National Institute of Mental Health.

Pearlin, Leonard I., Morton Lieberman, Elizabeth Menaghan, and Joseph Mullan. 1981. "The Stress Process." *Journal of Health and Social Behavior* 22:337–56.

Selye, Hans. 1982. "History and Present Status of the Stress Concept." Pp. 7–17 in *Handbook of Stress,* edited by L. Goldberger and S. Breznitz. New York: Free Press.

Thoits, Peggy A. 1981. "Undesirable Life Events and Psychophysiological Distress: A Problem of Operational Confounding." *American Sociological Review* 46:97–109.

———. 1983. "Dimensions of Life Events That Influence Psychological Distress: An Evaluation and Synthesis of the Literature." Pp. 33–103 in *Psychosocial Stress,* edited by H.B. Kaplan. New York: Academic Press.

Turner, R. Jay. 1983. "Direct, Indirect and Moderating Effects of Social Support on Psychological Distress and Associated Conditions." Pp. 105–55 in *Psychosocial Stress,* edited by H.B. Kaplan. New York: Academic Press.

Vinokur, Amiram and Melvin L. Seltzer. 1975. "Desirable versus Undesirable Life Events: Their Relationship to Stress and Mental Distress." *Journal of Personality and Social Psychology* 32:329–37.

Wheaton, Blair. 1988. "Life Transitions, Prior Role Problems and Mental Health: Where More Stress Is Stress Relief." Paper presented at meetings of the American Sociological Association, Atlanta.

———. In press. "Where Work and Family Meet: Stress across Social Roles." In *The Transmission of Stress between Work and Family,* edited by J. Eckenrode and S. Gore. Plenum.

Williams, Robin. 1960. *American Society.* New York: Knopf.

DISCUSSION QUESTIONS

1. What are the major components of the stress process model? Draw a visual representation that illustrates the relationships among these components.

2. How does Pearlin characterize the unique contributions of sociology to the study of stress? In what ways is his characterization similar to and different from Aneshensel's?

3. Apply Pearlin's model to a recent stressful experience you have had. What were the primary and secondary stressors? How did you cope? Did you receive support or assistance from others and, if so, how helpful was it? How did the stressful experience affect you in the short run? In the long run?

Peggy A. Thoits

Multiple Identities and Psychological Well-Being: A Reformulation and Test of the Social Isolation Hypothesis[†]

In this classic article, Peggy A. Thoits develops and tests an influential hypothesis about how and why role involvements affect mental health—the identity accumulation hypothesis. In addition to its substantive contributions to research on the social origins of mental health problems, Thoits' article serves as a model of systematic research into the validity of theoretically-derived hypotheses.

Of the several hypotheses which relate social conditions to mental disorder, the social isolation hypothesis has remained moderately popular since its initial statement by Robert Faris in 1934. Faris suggested with respect to schizophrenia that "any form of isolation that cuts the person off from intimate social relations for an extended period of time may possibly lead to this form of mental disorder" (1934: 157).

In a critical review, Clausen and Kohn (1954) raised several questions about the hypothesis: "What constitutes *sufficient* attenuation of interpersonal relationships to be called 'isolation'?...What [are] the distinguishable types of isolating experiences?...What are the differential consequences of attenuated social relationships in different situational contexts and for different temperamental types?...At what period or periods in the individual's life does the experience of isolation have the greatest effect?...Finally,...is isolation a symptom of already-developing illness; is it an essential condition for the subsequent development of illness; or is it, possibly, both symptomatic of the beginning of the illness and a cause of its further development?" (Clausen & Kohn, 1954, 145–46). As originally formulated, the isolation hypothesis does not adequately address these issues.

To address these questions, this paper attempts a reformulation of the hypothesis. This reformulation, termed the *identity accumulation hypothesis*, is then tested using individual-level data from the New Haven community survey (Myers et al., 1971). Finally, the implications of the identity accumulation hypothesis for current theory on the advantages of multiple roles are discussed and further directions for study are outlined.

Thoits, Peggy A. 1983. "Multiple Identities and Psychological Well-Being: A Reformulation and Test of the Social Isolation Hypothesis." *American Sociological Review* 48:174–187.

IDENTITY AND PSYCHOLOGICAL WELL-BEING

Faris's hypothesis was based in the symbolic interactionist tradition. Symbolic interactionism assumes that social interaction is essential to normal personality development and to appropriate social conduct. Interaction produces the social self, that part of the personality which links the individual to society and is an important intervening variable in human behavior. In particular, Mead (1934) described the process through which self-conceptions develop in interaction. The individual acquires a view of him/herself as an objective and meaningful social entity by taking the role of specific and then of generalized others.

For this paper, the process of taking the role of the generalized other has two important implications. First, it implies that the individual develops an awareness and an acceptance of the social positions he/she occupies in the community and larger society. Second, it suggests that the developed self must be a complex, semipermanent, organized structure.

In taking the role of the generalized other, the individual perceives that he/she has been placed by others into recognized and meaningful social categories, or social positions. Social positions are locations within systems of relationships (Linton, 1936; Merton, 1957). Attached to positions are sets of behavioral expectations, i.e., roles. Social positions are usually enacted in an array of reciprocal role relationships, what Merton terms the role-set (1957). When the individual assigns to him/herself the same positional designations and behaves as expected in role relationships with others, he/she can be said to have taken on a set of identities (Stryker, 1980; Stryker & Serpe, 1982, 1983). Consistent with Stryker, the self is conceptualized here as a set of discrete identities—self-definitions in terms of occupied social positions.

How is psychological well-being related to this multiple self? The key lies in identity enactment.

Identities are claimed and sustained in reciprocal role relationships. Role relationships are governed by behavioral expectations; the rights and duties of each interactant are normatively prescribed. Thus, *if one knows who one is (in a social sense), then one knows how to behave.* Role requirements give purpose, meaning, direction, and guidance to one's life. The greater the number of identities held, the stronger one's sense of meaningful, guided existence. The more identities, the more "existential security," so to speak. A sense of meaningful existence and purposeful, ordered behavior are crucial to psychological health, as many authors have pointed out, either explicitly or implicitly (cf. Frankl, 1959; Rose, 1962; Sarbin, 1968; Bart, 1974; Sieber, 1974). For example, Sieber has made a similar argument with regard to the benefits of role accumulation: "status and role alternatives afford a sense of *general status security*" (1974, 574, emphasis added). Multiple roles may produce "ego-gratification, namely, the sense of being appreciated or needed by diverse role partners" (Sieber, 1974, 576). Rose (1962, 539) describes the reverse case: "A depreciated or 'mutilated' self is a major factor in the development of a neurosis,...because an individual's ability to accept strongly held values of any kind and to act effectively to achieve those values is a function of his conception of himself." In other words, if one does not know who one is (in a social sense), or if one loses a valued identity, then one simply does not know how to behave. Not only may a profound sense of anxiety or depression be experienced, but severely disorganized behavior may result. In short, identity accumulation should enhance psychological well-being, and identity lack or loss should impair it. The direct relationship between identity accumulation and psychological well-being is termed here the "identity accumulation hypothesis."

A word is required at this point regarding role strain and role conflict. It has long been assumed that role strain and role conflict are normal consequences of multiple identities (Merton, 1957; Goode, 1960; Sarbin & Allen, 1968). Sieber (1974) points out that researchers and theorists have disregarded possible rewards from role accumulation, which may far outweigh tensions due to strain and conflict. He identifies several types of rewards: privileges, resources manipulable for further status enhancement, a sense of general status security, and ego-gratification (feelings of personal worth). Privileges and resources may be used to free the individual from constraining or overwhelming demands and to increase prestige, while sheer occupancy of multiple positions may enhance general feelings of security and a sense of personal worth, and buffer the effects of identity loss. However, it is possible that the relationship between multiple identities and well-being may not be additive but curvilinear. Beyond some optimal number of identities, role strains and conflicting demands may undermine the sense of orderly, purposeful existence and thereby decrease psychological well-being. This is an important question to explore empirically and will be attempted in the analysis to follow. An additive process will be described here, for simplicity in presentation.

Evidence which bears directly on the identity accumulation hypothesis is difficult to find. Indirect evidence is provided by studies of the incidence and prevalence of mental illness. Those who hold few social identities—the unmarried, the unemployed, the retired, housewives, those who live alone—have a greater risk of psychological disturbance than their more integrated counterparts (Gurin et al., 1960; Bradburn, 1969; Gove, 1972; Gove & Tudor, 1973; Radloff, 1975; Gove & Hughes, 1980). More directly, several studies show that small social networks and the lack of intimate relationships with a spouse or other primary group members are associated with the development of depression, more serious mental illness, or even death (Lowenthal, 1964; Miller & Ingham, 1976; Henderson et al., 1978; Roy, 1978; Berkman & Syme, 1979; Mueller, 1980). Furthermore, the death of a spouse (e.g., Clayton et al., 1972), social "exits" (Paykel, 1974), and significant role losses (Bart, 1974; Glassner et al., 1979) have proved more common in the lives of psychiatric patients prior to onset of illness compared to controls. Other studies of "major life events" (such as divorce, graduation, marriage, the start of a job) at least indirectly support the identity accumulation hypothesis. The majority of items listed on life events scales involve losses or gains of important social positions (Thoits, 1978, 1982): The more life events experienced, particularly undesirable life events, the more likely an individual is to become psycho-logically disturbed (Dohrenwend &Dohrenwend, 1974; Thoits, 1983).

In short, although the evidence is scattered and primarily indirect, there is support for the identity accumulation hypothesis in the literature. But further empirical testing is clearly required. Before turning to a test of the hypothesis, however, additional implications of the structure of multiple identities should be explored briefly.

IDENTITY ACCUMULATION AND COMMITMENT

Because identities are based upon role relationships that are relatively endur-ing and organized, the social self must also be a semipermanent and orga-nized structure (Rosenberg, 1979; Stryker & Serpe, 1982, 1983). But how are the various identities making up the social self organized? Stryker (1980) and Stryker & Serpe (1982, 1983) suggest that identities may be organized in a "salience hierarchy," where salience is the probability that a given identity will be invoked across a variety of situations. Salience, in turn, is determined by the amount of commitment an individual has to an identity. Commitment is "the degree to which the person's relationships to specified sets of others depends upon his or her being a particular kind of person, i.e., occupying a particular position in an organized structure of relationships and playing a particular role" (Stryker & Serpe, 1982, 207). Commitment is a function of the number, affective importance, and multiplexity (or overlap) of network ties that are formed by the person enacting an identity. In short, identities are hierarchically organized by degree of commitment, or what might be called their "network-embeddedness."

Other theorists have pointed to commitment as an ordering principle as well, but their conceptions of commitment differ somewhat from Stryker's. Multiple-role theorists (e.g., Goode, 1960; Sarbin, 1968; Coser, 1974) tradi-tionally have assumed that commitment depends upon the amount of time and energy invested in identity enactment (Marks, 1977). Underlying this assumption is a scarcity principle (Marks, 1977). The time and energy that people have available is limited; these limited resources must be differen-tially allocated among various roles. Identities are hierarchically organized, then, by the amount of time and energy committed to, or invested in, their enactment. Note that this conception of commitment differs from but is not incompatible with Stryker's. According to Stryker, the actor formulates net-work ties contingent upon certain identities. Time and energy limits may constrain those choices; extensive, intense, and multiplex ties may be initi-ated for only a few of the many identities a person sustains.

An alternative view of commitment is offered by Rosenberg (1979) and Marks (1977), who argue that commitment is a function only of the "psycho-logical centrality" or subjective importance accorded to a role or identity. Although time and energy investments generally tend to covary with the importance attached to an identity, it is possible to be highly committed to an identity but spend little time or effort enacting it (and vice versa). Thus, identities may be ordered simply by their relative subjective importance.

Interestingly, all of these theorists for the most part ignore or deemphasize an important sociological aspect of various positional identities, namely, their relative value or worth. Social positions are culturally ranked, i.e., they are differentially valued. Commitment to an identity (whether measured in network ties, invested time and energy, or subjective importance) should vary with the value or worth of the position upon which the identity is based (Goode, 1960). Cooley's (1902) looking-glass self notion is useful here. If self-evaluations depend upon the appraisals of others with whom one interacts—and a sizable body of research supports this proposition (Webster & Sobieszek, 1974)—and if others' appraisals are at least partially determined by the value of the position held (see Berger et al., 1977, for supporting evidence), then one's commitment to an identity should depend upon its degree of culturally or subculturally positive valuation. For the purposes of this discussion, then, identities making up the social self are assumed to be structured by the cultural ranking of positions held by an individual. Cultural ranking should determine the importance attached to various identities (subjective commitment), the amount of time and energy invested in each identity, and the extensiveness or complexity of network ties in which each identity is sustained (behavioral manifestations of commitment).

These considerations suggest that identities may be weighted by their cultural or subcultural rank, or by a variety of measures of subjective or behavioral commitment. Such weightings should enhance the predictiveness of the identity accumulation hypothesis and its implications for identity change. Specifically, the more valued a position, the more committed an individual will be to it, and therefore, the greater will be the psychological impact of its loss or gain.

But commitment may not be only a function of cultural or subcultural ranking. The sheer number of identities possessed by an actor should also have an effect upon identity commitment. However, this effect will differ depending upon the assumptions brought to bear upon how commitment is manifested behaviorally.

If one assumes that commitment is reflected in the amount of time and energy invested in identity enactment, and that available time and energy are naturally limited, then it is reasonable to infer that as the number of identities comprising the self increases, the individual's commitment to any one identity will decrease. On the other hand, as the number of identities decreases, commitment should increase: time and energy are available for investment. The greater the number of identities, the less the stake in any particular identity; the fewer the number of identities, the greater the stake in each one. A dramatic example of this principle is provided by the results of Zimbardo's well-known prison simulation (Haney et al., 1973; Zimbardo et al., 1973). This work demonstrates not only that identity (self-definition in terms of social position) emerges from role enactment (e.g., prisoner or guard), but that investment of time and energy is great when alternative identities are unavailable. It is important to note that high commitment to the prisoner identity in the simulation occurred despite the devalued nature of this position. Any identity, even a devalued one, provides existential security; if only one identity is available, commitment to it should be high despite its relative cultural worth.

The proposed inverse relationship between number of identities and degree of commitment has important implications for changes in psychological well-being. For ease in discussion, an actor who possesses few or no identities will be termed isolated. An actor who possesses many identities will be termed integrated.

According to the time and energy proposition, an integrated person is less committed, in general, to each of his/her identities than an isolated person. Therefore, an identity loss should have less psychological impact on the integrated actor. He/she has alternative sources of identity in which to reinvest newly released time and energy. A familiar example is the man who "loses himself in his work" after being left by his wife. The integrated individual retains social positions which make life meaningful and orderly. For the integrated, then, life's blows should be softened, or buffered, by other involvements.

The isolated individual, on the other hand, not only loses an identity to which he/she has been highly committed, but has few (perhaps no) remaining identities in which to reinvest. A familiar example is the newly widowed, traditional housewife who asks, "What have I left to live for?" For the isolated, life's blows should be magnified in impact due to the lack of other meaningful involvements.

Similar predictions may be made for the effects of identity gain. The integrated actor has less to gain from an added identity than the isolated actor; added identities should have decreasing "marginal utility" in terms of meaning and purpose. The isolated person, on the other hand, should experience significant benefit from an identity acquisition since it adds substantially to his/her purpose in life. Thus, for the integrated, the effects of identity losses and gains should be dampened somewhat, while for the isolated, both losses and gains should be amplified in impact.

However, if commitment is conceptualized in terms of network-embeddedness, a contradictory set of conditional hypotheses may be derived. Implicit in the time and energy proposition is an assumption that identities are independent of one another, i.e., that roles are segregated in time and space and that role partners do not overlap. Time and energy invested in one set of role relationships must be taken away from investment in others. Yet observation reveals that social roles are often nested within one another; the persons to whom one is attached due to being in one position are often the same as those with whom one interacts in other positions (Stryker & Serpe, 1983). For example, the overlap of individuals to whom one relates through marriage and through parenthood is usually considerable. To the degree that relationships are multiplex in nature, limited time and energy may be invested in several roles simultaneously. Such multiplex relationships not only maximize the efficient use of scarce time and energy resources, but should enhance the affective importance and meaningfulness of the identities involved. Friendships made and sustained by a married couple, for example, not only add to each spouse's set of identities, but reinforce the meaningfulness of the marriage itself. Embedded, multiplex relationships, then, should have quite different implications for the psychological well-being of isolated and integrated individuals.

It is reasonable to propose that the more identities possessed by an actor, the more likely he/she is to form multiplex (overlapping) ties to others. The fewer the identities, the less likely are multiplex relationships to develop. The interdependence of identities, and of the relationships predicated upon those identities, suggests that integrated individuals have both more to lose due to identity loss and more to gain from identity accumulation than isolated individuals. The effects of loss and gain should be multiplicatively greater for the integrated because the disruption or elaboration of interaction patterns is more extensive. Contrary to the implications of the time and energy proposition, network conceptualizations of commitment suggest that life's tragedies and triumphs should be amplified for the integrated and dampened for the isolated.

The contradictory implications of the time and energy conception and the network-embeddedness conception of commitment can be evaluated empirically. The analyses to follow examine the psychological impacts of identity changes conditional upon the number of initial identities that comprise a person's social self.

Several questions raised by Clausen and Kohn (1954) can now be answered. First, what constitutes a sufficient attenuation in interpersonal relationships to be called "isolation"? In this paper, isolation has been placed (implicitly) on a continuum of social involvement: the fewer identities claimed and validated in interaction, the more existentially insecure the individual, and the more psychological distress he/she will exhibit. Varying *degrees* of isolation should produce similarly varying amounts of disturbance.

What are the distinguishable types of isolating experiences? Clearly, losses of positional relationships are the primary isolating experiences in this reformulation. And, given that commitment to identities may vary due to their differential cultural worth, this statement can be further clarified: the more important the position, the more committed the individual should be to it, and therefore, the greater should be the psychological impact of its loss.

At what period or periods in the individual's life does the experience of isolation have the greatest effect? Following the implications of the time and energy proposition, because the isolated actor has few initial sources of social identity, he/she has both more to gain from identity acquisition and more to lose from identity loss than the integrated actor. Thus, isolation should have more of an effect during life cycle stages characterized by numerous position or role changes. The transition from adolescence to young adulthood may be especially beneficial to those with few identities; in this stage of life, one typically gains occupational, marital, and parental positions. Similarly, late middle age may be particularly difficult for those with few identities; children leave home, retirement impends, and relatives and friends die. However, following the implications of the network-embeddedness proposition, these life cycle periods should have greater impacts upon integrated actors than isolated actors.

Finally, is isolation a symptom of already developing illness; is it an essential condition for the subsequent development of illness; or is it, possibly, both symptomatic of the beginning of the illness and a cause of its further development? This reformulation has assumed that social interaction is essential to normal psychological development and ordered social conduct. Thus, isolation (a lack of involvement in role relationships) is an essential condition for the subsequent development of psychological disturbance. However, it is also reasonable to assume that psychological disturbance may in turn foster further isolation. Psychological disturbance may prevent the individual from fulfilling the few role obligations he/she may have and therefore may result in further position loss. Isolation, then, may be both symptomatic of the beginning of an illness and a cause of its further development, as Clausen and Kohn (1954) suggest.

The following sections describe the sample, procedures, and results of initial tests of the identity accumulation hypothesis and of the conditional effects of identity change.

METHODS

Sample

This study uses panel data from the New Haven community survey conducted by Myers and his associates (Myers et al., 1971, 1974). The sample consisted of 1,095 adult men and women selected at random from a community mental health center catchment area in metropolitan New Haven. A total of 938 individuals were interviewed in 1967. Two years later, 720 of the original cohort were reinterviewed. The analysis reported here is based on the reinterviewed sample of 720. This sample does not differ significantly from the original cohort within major categories of sociodemographic variables, with one exception: the under-30 age group dropped from 25 percent in 1967 to 19 percent in 1969 (Myers et al., 1974).

This study uses selected items from the panel survey data base, described in the following sections. It should be noted that the data provide information sufficient only for a test of the basic identity accumulation hypothesis and the hypotheses regarding the conditional effects of identity change. A measure of the intervening variable, a sense of meaningful, purposeful existence, or existential security, is not available, so it must be omitted from the analysis. Direct measures of cultural value or identity commitment are also not available, so identities cannot be weighted by their personal or cultural importance in this analysis.

Table 1 Mean Psychological Distress by Number of Identities at Time 1 and Time 2[a]

Number of Identities, Time 1 and Time 2	TIME 1			TIME 2		
	Mean Distress[b]	(St.D.)	N	Mean Distress[b]	(St.D.)	N
0	26.0	(–)	1	25.0	(–)	1
1	33.2	(10.8)	11	26.8	(9.9)	9
2	32.3	(9.5)	42	31.3	(12.7)	35
3	30.6	(9.5)	102	30.2	(9.8)	84
4	27.7	(7.5)	147	27.3	(6.7)	153
5	27.8	(8.2)	187	27.1	(7.1)	201
6	25.7	(6.2)	152	25.1	(6.5)	152
7	24.8	(4.9)	70	23.6	(3.7)	66
8	—	(–)	0	—	(–)	0
For Total Sample:	27.8	(8.0)	712	27.0	(7.7)	701

Mean Identities, Time 1: 4.67 (St.D. = 1.45)
Mean Identities, Time 2: 4.73 (St.D. = 1.38)

[a]Total Ns do not sum to 720 due to missing values on either identity accumulation or distress.
[b]Analysis of variance reveals significant differences between each subgroup: At Time 1, $F_{7,704} = 7.85, p < .001$; at Time 2, $F_{7,693} = 7.31, p < .001$. No significant deviations from linearity are found.

Measurement

1. Identity Accumulation

A sense of meaningful, purposeful existence is assumed to depend upon the number of positions held by an individual and validated in role relationships. Because data are limited with respect to specific numbers of role relationships enacted by individuals in the sample, identity accumulation will be measured here only as the sum of social positions held by the individual. The following social positions may be held: spouse, parent, employee, student, organizational member, church member, neighbor, and friend. Specifically, the identity accumulation variable is successively incremented by "1" if the respondent is married, has children, is employed, is in school, attends organizational meetings, attends church services, visits neighbors, and has two or more close friends. The identity accumulation variable ranges from 0 to 8 in value and is measured at two time points, 1967 and 1969.

2. Psychological Distress

Psychological distress is measured with an instrument developed by Macmillan (1957) and further modified by Gurin et al. (1960). The instrument consists of a list of 20 psychological and psychosomatic symptoms. The Likert-type responses to the items are reverse-coded and summed; scores range from 20 (little or no distress—i.e., psychological well-being) to 80 (high distress). The index was administered twice, in 1967 and in 1969. Cronbach's alpha is satisfactorily high for the index, approximately .84 or above at each time point.

Table 2 Regressions of Psychological Distress on Background Characteristics and Identity Accumulation, at Time 1 and Time 2[a] (N = 692)[b]

Equation	Female	Age	Education	Family Income	Identity Accumulation, Time 1	Identity Accumulation, Time 2	Change in Identity, Time 2–Time 1	Distress, Time 1	R^2
1. Distress at Time 1 regressed on:	.13***	-.14***	-.14***	-.12**	—	—	—	—	.068
2. Distress at Time 1 regressed on:	.08*	-.14***	-.12**	-.07†	-.19**	—	—	—	.099[c]
3. Distress at Time 2 regressed on:	.09*	-.08†	-.14**	-.09*	—	—	—	—	.042
4. Distress at Time 2 regressed on:	.05	-.10*	-.13**	-.03	—	-.21***	—	—	.081[d]
5. Distress at Time 2 regressed on:	.01	-.02	-.07†	-.002	-.10*	—	-.12***	.49***	.298

[a]Standardized regression coefficients are presented.

[b]N differs from total sample N due to omitted cases with missing values.

[c]Hierarchical tests for equations 1 and 2 indicate that identity accumulation adds significantly to explained variance in distress, $F_{1,686} = 24.03$, $p < .001$.

[d]Comparing equations 3 and 4, identity accumulation adds significantly to explained variance in distress, $F_{1,686} = 28.75$, $p < .001$.

†$p < .10$ *$p < .05$ **$p < .01$ ***$p < .001$.

Table 3 Mean Distress at Time 2 and Mean Change in Distress from Time 1 to Time 2 by Net Identity Change

Net Change in Identity (Identity Accumulation$_2$ – Identity Accumulation$_1$)		Mean Distress Time 2		Mean Change in Distress (Distress$_2$ – Distress$_1$)		N
		Mean[a]	(St.D.)	Mean[b]	(St.D.)	
	−4	42.0	(0)	13.0	(0)	1
Identity	−3	32.0	(14.1)	6.6	(10.6)	8
Loss	−2	27.4	(7.2)	−1.2	(8.4)	49
	−1	27.4	(8.5)	−.3	(7.6)	141
No Change	0	26.8	(7.8)	−.8	(7.9)	261
	+1	26.6	(6.9)	−1.0	(6.8)	163
Identity	+2	26.9	(7.0)	−1.6	(7.1)	58
Gain	+3	26.5	(4.0)	−5.2	(7.9)	11
	+4	27.0	(0)	−5.0	(0)	1
For total sample:		27.0	(7.7)	−.8	(7.6)	693
Mean Identity						
Change:	.07					
(St.D.):	(1.2)					

[a]Analysis of variance reveals no significant differences between subgroups.
[b]Analysis of variance reveals significant differences between subgroups, $F_{8,684} = 2.06$, $p < .05$.

3. Background Variables

Four sociodemographic variables are controlled in the analysis. These are age, sex, family income, and education. (Other sociodemographic variables such as marital status and occupation are not controlled, as they are reflected in the identity accumulation variable.) Sex is represented as a dummy variable, where female is coded 1. Age is measured in years. Family income and education are measured ordinally.

RESULTS: EFFECTS OF IDENTITY ACCUMULATION ON DISTRESS

Table 1 presents the mean psychological distress scores of individuals at each level of identity accumulation at Time 1 and Time 2. Few individuals possess the absolute minimum or maximum number of identities at either time point. For those possessing 1 to 7 identities, distress decreases steadily with level of identity accumulation, with one exception: at Time 2, persons with only one identity have lower distress scores than persons with two to five identities. However, this average value is based on a very small number of cases ($N = 9$). Analysis of variance reveals significant differences between subgroups at both time points and no significant deviations from linearity. In short, the greater the number of identities possessed, the less psychological distress. There is no significant curvilinear relationship between identity accumulation and distress, at least for the limited range of this identity accumulation variable.

Table 2 presents the results of regression analyses which assess the effects of identity accumulation and change in identity upon psychological distress at Time 1 and Time 2, while background variables are controlled. Equations 1 and 3 simply verify that background variables are related to distress in expected ways. Consistent with prior research females exhibit significantly higher distress levels than males, and distress decreases significantly with age, education, and family income (cf., Gurin et al., 1960; Gove & Tudor, 1973; Dohrenwend et al., 1980). Equations 2 and 4 examine the influence of identity accumulation on distress at Times 1 and 2, respectively, holding background factors constant. In each equation, identity accumulation significantly reduces distress, as predicted. Hierarchical tests for equations 1 and 2 and for 3 and 4 indicate that at each time point, identity accumulation adds significantly to explained variance in the dependent variable. We will return to equation 5 of Table 2 momentarily.

Table 3 indicates the relationship between identity change and distress. The more identities lost from Time 1 to Time 2, the greater the mean distress at Time 2 and the greater the increase in distress from Time 1 to Time 2. Conversely, the more identities gained over time, the very slightly less Time 2 distress and the greater the decrease in distress from Time 1 to Time 2. Analysis of variance indicates no significant differences between

Table 4 Regressions of Psychological Distress at Time 2 on Identity Accumulation at Time 1, Change in Identity, Prior Psychological Distress, and Identity-Change Interaction Terms[a] ($N = 693$)

Equation	Identity Accumulation, Time 1	Change in Identity, Time 1 to Time 2	Psychological Distress, Time 1	Multiplicative Gain Term[b]	Multiplicative Loss Term[c]	R^2
1. Distress at Time 2 regressed on:	−.10*	−.12***	.49***	—	—	.297
2. Distress at Time 2 regressed on:	−.09*	.07	.49***	−.11	.13[†]	.301[d]

[a]Background factors (age, sex, education, and family income) are controlled in each equation. Standardized regression coefficients are presented.
[b]Measured as: Net Identities Gained × Identity Accumulation $_1$.
[c]Measured as: Net Identities Lost × Identity Accumulation $_1$.
[d]The multiplicative terms add significantly to explained variation in distress, from a hierarchical test of equations 1 and 2: $F_{2,683} = 3.38, p < .05$.
†$p < .10$ * $p < .05$ ** $p < .01$ *** $p < .001$.

identity-change subgroups for mean distress at Time 2, but significant between-group differences for the distress change scores. No significant deviations from linearity for either distress variable are found by subgroup.

Return now to equation 5 in Table 2. Equation 5 examines the effect of identity change upon change in distress from Time 1 to Time 2, controlling for background factors. The more identities gained, the greater the reduction in distress ($\beta = -.12$, $p < .001$). The identity-change variable adds significantly to explained variance in distress at Time 2, as revealed by a hierarchical test not shown here ($F_{1,685} = 11.20$, $p < .001$). The results in Table 3 and for equation 5 in Table 2 clearly support the dynamic implications of the identity accumulation hypothesis.

The implications of the time and energy commitment proposition suggest that changes in identity will have greater psychological impacts for more isolated individuals than more integrated individuals. That is, gains will benefit and losses will harm isolated persons more than integrated persons. Conversely, the network-embeddedness conception of commitment suggests that changes in identity will have greater psychological impacts on more integrated than more isolated individuals. That is, gains will benefit and losses will harm integrated persons more than isolated persons. To examine the validity of these contradictory predictions, identity-change interaction terms were computed for respondents who had experienced net gains or net losses of identities over time. For persons experiencing net gain:

Number of Identities Gained $\times$ Identity Accumulation$_1$.

And for persons experiencing net loss:

Number of Identities Lost $\times$ Identity Accumulation$_1$. (Persons with no changes or a net change of zero receive a value of 0 on these variables.)

If the time and energy predictions are valid, there should be a positive relationship between the multiplicative gain term and change in psychological distress: for each gained identity, those with few initial identities should have less distress at Time 2 compared to those with many initial identities. There should be a negative relationship between the multiplicative loss term and change in distress: for each identity loss, those with fewer identities at Time 1 should have substantially increased distress at Time 2 compared to those with many identities. On the other hand, if the network-embeddedness predictions are valid, the signs of the interaction terms should be reversed. The multiplicative gain term should be negative, indicating reduced distress for the initially integrated with each identity gain, and the multiplicative loss term should be positive, indicating additional distress for the integrated with each identity loss, compared to the isolated. The multiplicative gain and loss terms were added hierarchically to equation 5 of Table 2. The results are shown in equation 2 of Table 4. (Equation 1 of Table 4 simply repeats the findings of the prior equation for comparative purposes here.)

The implications of the network-embeddedness propositions are supported in Table 4. Although the multiplicative gain term is nonsignificant, its sign indicates that for each identity gain, the distress of initially integrated actors is reduced more than that of initially isolated actors. The multiplicative loss term is significant and positive. For each identity loss, initially integrated actors are distressed more than are the initially isolated. The multiplicative terms add significantly to explained variation in distress, as revealed by a hierarchical test for equations 1 and 2 in Table 4. In short, integration at Time 1 does not lower but tends to *enhance* the psychological utility of identity gain; integration at Time 1 does not buffer but *exacerbates* the psychological impact of identity loss.

DISCUSSION AND CONCLUSIONS

In the preceding sections it was argued that social identities provide actors with existential meaning and behavioral guidance, and that these qualities are essential to psychological well-being and organized, functional behavior. It was shown that individuals who possess numerous identities do report significantly less psychological distress. No evidence of a curvilinear relationship between identity accumulation and distress was found, suggesting that multiple identity involvements do not necessarily result in role strain or role conflict, as has previously been argued (Goode, 1960; Sarbin & Allen, 1968). Moreover, change in identity was found inversely and significantly related to change in distress. Thus, social identity lack and identity loss do have important psychological consequences, as do identity possession and identity gain. Although the analysis here, of necessity, has focused on reported feelings of psychological distress, it could easily be extended in future research to more serious forms of disorder which indicate disorganized functioning.

It was argued also that the effects of identity change are not simply additive, but conditional upon the actor's relative degree of isolation or integration. Conditional, or interactive, effects can be derived from principles regarding the structure of multiple identities. Theorists generally have assumed that identities are hierarchically organized by differing degrees of subjective or behavioral commitment. In this paper, commitment is hypothesized to vary with the relative cultural or subcultural valuation of identities possessed by the actor. These cultural rankings should determine not only the subjective importance attached to each role, but the investment of time and energy in each role enactment, and the extensivity and complexity of network ties in which each identity is sustained. Unfortunately, due to data limitations, this hypothesis regarding the structure of identity commitments could not be tested directly.

However, the predictive utility of the time and energy investment and the network-embeddedness conceptions of commitment could be contrasted within the context of conditional effects. If the expenditure of time and energy in any one identity is inversely related to the number of identities possessed, then isolated actors should be more psychologically affected than integrated actors by identity gains and losses; the isolated actor has both more to lose and more to gain through change. If, on the other hand, the multiplexity of network relationships varies directly with the number of identities possessed, then integrated persons should be more psychologically affected by identity changes than isolated persons; the integrated actor has both more to lose and more to gain through change. The analysis indicated support for these latter predictions. The more identities possessed by individuals initially, the greater the distressing impact of subsequent identity loss and the greater the ameliorative impact of identity gain. These findings were replicated within broad age groupings related to position-expanding and position-contracting stages in the adult life cycle.

These conditional effects of identity change point strongly to the predictive utility of the network-embeddedness notion of commitment proposed by Stryker and Serpe (1982, 1983). Their conceptualization overcomes a major limitation of the more simplistic investment notion, namely, the implicit assumption that identities are mutually independent, so that time and energy spent in one role necessarily must be taken away from such expenditures in other roles. The network-embeddedness conception explicitly incorporates the possibility of interdependence among identities. Where role partners overlap in the same person or persons, scarce time and energy can be spent sustaining two or more identities simultaneously (thus reducing the possibility of role strain as well). Further, the network-embeddedness conception suggests a further specification of the conditional effects of identity change proposed in this paper. *Among actors whose identities are segregated, or independent*, identity changes should have greater impacts upon the relatively isolated than the integrated. *Among actors whose identities are nonsegregated, or overlapping*, identity changes should have greater impacts upon the relatively integrated than the isolated. Had measures of network structure been available in the data set employed here, so that respondents could have been partitioned into these classes, stronger interactions of identity change with the number of identities initially possessed might have been found.

The distinction between segregated and non-segregated identities pointed to by the network-embeddedness conception also helps specify the observations of Sieber (1974) and Marks (1977) regarding the expansive benefits of multiple roles and the expansive nature of subjective commitment. Sieber argues that the privileges, resources, and rewards of multiple roles can be parlayed by the actor into even more privileges, resources, and rewards, thus outweighing the possible effects of role conflict and role strain. For example, resources provided in one set of role activities (e.g., social contacts, company property, expense accounts, technical knowledge or skills) can be used to meet obligations in other roles; such expandable capital makes the person more valuable to other role partners. Multiple roles also provide legitimate excuses for failing to meet normal obligations; the competing demands of other roles may be cited. Finally, multiple roles buffer the actor against the consequences of role failure or role loss; the actor has other involvements upon which to fall back. To the extent that multiple roles are *segregated*, these postulated benefits should occur. The actor's resources will be valuable to others who do not share those resources themselves, the legitimacy of excuses cannot be checked, and the consequences of role failure or loss can be contained more within one sphere of activities. Such benefits should not be as probable under conditions of identity or role overlap.

Marks (1977) argues that subjective commitment to a role or identity can swell when one or more of four elements increase: spontaneous enjoyment of role performance, spontaneous loyalty to a role partner, anticipation of rewards from role enactment, or avoidance of punishment through role enactment. These elements are most likely to be affected when roles are *nonsegregated*. When role partners overlap in the same person or persons, the emotional intensity of those relationships and the loyalty felt toward those partners should increase (Stryker & Serpe, 1983). The cost of giving up each identity involved should also be increased. Thus, subjective commitment to identities should expand when those identities are enacted in multiplex relationships.

In short, the network-embeddedness conception of commitment has several advantages. First, consistent with the thesis that identities are claimed and sustained in relationships with others, it points to straightforward indicators of key concepts using the structure of network ties. Second, it neatly subsumes the time and energy expenditure and subjective importance conceptions of commitment. Finally, it points to conditions which help specify when multiplicative effects of identity accumulation might be expected. These advantages of the network-embeddedness conception of commitment should facilitate further work on the psychological effects of multiple identities.

References

Bart, Pauline 1974 "The sociology of depression." Pp. 139–57 in Paul Roman and Harrison Trice (eds.), Explorations in Psychiatric Sociology. New York: Science House.

Berger, Joseph, M. Hamet Fisek, Robert Z. Norman and Morris Zelditch 1977 Status Characteristics and Social Interaction. New York: Elsevier.

Berkman, Lisa and S. Leonard Syme 1979 "Social networks, host resistance, and mortality: a nine-year follow-up study of Alameda County residents." American Journal of Epidemiology 109:186–204.

Bradburn, Norman M. 1969 The Structure of Psychological Well-Being. Chicago: Aldine.

Clausen, John A. and Melvin L. Kohn 1954 "The ecological approach in social psychiatry." American Journal of Sociology 60:140–51.

Clayton, Paula J., James A. Halikas and William L. Maurice 1972 "The depression of widowhood." British Journal of Psychiatry 120:71–77.

Cooley, Charles Horton 1902 Human Nature and the Social Order. New York: Scribner's.

Coser, Lewis (with Rose Laub Coser) 1974 Greedy Institutions. New York: Free Press.

Dohrenwend, Barbara Snell and Bruce P. Dohrenwend 1974 Stressful Life Events: Their Nature and Effects. New York: Wiley.

Dohrenwend, Bruce P., Barbara S. Dohrenwend, Madelyn Schwartz Gould, Bruce Link, Richard Neugebauer, and Robin Wunsch-Hitzig 1980 Mental Illness in the United States: Epidemiological Estimates. New York: Praeger.

Faris, Robert E. L. 1934 "Cultural isolation and the schizophrenic personality." American Journal of Sociology 40:155–69.

Frankl, Viktor 1959 Man's Search for Meaning. Boston: Beacon Press.

Glassner, Barry, C. V. Haldipur and James Dessauersmith 1979 "Role loss and working-class manic depression." Journal of Nervous and Mental Disease 167:530–41.

Goode, William J. 1960 "A theory of role strain." American Sociological Review 25:483–96.

Gove, Walter S. 1972 "The relationship between sex roles, mental illness, and marital status." Social Forces 51:34–44.

Gove, Walter S. and Michael Hughes 1980 "Reexamining the ecological fallacy: a study in which aggregate data are critical in investigating the pathological effects of living alone." Social Forces 58:1157–77.

Gove, Walter and Jeannette F. Tudor 1973 "Adult sex roles and mental illness." American Journal of Sociology 78:50–73.

Gurin, Gerald, Joseph Veroff and Sheila Feld 1960 Americans View Their Mental Health. New York: Basic Books.

Haney, Craig, W. Curtis Banks and Philip Zimbardo 1973 "Interpersonal dynamics in a simulated prison." International Journal of Criminology and Penology 1:69–97.

Henderson, Scott, D. G. Byrne, P. Duncan-Jones, Sylvia Adcock, Ruth Scott and G. P. Steele 1978 "Social bonds in the epidemiology of neurosis: a preliminary communication." British Journal of Psychiatry 132:463–66.

Linton, Ralph 1936 The Study of Man. New York: Appleton-Century.

Lowenthal, Marjorie Fiske 1964 "Social isolation and mental illness in old age." American Sociological Review 29:54–70.

Macmillan, Allister M. 1957 "The Health Opinion Survey: technique for estimating prevalence of psychoneurotic and related types of disorder in communities." Psychological Reports 3:325–39.

Marks, Stephen 1977 "Multiple roles and role strain: some notes on human energy, time, and commitment." American Sociological Review 42:921–36.

Mead, George Herbert 1934 Mind, Self, and Society. Chicago: University of Chicago Press.

Merton, Robert K. 1957 Social Theory and Social Structure. Revised Edition. New York: The Free Press.

Miller, Patrick McC. and J. G. Ingham 1976 "Friends, confidants, and symptoms." Social Psychiatry 11:51–58.

Mueller, Daniel P. 1980 "Social networks: a promising direction for research on the relationship of the social environment to psychiatric disorder." Social Science and Medicine 14A:147–61.

Myers, Jerome, Jacob J. Lindenthal, and Max Pepper 1971 "Life events and psychiatric impairment." Journal of Nervous and Mental Disease 152:149–57.

—— 1974 "Social class, life events, and psychiatric symptoms: a longitudinal study." Pp. 191–205 in Barbara S. Dohrenwend and Bruce P. Dohrenwend (eds.), Stressful Life Events: Their Nature and Effects. New York: Wiley.

Paykel, Eugene S. 1974 "Recent life events and clinical depression." Pp. 134–63 in E.K.E. Gunderson and Richard H. Rahe (eds.), Life Stress and Illness. Springfield, IL: Charles C Thomas.

Radloff, Lenore 1975 "Sex differences in depression." Sex Roles 1:249–65.

Rose, Arnold M. 1962 "A social psychological theory of neurosis." Pp. 537–49 in Arnold M. Rose (ed.), Human Behavior and Social Processes. Boston: Houghton Mifflin.

Rosenberg, Morris 1979 Conceiving the Self. New York: Basic.

Roy, A. 1978 "Vulnerability factors and depression in women." British Journal of Psychiatry 133:106–110.

Sarbin, Theodore R. 1968 "Notes on the transformation of social identity." Pp. 97–115 in L. M. Roberts, N. S. Greenfield, and M. H. Miller (eds.), Comprehensive Mental Health: The Challenge of Evaluation. Madison: University of Wisconsin Press.

Sarbin, Theodore R. and Vernon L. Allen 1968 "Role theory." Pp. 488–567 in Gardner Lindsey and Elliot Aronson (eds.), The Handbook of Social Psychology, Vol. 1 (Second Edition). Reading, MA: Addison-Wesley.

Sieber, Sam D. 1974 "Toward a theory of role accumulation." American Sociological Review 39:567–78.

Stryker, Sheldon 1980 Symbolic Interactionism: A Social Structural Version. Palo Alto, CA: Benjamin/Cummings.

Stryker, Sheldon and Richard T. Serpe 1982 "Commitment, identity salience, and role behavior." Pp. 199–218 in William Ickes and Eric S. Knowles (eds.), Personality, Roles, and Social Behavior. New York: Springer-Verlang.

—— 1983 "Towards a theory of family influence in the socialization of children." In Alan C. Kerckhoff (ed.), Research in the Sociology of Education and Socialization, Vol. IV. Greenwich, CT: JAI Press (in press).

Thoits, Peggy A. 1978 Life Events, Social Integration, and Psychological Distress. Doctoral dissertation, Sociology Department, Stanford University, Stanford, California.

—— 1982 "Conceptual, methodological, and theoretical problems in studying social support as a buffer against life stress." Journal of Health and Social Behavior 23:145–59.

—— 1983 "Dimensions of life events as influences upon the genesis of psychological distress and associated conditions: an evaluation and synthesis of the literature." In Howard B. Kaplan (ed.), Psychosocial Stress: Trends in Theory and Research. New York: Academic Press (forthcoming).

Zimbardo, Philip G., Craig Haney, W. Curtis Banks, and David Jaffe 1973 "A Pirandellian prison: the mind is a formidable jailer." New York Times Magazine April 8:38–60.

DISCUSSION QUESTIONS

1. According to Thoits, why are role relationships important to mental health? What do we gain from those relationships?

2. What is the identity accumulation hypothesis? What does it predict regarding the effects of multiple role involvements on mental health?

3. Thoits distinguishes between the "time and energy" conceptualization of role commitments and the "network-embeddedness" conceptualization. Which receives greatest support from her analysis?

4. What questions does Thoits' analysis raise but not answer? What might be a fruitful direction for future research on roles and mental health?

R. Jay Turner, Blair Wheaton, and Donald A. Lloyd

The Epidemiology of Social Stress[†]

R. Jay Turner and colleagues introduce a major debate within sociological research on stress: whether differences in mental health based on social statuses (gender, occupational prestige, marital status, and age) reflect differences in exposure to stressful life experiences or differences in vulnerability to stress. For purposes of their analysis, they developed a much more comprehensive measure of stressful life experiences than those used in prior research. This measure allows them to present persuasive evidence that group differences in stress exposures are major determinants of group differences in mental health.

Much of the research conducted by sociologists of mental health begins with the long established associations between mental health problems and socio-economic status (Dohrenwend & Dohrenwend, 1969; Faris & Dunham, 1939; Hollingshead & Redlich, 1958), marital status (Gove, 1972; Gurin, Veroff, & Feld 1960; Turner, Dopkeen, & Labreche, 1970) and, more recently, gender (Al-Issa, 1982; Nolen-Hocksema, 1987; Weissman & Klerman, 1977). It has usually been assumed that there are important etiological messages to be found within these established links, but the exact nature of these messages has been the subject of considerable debate.

Since the pioneering work of Faris and Dunham (1939) on social class and mental illness, it has been generally acknowledged that the interpretation of social epidemiologic observations must confront two competing classes of explanation—the *social causation hypothesis* and the *social selection hypothesis* (Dohrenwend & Dohrenwend, 1969; Turner & Wagenfeld, 1967). The question is whether, and the extent to which, these relationships arise from variations in the environmental experiences of individuals of differing social statuses, or alternatively, they reflect the workings of a quasi-open society that sifts and sorts individuals into different social locations and positions based, in part, on physical and mental health, levels of social competence and so on. As Aneshensel (1992) has recently noted, with the apparent exception of schizophrenia, evidence indicates that social causation processes are of greater significance than social selection processes in relationships between social class and mental health (Dohrenwend et al., 1992; Eaton, 1986; Liem & Liem, 1978; Wheaton, 1978). A similar conclusion seems justified with respect to mental health and marital status (Gove, 1972). In the case of gender, evidence supports the social causation hypothesis and is contrary to the argument that the elevated levels of distress and disorder observed among women are genetically or biologically driven (Nolen-Hocksema, 1987).

Turner, R. Jay, Blair Wheaton, and Donald A. Lloyd. 1995. "The epidemiology of social stress." *American Sociological Review* 60: 104–125.

Researchers who have interpreted the available evidence to mean that social stratification and other structural factors may be causally significant for mental health have focused attention on the questions of how these structural factors influence individual health and under what circumstances such effects are made more or less intense (House & Mortimer, 1990). On the assumption that patterned differences in social experiences and in the acquisition of social and developmental resources are likely to be implicated, a number of hypotheses about the role of psychosocial factors have been suggested. These hypotheses focus on differences in the social experiences and circumstances of individuals, as well as on differences in relevant personal and social resources, that could contribute to psychological distress or mental illness and that vary systematically across social statuses (e.g., sex, age, marital status, etc.).

Until a dozen or so years ago a principal focus of research on social status contingencies in mental health was on stressful life events, which had been repeatedly shown to be associated with physical and mental health (Dohrenwend & Dohrenwend, 1974; Jemmott & Locke, 1984; Jenkins, 1976). The appealing hypothesis was that the elevated levels of psychological distress and disorder observed among people in low status groups may be substantially attributable to their greater exposure to stressful life events (Dohrenwend & Dohrenwend, 1969; Kohn, 1972). The plausibility of this hypothesis, then and now, rests on the assumption that variations in exposure to stress influence mental well-being, rather than the reverse. While it has been shown that mental health status can influence subsequent experiences of stressful events (Turner & Noh, 1988), it is clear that a substantial proportion of this causal link is in the opposite direction—from social stress to mental health status (Thoits, 1983).

This general perspective has recently been revitalized by Pearlin (1989), who compellingly argued the need for careful and comprehensive attention to the structural contexts of people's lives. In his view, stressful events and life circumstances are rooted in these structural contexts, and thus, there is a basis for assuming that variations in exposure to stress arise substantially out of contemporaneous and developmental conditions of life. Pearlin's treatment of the social context of stressful experiences is not limited to the realm of stressful life events, but includes the ongoing and difficult conditions of daily life that are now usually termed chronic stressors (Pearlin, 1989; Pearlin & Schooler, 1978; Wheaton, 1994). To the extent that important differences in stress-relevant social conditions or contexts tend to be defined by one's gender, socioeconomic, and marital statuses, the hypothesis indeed seems to follow that observed relationships between these social statuses and mental health must, to some extent, be attributable to status variations in exposure to stress. The observation of clear associations between the levels of stress one experiences and one's social status location would be consistent with this social causation hypothesis.

As we interpret the recent history of the study of stress and mental health, an important transition in the dominant perspective emerged during the late 1970s and early 1980s. This new view was apparently based on somewhat fateful interpretations of two types of evidence. First, cumulative results indicated that the correlations observed between measures of stressful life events and indices of mental health and well-being varied from less than .10 to little more than .30, suggesting that the variance accounted for by differences in stress exposure is less than 10 percent and is thus of rather trivial practical significance (Rabkin & Struening, 1976; Thoits, 1983). This conclusion was supported by the finding, first reported by Kessler (1979; Kessler & Cleary, 1980) but later confirmed by others (Aneshensel, 1992; Thoits, 1987), that differential exposure to stressful life events is substantially less important than differential vulnerability to stress in determining the relationships between mental health and social class, gender, and marital status.

These observations appropriately encouraged the ensuing widespread efforts to understand the origins of differential vulnerability to stress (Aneshensel, 1992). A less propitious consequence, we believe, has been the encouragement of a widespread habit of thought that social stress is of only minimal significance for understanding variations in psychological distress and psychiatric disorder.

In our view, the hypothesis that level of social stress is an important determinant of mental health status has never been effectively tested because we have yet to adequately measure variations in stress exposure. If we are correct, the question of the relative contributions of variations in exposure to stress and differences in vulnerability to stress to the social distribution of mental health must be left open. This is because unmeasured differences in stress exposure across social statuses parade within research findings as vulnerability differences. Clearly, research is required that indexes social stress in a more comprehensive way than typical life event inventories have allowed.

In this paper we employ an estimate of stress exposure that is more comprehensive than has been typical—we add indices for the presence of continuous, ongoing stressors and of exposure to major traumas over the life course, and we present distributions of stressful experiences thus indexed by sex, age, marital status, and occupational level. Before reporting findings on the epidemiology of life stress, we will present evidence that challenges the often repeated conclusion—that exposure to stress accounts for only a very modest proportion of mental health variability.

METHOD

Our data came from face-to-face interviews conducted in 1990 and 1991 with 1,393 adult residents of metropolitan Toronto. Eligible subjects were all individuals 18 to 55 years of age living in their principal residence, who were fluent in English and physically and mentally capable of responding to the questionnaire. This age range was selected to correspond to the ages that incur substantial risks for psychiatric and substance abuse problems, which are central dependent variables within the larger study, and to allow us to use the same assessment procedures for all subjects. The sampling process was aided by a 1989 household enumeration conducted by Statistics Canada to develop a sampling frame for the Ontario Health Study. We were provided with a nonoverlapping representative sample of addresses selected from each borough in proportion to the 1986 population census. Success rate in interviewing the selected subjects was 77 percent which, we believe, indicates the sample is reasonably representative.

MEASURES

Life Stress

Life stress is indexed in this study in terms of stressful life events, enduring or chronic stressors, and major lifetime traumas. *Stressful life events* were assessed using a 34-item checklist of negative events common to many life events indices (Henderson, Byrne, & Duncan-Jones, 1981; Holmes & Rahe, 1967; Sarason, Johnson, & Siegel, 1978). (Items are presented in Appendix A.) Because each reported event required an additional series of probing questions, we placed limits on the number of events included in the checklist to keep interviews at an acceptable length. Respondents were asked to indicate which of the 34 events they had experienced personally during the 12 months preceding the interview. For 21 of the events, they were also asked whether their spouse or partner had experienced the event. For 18 events they were also asked if their children experienced the event, and for 7 events, respondents were asked to consider other relatives and friends. Respondents indicated the month in which each stressful event began and the month in which it ended. To assist this process, a calendar for the previous 12-month period was used during the interview. Respondents were encouraged to place significant dates, such as holidays and birthdays, on the calendar and then to identify the months in which each reported stressful event began and ended.

Enduring or chronic stressors were measured by a 51-item inventory developed by Wheaton (1991, 1994; see Appendix A). The items fall into nine areas—financial issues, general or ambient problems, work, marriage and relationship, parental, family, social life, residence, and health. These items are subjectively reported life conditions and situations. Wheaton (1991, 1994) has argued that these stressors are inherently subjective, and that measurement approaches should take this into account. The advantage of using subjective reports of chronic stress is that they allow shorthand reference to an array of possible objective social realities that would be impractical to measure directly, and more importantly, they typically reflect realities that most would consider objectively stressful.

With respect to major lifetime *traumas*, we distinguished between those occurring before adulthood (8 items) and those that may have occurred at any time during the respondent's lifetime (12 items, see Appendix A). Items from the "any time" list were considered to be childhood/adolescent traumas when they occurred before age 23.

Indexing Social Statuses

As noted, sex, marital status, and socioeconomic status, along with age, have been reliably linked with variations in mental health, and for decades these links have been a major basis for hypotheses and research aimed at understanding the social determinants of mental disorder and well-being.

We group our subjects into four age *categories*: 18–25, 26–35, 36–45, and 46–55. The rationale for these particular groupings is limited to their intuitive appeal and the need for large enough numbers in each age category to assure stable estimates of variations in both exposure to stress and mental health status. In the regression analyses, age is employed as a continuous variable, and the square of age is also included to test for curvilinear effects (Mirowsky & Ross, 1992).

Three *marital status categories* are distinguished: never married, currently married, and previously married. "Previously married" includes a small number of widowed with the separated and divorced to achieve an adequate subsample size.

We have operationalized socioeconomic status in terms of *occupational prestige level*. The jobs of all employed respondents (including those temporarily laid off) and of the spouses of currently married respondents were coded according to Hollingshead's (1957) seven occupational prestige categories. Nonemployed subjects were assigned the score for their last job held. The occupational prestige level assigned for a respondent was for either his or her own job or the spouse's job, whichever was higher. While this procedure presumably yields an elevated socioeconomic class distribution compared to other operationalizations, we believe it to be an accurate estimate of each respondent's position in the social hierarchy and the conditions of life he or she experiences. To maintain adequate subsample sizes, subjects in the semiskilled and unskilled job prestige categories were combined.

Mental Health Measures

Because of the visibility of depression in social epidemiological literature, we focus on two depression measures as primary outcomes of stress. *Depressive symptomatology* is assessed by administering the Center for Epidemiologic Studies Depression Scale (CES-D), a widely used and highly reliable index of depressive symptomatology (Devins & Orme, 1985; Radloff, 1977). *Major depressive disorder* was defined in terms of the *Diagnostic and Statistical Manual of Mental Disorders* of the American Psychiatric Association (1987, vers. 3 rev.). The occurrence of this disorder was estimated utilizing the Michigan revision of the Composite International Diagnostic Interview (CIDI) (World Health Organization [WHO], 1990; Robins et al., 1988). Evidence of excellent inter-rater reliability (Wittchen et al., 1991) and good test-retest reliability (Wacker, Battegay, Mullejans, and Schlosser, 1990) is available for the CIDI, as is evidence for validity based on concordance with clinical diagnoses (Janca, Robins, Cottler, & Early, 1992; Spengler & Wittchen, 1989).

Table 1 Mean Depressive Symptom Scores and One-Year Prevalence Rates for Major Depressive Disorder by Social Status Variables: Residents of Toronto, Ontario, Ages 18–55, 1990–1991

Social Status Variables	Mean Depressive Symptom Score[a]	N[c]	One-Year Prevalence Rate of Major Depressive Disorder[b] (Percent)	N[c]
Sex				
Male	10.21	603	7.7	604
Female	13.10	788	12.9	789
p-value[d]		<.001		.002
Age				
18–25	15.14	304	18.4	304
26–35	10.92	470	9.8	471
36–45	11.09	393	7.2	393
46–55	9.15	224	4.7	225
p-value[d]		<.001		<.001
Marital Status				
Married	9.98	673	6.6	675
Previously married	14.22	171	11.5	171
Never married	13.70	547	15.8	547
p-value[d]		<.001		<.001
Occupational Prestige				
Major professional	9.16	158	4.1	158
Lesser professional	10.53	317	7.5	317
Minor professional	11.14	257	8.6	258
Clerical/sales	13.36	378	14.2	378
Skilled/manual	10.41	97	4.9	98
Semi skilled/ unskilled	14.24	165	18.3	165
p-value[d]		<.001		<.001
Total	11.79	1,391	10.6	1,393

[a] Depressive symptom score is the score on the CES-D (Radloff, 1977).

[b] Rates of major depressive disorder are based on diagnostic algorithms derived from the *Diagnostic and Statistical Manual of Mental Disorders* (American Psychiatric Association 1987, vers. 3 rev.) and applied to responses measured using the Michigan revision of the Composite International Diagnostic Interview (CIDI) (WHO, 1990).

[c] Nineteen cases are missing for the occupation categories, and two additional cases are missing for the CES-D measure, due to nonresponses to the relevant questions.

[d] The *p*-values shown indicate significant group mean differences in depressive symptoms according to one-way ANOVA tests, and in group-specific rates of depression according to chi-square tests. Two-tailed tests of significance are used in both sets of results.

RESULTS

Social Status Characteristics and Mental Health Status

Prior to examining the epidemiology of social stress, we verified that the typical distributions of mental health status we seek to understand were, in fact, observable in our data. Table 1 presents mean depressive symptom (CES-D) scores and one-year prevalence rates of major depressive disorder (the proportion of respondents experiencing the disorder over the year preceding the interview) by sex, age, marital status, and occupational prestige level. Both sets of comparisons quite uniformly replicate the distributions reported over several decades based on studies of treated and untreated populations with respect to sex, marital status, and socioeconomic status. Women report substantially higher levels of both depressive symptoms and major depressive disorder than do men, while the married, on average, experience substantially lower levels than do the never or previously married.

With respect to occupational prestige, our measure of SES, the expected linear pattern is observed. Increasing levels of occupational prestige are associated with decreasing levels of depressive symptoms and decreasing rates of major depressive disorder. However, this pattern is interrupted in both instances by substantially deviant scores in the skilled-manual category. Because 75 percent of subjects in this category were men, the possibility that these deviant scores may be an artifact of sex composition had to be considered. Separate analyses, however, revealed that the pattern is at least

Table 2 Bivariate Correlation Coefficients and Multivariate Beta Coefficients from the Regression of the Depressive Symptom Score (OLS) and One-Year Major Depressive Disorder (Logistic) on Five Stress Indices: Residents of Toronto, Ontario, Ages 18–55, 1990–1991

Stress Index	Depressive Symptom Score		One-Year Major Depressive Disorder	
	r	ß	r	ß
Recent Life Events				
Events to self	.291***	.153***	.297***	.193***
Events to others	.198***	.089***	.210***	.117***
Chronic Stress	.456***	.396***	.353***	.270***
Lifetime Trauma				
Adult trauma	.019	−.087***	−.002	−.092
Childhood trauma	.234***	.037	.237***	.060
R^2	—	.247	—	.155‡
Number of Cases	1,391		1,393	

*$p < .05$ **$p < .01$ ***$p < .001$ (two-tailed tests)

‡Pseudo R^2 = Explained SS/(Explained SS + 3.29 N) (Aldrich & Nelson, 1984).

as pronounced among women as among men. It is assumed that these low levels of distress and disorder found in the skilled-manual category are real and deserve additional research. We return to this matter below.

A second preliminary issue involved confirming that the widely reported relationship between life stress and mental health status is observed in our data set and evaluating the conventional wisdom that the quantity of stress experienced is of only minimal explanatory significance. Table 2 presents the results of bivariate correlation and multiple OLS or logistic regression analyses assessing the associations between life stress index scores and both depressive symptoms and one-year major depressive disorder. Interestingly, the correlations between "events to self" and depressive symptoms (.29) and major depressive disorder (.30) approximate the relationships typically reported in the literature and account for less than 9 percent of the variation (Rabkin & Struening, 1976). However, when the independent contributions of all categories of assessed stressors are considered together, including measures of current chronic stress and past traumas, the magnitude of these associations jumps dramatically. This is especially true for depressive symptoms, where the variability accounted for is about 2.5 times the upper range of previous reports that have considered only stressful events.

With respect to chronic stress, not only are the results consistent with prior evidence linking persistent stressors to psychological distress (e.g., Liem & Liem, 1978; Ross & Huber, 1985), but they support the contention that chronic stress may be of primary significance (Pearlin & Lieberman, 1979; Wheaton, 1991). Adult trauma scores also contribute significantly and independently to depressive symptomatology, but the coefficient is negative, indicating that higher trauma scores are associated with lower levels of depression. Since these scores are not adjusted for time at risk, this apparently anomalous finding can be resolved by considering the fact that the likelihood of ever having experienced an adult trauma naturally increases with age, and age is generally related to less depression up to the age limit in our data. Although the net effect of childhood traumas is not significant, they are clearly correlated with depressive symptoms in later life. The absence of strong direct effects suggests that the consequences of major childhood stressors tend to be transmitted by other stressors in this equation, which act as intervening variables. For example, being abused by a parent or losing a parent during childhood may increase risk of interpersonal difficulties and hence relationship strains in adulthood.

It is worth emphasizing that, while it is clear that this is an unusually comprehensive effort to assess stress exposure, it cannot be claimed that we have yet adequately estimated variations in social stress. Thus, we conclude that social stress may be a considerably more powerful determinant of health and well-being than is generally assumed, and that the hypothesis that differences in stress exposure across social structures and contexts partially account for mental health differences remains a tenable one. It is to this latter issue that we now turn.

Table 3 Standard Scores for Levels of Exposure to Stress by Social Status Variables: Residents of Toronto, Ontario, Ages 18–55, 1990–1991

Social Status Variables	N	Stressful Life Events				Chronic Stress (5)	Operant Burden (6)	Cumulative Burden (7)
		Self (1)	Others (2)	Total (3)	Operant Events (4)			
Sex								
Male	604	−.005	−.061	−.038	−.078	−.064	−.087	−.055
Female	789	.004	.051	.032	.065	.053	.072	.046
p-value[a]			.037		.008	.029	.003	.046
Age								
18–25	304	.313	.104	.284	.114	.101	.132	.253
26–35	471	−.020	−.087	−.064	−.054	−.017	−.044	−.030
36–45	393	−.179	.009	−.124	−.003	.053	.031	−.061
46–55	225	−.180	−.014	−.138	−.076	−.217	−.180	−.254
p-value[a]		<.001		<.001	.029	.002	<.001	<.001
Marital Status								
Married	675	−.204	.015	−.139	−.041	−.117	−.097	−.173
Previously married	171	.290	−.028	.193	.213	.457	.412	.402
Never married	547	.213	−.014	.145	.005	.052	.035	.143
p-value[a]		<.001		<.001		<.001	<.001	<.001
Occupational Prestige[b]								
Major professional	158	−.142	−.090	−.153	−.155	−.241	−.243	−.281
Lesser professional	317	−.084	.048	−.034	−.020	−.083	−.063	−.064
Minor professional	258	.072	.026	.067	.001	.077	.048	.106
Clerical/sales	378	−.062	.060	−.010	.012	.072	.052	.017
Skilled/manual	98	.137	−.061	.064	.105	.062	.103	.176
Semi skilled/unskilled	165	.225	−.094	.109	.123	.126	.153	.120
p-value[a]		.002		<.001		.003	.004	<.001

[a]The p-values shown indicate significant group mean differences in stress exposure according to oneway ANOVA tests (two-tailed).

[b]Nineteen cases are missing for the occupation categories due to nonresponse on the relevant questions. The total N for sex, age, and marital status categories is 1,393; for occupational prestige, 1,374.

For each comparative analysis, Table 3 presents seven separate sets of distributions. Within each distribution, these scores have been standardized to a mean of 0 and a standard deviation of 1. Columns 1 through 3 present summary measures that distinguish recent stressful life events occurring to the respondent, to significant others, and a combined total of stressful events reported for the preceding 12 months. Column 4, "operant events," reflects life event checklist data, combining reports of ongoing life events and of very recent eventful stressors. Based on evidence suggesting that event checklists may confound information on discrete stressful events and more chronic stressors (Avison & Turner, 1988; Turner & Avison, 1992), we asked respondents to provide information on the starting and ending points of each reported stressor. Operant events include those events reported as occurring in the same month or the month preceding the interview, plus all those that continued into this period, regardless of when they began.

The chronic stress distributions (column 5) are based on a count from Wheaton's (1991) 51-item inventory. This provides, we believe, the most comprehensive assessment of role-related stresses and other long-term life difficulties so far available.

Information on stressful experiences across measuring instruments is shown in columns 6 and 7. The most important of these results are in column 6, "operant burden." We believe these results represent the best and most complete estimates of contemporary (i.e., recent and ongoing) exposure to stress. These scores combine "operant events" and "chronic stress" data from the preceding two columns (standardized scores are used to achieve equal weighting). The resulting sums were then restandardized. "Cumulative burden" reflects all three domain of stress exposure. Specifically, it is the restandardized sum of standardized scores for total stressful life events, chronic stress, and lifetime traumas. The lifetime trauma score consists of the sum of standardized childhood and adult trauma scores, with the adult scores age-adjusted to control for variations in time at risk. We will comment on the results for cumulative burden following the remainder of our discussion of Table 3.

Sex and Social Stress

Most previous studies have considered only stressful events experienced personally by the respondent, sometimes including stressful events occurring to someone close to the respondent. These measurement approaches are represented in columns 1 and 3 of Table 3 and offer no evidence for a sex difference in stress exposure. However, the fact that higher levels are observed among women when only events occurring to significant others are considered is consistent with the argument that women tend to have a wider domain of social concern and that they may bear an emotional "cost of caring," as some evidence has suggested (Kessler & McLeod, 1984; Turner & Avison, 1989).

The central point here is that when we consider only the stressful event checklist data and treat such data in the conventional way, our findings quite closely conform to previous findings—they contradict the hypothesis that different levels of exposure to stressful events is implicated in the observed sex differences in mental health. However, where estimates of stress exposure take account of the enduring character of some eventful stressors and/or of both role-related and other long-term chronic stresses, a different picture emerges. Whether the operant events or chronic stress measures are considered separately or the two are combined into our best estimate of stress exposure (operant burden), women report experiencing significantly higher levels of recent and ongoing stress than do men. Thus, when more than the number of reported events is taken into account, the hypothesis remains tenable that gender differences in mental health status may at least partially arise from the tendency for women to experience higher levels of social stress. It is worth pointing out that gender differences are especially apparent in the area of operant burden, denoting the importance of current stresses, and are less apparent for cumulative burden.

Age and Social Stress

Almost all previous studies have found younger subjects to experience higher levels of stressful life events. Table 3 supports this conclusion, whether only stressful life events are counted or more comprehensive estimates of stress exposure are employed. Interestingly however, the magnitude of the elevation of stress observed among the young is most pronounced where only event counts are used as estimators (columns 1 and 3), and only minimal differences occur among the remaining age categories. In fact, the age differences in exposure to stressful life events look strikingly similar to the negative decelerating curve we observed for age differences in depression. In contrast, when chronic stress is considered, age differences in stress are more linear: There is a more modest elevation in life stress for the young, along with evidence that those in the oldest age grouping (46–55) experience significantly lower levels of stress than their younger counterparts ($p < .05$). This same pattern is also observed for operant burden (chronic stress and operant events combined, column 6), although the stress advantage found for the oldest category falls slightly short of the usual criterion for statistical significance ($p < .10$).

This set of results is consistent with both prior evidence and expectations based on age variations in mental health status. As shown in Table 1, high levels of depressive symptoms and major depressive disorder are most frequent in the youngest age group and least frequent among respondents over 45, precisely matching the observed age distribution of stress exposure.

The observed age distributions of social stress, variously indexed, suggest, but do not demonstrate directly, the potential utility of stress exposure differences in understanding age differences in mental health.

Stress and Marital Status

As in the case of age, the typical finding that married persons have a significant advantage with respect to stressful life events is mirrored in our data (columns 1 and 3). Moreover, the estimates that take account of more enduring stresses or life difficulties (columns 4 to 6) provide additional support for this widely accepted association. However, the uniformity of findings on married persons, regardless of how stress exposure is estimated, is not matched in the various contrasts between the previously married and never married persons. While the life event data reveal little difference in stress exposure across these two categories, a clear difference is displayed for chronic stress, on operant events where account is taken of more enduring stressful occurrences, and when these two stress assessments are combined (operant burden, column 6). Based on these measures, the previously married report substantially higher levels of social stress than do the never married. While this difference may arise partially from the tendency for older individuals to experience more chronic stressors, it also reflects, we believe, the fact that separated and divorced individuals tend to confront a disproportionate number of persistent life problems.

Whatever the relative exposure to, and significance of, eventful versus chronic stresses across marital statuses, it is clear that the consistently observed association between marital status and risk for both depressive symptoms and depressive disorder is replicated by its association with level of social stress. The conclusion is therefore warranted that differences in exposure to stress may contribute to the documented differences in mental health risk by marital status.

Social Class and Social Stress

The bottom portion of Table 3 presents the indices of stress exposure by occupational prestige level. The results in columns 1 and 3 suggest one explanation for the inconsistency of prior reports on the association between stressful life events and socioeconomic status. Both distributions of stressful life events for self and total stressful events are generally linear, with the lowest stress levels found in the highest occupational category, but the contrasts based on events to self are statistically significant, while those for total stressful events are not. The hypothesized linear distribution by social class is observed for the operant burden index (column 6) and is generally found where only the Wheaton (1991) chronic stress index is used (column 5). Notwithstanding the ambiguity of findings when only stressful life events are considered, these results support the conclusion that exposure to stress tends to occur differentially for those differently situated in the social hierarchy. Moreover, they are consistent with the criticism of findings on social class for failing to consider the tendency for many stressors in the lower class to be more enduring or chronic in nature (Liem & Liem, 1978). Thus, the hypothesis that stress differences contribute to class differences in mental health status remains tenable.

Earlier we noted that the observed linear pattern of depressive symptoms and depressive disorder by occupational status were interrupted by substantially deviant results in the skilled-manual occupational category. The absence of a similar deviation within the social stress distribution indicates that stress differences are unlikely to be implicated in those deviant scores. Parenthetically, we have shown elsewhere that the SES distribution of both social support and self-esteem precisely mirror those for depressive symptoms and disorders, including the deviation from linearity at the skilled-manual level (Turner, 1992; Turner & Marino, 1994). Apparently, differences in stress mediators rather than differences in levels of stress exposure account for this distinctive observation.

Cumulative Stress Burden

So far, we have not commented on column 7 of Table 3, which presents estimates of social stress that include total stressful life events, chronic stress, and a lifetime trauma score. We call this "cumulative burden." This operationalization of stress exposure differs from the others in its focus on cumulative, rather than contemporary, stressful experiences. The similarity of these cumulative burden distributions in column 7 with the operant burden distributions in column 6 suggests some degree of stability and continuity in stress experiences over the life course. Presumably, the social contexts or roots that are associated with elevated risk for major traumas are also relevant to eventful and enduring stress experiences.

Stress Exposure and Mental Health

The results presented to this point have addressed the plausibility of the hypothesis that differences in exposure to stress play a significant role in explaining epidemiological variations in mental health status. We have suggested that if distributions of social stress complement established distributions of depressive symptoms and depressive disorder preliminary support for this hypothesis would be established. Such support is clearly revealed in Table 3. Our results also lend credibility to the two assumptions that largely motivated these analyses: (1) that variations in exposure to social stress substantially arise out of developmental and contemporary conditions of life; and (2) that one's gender and age and one's occupational and marital statuses effectively define important differences in such conditions of life. However, we have not yet provided an estimate of the magnitude of the contribution that stress exposure makes toward variance in mental health status. It is to this issue that we now turn.

Given the current visibility of the differential vulnerability hypothesis and the tendency for researchers to favor such explanations, we must account for possible social status variations in *responsiveness* to social stress. A direct assessment of this issue involves testing interactions between exposure to stressful life events and social status and, where interactions are found, decomposing status differences in mental health into portions attributable to differences in stress exposure, and to differential vulnerability to the same level of exposure by sex, age, marital status, and occupation (Iams & Thornton, 1975; Jones & Kelley, 1984).

We tested interactions between each of the four status dimensions and our most complete estimate of recent and ongoing stress exposure (operant burden) for both depressive symptoms and major depressive disorder. Of the eight interactions tested, only the one between sex and operant burden in predicting depressive symptoms was significant at the .05 level. Repeating these analyses with controls produced the same result—only the interaction with sex was significant. Thus, in seven of the eight cases, and regardless of whether the other social status variables were controlled, our results fail to support the differential vulnerability hypothesis. This is notable in the context of the tendency of researchers to focus primary attention on ascertaining the determinants of differential vulnerability to stress (Aneshensel, 1992).

Table 4 summarizes estimates of the magnitude of the contributions of stress exposure toward explaining observed social status distributions of depressive symptoms and major depression. Depressive symptoms and major depressive disorder were regressed on the four social status variables. We then estimated equations in which each component, and then the combined components, of the operant burden of stress were added separately. This procedure allows examination of whether and how current chronic stress and still operant stressful life events combine in their effects as total operant burden. In addition, it reveals the extent to which either chronic stress or operant life events offers the principal explanation for variations in mental health across each status variable. As noted earlier, we regard operant burden as the best estimate of contemporary stress exposure, but there may be instances in which one type of stress is most clearly implicated in status differences in mental health, and our analyses should be sensitive to this possibility.

The left panel of Table 4 shows the results of bivariate analyses of each social status variable with controls for stress added in each successive equation. These results are of particular interest because most previous studies have considered only one of these mental health correlates at a time. Thus, this panel indicates the extent of the contribution of exposure to stress in accounting for the relationships at issue as they have most typically been observed. The right panel shows the results when the effects of the other social status variables are considered simultaneously, with controls for stress added in the same sequence. In each analysis, first chronic stress is controlled, then operant stressful events, and finally the combination of the two as operant stress burden. Comparisons between the left and right panels indicate the effect of controlling on other social status variables. Thus, Table 4 allows us to evaluate the effect of each risk factor, controlling for both stress exposure differences and the effects of prior or intervening risk factors.

The top left panel shows a female-male difference on depressive symptoms (CES-D scores) of .31 standard deviations, quite typical of such differences in the existing literature. Controlling in turn for chronic stress, operant events,

Table 4 Metric Coefficients for Regression of Depressive Symptoms[a] (OLS) and Major Depressive Disorder (Logistic) on Social Status Variables and on Combinations of Recent Exposure to Stress: Residents of Toronto, Ontario, Ages 18–55, 1990–1991

Social Status Variables	Bivariate (1)	Controlling for Stress as Measured by:			Other Social Status Variables Controlled (5)	Controlling for Other Social Status Variables and Stress as Measured by:		
		Chronic Stress (2)	Operant Events (3)	Operant Burden (4)		Chronic Stress (6)	Operant Events (7)	Operant Burden (8)
Depressive Symptoms[a]								
Female	.31***	.25***	.27***	.24***	.30***	.26***	.27***	.24***
Age	–.10***	–.10***	–.10***	–.10***	–.08***	–.09***	–.08***	–.08***
Age^2	.001***	.001***	.001***	.001***	.001***	.001***	.001***	.001***
Previously married	.45***	.20*	.38***	.22**	.41***	.17	.34***	.20*
Never married	.40***	.32***	.38***	.34***	.12	.09	.14*	.12
Occupational prestige	.15***	.10***	.13***	.10***	.08**	.05*	.06*	.05*
Major Depressive Disorder								
Female	.57**	.51**	.50**	.47	.64**	.60**	.58**	.56**
Age	–.15*	–.15*	–.16*	–.16*	–.11	–.11	–.11	–.11
Age^2	.002	.001	.002	.002	.001	.001	.001	.001
Previously married	.61	.21	.47	.23	.56	.14	.40	.16
Never married	.98***	.93***	.97***	.95***	.39	.36	.40	.40
Occupational prestige	.38***	.33***	.36***	.33***	.26**	.20	.24*	.20

[a]From standardized CES-D scores.

$p < .05$ $p < .01$ $p < .001$ (two-tailed tests).

and operant burden shows that both chronic stress and operant events contribute to the explanation of male-female differences. The effect drops to .25 when controlling for chronic stress only, to .27 when controlling for operant events only, and to .24 when controlling for total operant burden. This latter figure, and that shown in column 8 where other demographic factors are controlled, were estimated by means of the decomposition procedure described above which controlled for differential vulnerability. This reduction in effect indicates that operant stress burden explains about 23 percent of the sex difference in depressive symptoms.

In the absence of evidence for other differential responses to estimated levels of operant stress burden, all other entries in Table 4 simply reflect the effect of each social status variable when various indices of stress exposure are controlled. There is a large difference in depressive symptoms between previously married respondents and the currently married ($b = .45$). While both types of stress have some role in explaining this difference, it is primarily chronic stress differences that account for the higher depressive symptoms among the previously married. This is consistent with hypotheses focusing on the built-in strains and difficulties of this role. Note that stress exposure differences account for about 50 percent of the effect ($b = .22$ in the final model). The picture for never married respondents is quite different: Much less of the difference between them and married respondents is due to stress exposure ($b = .32$ when controlling for chronic stress; $b = .40$ when uncontrolled). Still, controlling for chronic stress leads to a 20 percent reduction in effect. It is clear from looking at the right panel that much of the difference in depressive symptoms between never married and currently married respondents disappears when considering all social status variables simultaneously, even before controlling for stress ($b = .12$, not significant). This indicates a probable influence of age differences on the initial bivariate findings. That is, most of the initial difference in depressive symptoms may be due to the fact that never married respondents tend to be younger than currently married respondents, and increased depression is associated with youth. Thus, controlling for age is crucial for understanding the importance of marital status to mental health. With age controlled, the previously married–currently married difference persists.

For occupational status, differences in stress exposure account for 33 percent of the initial uncontrolled effect on depressive symptoms and 38 percent when other risk factors are controlled. Again, chronic stress plays a strong role in explaining these differences since the addition of operant events yields no further reduction in the coefficient.

Age differences in depressive symptoms are more independent of stress exposure than any other social status variable. Table 4 shows that controlling for stress does nothing to explain differences by age. This is, in effect, consistent with the conclusion in Mirowsky and Ross (1992) that there are life cycle influences on mental health.

In summary, then, for depressive symptoms, differences in levels of exposure to stress account for between 23 and 50 percent of observed differences in mental health by sex, marital status, and occupation. Stress exposure did not account for differences in depressive symptoms by age.

The right panel of Table 4 shows that controlling for other social status variables has little influence on the impact of sex, age, and previous marriage on depressive symptoms, but has a large impact on the influence of being never married (as noted above) and of occupational prestige. About 50 percent of the differences in depressive symptoms by occupation disappears when controls for other social status variables are used. This indicates, we believe, the joint associations of age with higher occupational levels and lower depression. This is because as we scored occupational prestige it is not confounded with gender, and its relationship with the previously married versus currently married comparison is minimal. Significantly, then, controlling for age differences may be crucial in properly specifying the effects of other social status variables.

The bottom panel of Table 4 reports our results for major depressive disorder. In general, these results resemble those for depressive symptoms, except that the influence of exposure to stress is generally somewhat less. Still, variations in operant burden clearly contribute toward explaining sex differences in major depressive disorder, and explain some of the differences by occupational prestige and marital status, where chronic stress plays a primary role. It is interesting that in comparison to the results for depressive symptoms, results for major depressive disorder show that the effects of occupational prestige persist somewhat more clearly when other status variables are controlled. For major depressive disorder only about 31 percent of the effect of occupation is explained by other status variables. This suggests that occupational status is at least as important for understanding differences in the occurrence of more serious mental health problems as it is for understanding differences in psychological distress.

SUMMARY AND CONCLUSIONS

We have addressed two hypotheses—that social stress is an important determinant of mental health status and that sex, age, marital status, and social class affect mental health and well-being partly because of social status differences in exposure to stress. We argued that the stress hypothesis has not been effectively tested because wholly adequate measurement of stress exposure remains to be achieved. For the same reason, we suggested that the importance of stress itself for explaining the epidemiology of mental health has been prematurely foreclosed by researchers in favor of focusing on social status differences in vulnerability to stress.

Our purpose has not been to disprove or even to challenge the differential vulnerability hypothesis. Rather, we simply proposed that social stress may be substantially more important as a determinant of mental health than currently supposed and that the role of stress in explaining variations in mental health by sex, age, marital status, and socioeconomic status remains to be established. We made a more comprehensive effort to estimate stress exposure than has been typical, and argued that findings indicating that the social distribution of stress complements the distributions for depressive symptoms and major depressive disorder would provide preliminary support for the stress exposure hypothesis.

Based on "operant burden," which we believe to be the best available estimate of current and recent stressful experiences, we found that stress distributions corresponded very closely with those observed for depression across sex, age, marital status, and occupation. These findings are consistent with the hypothesis that differences in mental health arise, at least in part, from systematic differences in the quantity and/or nature of stress experienced by individuals differentially situated in the social system. Evaluation of the magnitude of the contributions of stress to these distributions indicated substantial effects of stress on differences in mental health by occupational status, large effects relating to the risk status of previously married, and at least a notable contribution to the gender-mental health relationship.

Our findings suggest that the widely held conclusion that social status differences in vulnerability to stress are more consequential than differences in levels of stress exposure may be premature. We argue that the importance of differential vulnerability has been overestimated to the degree that differential exposure to stress has been underestimated, because unmeasured group differences in stress exposure parade within research findings as vulnerability differences. Our results suggest that differential exposure to stress by social status deserves renewed attention, with the provision that a broader array of stressful experiences must be measured.

APPENDIX A. SOCIAL STRESS INDICATORS

I. Life Events

Each life event index is a simple count from the number of positive responses to the following 34 items. Events to self indicate events that occurred to the respondent during the preceding 12 months. Events to others are the number from subsets of these events that occurred to the respondent's spouse or partner, children, and relatives or close friends.

A. I'd like to ask about some things that happened to you or to anyone close to you (that is your spouse/partner, children, relatives or close friends). Please tell me which of the following experiences happened to you or someone close to you in the past 12 months.

　　1. Was there a serious accident or injury?

　　2. Was there a serious illness?

　　3. Did a child die?

　　4. Did a spouse/partner die?

    5. Was there trouble with the law?

    6. Did anyone have something taken from them by force (robbed)?

    7. Was anyone beaten up or physically attacked?

B. Now, I'd like to ask you just about your family. Please tell me which of the following occurred to you, your spouse/partner, or children in the past 12 months.

    8. Was there an unwanted pregnancy?

    9. Was there an abortion or miscarriage?

   10. Did a close friend die?

   11. Was there a marital separation or divorce?

   12. Lost a home due to fire, flood, or other disaster?

   13. Was fired or layed off?

   14. Had a business that failed?

   15. Had a major financial crisis?

   16. Was accused or arrested for a crime?

   17. Failed school or training program?

   18. Dropped out of school?

C. Now, I'd like to ask you about some things that happened to you or your spouse/partner. Please tell me which of the following occurred to you or to your spouse in the past 12 months.

   19. Experienced a change of job for a worse one?

   20. Was demoted at work or took a cut in pay?

   21. Was sued by someone?

D. Now, I'd like to ask about some things that happened to you personally. Please tell me which of the following experiences you have had in the past two months?

   22. Went on welfare?

   23. Went on strike?

   24. Found out partner was having an affair?

   25. A romantic relationship ended?

   26. A close relationship ended?

   27. Partner found out about affair?

   28. Increased arguments with your partner?

   29. Moved to a worse residence or neighborhood?

   30. Moved out of city or area?

31. Had drivers license taken away?
32. Had your house or car broken into?
33. Had a child move back into the house?
34. Had a child move out of the house?

II. Chronic Stress

Some of the following 51 items form multi-item indices for chronic stress experienced in specific social roles or domains of life. Following the results of factor and internal reliability analyses of the intended subscales, five standard scores based on empirically-selected items (themselves scored: not true = 0; somewhat true = 1; very true = 2) were calculated. The 23 remaining items, dichotomized between not true (scored 0) and somewhat true or very true (scored 1) were individually standardized to Z-scores. The restandardized sum of the 28 standard scores forms a final estimate of chronic stress that equally weights contributions from the spectrum of roles and situations reflected in the items below.

Now, I'll describe some situations that sometimes come up in people's lives. I'd like you to tell me if these things are not true, somewhat true, or very true for you at this time.

1. You're trying to take on too many things at once.
2. There is too much pressure on you to be like other people.
3. Too much is expected of you by others.
4. You don't have enough money to buy the things you or your kids need.
5. You have a long-term debt or loan.
6. Your rent or mortgage is too much.
7. You don't have enough money to take vacations.
8. You don't have enough money to make a down payment on a home.
9. You have more work to do than most people.
10. Your supervisor is always monitoring what you do at work.
11. You want to change jobs or career but don't feel you can.
12. Your job often leaves you feeling both mentally and physically tired.
13. You want to achieve more at work but things get in the way.
14. You don't get paid enough for what you do.
15. Your work is boring and repetitive.
16. You are looking for a job and can't find the one you want.
17. You have a lot of conflict with your partner.
18. Your relationship restricts your freedom.

19. Your partner doesn't understand you.

20. Your partner expects too much of you.

21. You don't get what you deserve out of your relationship.

22. Your partner doesn't show enough affection.

23. Your partner is not committed enough to your relationship.

24. Your sexual needs are not fulfilled by this relationship.

25. Your partner is always threatening to leave or end the relationship.

26. You wonder whether you will ever get married.

27. You find it is too difficult to find someone compatible with you.

28. You have a lot of conflict with your ex-spouse.

29. You don't see your children from a former marriage as much as you would like.

30. You are alone too much.

31. You wish you could have children but you cannot.

32. One of your children seems very unhappy.

33. You feel your children don't listen to you.

34. A child's behavior is a source of serious concern to you.

35. One or more children do not do well enough at school or work.

36. Your children don't help around the house.

37. One of your children spends too much time away from the house.

38. You feel like being a housewife is not appreciated.

39. You have to go to social events alone and you don't want to.

40. Your friends are a bad influence.

41. You don't have enough friends.

42. You don't have time for your favorite leisure time activities.

43. You want to live farther away from your family.

44. You would like to move but you cannot.

45. The place you live is too noisy or too polluted.

46. Your family lives too far away.

47. Someone in your family or a close friend has a long-term illness or handicap.

48. You have a parent, a child, or a spouse or partner who is in very bad health and may die.

49. Someone in your family has an alcohol or drug problem.

50. A long-term health problem prevents you from doing the things you like to do.

51. You take care of an aging parent almost every day.

III. Major Traumatic Events

We distinguish two phases of the life course to estimate exposure to major life events: childhood and adulthood. These events are not limited to occurrence within the year before interview. Simultaneously considering the distinct lists of childhood and lifetime traumas below, we counted all occurrences prior to the age of 23 as the number of childhood traumatic events, and items endorsed as occurring at age 23 or later were counted as adult traumas. Each score represents a simple count of these events that last occurred in one or the other life phase.

A. Childhood Traumas

Now, I'd like to ask about some things that may have happened to you while you were a child or a teenager, before you moved out of the house.

1. Did you ever have a major illness or accident that required you to spend a week or more in the hospital?
2. Did your parents get a divorce?
3. Did you have to do a year of school over again?
4. Did your father or mother not have a job for a long time when they wanted to be working?
5. Did something happen that scared you so much you thought about it for years after?
6. Were you ever sent away from home because you did something wrong?
7. Did either of your parents drink or use drugs so often or so regularly that it caused problems for the family?
8. Were you regularly physically abused by one of your parents?

B. Lifetime Traumas

Now, I'd like to ask you about some events that could have happened at any time in your life. Please tell us if any of these things have happened, and how old you were.

1. Have you ever been divorced or ended a relationship with someone you were still in love with?
2. Has one of your parents died?
3. Has a spouse, child or other loved one died?
4. Have you ever seen something violent happen to someone or seen someone killed?
5. Have you ever been in a major fire, flood, earthquake, or other natural disaster?
6. Has you ever had a serious accident, injury, or illness that was life threatening or caused long-term disability?

7. Has one of your children ever had a near fatal accident or life-threatening illness?

8. Have you ever been in combat in a war, lived near a war zone or been present during a political uprising?

9. Have you ever discovered your spouse or partner in a close relationship was unfaithful?

10. Have you ever been physically abused by your current or a previous spouse or partner?

11. Has your spouse, partner, or child been addicted to alcohol or drugs?

References

Al-Issa, Ihsan. 1982. "Gender and Adult Psychopathology." Pp. 83–110 in *Gender and Psychopathology*, edited by I. Al-Issa. New York: Academic.

Aneshensel, Carol S. 1992. "Social Stress: Theory and Research." *Annual Review of Sociology* 18:15–38.

Avison, William R. and R. Jay Turner. 1988. "Stressful Life Events and Depressive Symptoms: Disaggregating the Effects of Acute Stressors and Chronic Strains." *Journal of Health and Social Behavior* 29:253–64.

Devins, Gerald M. and Carolee Orme. 1985. "Center for Epidemiological Studies Depression Scales." Pp. 144–60 in *Test Critiques*, vol. 2, edited by D. J. Keyser and R. C. Sweetland. Kansas City, MO: Test Corporation of America.

Dohrenwend, Barbara S. and Bruce P. Dohrenwend. 1974. "Overview and Prospects for Research on Stressful Life Events." Pp. 313–31 in *Stressful Life Events: Their Nature and Events*, edited by B. S. Dohrenwend and B. P. Dohrenwend. New York: John Wiley.

Dohrenwend, Bruce P. and Barbara S. Dohrenwend. 1969. *Social Status and Psychological Disorder: A Causal Inquiry*. New York: John Wiley.

Dohrenwend, Bruce P., Itzhak Levan, Patrick E. Shrout, Sharon Schwartz, Guedalia Naveh, Bruce G. Link, Andrew E. Skodol, and Ann Stueve. 1992. "Socioeconomic Status and Psychiatric Disorders: The Causation-Selection Issue." *Science* 255:946–52.

Eaton, William W. 1986. *The Sociology of Mental Disorders*. 2d ed. New York: Praeger.

Faris, Robert E. L. and H. Warren Dunham. 1939. *Mental Disorders in Urban Areas*. New York: Hafner.

Gove, Walter 1972. "The Relationship between Sex Roles, Mental Illness and Marital Status." *Social Forces* 51:34–44.

Gurin, Gerald, Joseph Veroff, and Sheila Feld. 1960. *Americans View Their Mental Health: A Nationwide Survey*. New York: Basic Books.

Henderson, Scott, D. G. Byrne, and Paul Duncan-Jones. 1981. *Neurosis and the Social Environment*. New York: Academic Press.

Hollingshead, August B. 1957. *Two Factor Index of Social Position*. New Haven, CT: A. B. Hollingshead.

Hollingshead, August B. and Frederick C. Redlich. 1958. *Social Class and Mental Illness: A Community Study*. New York: Wiley.

Holmes, Thomas H. and Richard H. Rahe. 1967. "The Social Readjustment Rating Scale." *Journal of Psychosomatic Research* 11:213–18.

House, James S. and Jeylan Mortimer. 1990. "Social Structure and the Individual: Emerging Themes and New Directions." *Social Psychology Quarterly* 53:71–80.

Iams, Howard M. and Arland Thornton. 1975. "Decomposition of Differences: A Cautionary Note." *Sociological Methods and Research* 3:341–52.

Janca, Aleksandar, Lee N. Robins, Linda B. Cottler, and T. S. Early. 1992. "Clinical Observation of CIDI Assessments: An Analysis of the CIDI Field Trials—Wave II at the St. Louis Site." *British Journal of Psychology* 160:815–18.

Jemmott, John B., III and Steven E. Locke. 1984. "Psychosocial Factors, Immunologic Mediation, and Human Susceptibility to Infectious Diseases: How Much Do We Know?" *Psychological Bulletin* 95:78–108.

Jenkins, David C. 1976. "Recent Evidence Supporting Psychologic and Social Risk Factors for Coronary Disease." *New England Journal of Medicine* 294:987–94, 1033–38.

Jones, F. L. and Jonathan Kelley. 1984. "Decomposing Differences between Groups: A Cautionary Note on Measuring Discrimination." *Sociological Methods and Research* 12:323–43.

Kessler, Ronald C. 1979. "A Strategy for Studying Differential Vulnerability to the Psychological Consequences of Stress." *Journal of Health and Social Behavior* 20:100–08.

Kessler, Ronald C. and Paul D. Cleary. 1980. "Social Class and Psychological Distress." *American Sociological Review* 45:463–78.

Kessler, Ronald C. and Jane D. McLeod. 1984. "Sex Differences in Vulnerability to Undesirable Life Events. *American Sociological Review* 49:620–31.

Kohn, Melvin L. 1972. "Class, Family and Schizophrenia: A Reformulation." *Social Forces* 50:295–313.

Liem, Ramsay and Joan Liem. 1978. "Social Class and Mental Illness Reconsidered: The Role of Economic Stress and Social Support." *Journal of Health and Social Behavior* 19:139–56.

Mirowsky, John and Catherine E. Ross. 1992. "Age and Depression." *Journal of Health and Social Behavior* 33:187–205.

Nolen-Hoeksema, Susan. 1987. "Sex Differences in Unipolar Depression." *Psychological Bulletin* 101:259–82.

Pearlin, Leonard I. 1989. "The Sociological Study of Stress." *Journal of Health and Social Behavior* 30:241–56.

Pearlin, Leonard I. and Morton A. Lieberman. 1979. "Social Sources of Emotional Distress." Pp. 17–48 in *Research in Community and Mental Health,* edited by R. Simmons. Greenwich, CT: JAI Press.

Pearlin, Leonard I. and Carmi Schooler. 1978. "The Structure of Coping." *Journal of Health and Social Behavior* 19:2–21.

Rabkin, Judith G. and Elmer L. Struening. 1976. "Life Events, Stress, and Illness." *Science* 194:1013–20.

Radloff, Lenore S. 1977. "The CES-D Scale: A Self-Report Depression Scale for Research in the General Population. *Applied Psychological Measurement* 1:385–401.

Robins, Lee N., John Wing, Hans -Ulrich Wittchen, John E. Helzer, Thomas Babor, Jay Burke, Ann Farmer, Assen Jablenski, Roy Pickens, Darrel Regier, Norman Sartorius, and Leland Towle. 1988. "The Composite International Diagnostic Interview: An Epidemiologic Instrument Suitable for Use in Conjunction with Different Diagnostic Systems and in Different Cultures." *Archives of General Psychiatry* 45:1069–77.

Ross, Catherine E. and Joan Huber. 1985. "Hardship and Depression." *Journal of Health and Social Behavior* 26:312–27.

Sarason, Irwin G., James H. Johnson, and Judith M. Siegel. 1978. "Assessing the Impact of Life Changes: Development of the Life Experiences Survey." *Journal of Consulting and Clinical Psychology* 46:932–46.

Spengler, P. and H. U. Wittchen. 1989. "Procedural Validity of Standardized Symptom Questions for the Assessment of Psychotic Symptoms: A Comparison of the CIDI with Two Clinical Methods." *Comprehensive Psychiatry* 29:309–22.

Thoits, Peggy A. 1983. "Dimensions of Life Events that Influence Psychological Distress: An Evaluation and Synthesis of the Literature." Pp. 33–103 in *Psychosocial Stress: Trends in Theory and Research*, edited by H. Kaplan. New York: Academic Press.

———. 1987. "Gender and Marital Status Differences in Control and Distress: Common Stress Versus Unique Stress Explanations." *Journal of Health and Social Behavior* 28:7–22.

Turner, R. Jay. 1992. "Epidemiologic Aspects of the Stress Process." 1992. Rema Lapouse Award Lecture, presented at the annual meeting of the American Public Health Association, November, Washington, DC.

Turner, R. Jay and William R. Avison. 1989. "Gender and Depression: Assessing Exposure and Vulnerability to Life Events in a Chronically Strained Population." *The Journal of Nervous and Mental Disease* 177:443–455.

———. 1992. "Sources of Attenuation in the Stress-Distress Relationship: An Evaluation of Modest Innovations in the Application of Event Checklists." Pp. 265–300 in *Research in Community and Mental Health*, edited by J. Greenley and P. Leaf. Greenwich, CT: JAI Press.

Turner, R. Jay and Franco Marino. 1994. "Social Support and Social Structure: A Descriptive Epidemiology." *Journal of Health and Social Behavior* 35:193–212.

Turner, R. Jay, Leslie S. Dopkeen, and Gary P. Labreche. 1970. "Marital Status and Schizophrenia: A Study of Incidence and Outcome." *Journal of Abnormal Psychology* 76:110–16.

Turner, R. Jay and Morton O. Wagenfeld. 1967. "Occupational Mobility: An Assessment of the Social Causation and Social Selection Hypothesis." *American Sociological Review* 32:104–13.

Turner, R. Jay and Samuel Noh. 1988. "Physical Disability and Depression: A Longitudinal Analysis." *Journal of Health and Social Behavior* 29:263–77.

Wacker, H. R., R. Battegay, R. Mullejans, and C. Schlosser. 1990. "Using the CIDI-C in the General Population." Pp. 138–43 in *Psychiatry: A World Perspective*, edited by C. N. Stefains, A. D. Rabavilas, and C. R. Soldatos. New York: Elsevier Science Publishers.

Weissman Myrna M. and Gerald L. Klerman. 1977. "Sex Differences and the Epidemiology of Depression." *Archives of General Psychiatry* 34:98–111.

Wheaton, Blair. 1978. "The Sociogenesis of Psychological Disorder: Reexamining the Causal Issues with Longitudinal Data." *American Sociological Review* 43:383–403.

———. 1991. "The Specification of Chronic Stress: Models and Measurement." Paper presented at an annual meeting of the Society for the Study of Social Problems, August, Cincinnati, OH.

———. 1994. "Sampling the Stress Universe." Pp. 77–114 in *Stress and Mental Health: Contemporary Issues and Prospects for the Future*, edited by W. Avison and I. Gotlib. New York: Plenum.

Wittchen, Hans -Ulrich, Lee N. Robins, Linda B. Cottler, Norman Sartorius, Jay D. Burke, Darrel A. Regier, and Participants in the Multicenter WHO/ADAMHA Field Trials. 1991. "Cross-Cultural Feasibility, Reliability and Sources of Variance in the Composite International Diagnostic Interview (CIDI)." *British Journal of Psychiatry* 159:645–53.

World Health Organization (WHO). 1990. *Composite International Diagnostic Interview.* Version 1.0. Geneva, Switzerland: World Health Organization.

DISCUSSION QUESTIONS

1. Why was it so important to Turner and colleagues that their measures of stress exposure be comprehensive? How might their results differ if their measures failed to include stressful life experiences common to people who are not married or who hold low prestige jobs?

2. Summarize the main conclusions that can be derived from the data in each of the tables the authors present. What does each step in the analysis tell us? How do the different steps in the analysis fit together?

3. Try to develop a measure of stress that is appropriate to college-age populations. Which of the items from Turner et al.'s measures would you retain? Which would you delete? What would you add?

Roles, Social Statuses, and Mental Health

John Mirowsky and Catherine E. Ross

Sex Differences in Distress: Real or Artifact?[†]

On average, women report higher levels of psychological distress than men, higher rates of depression and anxiety, and lower rates of substance use and antisocial personality disorder. Sociologists have actively debated the origins of those differences since the 1970s. In 1973, Gove and Tudor presented a "sex role" theory which proposed that women experience more mental illness than men because their positions in society are more frustrating and less satisfying. They rest their argument on five points: (1) "most women are restricted to a major societal role—housewife, whereas most men occupy two such roles, household head and worker," (2) "it seems reasonable to assume that a large number of women find their major instrumental activities—raising children and keeping house—frustrating," (3) "the role of housewife is relatively unstructured and invisible," (4) "even when a married women works, she is typically in a less satisfactory position than the married male," and (5) "the expectations regarding women are unclear and diffuse (pp. 814–815)." In 1976, Dohrenwend and Dohrenwend countered that women do not experience more mental illness than men; they simply experience different kinds of mental illness. In this selection, John Mirowsky and Catherine E. Ross bring the debate up-to-date with more recent evidence and arguments.

American surveys find that women report higher average levels of depression and anxiety than men (Aneshensel, 1992; Mirowsky & Ross, 1986). What explains these sex differences in reports of distress? One possibility is that women genuinely suffer greater distress than men. If so, the difference in distress reflects and reveals women's relative disadvantage in American society. Another possibility is that women may simply express their emotions more freely than men, and thus appear more distressed. Or, women may respond to stressors with somewhat different emotions than men. Thus, if surveys ask more questions about responses typical of women than about those typical of men, women may falsely appear more distressed.

Mirowsky, John and Catherine E. Ross. 1995. "Sex Differences in Distress: Real or Artifact?" *American Sociological Review* 60:449–468.

DISTRESS AND FEMALE DEPRESSION

Theories of gender inequality, gender roles, or gender-based exposure to social stressors explain women's elevated distress as the consequence of inequality and disadvantage (Gove & Tudor, 1977; Pearlin, 1989; Ross & Huber, 1985). According to the *structured-strain* view, different positions in the social structure expose individuals to different amounts of hardship and constraint. Women's positions at work and in the family disadvantage them compared to men because of their greater burden of demands and limitations. This burden creates stress and frustration and is manifested in higher levels of distress.

Two alternative views say that women simply express themselves differently than men, thus creating a false impression of greater distress (Nolen-Hoeksema, 1987). According to the *response-bias* view, women express all emotions more freely than men. According to this view, women are more aware than men of their emotions, they are also more likely to talk about emotions to others, to be open and expressive, and to think that discussing personal well-being is acceptable rather than stigmatizing. Thus, when women and men are questioned about depression and anxiety the women report it more frequently. Alternatively, the *gendered-response* theory says women respond to the ubiquitous stress of life with somewhat different emotions than men. In particular, women might feel anxious and depressed where men might feel agitated and angry. If surveys ask more questions about types of distress typical of women than about those typical of men, then women may falsely appear more distressed.

Testing Response-Biases and Gendered-Responses

Female expressiveness may mask the distinction between feminine and masculine types of distress. Women may report greater hostility and anger than men simply because women more freely report their emotions. Thus, the failure to find clear evidence of gendered responses may be seen as evidence of response bias. While this may seem like a reasonable interpretation, it reveals a possible circularity in the arguments against genuine sex differences in distress: If men *do* report more anger than women, then women's greater depression and anxiety is dismissed as the "feminine response" to burdens and frustrations shared equally with men (gendered response); if men *do not* report more anger than women do, then men's lower distress is dismissed as "masculine stoicism" and reserve about burdens and frustrations shared equally with women (response bias). Any true tests of the response-bias and gendered-response hypotheses must avoid this circularity. It must be possible to accept or reject each hypothesis independently.

Independent tests require explicit measures and adjustments for expressiveness, and the examination of various forms of distress. We measure expressiveness directly by asking people whether they keep their emotions to themselves, and indirectly by assessing the tendency to report both positive and negative emotions (an unobtrusive latent factor). We examine various outcomes, including depressed mood (sadness), positive mood (happiness), anxiety, anger, malaise, and physiological symptoms (aches).

Accepting the response-bias perspective requires that we find support for all three of the following hypotheses:

H$_1$: Women are more likely than men to express their feelings.
H$_2$: Expressiveness increases reports of distress.
H$_3$: Adjustment for the tendency to express emotions explains sex differences in distress (the effect of sex on distress becomes insignificant with adjustment for response tendencies).

Accepting the gendered-response perspective requires that we find support for both of the following hypotheses:

H$_4$: Women have higher levels of depression; men have higher levels of anger.
H$_5$: People with higher levels of anger have lower levels of depression.

METHODS

Sample

This research draws on a fall 1990 telephone survey of a national probability sample of U.S. households. Sampling followed the Waksberg-Mitofsky random-digit dialing procedure, which ensures the inclusion of unlisted numbers (Waksberg, 1978). The interviewers called primarily during evenings and weekends. Unanswered working numbers were called back 10 times before being dropped. Non-household numbers were dropped (businesses, dorms, etc.). In each household the adult (18 years old or older) with the most recent birthday was selected as respondent. (This is an efficient way to randomly select a respondent within the household [O'Rourke & Blair, 1983]). Up to 10 callbacks were made to selected respondents who could not be interviewed immediately. Of the selected respondents, 82.3 percent completed interviews, yielding a total of 2,031 respondents (1,282 females and 749 males), ranging in age from 18 to 90.

Measures

Distress is measured using six indexes representing sadness, happiness, anger, anxiety, malaise, and aches. For each symptom of distress, respondents were asked, "On how many of the past 7 days have you...?" Responses are coded from 0 to 7, from never experiencing the symptom to experiencing it every day. Each index represents the mean frequency of its component items. *Sadness* averages the frequency of feeling sad, lonely, and unable to shake the blues (α = .82). *Happiness* averages the frequency of feeling happy, feeling hopeful about the future, and enjoying life (α = .79). *Anxiety* averages the frequency of worrying a lot about little things, feeling tense or anxious, and feeling restless (α = .82). *Anger* averages the frequency of feeling annoyed with things or people, feeling angry, and yelling at someone (α = .71). *Malaise* averages the frequency of feeling everything is an effort, feeling that you just can't get going, having trouble keeping your mind on what you are doing, and having trouble getting to sleep or staying asleep (α = .73). *Aches* averages the frequency of having aches and pains, having headaches, and feeling weak all over (α = .60).

Although some researchers invoke emotional expressiveness as an explanation of sex differences in measured distress, we know of none who has measured expressiveness and shown that sex differences in distress vanish when controlling for it. Part of the reason no one has done this may be that differences in the willingness to express emotions are easier to imagine than to measure. Our analyses below take two approaches to assessing possible response bias: one self-evident and the other unobtrusive.

The first measure is a *self-evident question* about how much the respondent agrees with the statement, "I keep my emotions to myself." The responses indicate self-evaluated emotional reserve (called "reserve" for short). The response categories are "strongly disagree" (coded –2), "disagree" (coded –1), "agree" (coded 1), and "strongly agree" (coded 2). (Six women and 2 men said "don't know" and were coded 0). This measure is simple and direct. However, it has several disadvantages. Someone who is circumspect about emotions may be disinclined to say so. Or people may be unaware of their own emotional expressiveness compared to others'. On the other hand, people who are wary of sharing emotions with friends and acquaintances may be relieved to report them as an anonymous respondent. Perhaps more to the point, the conscious restraint of one's emotions may indicate a heightened level of disturbing emotion, a dysfunctional coping strategy, or a sense of needing to tell someone.

The second measure is an *unobtrusive latent factor* implicit in the reports of positive and negative moods (happiness and sadness). In this crossed 2 × 2 measurement, people who report more of both emotions are considered more emotionally expressive. We call the factor "expression" for short. The model defines expression and depression as crosscutting factors, each indicated by reports both of sadness and of happiness: Expression increases reports of happiness and of sadness net of the level of depression, whereas depression increases reports of sadness and *decreases* reports of happiness net of the level of expression.

Female is a dummy variable representing sex, coded 1 for females and 0 for males.

Sociodemographic variables are adjusted in some of the models. *Age* is coded in number of years. *Minority status* is coded 0 for non-Hispanic whites and 1 for others. *Marital status* is coded 1 for married or living together as married and 0 otherwise. *Education* is coded as the number of completed years of formal schooling.

ANALYSIS AND RESULTS

The analysis has three parts. The first part describes sex differences in the *degree* of emotional expression and tests the *response-bias* hypothesis. The second part describes sex differences in the *type* of emotional expression and tests the *gendered-response* hypothesis. The third part analyzes the impact of sex differences in the degree and type of emotional expression on regression estimates of the sex difference in distress. The introduction to the results in each part explains the reasoning behind its models and analyses.

Analysis 1: Response Bias and Female Expressiveness

Analysis 1 explores the possibility that women seem more depressed than men because women report their emotions more freely.

Self-evident appraisal of expressiveness. The statement, "I keep my emotions to myself," voices emotional reserve—the self-perceived restraint of emotional expression. Cross-tabulating the responses by sex shows that more men than women claim to keep emotions to themselves. Sixty-eight percent of the men either agree or strongly agree with the statement, compared to 50 percent of the women. Thus, in our sample men are 1.360 times more likely than women to say they keep emotions to themselves. (Alternatively, the odds of agreeing with the statement are 2.125 times greater for men than for women.) The men's average score exceeds the women's by about a third of a standard deviation. Both the chi-square test of the cross-tabulation and the *t*-test of the difference in mean scores are statistically significant at $p < .001$.

Does male reserve account for the fact that men report being depressed less often than women? No. We find that people who claim to keep emotions to themselves report *more* days of depressed mood, not fewer. The sadness index from the CES-D averages the number of days from the previous week the respondent reported feeling sad, lonely, and blue. Figure 1 shows that mean scores for sadness *increase* with self-reported emotional reserve. People who strongly agree that "I keep my emotions to myself" average more than twice the frequency of sadness than people who disagree. Women are sadder than men within each category of emotional reserve.

This simple analysis suggests that male reserve cannot account for sex differences in depression. In fact, if the only difference between the sexes were that men had greater emotional reserve, men would be sadder than women because people who say they keep their emotions to themselves report *more* sadness than others, not less.

Unobtrusive appraisal of expressiveness. The crosscutting factor model indicates that women express emotions more freely than do men, but also that they are more depressed than men. The main difference in results between our two measures is that the unobtrusive factor relates to measures of distress more as one would expect for an index of emotional expressiveness. With the direct question about emotional reserve, people who claim to be the

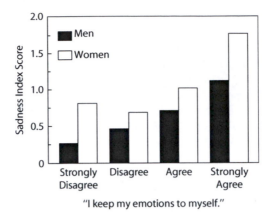

Figure 1 Relationship between Sadness Index Score and Emotional Reserve[a]
[a]Sadness increases with emotional reserve. Women are sadder than men in each category.

most reserved actually report *more* days of sadness than others, not fewer. By definition, people with low scores on the expression factor report *fewer* days of sadness, and fewer of happiness.

The basic model shows the logic behind the crosscutting factor model in its simplest and clearest form. The effect of being female on expressiveness is .170 (row 1, column 3 of Table 1). The effect of being female on depression is .182 (row 1, column 2 of Table 1). According to the model, women feel more depressed than men, and they express their feelings more freely.

In these data women report about the same frequency of happiness as men. (Women actually report slightly more happiness than men, but the difference is not statistically significant [p = .422]). How can women be sadder than men but not less happy? The model says that the *apparent* inconsistency reflects the presence of the crosscutting expression factor. Depression shifts women's balance of emotions away from happiness toward sadness, but greater emotional expressiveness means they report more happiness than men do at the same level of depression.

Interestingly, the basic crosscutting factor model shows no direct effect of self-evaluated reserve on the expression of positive and negative emotions. As in the simple analysis of Figure 1, depression increases with emotional reserve (b = .165, row 2, column 2 of Table 1). Again, our results imply that men would report more depression than would women if the sexes differed only in emotional reserve.

Analysis 2: "Masculine" and "Feminine" Types of Distress

Surveys might give a false impression by asking mostly about feminine types of distress. The analyses up to this point have concentrated on feelings of depression. By that measure women exhibit more distress than men. Does the relationship hold for more "masculine" forms of distress? The *escalating anger* model and the *hierarchical distress* model address this question.

Table 1 Metric Coefficients from the Basic Crosscutting Factor Model[a] Testing Sex Differences in Depression and Emotional Expressiveness: U.S. Men and Women Ages 18 to 90, 1990

	Dependent Variables		
Independent Variables	(1) "I keep my emotions to myself."	(2) Depression Factor[b]	(3) Expression Factor[b]
(1) Female	−.442*** (−8.531)	.182** (3.095)	.170*** (4.729)
(2) "I keep my emotions to myself."	—	.165*** (6.934)	.000[c]

*$p < .05$ **$p < .01$ ***$p < .001$ (two-tailed tests)
[a]EQS Model (Bentler 1989): $N = 2,027$; $\chi^2 = .001$; d.f. = 1; $p = .978$; normed fit = 1.000; nonnormed fit = 1.009; comparative fit = 1.000.
[b]The depression and expression factors are both indicated by a three-item index of sadness and a three-item index of happiness. The metric loadings of the indexes on the depression factor are fixed to +1 and −1 respectively. The metric loadings on the expression factor are both fixed to +1. The regression residuals of the depression and expression factors have a covariance of −.284 ($t = −12.539$).
[c]The parameter is fixed to zero. When freed it is not significantly different from zero.
Note: Numbers in parentheses are *t*-values.

Sex and escalating anger. Do women get depressed and men get angry? Gendered-response theory suggests that the answer is yes, but our data indicate that the answer is no. Table 2 shows the escalating anger model. Three reports indicate the level of anger: feeling annoyed with things or people, feeling angry, and yelling at someone. The results show that women are angrier than men and are more likely to express their anger by yelling.

Anger has another thing in common with depression, in addition to showing higher levels among women than among men: People who say they keep emotions to themselves report feeling angry more frequently than others— not less.

Sex and the hierarchy of distress. Various measures of distress are positively correlated with each other. Depression, anxiety, anger, and physical symptoms correlate positively and significantly. Positive mood correlates negatively with all psychophysiological measures of distress. Thus, people who feel sad, for example, also tend to feel unhappy, anxious, angry, depleted, and ill.

Analysis 3: Adjusted Regressions

Response bias and gendered response. Response-bias theory implies that adjusting for emotional reserve and expression will eliminate or greatly reduce the estimated effect of sex on levels of distress. Table 3 shows six sets of regressions. The first in each set regresses an index of distress on sex adjusting for age, minority status, marital status, and education. The second adjusts also

Table 2 Metric Regression Coefficients and Factor Loadings for the Escalating-Factor Model[a] Testing Sex Differences in Anger: U.S. Men and Women Ages 18 to 90

	Dependent Variables			
Independent Variables	Anger Factor	Annoyed	Angry	Yelled
Female	.146**			.534***
	(2.844)			(5.945)
Marriage				.358***
				(4.396)
Age	−.021***			
	(−8.774)			
Education				−.070***
				(−4.549)
"I keep emotions to myself."	.050**			
	(2.513)			
Anger factor		1.817***	1.000[b]	1.000[b]
		(7.372)		
		(3.315)		
Annoyed			.305***	
			(8.597)	
Angry				.374***
				(7.809)

*$p < .05$ **$p < .01$ ***$p < .001$ (two-tailed tests)

[a]EQS Model (Bentler 1989): $N = 2,031$; $\chi^2 = 11.557$; d.f. = 10; $p = .316$; normed fit = .994; nonnormed fit = .998; comparative fit = .999. This model meets the criteria that (a) all of the coefficients have two-tailed p-values of .10 or less and that (b) a Lagrange multiplier test indicates the overall fit cannot be improved by freeing any of the parameters fixed to 0, +1, or −1. The table does not show the regression of keeping emotions to oneself because it is the same as in the first column in Table 2a.

[b]Coefficients without t-values are fixed to the values shown. Blanks represent coefficients fixed to zero.

Note: A t-values in parentheses (t) measures the coefficient's standard-error distance from 0; A t-value in brackets $\{t\}$ measures its standard-error distance from the theoretical metric loading of +1.

for the expression index (*Expression = (Sadness + Happiness)/2*), and the third adds adjustment for keeping emotions to oneself. The first row of Table 3 shows the effect of being female on each type of distress, first without and then with the adjustments for expressiveness and reserve. For the five negative emotions the effect of sex gets smaller with adjustment for the expression index, but it gets larger with adjustment for emotional reserve. Only the effect of being female on sadness is smaller with the two adjustments than without them, but still it remains quite significant. For happiness, the effect of sex changes sign when adjustment for the expression index is added, from positive but very nonsignificant to negative and nearly significant for a two-tailed test (or significant for a one-tailed test; $t = −1.937$). The negative effect of being female on happiness becomes more negative and more statistically

Table 3 Metric Coefficients for the Regression of Six Indexes of Distress on Sex and Sociodemographic Variables, without and with Adjustment for Expressiveness and Emotional Reserve: U.S. Men and Women Ages 18 to 90, 1990

Independent Variables	Sadness			Happiness			Anger		
	Model 1	Model 2	Model 3	Model 1	Model 2	Model 3	Model 1	Model 2	Model 3
Female	.234***	.127*	.198***	.048	-.118+	-.188**	.387***	.337***	.413***
	(3.447)	(2.076)	(3.153)	(.635)	(-1.937)	(-3.056)	(5.251)	(5.092)	(5.468)
Age	-.002	-.005**	-.005**	.009***	.005**	.006**	-.033***	-.033***	.034***
	(-.960)	(-2.582)	(-3.021)	(4.196)	(2.882)	(3.339)	(-15.547)	(-15.603)	(-15.759)
Minority	.073	.022	.030	.069	-.010	-.018	.090	.086	.090
	(.833)	(.275)	(.378)	(.706)	(-.132)	(-.238)	(.950)	(.897)	(.941)
Married	-.527***	-.497***	-.458***	.446***	.492***	.452***	.004	.007	.027
	(-7.776)	(-8.154)	(-7.516)	(5.870)	(8.141)	(7.485)	(.058)	(.095)	(.370)
Education	-.067***	-.064***	-.060***	.059***	.064***	.061**	-.015	-.014	-.013
	(-5.214)	(-5.501)	(-5.222)	(4.076)	(5.584)	(5.298)	(-1.049)	(-1.025)	(-.891)
Expression Index		.785***	.784***		1.220***	1.221***		.073+	.073+
		(21.788)	(21.924)		(34.157)	(34.475)		(1.687)	(1.675)
"I keep my emotions to myself."			.149***			-.539***			.077
			(5.682)			(-5.885)			(2.413)
Intercept	1.960	-.518	-.623	4.328	.475	.582	3.000	2.769	2.715
R²	.053	.234	.246	.032	.388	.398	.117	.118	.121

(continued)

Table 3 Continued

Independent Variables	Anxiety			Malaise			Aches		
	Model 1	Model 2	Model 3	Model 1	Model 2	Model 3	Model 1	Model 2	Model 3
Female	.584***	.546***	.626***	.294***	.273***	.327***	.298***	.284***	.302***
	(5.650)	(5.284)	(5.963)	(4.528)	(4.206)	(4.954)	(4.823)	(4.587)	(4.798)
Age	-.021***	-.022***	-.002***	-.001	-.002	-.002	.005***	.005**	.005**
	(-6.951)	(-7.283)	(-7.584)	(-.574)	(-.859)	(-1.174)	(2.974)	(2.775)	(2.653)
Minority	-.166	-.185	-.175	-.035	-.045	-.039	-.080	-.086	-.084
	(-1.284)	(-1.391)	(-1.326)	(-.413)	(-.536)	(-.464)	(-1.001)	(-1.082)	(-1.055)
Married	-.306**	-.296**	-.250*	-.374***	-.341***	-.310***	-.280***	-.277***	-.266***
	(-5.361)	(-2.881)	(-2.425)	(-5.361)	(-5.289)	(-4.799)	(-4.559)	(-4.495)	(-4.293)
Education	-.007***	-.076***	-.072***	-.109***	-.109***	-.106***	-.094***	-.094***	-.093***
	(-3.936)	(-3.888)	(-3.680)	(-8.853)	(-8.832)	(-8.624)	(-8.084)	(-8.043)	(-7.949)
Expression Index		.280***	.279***		.155***	.154***		.099**	.099**
		(4.627)	(4.621)		(4.071)	(4.063)		(2.733)	(2.725)
"I keep my emotions to myself."			.174***			.117***			.041
			(3.930)			(4.191)			(1.534)
Intercept	4.164	3.279	3.156	2.588	2.028	2.016	2.072	1.758	1.729
R²	.045	.055	.062	.065	.072	.080	.065	.069	.070

*p < .05 **p < .01 ***p < .001 (2-tailed tests)
†p < .05 (one-tailed tests)
Note: Numbers in parentheses are t-values.

significant with the added adjustment for keeping emotions to oneself. Overall, the regressions show that, adjusting for expressiveness, women are more distressed than men on all six measures, and that adjusting for reserve increases the estimated differences.

Gendered-response theory has implied that women's distress would most exceed men's when measured as sadness and unhappiness and least when measured as anger. Our regressions show just the opposite. Sex differences are smallest for sadness and happiness, and the sex difference in anger is twice as large as that for sadness and happiness. Sex has its largest effect on anxiety. In terms of days per symptom per week, the gender gap in anxiety and anger far exceeds that in sadness and unhappiness.

A measure of relative frequency shows that women experience symptoms of distress roughly 30 percent more often than men. Taking the regression coefficient for sex as a percentage of the mean symptom score among men shows roughly the percentage increase in the frequency of symptoms for women as compared to men. For example, Table 3 shows that the adjusted effect of being female on the frequency of sadness is .198. The mean frequency of sadness for men is .680 days per symptom per week. Thus, adjusting for emotional reserve and expressiveness, women are sad about 29.1 percent more frequently than men (100[.198/.680] = 29.1). The outline below shows the adjusted rate fractions for the six indexes in Table 3 and for the composite indexes that represent higher-order factors up to the level of general distress.

Distress 29.4 percent
    Emotional Distress 25.7 percent
        Depression 19.8 percent
            Sadness 29.1 percent
            Happiness –3.3 percent
        Agitation 29.5 percent
            Anger 28.7 percent
            Anxiety 30.5 percent
    Physical Distress 36.6 percent
        Malaise 37.6 percent
        Aches 35.2 percent

DISCUSSION

Response Bias

For two decades researchers have debated whether sex differences in reported psychophysiological distress are real or an artifact of differences in the expression of emotions (Cooperstock & Parnell, 1975; Gove, 1993; Gove &

Clancy, 1975; Ritchey et al., 1993; Seiler, 1975). Most available evidence indicates that sex differences in distress are not due to reporting tendencies. In some cases the response tendency is not correlated with distress, and in others it is not correlated with sex or is correlated in the wrong direction (Clancy & Gove, 1974; Gove & Geerken, 1977; Gove, McCorkel, Fain, & Hughes, 1976; Ross & Mirowsky, 1984). However, few studies examine all the links necessary to determine whether response tendencies bias the observed association between sex and distress. Furthermore, previous studies measure tendencies such as yea-saying and giving socially desirable responses that do not appear to represent expressiveness. Some researchers still maintain that sex differences in distress are due to reporting differences. For instance, a recent study of the homeless interpreted the higher reports of physical and psychological symptoms by the women as due to a "tendency for women to perceive and report symptoms more freely and for men to underreport" (Ritchey et al., 1991, p.45).

The response-bias hypothesis makes three claims: (1) that women express their emotions more freely than men, (2) that expressiveness increases the reporting of symptoms, and (3) that adjusting for expressiveness eliminates the association between sex and distress. Our results support the first proposition—that women are more expressive than men. Women score higher on both indicators of potential response bias: the unobtrusive sum of both positive and negative mood and disagreement with the self-evident statement that, "I keep my emotions to myself." Our results support the second claim for the unobtrusive expression factor but not for the direct question about emotional reserve. Scores on all six indexes increase with the expression factor (although not quite significantly for anger), but they also increase the more that respondents claim to keep emotions to themselves. Our results contradict the third proposition for both measures. The estimated effect of sex on the measures of negative mood remains quite significant after adjusting for the expression of positive and negative mood. And adjusting for self-reported reserve actually increases the estimated effect of sex on all six measures. Broadly speaking, the effect of sex on measures of distress diminishes somewhat with adjustment for emotional expression, but it does not vanish.

Reserve and expressiveness are distinct traits with distinct relationships to measures of distress, although women are more expressive than men by both standards. As a measure, asking people if they keep emotions to themselves has the advantage of simplicity and directness. However, people who say they keep emotions to themselves actually report more symptoms than others, not fewer. The expression factor that crosscuts the depression factor behaves more as one would expect of a measure of emotional expressiveness. By definition the expression factor increases the reported frequency of both positive and negative mood. The expression factor also increases the reported frequency of anger, anxiety, malaise, and aches (although the anger coefficient was not significant in the hierarchical factor model). Interestingly, models indicate that self-evaluated reserve does not significantly affect the unobtrusive expression factor. Regardless of which is a better measure, neither reserve nor expressiveness explains the observed sex difference in distress.

Masculine and Feminine Distress

Freudian ideas about the psychodynamics of depression, coupled with contemporary ideas about sex-role socialization, suggest the possibility of gendered response to stress (Rosenfield, 1980). According to the theory, frustration naturally produces hostility and anger. However, women learn to repress those feelings as they are contrary to nurturing and supportive feminine roles. Repressing hostility and anger toward others redirects punishment inward, producing depression. If true, this dynamic raises the possibility that men and women differ only in the *type* of distress and not in the *amount* of it. In theory, men become angry; women become depressed. In fact, women become angry as well as depressed. Depression is anger's companion: not its substitute.

The gendered-response explanation of women's greater reported distress assumes three things that all appear to be false. First, the explanation assumes that the recognition and expression of one's anger reduces depression. However, our results show that sadness, malaise, and the other indexes of distress all correlate positively with reported anger, not negatively. Anger can be viewed as one manifestation of distress on a par with sadness, unhappiness, anxiety, malaise and aches. Second, the gendered-response view assumes that women feel less angry toward others than do men. On the contrary, our results show that women feel more angry toward others. Thus, our results confirm those of earlier studies showing that women report greater anger, hostility, and manifest irritation than do men (Conger et al., 1993; Frank, Carpenter, & Kupfer, 1988; Gove, 1978). It assumes that women feel less angry toward others than men at any given level of distress. However, the escalating anger model shows that women are more likely to yell at someone than men who are equally angry. Thus, our results contradict the idea that men and women suffer equal frustration but transform it into different emotions. By all our measures, women suffer more distress than men.

Related Issues

Alcoholism, Drug Abuse, and Antisocial Behavior. Our analysis examines sex differences in *distress.* A focus on misery and suffering seems justified on its own, without reference to other values. It is worse to feel distressed, sad, lonely, worried, tense, anxious, angry, annoyed, run down, and unable to concentrate or to sleep than to feel happy, hopeful about the future, and to enjoy life. However, disorder may take behavioral forms as well as emotional ones. The distinction raises the possibility that gendered responses may occur across realms of disorder, even though they do not occur within the emotional realm (Horowitz & White, 1987). In other words, women and men may experience equal levels of frustration and hardship that produce emotional problems in women and behavioral problems in men. In particular, surveys of the general population find that women qualify for psychiatric diagnoses of affective disorders more frequently than men, whereas men qualify for diagnoses of alcoholism and drug abuse more frequently than women (Aneshensel, Rutter, & Lach-enbruch, 1991). Gove and Tudor (1977) argue that symptoms or diagnoses from different realms should *not* be combined—that they represent inherently distinct phenomena that may be interrelated but should not be confounded. Indeed, research shows that some stressors associated with depression and anxiety differ from those associated with alcoholism and drug abuse (Aneshensel et al., 1991). However, the possibility remains that women feel more distressed than men because the men transform their frustrations into behavioral disorder.

The possibility of cross-realm gendered responses extends to a broader arena then the question addressed in our analysis. Do women merely appear more distressed than men because the men convert distress into other realms of disorder? This question is beyond the scope of the data analyzed here, but conceptual distinctions and empirical observations suggest that the answer is no. Conceptually, problems like alcoholism, drug abuse, and antisocial behavior are not in themselves distress. If men escape distress by that route then the sex difference in distress is genuine, not false. Empirically, though, alcoholism, drug abuse, and antisocial behavior probably produce more distress than they avoid. If men were not as inclined toward behavioral disorder, the gender gap in distress might be even larger.

What pacifier for frustration not included in our study might possibly explain men's lower distress? Alcoholism and drug abuse are the chief candidates. Clearly, men drink more heavily and use illegal drugs more frequently than women. However, women actually may depend on drugs for emotional relief more frequently than men. Women use *prescribed* psychoactive drugs far more than men—over *one woman in 5* compared to less than one man in 10 (Verbrugge, 1985). The fact that women use psychoactive drugs on the advice of their doctors, whereas men use psychoactive drugs on their own authority, is a legal distinction. It makes it appear that men have more *problems* with psychoactive drugs even if women use them more often.

It is uncertain whether men use drugs to cope more frequently than women do. It is clear that alcoholism and drug abuse are temporary and counterproductive escapes at best. For cross-realm gendered response to explain women's greater distress, some behavioral disorder characteristics of men must reduce distress. If the disorder does not lower distress, then it cannot account for lower male levels of distress. On this count, there seems little or no support for such a cross-realm gendered response. For the most part, studies find that distress increases with increased levels of antisocial behavior, alcoholism, and drug abuse, which are the main problems found more commonly in men than in women (Boyd et al., 1984; Dohrenwend, Dohrenwend, Shrout, Egri, & Mendelsohn, 1980; Endicott & Spitzer, 1972). Alcoholism, drug abuse, and antisocial personality multiply the odds of a major depressive episode by 4.1, 4.2, and 5.1 respectively (Boyd et al., 1984). In sum, there is no evidence that men's use of alcohol or illegal drugs explains men's lower distress levels as an artifact of sex differences in the expression of problems. Heavy drinking and drug abuse probably do not protect men from feeling distressed.

Conclusion

We find that women experience distress about 30 percent more frequently than men. Women's extra burden of distress cannot be dismissed as mere bias due to greater expressiveness or to a "feminine" rather than "masculine" emotional response.

References

Aneshensel, Carol S. 1992. "Social Stress: Theory and Research." *Annual Review of Sociology* 18: 15–38.

Aneshensel, Carol S., Carolyn M. Rutter, and Peter A. Lachenbruch. 1991. "Social Structure, Stress, and Mental Health: Competing Conceptual and Analytic Models" *American Sociological Review* 56:166–78.

Bentler, Peter M. 1989. *EQS Structural Equations Program Manual*. Los Angeles, CA: BMDP.

Boyd, Jeffrey H., Jack D. Burke, Ernst Gruenberg, Charles E. Holzer, Donald S. Rae, Linda K. George, Marvin Karno, Roger Stolzman, Lary McEnvoy, and Gerald Nestadt. 1984. "Exclusion Criteria of DSM-III: A Study of Co-Occurrence of Hierarchy-Free Syndromes." *Archives of General Psychiatry* 41:983–89.

Clancy, Kevin and Walter R. Gove. 1974. "Sex Differences in Mental Illness: An Analysis of Response Bias in Self-Reports." *American Journal of Sociology* 80:205–15.

Conger, Rand D., Frederick O. Lorenz, Glen H. Elder, Ronald L. Simons, and Xiaojia Ge. 1993. "Husband and Wife Differences in Response to Undesirable Life Events." *Journal of Health and Social Behavior* 34:71–88.

Cooperstock, Ruth and Penny Parnell. 1975. Comment on Clancy and Gove. *American Journal of Sociology* 81:1455–57.

Dohrenwend, Bruce P., & Barbara Snell Dohrenwend. 1976. "Sex Differences and Psychiatric Disorders." *American Journal of Sociology* 81:1447–1454.

Dohrenwend, Bruce, Barbara S. Dohrenwend, Patrick E. Shrout, Gladys Egri, and Frederick S. Mendelsohn. 1980. "Nonspecific Psychological Distress and Other Dimensions of Psychopathology." *Archives of General Psychiatry* 37:1229–36.

Endicott, Jean and Robert L. Spitzer. 1972. "What! Another Rating Scale? The Psychiatric Evaluation Form." *The Journal of Nervous and Mental Disease* 154:88–104.

Frank, Ellen, Linda L. Carpenter, and David Kupfer. 1988. "Sex Differences in Recurrent Depression: Are There Any That Are Significant?" *American Journal of Psychiatry* 145:41–5.

Gove, Walter R. 1978. "Sex Differences in Mental Illness among Adult Men and Women: An Evaluation of Four Questions Raised Regarding the Evidence on the Higher Rates of Women." *Social Science and Medicine* 12B:187–98.

———. 1993. "Higher Rates of Physical Symptoms among Homeless Women Do Not Appear to be Due to Reporting Bias: A Comment on Ritchey et al." *Journal of Health and Social Behavior* 34:178–81.

Gove, Walter R. and Kevin Clancy. 1975. "Response Bias, Sex Differences, and Mental Illness: A Reply." *American Journal of Sociology* 81:1463–72.

Gove, Walter R. and Michael R. Geerken. 1977. "Response Bias in Surveys of Mental Health: An Empirical Investigation." *American Journal of Sociology* 82:1289–1317.

Gove, Walter R., James McCorkel, Terry Fain, and Michael D. Hughes. 1976. "Response Bias in Community Surveys of Mental Health: Systematic Bias or Random Noise?" *Social Science and Medicine* 10:497–502.

Gove, Walter R., & Jeannette F. Tudor. 1973. "Adult Sex Roles and Mental Illness." *American Journal of Sociology* 78:812–835.

Gove, Walter R. and Jeanette Tudor. 1977. "Sex Differences in Mental Illness: A Comment on Dohrenwend and Dohrenwend." *American Journal of Sociology* 82:1327–35.

Horowitz, Allan and Helene Raskin White. 1987. "Gender Role Orientations and Styles of Pathology among Adolescents." *Journal of Health and Social Behavior* 28:158–70.

Mirowsky, John and Catherine E. Ross. 1986. "Social Patterns of Distress." *Annual Review of Sociology* 12:23–45.

Nolen-Hoeksema, Susan. 1987. "Sex Differences in Unipolar Depression: Evidence and Theory." *Psychological Bulletin* 101:259–82.

O'Rourke, Diane and Johnny Blair, 1983. "Improving Random Selection in Telephone Surveys." *Journal of Marketing Research* 20:428–32.

Pearlin, Leonard I. 1989. "The Sociological Study of Stress." *Journal of Health and Social Behavior* 30:241–56.

Ritchey, Ferris J., Mark LaGory, and Jeffrey Mullis. 1991. "Gender Differences in Health Risks and Physical Symptoms among the Homeless." *Journal of Health and Social Behavior* 32:33–48.

———. 1993. "A Response to the Comments of Walter R. Gove on Gender Differences in Health Risks and Physical Symptoms among the Homeless." *Journal of Health and Social Behavior* 34:182–85.

Rosenfield, Sarah. 1980. "Sex Differences in Depression: Do Women Always Have Higher Rates?" *Journal of Health and Social Behavior* 21:33–42.

Ross, Catherine E. and Joan Huber. 1985. "Hardship and Depression." *Journal of Health and Social Behavior* 26:312–27.

Ross, Catherine E. and John Mirowsky. 1984. "Components of Depressed Mood in Married Men and Women." *American Journal of Epidemiology* 119:997–1004.

Seiler, Lauren H. 1975. "Sex Differences in Mental Illness: Comment on Clancy and Gove's Interpretations." *American Journal of Sociology* 81:1458–62.

Verbrugge, Lois M. 1985. "Gender and Health: An Update on Hypotheses and Evidence." *Journal of Health and Social Behavior* 26:156–82.

Waksberg, Joseph. 1978. "Sampling Methods for Random Digit Dialing." *Journal of the American Statistical Association* 73:40–46.

DISCUSSION

1. Mirowsky and Ross conclude that women suffer more distress than men. What evidence and arguments do they present to support their conclusion? How convincing do you find their evidence? Do you agree with

their assertion that alcohol abuse should not be considered an indicator of distress?

2. How do Mirowsky and Ross's arguments relate to earlier selections on the measurement of mental health in community studies? Would you expect different results if they had used different measures of distress or if they had used measures of mental disorders?

3. How might the explanations that Mirowsky and Ross propose for sex differences in distress apply to other social statuses, such as race/ethnicity or marital status?

Robin W. Simon

Revisiting the Relationships among Gender, Marital Status, and Mental Health[†]

Gender differences in the effects of marriage on mental illness are at the heart of Gove and Tudor's sex-role theory. Robin Simon interrogates their claims with more recent data that are of better quality than those available in the 1970s. She asks: After all of women's advances since the 1970s, does marriage still confer a mental health advantage to men over women? In the process, she introduces an important distinction in the sociological study of mental health: that between social causation processes and social selection processes.

INTRODUCTION

It has been 30 years since Gove (1972; Gove & Tudor, 1973) introduced his influential sex-role theory of mental illness, which argued that the female preponderance of psychological distress in the United States since World War II is due to the unrewarding and stressful nature of women's social roles in contemporary U.S. society. His theory rested on the assumption that marriage is advantageous for men's mental health but disadvantageous for women's. The evidence Gove used to support his theory was based on a review of 17 studies conducted since World War II, which found that women have higher rates of mental illness only among the married and that in all other marital statuses men's distress exceeds women's. Although Gove's article shaped the course of decades of theory and research on gender and mental health, it has been the subject of debate—with some of the most trenchant commentary appearing in this very journal (see Dohrenwend & Dohrenwend, 1976). Two main criticisms are at the center of this debate.

Simon, Robin W. 2002. "Revisiting the Relationships among Gender, Marital Status, and Mental Health." *American Journal of Sociology* 107:1065–1096.

First, Gove relied on cross-sectional studies, which made it impossible to adjudicate between his social-causation hypothesis and the alternative social-selection hypothesis, which argues that men and women differentially select into and out of marriage on the basis of their mental health status. Critics have argued that gender differences in distress among the married and the unmarried may reflect selection factors whereby emotionally healthy men are more likely to select into marriage and emotionally healthy women are more likely to select out of marriage, in the first place. Second, Gove drew conclusions from studies that include female types of emotional problems, such as depression, and exclude male types of emotional problems, such as substance abuse. According to the Dohrenwends (1976), studies based on psychological problems that are more common among females are likely to overestimate women's distress and underestimate men's. Unfortunately, these methodological and conceptual limitations are evident in much subsequent research on the relationships among gender, marital status, and mental health (Aneshensel, 1992; Aneshensel, Rutter, & Lachenbruch, 1991; Lennon, 1987; Simon, 1998).

However, in addition to these methodological and conceptual criticisms, Gove's thesis is debated on substantive grounds. Even if his central assumption was correct in the 1970s, scholars question its accuracy at the close of the 20th century, given social changes that have occurred over the last quarter of the century in men's and women's social roles, as well as in marital patterns in the United States. In fact, despite a wealth of research on this topic, scholars continue to disagree about the consequences of marriage for men's and women's mental health.

In this article, I revisit the relationships among gender, marital status, and mental health in the United States using two waves of panel data from a recent national sample, with special attention given to the types of emotional problems associated with both males and females. Overcoming the limitations of previous work, I assess whether marriage is currently emotionally advantageous for men and disadvantageous for women, as well as question the wisdom of focusing exclusively on social roles for explaining gender differences in psychological distress among adults.

BACKGROUND

Research on the Relationships among Gender, Marital Status, and Mental Health

Since Gove's publication, dozens of studies have examined gender differences in mental health by focusing on self-reports of emotional problems in the nontreated (i.e., the general) population. Most of this research is based on cross-sectional data from community samples of individuals who report the frequency or intensity in which they experience psychological symptoms such as nonspecific distress, anxiety, and depression. What does the plethora of studies find with respect to Gove's theoretical and substantive claims? Overall, the past 30 years of research has produced three main findings regarding the relationships among gender, marital status, and mental health.

First, in contrast to Gove's argument that marriage is beneficial for men's mental health and detrimental for women's, research consistently indicates that marriage is associated with enhanced mental health for men *and* women. Studies that have focused on marital-status differences in well-being among men and among women (i.e., marital status within gender analyses) show that regardless of gender, married people enjoy better mental health than unmarried (including never and formerly married) persons (Kessler & McRae, 1984; Pearlin & Johnson, 1977; Thoits, 1986; Waite & Gallagher, 2000). However, while studies based on cross-sectional data are informative, they cannot be used to rule out the alternative social-selection hypothesis that mentally ill persons are less likely to get married in the first place. Subsequent longitudinal studies that have examined this issue find that social causation and selection processes are at work, and that mental health is a consequence as well as a cause of marital status (Booth & Amato, 1991; Mastekaasa, 1992).

Second, and again in contrast to Gove's claims, research consistently indicates that women report more mental health problems than men, irrespective of marital status. Studies that have focused on gender differences in psychological well-being among the married and among the unmarried (i.e., gender within marital-status analyses) find that women report greater distress than comparable men in *all* marital-status categories (Fox, 1980; Radloff, 1975; Warheit et al., 1976). However, because most of these studies are based on emotional problems typically experienced by females and do not consider emotional problems typically experienced by males, it is likely that they overestimate women's distress and underestimate men's (Aneshensel et al., 1991; Dohrenwend & Dohrenwend, 1976; Horwitz, White, & White, 1996b; Lennon, 1987; Simon, 1998).

Third, research has been less consistent with regard to the *interaction* between gender and marital status and whether the mental health advantage of marriage is greater for men. While several studies suggest that men derive more emotional benefit from marriage (Aneshensel et al., 1991; Kessler & McRae, 1984; Menaghan, 1989), others imply that women are the true mental health beneficiaries of marriage (e.g., Thoits, 1986). However, here again, because most of these studies are based on cross-sectional data and types of psychological problems typically experienced by females, they provide limited insight into whether marriage (or the lack thereof) actually has different emotional consequences for women and men.

Research that has examined the impact of marital transitions with longitudinal data has also produced inconsistent results. Some studies find that divorce and widowhood are more harmful for men (Umberson, Wortman, & Kessler, 1992), while others show that women are more distressed by marital loss (Aseltine & Kessler, 1993; Menaghan & Lieberman, 1986; Simon & Marcussen, 1999). The handful of studies that have assessed the effects of marital gain indicate that marriage reduces the distress of men and women, but that there are no sex differences in the emotional benefits of marriage (Horwitz et al., 1996b; Simon & Marcussen, 1999). Moreover, in a recent study based on the National Survey of Families and Households, Marks and Lambert (1998) show that individuals who transitioned out of marriage report more, while people who transitioned into marriage report less, depressive symptoms than continuously married persons. Marks and Lambert also find that while marital loss is more depressing for women, there are no gender differences in the impact of marital gain. However, while informative, this study provides no insight into whether persons who transitioned into marriage are less depressed than unmarried, including never and previously married, people.

On the basis of their extensive review of studies on this topic, Waite and Gallagher (2000) recently concluded that the mental health benefits of marriage currently apply equally to women and men (also see Waite, 1995). However, once again, because most of these studies include emotional problems common among females and exclude those common among males, they also provide an incomplete picture of the relationships among gender, marital status, and mental health (for exceptions, see Horwitz et al., 1996b; Riessman & Gerstel, 1985; Riessman, 1990).

It is important to acknowledge the many contributions feminist scholars have made to theory and research on this topic. For example, in her early discussion of the future of marriage, Bernard (1972) also argued that marriage is emotionally advantageous for men and disadvantageous to women, which she attributed to gender inequality in power and authority in both the family and society. While feminist scholars continue to stress the linkages between families and wider systems of male domination for understanding gender inequality in a variety of contexts, they now criticize the early emphasis on sex roles and sex-role socialization in favor of explanations that emphasize micro- and macroprocesses of categorization and stratification by gender (see Ferree, 1990; Ferree, Lorber, & Hess, 1999; Lopata & Thorne, 1978; Osmond & Thorne, 1990; Reskin, 1988; Risman, 1987; Stacey, 1993; Stacey & Thorne, 1985; West & Zimmerman, 1987). According to the new gender theory, gender is a lifelong process that reflects and reproduces structural differentiation in which males have material and ideological advantages over females. However, although feminist scholars now argue that gender is socially constructed and that a variety of gendered roles offer rewards and costs to women *and* men, an implication of the new gender theory is that the emotional benefits of marriage continue to be fewer for women in light of pervasive structural inequality and female subordination in contemporary American society (England, 2000; Thompson & Walker, 1989).

Ironically, although the past few decades of research have provided little empirical support for Gove's sex-role theory of mental illness, theories which argue that differences in the nature of men's and women's social roles are the primary determinants of gender differences in mental health continue to dominate sociological research on gender and mental health. However, while role explanations are compelling and have advanced our understanding of some linkages between social structure and individual well-being, or what Mills (1959) called the "intersections of social structure and biography,"

THE FUTURE OF MARRIAGE

The following quote from Jessie Bernard's book, *The Future of Marriage*, first published in 1972, illustrates a common feminist outlook on marriage at the time. It also brings life to past and current claims about the differences in life prospects for men and women as they relate to mental health.

"Strictly speaking, we cannot speak of marriage as the 'cause' of the dismal mental-health status of wives, for the evidence is not clinical but statistical in nature. The two are not identical. The statistical approach tries to discover relationships and associations among factors. If these relationships and associations are close, some kind of causal pattern is inferred even though it cannot be demonstrated in each individual case.

A classic illustration of the difference between the clinical and the statistical or epidemiological approach is that of cigarette smoking. Most of the scientific evidence on the pathogenic effects was statistical or epidemiological rather than clinical. And for the layman such evidence is often confusing. Here is John Doe who has been smoking cigarettes for seventy years, still hale and hearty, at eighty-five. So what's wrong with cigarettes? All right, says the epidemiologist, John Doe is lucky, a "deviant case," "a chance error" who represents the one case in a thousand that escapes the pathological effects. Similarly, not everyone exposed to plagues or epidemics dies. Not everyone in tuberculosis areas contracts the disease. Nor do all women exposed to the destructive aspects of marriage as now structured become depressed or develop mental health impairments or show symptoms of psychological distress. Still, it is worthwhile to inaugurate public health programs even though not everyone is susceptible to the pathogenic factor; and it is worthwhile to see what can be done about the wife's marriage even though not all wives are vulnerable to its depredations.

It is not necessarily the magnitude of the statistical differences between the mental health of married and single women or between married men and married women that is so convincing; it is, rather, the consistency of the differences. No one difference or even set of differences by itself would be definitive; but the cumulative effect of so many is. The poor mental health of wives is like a low-grade infection that shows itself in a number of scattered symptoms, no one of which is critical enough to cause an acute episode. And so, therefore, it is easy to ignore. Or to dismiss. Or to blame on women themselves. There must be something wrong with them if they are psychologically so distressed.

But even those who blame women themselves for their psychological malaise and see it is an inability on their part to cope with the demands of marriage or to come to terms with their destiny finally have to concede that the way the social world is organized may have something to do with their plight. (pp. 36–37)"

Bernard, Jessie. 1972. *The Future of Marriage*. New York: The World Publishing.

epidemiological evidence over the past quarter of a century, coupled with recent findings on adolescents, calls into question the wisdom of focusing exclusively on social roles for explaining gender differences in mental health among adults in the United States today.

Evidence of Male and Female Types of Emotional Problems

Epidemiological research on both lifetime and recent prevalence rates of mental disorders consistently demonstrates that while women have higher rates of affective and anxiety disorders (and their psychological corollaries of nonspecific distress, anxiety, and depression), men have higher rates of antisocial personality and substance abuse dependence disorders (and their psychological corollaries of antisocial behavior and drug/alcohol problems; Dohrenwend et al., 1980; Meyers et al., 1984; Robins et al., 1984; Robins & Regier, 1994). In fact, epidemiologists have concluded that when male and female types of psychiatric disorders and psychological problems are all considered, there are no gender differences in overall rates of mental illness among adults in the United States today.

Moreover, research on adolescent mental health documents that gender differences in specific types of emotional problems emerge prior to the acquisition of adult social roles. Studies that compare boys and girls in early, middle, and late adolescence reveal that girls report more symptoms of distress, anxiety, and depression, while boys report more antisocial behavior and substance problems (Avison & McAlpine, 1992; Gore, Aseltine, & Colten, 1992).

Finally, and consistent with epidemiological studies, findings from the National Co-Morbidity Study (Kessler et al., 1993, 1994) indicate that there are no gender differences in the overall prevalence of mental disorders but that there are gender differences in the prevalence of specific types of disorders. Consistent with the recent research on adolescents, the National Co-Morbidity Study also reveals that female's greater self-reported feelings of depression and male's greater self-reports of substance problems begin to appear in adolescence—before they have assumed their adult social roles (also see Avison & McAlpine, 1992; Gore et al., 1992).

To the extent that gender differences in the prevalence of specific emotional problems are evident in adolescence—as this recent research indicates—we cannot continue to attribute gender differences in mental health in adulthood solely to differences between men's and women's roles in society. Rather, gender differences in mental health among adults in the United States should be reinterpreted as a function of gender-linked emotional socialization, which predisposes males and females to respond to stress throughout the entire life course with sex-typical emotional problems (Aneshensel, 1992; Aneshensel et al., 1991; Horwitz et al., 1996b; Lennon, 1987; Rosenfield, Vertefuille, & McAlpine, 2000; Simon, 1998).

Drawing on insights from the sociology of emotion, I argue that embodied in U.S. emotional culture are beliefs about the "proper" emotional styles of males and females, as well as norms that specify "appropriate" feeling and expression for men and women (Gordon, 1981, 1989; Hochschild, 1975, 1979; Simon & Kanellakos, 2001; Smith-Lovin, 1995; Thoits, 1989). A consequence of gender-linked emotional socialization is that females learn to express distress through internalizing emotional problem, such as depression, while males learn to express distress vis-à-vis externalizing emotional problems, such as substance abuse. Insofar as males and females manifest distress with different types of emotional problems, role arguments are most useful for explaining differences in mental health among men and among women (i.e., *within* gender variation), whereas socialization arguments are most useful for explaining *gender differences* in mental health among persons who hold the same configuration of social (including marital) statuses (i.e., *between* gender variation).

I also argue that in order to more fully understand the relationships among gender, marital status, and mental health in the United States today, studies must simultaneously (*a*) include the types of emotional problems associated with males *and* females, (*b*) be based on cross-sectional *and* longitudinal analyses of recent national data, (*c*) examine the emotional impact of marital loss and marital gain on men and women compared to their stably married *and* stably unmarried counterparts, and (*d*) investigate the alternative hypothesis that women differentially select into and out of marriage on the basis of their mental health status. Such an analysis is critical not only for conceptual, methodological, and theoretical reasons, but also on substantive grounds. Historical changes in men's and women's social roles over the last quarter of the 20th century have resulted in changes in marital patterns among males and females in the United States (Oppenheimer, 1994; Spain & Bianchi, 1996). Therefore, since the time Gove introduced his sex-role theory of mental illness, changes may have occurred in the nature, meaning, and significance of marriage and the consequences of marital status for men's and women's mental health.

In this article, I overcome the conceptual and methodological limitations of previous work on this topic by revisiting the relationships among gender, marital status, and mental health using panel data from a recent national sample of adults, with special attention given to the types of emotional problems associated with males and females in the United States. Consistent with emotional-socialization arguments, I hypothesize that (1) in all marital statuses women report more depression than men and men report more substance abuse than women. Consistent with role theoretical claims, I also hypothesize that (2) married people report fewer symptoms of depression and substance problems than the unmarried, net of other factors. Moreover, I hypothesize that (3) marital loss has harmful, while marital gain has beneficial, consequences for men's *and* women's mental health. Insofar as males and females respond to stress with sex-typical emotional problems, I further hypothesize that (4) when there are gender differences in the impact of marital transitions, the greater impact on men or women will be evident only for symptoms associated with their gender. Finally, I investigate—for the first time with recent national data—whether alcohol-abusing men are more likely to select out of marriage, and depressed women are more likely to select into marriage, than their nondistressed counterparts. Overall, in addition to contributing to our understanding of the relationships among gender, marital status, and mental health in the United States today, by examining social-causation and social-selection hypotheses, my research sheds new light on whether marriage (or the lack thereof) is a cause or consequence of mental illness and whether there are gender differences in the selection into and out of marriage on the basis of mental health.

METHODS

Data

I conducted my analyses on two waves of data from the National Survey of Families and Households (NSFH), which is based on a recent national probability sample of adults in the United States (Sweet & Bumpass, 1996). The first wave of interviews (time 1) was administered in 1987–88 with individuals ages 19 and over from 13,017 households, which included an oversampling of minorities and single parents. The response rate at time 1 (T1) was 74 percent. The second wave of interviews (time 2) was administered in 1992–94 with 10,005 respondents. Excluding people who had died ($N = 763$), the response rate at time 2 (T2) was 82 percent. Logistic regression analyses (not shown) indicate that several factors measured at T1 significantly predict attrition by T2, including marital and employment status, gender, age, race, education, household income, and depression. People who were unmarried and unemployed at T1 were more likely to leave the study, as were men, older people, nonwhites, persons with lower levels of education, and persons with higher levels of income and depression. Due to oversampling at T1, the panel contains relatively high proportions of racial minorities and single parents; however, the sample may underrepresent the unmarried and unemployed, as well as men, older persons, people with lower levels of education, and persons with higher levels of income and depression. Results of analyses, especially those based on people who are stably unmarried or who had a marital gain between T1 and T2, should be interpreted with some caution in light of the greater attrition of respondents who were unmarried at T1.

Measures

Depression. The NSFH includes 12 items from the Center for Epidemiological Studies Depression Scale (CES-D), a commonly used measure of depressed mood that has high construct validity and internal consistency (Radloff, 1977). At T1 and T2, respondents were asked how many days in the past week: "you were bothered by things that usually don't bother you?," "you felt lonely?," "you felt you could not shake off the blues, even with the help of your family or friends?," "your sleep was restless?," "you felt depressed?," "you felt that everything you did was a effort?," "you felt fearful?," "you had trouble keeping your mind on what you were doing?," "you talked less than usual?," "you did not feel like eating, your appetite was poor?," "you felt sad?," and "you could not get going?" Item responses (zero–seven days) were summed. Scores on these measures range from 0–81 (chronbach's α = .93).

Alcohol abuse. The NSFH includes one measure of alcohol abuse at T1 and two measures of alcohol abuse at T2. The T1 measure of alcohol abuse is based on a question that asked respondents whether they had a drinking problem (yes = 1). The first measure of alcohol abuse at T2 is based on a question that asked respondents the number of days in the previous month they had five or more drinks. Scores on this measure range from 0–30 days. I also computed a second measure of alcohol consumption at T2 by multiplying the number of days in the past month the respondent had a drink by the number of drinks he or she reported having on those days (see Berkman & Breslow, 1983; Umberson et al., 1996). Scores on this measure range from 0–360. Because results for both of the T2 measures are very similar, I report only those for alcohol abuse since it is most similar to the T1 measure.

In this article, I investigate the relationships among gender, marital status, and mental health *at T2* as well as *over time*. I therefore computed two sets of martial-status variables.

Stable marital status. In order to examine marital-status differences in distress at a *single point in time,* I computed four dummy marital-status variables based on respondents whose marital status was stable over the study period. "Married" (coded "1") consists of persons who were married at T1 and T2, "never married" (coded "1") is based on respondents who had never married, "separated or divorced" (coded "1") consists of people who were separated or divorced at both points in time, and "widowed" (coded "1") is based on individuals who were widows at each interview.

Marital transition status. In order to examine the impact of marital loss and marital gain on individuals' mental health *between T1 and T2,* I computed two dichotomous marital-transition status variables. Similar to Marks and Lambert's study (1998), my measure of "marital loss" is based on respondents who were stably married (coded "0") or who had a marital loss (coded "1") during the five-year study period. However, unlike their study that compares individuals who had a marital gain to stably married persons, my measure of "marital gain" consists of (and compares) stably unmarried people (coded "0") and those who had a marital gain (coded "1").

Control variables. All analyses include a dichotomous variable for gender (female = 1). To control for sources of variation in depression and alcohol abuse other than gender and marital status, analyses also include respondent's age, race, education, and household income, as well as their employment and parental status (all measured at T2). I measure age and education in years; income in dollars; and race, employment, and parental status as dichotomous variables (nonwhite = 1, employed = 1, parent = 1). Furthermore, because some authors report a nonlinear relationship between age and depression (Mirowsky & Ross, 1992), the analyses include a term for age-squared. Finally, to assess gender differences in distress among respondents whose marital status was stable, as well as among those who experienced a marital transition during the study, I computed gender interactions for all (i.e., both sets) of the marital-status variables.

Analysis Sample and Data Analysis

Excluding respondents whose marital status was ambiguous at T1 or T2 and who did not have complete information on all analytic variables, the analysis sample is based on 8,161 individuals. I conduct two different sets of analyses. The first set is cross-sectional and assesses the associations between marital status and depression and alcohol abuse at T2 among respondents whose marital status was stable throughout the study period ($N = 6,612$). The second set of analyses is longitudinal and assesses the effects of marital loss and marital gain on change in depression and alcohol abuse between T1 and T2. For clarity of interpretation, the marital transition analyses are conducted on two subsamples composed of (1) stably married respondents ($N = 4,125$) and those who had experienced a marital loss ($N = 629$), and (2) the stably unmarried ($N = 2,487$) and persons who had experienced a marital gain ($N = 920$).

RESULTS

Gender Differences in the Associations between Marital Status and Mental Health

The first set of analyses focus on gender and marital-status differences in mental health among persons whose marital status was stable over the study period. Table 1 contains results of dummy-variable analyses in which respondent's levels of depression and alcohol abuse at T2 are regressed on two sets of variables. In order to assess variation in distress among the stably unmarried, I include three dummy variables that consist of never married, separated or divorced, and widowed persons; the stably married are the reference category. Although these analyses are cross-sectional, they go beyond those in previous studies because they are conducted on a national sample of men and women who have been in their current marital status for a minimum of five years and include male- and female-typical problems. A number of findings are evident in Table 1.

Consistent with previous cross-sectional research on depression and my first hypothesis, model 1 indicates that women report significantly more symptoms of depression than men, even after controlling for sociodemographic variables, as well as employment, parental, and marital status. Model 1 further shows marital-status differences in depression; consistent with my

Table 1 Unstandardized Coefficients from Regressions of Depression and Alcohol Abuse on Gender, Marital Status, and Control Variables among Respondents Whose Marital Status Was Stable

	Depression		Alcohol Abuse	
	Model 1	Model 2	Model 3	Model 4
Female (0, 1)	2.84***	2.56***	−1.03***	−.81***
	(.39)	(.47)	(.06)	(.08)
Age	.78	.70	−.06	−.03
	(.88)	(.88)	(.15)	(.15)
Age²	−.19*	−.19*	−.02	−.02
	(.08)	(.08)	(.01)	(.01)
Nonwhite (0, 1)	1.86***	1.82***	−.30***	−.29***
	(.46)	(.47)	(.08)	(.08)
Education	−.55***	−.55***	−.07***	−.07***
	(.07)	(.07)	(.01)	(.01)
Household income	−.20***	−.20***	−.01	−.01
	(.06)	(.06)	(.01)	(.01)
Employed (0, 1)	−3.58***	−3.61***	−.06***	−.02
	(.43)	(.43)	(.07)	(.07)
Parent (0, 1)	.63	.50	−.23*	−.17*
	(.48)	(.50)	(.08)	(.08)
Never married (yes = 1)	3.03***	2.24***	.34***	.57***
	(.64)	(.90)	(.11)	(.15)
Separated/Divorced (yes = 1)	4.27***	3.89***	.39***	1.15***
	(.57)	(1.05)	(.09)	(.18)
Widowed (yes = 1)	1.60*	1.80	.49***	1.28***
	(.80)	(1.84)	(.13)	(.31)
Female × never married	...	1.34	...	−.36*
		(1.08)		(.18)
Female × separated/divorced	...	.58	...	−1.07***
		(1.22)		(.20)
Female × widowed	...	−.10	...	−.99**
		(1.95)		(.32)
Adjusted R²	.08	.08	.06	.06

Note: Numbers in parentheses are SEs. The married are the reference (i.e., omitted) category. N = 6,612.
*P < .05, two-tailed tests.
**P < .01.
***P < .001.

second hypothesis, stably never married, separated or divorced, and widowed persons report significantly more depressive symptoms than the stably married, net of these other factors. However, although Gove (and others) claimed that being unmarried is associated with more distress for men and less distress for women, model 2 reveals that the associations between marital status and depression do not significantly differ for women and men.

In other words, unmarried men are not significantly more depressed than unmarried women.

Moreover, consistent with prior work and my first hypothesis, model 3 indicates that regardless of sociodemographic factors, as well as employment, parental, and marital status, men report significantly more alcohol abuse than women. Model 3 further shows marital-status differences in alcohol abuse. Consistent with my second hypothesis, stably never married, separated or divorced, and widowed persons report significantly more alcohol problems than stably married people, net of these other factors. However, and in contrast to depression, the associations between marital status and alcohol abuse significantly differ for men and women. Consistent with Gove's sex-role theory of mental illness, model 4 reveals that unmarried men report more drinking problems than unmarried women.

In sum, these analyses provide support for emotional-socialization arguments, which claim that males and females manifest psychological distress with different types of emotional problems. Regardless of marital status, women report more depression than men and men report more alcohol abuse than women. At the same time, these analyses provide support for role-theoretical claims that marital roles are associated with enhanced mental health. Net of other factors, stably unmarried persons report more symptoms of depression and more alcohol problems than stably married people. Finally, these analyses provide mixed support for Gove's sex-role theory of mental illness. Although there are no significant gender differences in the associations between marital status and depression, being unmarried is more closely associated with alcohol abuse for men than for women. Together, these findings strongly suggest that the benefits of marriage for depression apply equally to women and men, whereas the benefits of marriage for alcohol abuse are greater for men than for women.

However, while these cross-sectional analyses shed light on the relationships among gender, marital status, and mental health at a single point in time in a recent nationally representative sample of adults, they do not provide answers to other important questions regarding the relationships among gender, marital transitions, and mental health over time. For example, are there gender differences in the mental health consequences of marital transitions? If so, is the greater impact of a marital transition on men or women evident only for sex-typical emotional problems? Relatedly, are there gender differences in the causes of marital transitions? If so, are depressed women more likely and alcohol-abusing men less likely to become and remain married in the first place? To answer these questions, I now turn to longitudinal analyses.

Gender Differences in the Mental Health Consequences of Marital Transitions

Although Gove did not explicitly theorize about the mental health consequences of marital transitions for men compared to women, an implication

Table 2 Unstandardized Coefficients from Regressions of Depression and Alcohol Abuse on Gender and Marital Loss Among Respondents Who Were Married at T1

	Depression		Alcohol Abuse	
	Model 1[a]	Model 2[a]	Model 3[a]	Model 4[a]
Female (0, 1)	2.25*** (.40)	1.86*** (.43)	−.82*** (.08)	−.81*** (.08)
T1 depression/alcohol abuse[b]	.33*** (.01)	.33*** (.01)	1.60*** (.30)	1.59*** (.30)
Marital loss from separation/ divorce (yes = 1)	5.59*** (.70)	3.70*** (1.02)	.44*** (.12)	.62*** (.18)
Marital loss from widowhood (yes = 1)	4.23*** (1.10)	2.80 (2.42)	.07 (.20)	−.47 (.43)
Female × marital loss from separation/divorce	...	3.43*** (1.34)	...	−.31 (.24)
Female × marital loss from widowhood	...	1.89 (2.66)	...	.65 (.47)
Adjusted R^2	.18	.19	.06	.06

Note: Numbers in parentheses are SEs. The stably married are the reference category. $N = 4,754$.
[a]Each model controls for sociodemographic variables including age, race, education, and household income, as well as respondent's employment and parental status at T2.
[b]Respondent's level of depression at T1 is included in the depression models and whether they reported alcohol problems at T1 is included in the alcohol abuse models.
*$P < .05$, two-tailed tests.
**$P < .01$.
***$P < .001$.

of his sex-role theory that has received some scholarly attention is that marital loss is more harmful, and conversely, marital gain is more beneficial, for men's than women's mental health. To investigate these possibilities for the first time with male and female types of emotional problems in a national sample, Table 2 focuses on the impact of marital loss, and Table 3 focuses on the impact of marital gain, on women and men.

Tables 2 and 3 present the results of dummy variable analyses in which I regress respondent's level of depression and alcohol abuse at T2 on two sets of variables. In order to assess variation in emotional distress among persons who experienced a marital loss, I include two dummy variables in Table 2 analyses that consist of people who became separated or divorced and widowed; in these analyses, the stably married are the omitted category. To assess variation in mental health among people who had a marital gain, I include three dummy variables in Table 3 analyses that consist of previously never married, separated or divorced, and widowed persons; the stably unmarried are the reference category in these analyses. Because the purpose of these analyses is to assess whether change in mental health between T1 and T2 is a function of change in marital status during this time frame, these models all include respondent's level of distress at T1. While not shown, all models also include sociodemographic variables examined earlier, as well

Table 3 Unstandardized Coefficients from Regressions of Depression and Alcohol Abuse on Gender and Marital Gain among Respondents Who Were Unmarried at T1

	Depression		Alcohol Abuse	
	Model 1[a]	Model 2[a]	Model 3[a]	Model 4[a]
Female (0, 1)	2.10*** (.58)	2.41*** (.71)	−1.28*** (.11)	−1.42*** (1.33)
T1 depression/alcohol abuse[b]	.29*** (.01)	.29*** (.01)	2.62*** (.33)	2.61*** (.33)
Marital gain from previously never married (yes = 1)	−3.88*** (.86)	−3.38*** (1.16)	−.24 (.16)	−.34 (.22)
Marital gain from previously separated/divorced (yes = 1)	−2.65** (.86)	−2.08 (1.34)	−.28 (.16)	−.67** (.25)
Marital gain from previously widowed (yes = 1)	−3.80 (2.38)	−3.22 (3.90)	−.22 (.45)	−1.05 (.74)
Female × marital gain from previously never married	...	−.98 (1.54)	...	.21 (.29)
Female × marital gain from previously separated/divorced	...	−.92 (1.67)	...	.64* (.32)
Female × marital gain from previously widowed	...	−.87 (4.92)	...	1.30 (.93)
Adjusted R^2	.18	.18	.09	.09

Note: Numbers in parentheses are SEs. The stably unmarried are the reference category. N = 3,407.
[a]Each model controls for sociodemographic variables including age, race, education, and household income, as well as respondent's employment and parental status at T2.
[b]Respondent's level of depression at T1 is included in the depression models and whether they reported alcohol problems at T1 is included in the alcohol abuse models.
*$P < .05$, two-tailed tests
**$P < .01$.
***$P < .001$.

as respondent's employment and parental status at T2. There are several noteworthy findings in these tables.

Model 1 of Table 2 indicates, not surprisingly, that respondent's symptoms of depression at T1 significantly predict their symptoms at T2. Moreover, and consistent with longitudinal studies (e.g., Horwitz et al., 1996b; Menaghan & Lieberman, 1986) and my third hypothesis, the loss of the spousal role increases depression. Compared to the stably married, persons who had a marital loss from either separation and divorce or widowhood reported a significant increase in depressive symptoms between T1 and T2. However, there is no support for the argument that a marital loss is more depressing for men. In fact, model 2 reveals that women are significantly more depressed by separation and divorce. That is, that advantages of being married and disadvantages of becoming unmarried are greater for women when considering depression.

If men are more distressed by marital loss—as Gove's sex-role theory implies—their mental health disadvantage should be evident when a male-typical emotional problem is examined. Turning to alcohol abuse, model 3 indicates (again, not surprisingly) that respondent's alcohol abuse at T1 significantly predicts their alcohol abuse at T2. Moreover, and consistent with previous work (e.g., Horwitz & White, 1991; Horwitz et al., 1996b) and my third hypothesis, the loss of the spousal role increases alcohol problems. Compared to the stably married, persons who had a marital loss from separation and divorce (but not from widowhood) reported a significant increase in alcohol abuse between T1 and T2. However, there is no indication in model 4 that marital loss is more distressing for men, with respect to alcohol abuse. That is, the advantages of being married and disadvantages of becoming unmarried for alcohol abuse apply to women *and* men.

In short, while marital loss is distressing, there is no evidence in this national sample of adults to support the hypothesis that marital loss is more distressing for men, even when a male-typical emotional problem is examined. On the contrary, the above analysis indicates that women are actually more depressed by separation and divorce. However, while these analyses are informative, it is also useful to assess the psychological impact of a marital gain compared to being *continuously unmarried,* as well as gender differences in the mental health consequences of marital gain. Although Gove's sex-role theory implies that the emotional advantages of marital gain are greater for men, this hypothesis has, to date, not been examined with male and female types of emotional problems in a national sample.

Consistent with my third hypothesis, model 1 of Table 3 shows that marital gain reduces depression, though significantly so only for certain groups of people. Compared to the stably unmarried, previously never-married people who married and formerly separated or divorced persons who remarried reported a significant decrease in depressive symptoms between T1 and T2. Moreover, model 2 shows that the emotional advantages of marital gain are *not* significantly greater for men than for women. Although negative in sign, the interaction terms for gender and each marital gain dummy variable are not significant—at least not for this manifestation of emotional distress. In contrast to the implications of Gove's early sex-role theory, these findings clearly indicate that the benefits of marital gain for depression apply equally to women and men.

Turning to alcohol abuse, model 3 shows that marital gain does not reduce this type of emotional distress. In contrast to my third hypothesis, people who experienced a marital gain do not report a significant decrease in alcohol abuse relative to stably unmarried persons. However, model 4 reveals that the modest reduction in alcohol abuse among previously separated and divorced persons who remarried is significantly greater for men than for women. This finding is consistent with the implications of Gove's thesis and indicate that the benefits of marital gain for alcohol abuse— a male type of emotional problem—are greater for men than for women. This finding is also consistent with my fourth hypothesis, which states that when there are gender differences in the impact of marital transitions, the greater impact on men or women will be evident only for sex-typical emotional problems.

In brief, there is evidence in this national sample of adults that marital gain is emotionally beneficial for certain groups of people (i.e., previously never married, as well as formerly separated or divorced persons) and for certain types of emotional problems (i.e., feelings of depression). Moreover, there appears to be some support for the notion that the psychological advantages of marital gain are greater for men. While there are no significant gender differences in the benefits of marital gain for symptoms of depression, the modest benefits of remarriage among persons who had previously been separated or divorced are significantly greater for men, with respect to alcohol abuse.

Taken together, these longitudinal results provide support for both role and emotional socialization explanations of the relationships among gender, marital transitions, and mental health. While marital loss has negative consequences for individuals' mental health, marital gain has positive consequences for their emotional well-being. Moreover, when there are gender differences in the psychological impact of marital transitions, their greater impact on men or women is only evident for sex-typical emotional problems. The greater negative emotional impact of marital loss on women is evident for depression, whereas the greater positive emotional impact of marital gain on men is evident for alcohol abuse. However, beyond providing evidence for these two distinct though complimentary theoretical explanations, my findings also provide additional support for recent claims that the emotional advantages of being or becoming married—and the emotional disadvantages of being or becoming unmarried—apply to men *and* women.

Gender Differences in the Causes of Marital Transitions

Having examined gender differences in the consequences of marital loss and marital gain for male and female types of emotional problems, I now examine a final, yet pivotal, set of issues. That is, I assess whether individuals who have mental health problems are less likely than those who do not to either remain or become married in the first place. I also assess whether men and women differentially select out of or into marriage on the basis of their mental health status. Since men and women manifest distress with different types of emotional problems, it is possible that depressed women and alcohol-abusing men are less likely than their nondistressed counterparts to either become or remain married.

Table 4 presents the results of logistic regression analyses in which I regress whether respondents had experienced a marital transition during the study period on two sets of variables. Models 1 and 2 assess the determinants of marital loss. Because widowhood is a marital loss over which people have little, if any, control, these analyses exclude respondents who lost their spouse through death ($N = 173$) and are, therefore, based on stably married persons and those who had separated or divorced by T2. Models

Table 4 Unstandardized Coefficients from Logistic Regressions of Marital Loss and Marital Gain on Gender, Depression, Alcohol Abuse, and Control Variables at T1

	Marital Loss[a]		Marital Gain[b]	
	Model 1	Model 2	Model 3	Model 4
Female (0, 1)	−.14	−.07	−.30**	−.36
	(.11)	(.77)	(.10)	(1.38)
Age	−.05***	−.05***	.06***	−.03***
	(.01)	(.01)	(.00)	(.01)
Nonwhite (0, 1)	.47***	.25	−.89***	−.75***
	(.12)	(.18)	(.10)	(.16)
Education	−.05**	−.05*	.02	.02
	(.02)	(.03)	(.02)	(.03)
Household income	−.00	−.00	.13**	.4
	(.02)	(.02)	(.05)	(.05)
Employed (0, 1)	.01	−.44*	.35**	.61**
	(.13)	(.22)	(.11)	(.20)
Parent (0, 1)	−.05	−.05	.37***	.72***
	(.11)	(.16)	(.10)	(.22)
Depression	.13***	.17***	.02	.01
	(.04)	(.04)	(.02)	(.04)
Alcohol problems	.85**	.60	−.22	−.45
	(.32)	(.37)	(.27)	(.32)
Female × depression	...	−.01	...	.00
		(.01)		(.05)
Female × alcohol problems	...	1.28	...	.76
		(.75)		(.58)
Adjusted R^2	.07	.07	.15	.15

Note: Numbers in parentheses are SEs. All variables included in these analyses are based on information obtained at T1.
[a]The marital loss analyses exclude the 173 respondents who were widowed between T1 and T2. $N = 4{,}581$.
[b]$N = 3{,}407$.
*$P < .05$, two-tailed tests.
**$P < .01$.
***$P < .001$.

3 and 4 assess the determinants of marital gain and are based on all stably unmarried persons and all respondents who had a marital gain by T2.

While Gove's sex-role theory of mental illness argues that marital status— and, by extension, marital transitions—have different consequences for men's and women's mental health, the alternative hypothesis is that men and women differentially select out of and into marriage on the basis of their prior mental health status. Recall that since his article first appeared in the literature, scholars have argued that men who have mental health problems may "select out" of marriage, whereas women who have mental health problems may "select into" marriage, in the first place. Thus, rather than attributing gender differences in the relationships between marital status and mental health to social causation processes—as Gove's theory does—it is possible that social selection processes actually account for gender differences in these relationships. In Table 4 I examine this alternative social-selection hypothesis with respect to marital loss and marital gain for male and female types of emotional problems. A number of findings are evident in this final table.

First, model 1 indicates that respondent's age, race, and education all predict whether they had a marital loss through separation or divorce. Consistent with demographic research, younger, nonwhite, and less-educated persons are significantly more likely to become separated and divorced than older, white, and more-educated people. Interestingly, and in contrast to some demographic research, neither respondent's employment nor parental status predicts marital loss. Moreover, prior mental health status predicts marital loss. Consistent with social-selection arguments (Booth & Amato, 1991; Mastekaasa, 1992), persons who reported symptoms of depression and alcohol problems at T1 are significantly more likely to have separated and divorced by T2 than persons who did not report these problems. However, while these findings provide support for social-selection arguments, it is also possible to interpret them from a social-causation framework; these respondents may have reported more depression and drinking problems at T1 because they were already experiencing stress that precipitates separation and divorce (see Menaghan, 1985). Although my data unfortunately do not allow me to adjudicate which, if any, of these interpretations is more accurate for marital loss, there is no indication in model 2 that men and women differentially select out of marriage on the basis of their mental health status.

Second, model 3 indicates that respondent's age, race, household income, and gender predict whether they had a marital gain. Consistent with demographic research, younger and white persons, as well as those with higher household income and men, are significantly more likely to marry (and remarry) than older and nonwhite people, those with lower household income, and women. Moreover, and in contrast to marital loss, respondent's employment and parental status predict whether they had a marital gain; parents and employed persons are significantly more likely to get married (or remarried) than nonparents and nonemployed people. Model 3 further shows that neither depression nor drinking problems predict marital gain. Thus, there is no support for social-selection arguments of the relationship between marital status and mental health with respect to marital gain. Last, and most relevant for this article, model 4 reveals that there are no gender differences in the selection into marriage on the basis of prior mental health.

Overall, these concluding analyses indicate that social-selection and social-causation processes underlie the relationship between marital loss and mental health. Persons who separated or divorced by T2 reported more depression and drinking problems at T1 than those who remained married.

However, while these individuals' symptoms may have contributed to their subsequent loss, it is possible that they also reflected marital difficulties that typically precede separation and divorce. In contrast, social causation processes alone appear to account for the relationship between marital gain and mental health since individuals' symptoms at T1 did not play a role in whether they got married (or remarried) by T2. Finally, there is no evidence to support the hypothesis that men and women differentially select out of or into marriage on the basis of their mental health, and this finding holds for female and male types of emotional problems. Depressed women and alcohol-abusing men are neither more nor less likely to remain or become married.

CONCLUSIONS AND DISCUSSION

For three decades, sociologists have debated about the consequences of marriage for men's and women's mental health. Results of cross-sectional analyses provided support for emotional-socialization arguments, which claim that males and females respond to stress and manifest distress with different types of emotional problems. At the same time, these analyses provided support for role-theoretical claims that marriage is associated with enhanced mental health.

Results of longitudinal analyses provided further support for role-theoretical claims that social roles in general, and marital roles in particular, have consequences for mental health. Marital loss increases, whereas marital gain decreases, emotional distress—though these relationships are statistically significant only for certain groups of people and for certain types of emotional problems. These analyses also indicated that when there are gender differences in the emotional impact of marital transitions, their greater impact on men or women is evident only for sex-typical emotional problems. These findings suggest that women's symptoms of depression and men's alcohol problems are *functional equivalents* and that there is a relationship between marital status and externalizing emotional problems for men that was unarticulated in prior theory and research.

The last set of analyses investigated, for the first time with national data, the alternative social-selection hypothesis, which claims that individuals who have mental health problems are less likely than those who do not to either remain or become married. These analyses also examined whether there are gender differences in the causes of marital transitions and if distressed men select out of, while distressed women select into, marriage. Results for marital loss indicated that married respondents who subsequently separated and divorced report more depression and alcohol problems at T1 than those who remained married. However, I interpreted these results as providing support for *both* social selection and social causation hypotheses of the relationship between marital status and mental health. While it is likely that married people's depression or alcohol abuse contribute to marital problems and precipitate marital dissolution, it is equally likely that their distress reflects extant marital problems that typically precede separation and divorce (Riessman, 1990). These findings strongly suggest that social-selection and social-causation processes are complex and that the direction of causality of the relationship between marital loss and mental health cannot easily be disentangled—even in longitudinal research (Horwitz & White, 1991; Horwitz et al., 1996a; Mastekaasa, 1992; Menaghan, 1985, 1989; Menaghan & Lieberman, 1986).

In contrast to marital loss, results for marital gain provided support for only social-causation arguments since unmarried respondents' mental health status had no bearing on whether they subsequently married. It thus appears that distressed persons are not more likely to select out, and emotionally healthy people are not more likely to select into, marriage—at least not with respect to depression and alcohol abuse. Finally, there was no evidence to support the notion that men and women differentially select out of and into marriage on the basis of their mental health. That is, depressed women and alcohol-abusing men are neither less nor more likely to have remained or become married than nondepressed women and nonalcohol abusing men.

Taken as a whole, my analyses do not support Gove's early sex-role theory of mental illness, which claimed that marriage is emotionally advantageous for men and disadvantageous for women. My analyses also do not support the implications of the new gender theory, in which the psychological benefits of marriage are thought to be fewer for women than for men. On the contrary, my findings indicate that the emotional benefits of being married, and emotional costs of being unmarried, apply to women and men in the United States today. However, even though Gove's sex-role theory does not apply to contemporary women and men, my results do not imply and cannot speak to its accuracy earlier in the 20th century when the historical conditions under which he derived his hypotheses were in place. Indeed, Gove's theory was intended to be a *historically specific* theory about the nature and consequences of men's and women's marital roles from World War II through the 1970s—a historical period in which men's and women's roles both within and outside of marriage were more narrowly defined than they are today.

My research provides an opportunity to take stock of the nature, meaning, and significance of marriage for men and women at the close of the 20th century. The last 30 years have been a period of tumultuous social change in men's and women's roles and in marital patterns in the United States. There is currently greater involvement of men and women in both the family and workplace, as well as greater fluidity of marital status over the life course of males and females, respectively. Corresponding to these role-related changes are changes in the cultural meaning of marriage;

while marriage was once perceived as a permanent bond that was broken by death, it is now viewed as a temporary bond that could be severed through separation and divorce. Although I cannot say that these social changes have altered the consequences of marriage for men's and women's mental health, my results provide further evidence for recent claims (Waite, 1995; Waite & Gallagher, 2000) that the emotional advantages of marriage apply *equally* to men and women. My results also suggest that there is currently gender equality in the emotional costs of marital loss and the emotional benefits of marital gain—with the exception of separation and divorce. The emotional disadvantages of separation and divorce are greater for women with respect to depression, whereas the emotional benefits of marital gain among the previously separated and divorced are greater for men with respect to alcohol abuse.

References

Aneshensel, Carol S. 1992. "Social Stress: Theory and Research." *Annual Review of Sociology* 18:15–38.

Aneshensel, Carol S., Carolyn M. Rutter, and Peter A. Lachenbruch. 1991. "Social Structure, Stress, and Mental Health: Competing Conceptual and Analytic Models." *American Sociological Review* 56:166–78.

Aseltine, Robert H., and Ronald C. Kessler. 1993. "Marital Disruption and Depression in a Community Sample." *Journal of Health and Social Behavior* 34:237–51.

Avison, William, and Donna McAlpine. 1992. "Gender Differences in Symptoms of Depression among Adolescents." *Journal of Health and Social Behavior* 33:77–96.

Berkman, Lisa F., and Lester Breslow. 1983. *Health and Ways of Living: The Alameda County Study.* New York: Oxford Press.

Bernard, Jessie. 1972. *The Future of Marriage.* New York: Bantam Books.

Booth, Alan, and Paul Amato. 1991. "Divorce and Psychological Stress." *Journal of Health and Social Behavior* 32:396–407.

Dohrenwend, Bruce P., and Barbara S. Dohrenwend. 1976. "Sex Differences in Psychiatric Disorders." *American Journal of Sociology* 81:1447–54.

Dohrenwend, Bruce P., Patrick E. Shrout, Gladys Egri, and Frederick S. Mendelsohn. 1980. "Non-specific Psychological Distress and Other Dimensions of Psychopathology." *Archives of General Psychiatry* 37:1229–36.

England, Paula. 2000. "Marriage, the Costs of Children, and Gender Inequality." Pp. 320–42 in *The Ties that Bind: Perspectives on Marriage and Cohabitation,* edited by Linda J. Waite. New York: Aldine de Gruyter.

Ferree, Myra Marx. 1990. "Beyond Separate Spheres: Feminism and Family Research." *Journal of Marriage and the Family* 52:866–84.

Ferree, Myra Marx, Judith Lorber, and Beth B. Hess, eds. 1999. *Revisioning Gender.* Thousand Oaks, Calif.: Sage.

Fox, W. John. 1980. "Gove's Specific Sex-Role Theory of Mental Illness: A Research Note." *Journal of Health and Social Behavior* 21:260–67.

Gordon, Steven L. 1981. "The Sociology of Sentiment and Emotion." Pp. 562–92 in *Social Psychology: Sociological Perspectives*, edited by Morris Rosenberg and Ralph H. Turner. New York: Basic Books.

———. 1989. "The Socialization of Children's Emotions: Emotional Culture, Competence, and Exposure." Pp. 319–49 in *Children's Understanding of Emotion*, edited by Carolyn Saarni and Paul Harris. New York: Cambridge University Press.

Gore, Susan, Robert H. Aseltine, Jr., and Mary Ellen Colten. 1992. "Social Structure, Life Stress, and Depressive Symptoms in a High School Aged Population." *Journal of Health and Social Behavior* 33:97–113.

Gove, Walter R. 1972. "The Relationship between Sex Roles, Marital Status and Mental Illness." *Social Forces* 51:34–44.

Gove, Walter, and Jeanette F. Tudor. 1973. "Adult Sex Roles and Mental Illness." *American Journal of Sociology* 78:50–73.

Hochschild, Arlie R. 1975. "Attending to, Codifying, and Managing Feelings: Sex Differences in Love." pp. 225–62 in *Feminist Frontiers: Rethinking Sex, Gender, and Society*, edited by Laurel Richardson and Verta Taylor. Reading, Mass.: Addition-Wesley.

———. 1979. "Emotion Work, Feeling Rules, and Social Structure." *American Journal of Sociology* 85:551–75.

Horwitz, Allan V., and Helen Raskin White. 1991. "Becoming Married, Depression, and Alcohol Problems among Young Adults." *Journal of Health and Social Behavior* 32:221–37.

Horwitz, Allan V., Helen Raskin White, and Sandra Howell-White. 1996a. "Becoming Married and Mental Health: A Study of a Cohort of Young Adults." *Journal of Marriage and the Family* 58:895–907.

———. 1996b. "The Use of Multiple Outcomes in Stress Research: A Case Study of Gender Differences in Responses to Marital Dissolution." *Journal of Health and Social Behavior* 37:278–91.

Kessler, Ronald C., and James A. McRae. 1984. "Trends in the Relationships of Sex and Marital Status to Psychological Distress." *Research in Community and Mental Health* 4:109–30.

Kessler, Ronald C., Katherine A. McGonagle, Marvin Schwartz, Dan G. Blazer, and Christopher B. Nelson. 1993. "Sex and Depression in the National Co-Morbidity Survey I: Lifetime Prevalence, Chronicity, and Recurrence." *Journal of Affective Disorders* 25:85–96.

Kessler, Ronald C., Katherine A. McGonagle, Shanyang Zhao, Christopher B. Nelson, Michael Hughes, Suzanne Eshleman, Hans-Urlich Wittchen, and Kenneth S. Kendler. 1994. "Lifetime and 12-Month Prevalence of DSM-III-R Psychiatric Disorders in the United States." *Archives of General Psychiatry* 51:8–19.

Lennon, Mary Clare. 1987. "Sex Differences in Distress: The Impact of Gender and Work Roles." *Journal of Health and Social Behavior* 28:290–305.

Lopata, Helena, and Barrie Thorne. 1978. "On the Term 'Sex Roles'." *Signs* 3:718–21.

Marks, Nadine F., and James David Lambert. 1998. "Marital Status Continuity and Change among Young and Midlife Adults: Longitudinal Effects on Psychological Well-Being." *Journal of Family Issues* 19:652–86.

Mastekaasa, Arne. 1992. "Marriage and Psychological Well-Being: Some Evidence on Selection into Marriage." *Journal of Marriage and the Family* 54:901–11.

Menaghan, Elizabeth G. 1985. "Depressive Affect and Subsequent Divorce." *Journal of Family Issues* 6:296–306.

———. 1989. "Role Changes and Psychological Well-Being: Variations in Effects by Gender and Role Repertoire." *Social Forces* 67:693–714.

Menaghan, Elizabeth G., and Morton A. Lieberman. 1986. "Changes in Depression Following Divorce: A Panel Study." *Journal of Marriage and the Family* 48:319–28.

Meyers, Jerome K., Myrna M. Weissman, Gary L. Tischler, Charles E. Holzer, Philip J. Leaf, Helen Orvaschel, James C. Anthony, Jeffrey H. Boyd, Jack D. Burke, Jr., Morton Kramer, and Roger Stoltzman. 1984. "Six-Month Prevalence of Psychiatric Disorders in Three Communities." *Archives of General Psychiatry* 41:959–67.

Mills, C. Wright. 1959. *The Sociological Imagination*. New York: Oxford University Press.

Mirowsky, John, and Catherine E. Ross. 1992. "Age and Depression." *Journal of Health and Social Behavior* 33:187–205.

Oppenheimer, Valerie K. 1994. "Women's Rising Employment and the Future of the Family in Industrialized Societies." *Population and Development Review* 20:293–342.

Osmond, Marie Withers, and Barrie Thorne. 1990. "Feminist Theories: The Social Construction of Gender in Families and Society." In *Sourcebook of Family Theories and Methods: A Contextual Approach* (pp. 623–626), edited by Pauline Boss et al. New York: Plenum.

Pearlin, Leonard, and Joyce Johnson. 1977. "Marital Status, Life Strains, and Depression." *American Sociology Review* 42:704–15.

Radloff, Lenore S. 1975. "Sex Differences in Depression: The Effects of Occupation and Marital Status." *Sex Roles* 1:249–65.

———. 1977. "The CES-D Scale: A Self-Reported Depression Scale for Research in the General Population." *Applied Psychological Measurement* 1:385–401.

Reskin, Barbara. 1988. "Bringing the Men Back In: Sex Differentiation and the Devaluation of Women's Work." *Gender and Society* 2:58–81.

Riessman, Catherine Kohler. 1990. *Divorce Talk: Women and Men Make Sense of Personal Relationships*. New Brunswick, N.J.: Rutgers University Press.

Riessman, Catherine Kohler, and Naomi Gerstel. 1985. "Marital Dissolution and Health: Do Males or Females Have Greater Risk?" *Social Science and Medicine* 20:627–35.

Risman, Barbara. 1987. "Intimate Relationships from a Micro-Structural Perspective: Men Who Mother." *Gender and Society* 1:6–32.

Robins, Lee N., John E. Helzer, Myrna M. Weissman, Helen Orvaschel, Earnest Gruenberg, Jack D. Burke, and Darrel A. Rieger. 1984. "Lifetime Prevalence of Specific Psychiatric Disorders in Three Sites." *Archives of General Psychiatry* 41:949–58.

Robins, Lee N., and D. A. Regier, eds. 1994. *Psychiatric Disorders in America: The Epidemiologic Catchment Area Study*. New York: Free Press.

Rosenfield, Sarah, Jean Vertefuille, and Donna McAlpine. 2000. "Gender Stratification and Mental Health: Dimensions of the Self." *Social Psychology Quarterly* 63:208–23.

Simon, Robin W. 1998. "Assessing Sex Differences in Vulnerability among Employed Parents: The Importance of Marital Status." *Journal of Health and Social Behavior* 39:38–54.

Simon, Robin W., and Leda E. Kanellakos. 2001. "Examining Emotion Culture in the U.S.: Is There Any Truth to Gender Stereotypes in Emotional Experience and Expression in the GSS?" Paper presented at the Annual Meetings of the American Sociological Association, Anaheim, California.

Simon, Robin W., and Kristen Marcussen. 1999. "Marital Transitions, Marital Beliefs, and Mental Health." *Journal of Health and Social Behavior* 40:111–25.

Smith-Lovin, Lynn. 1995. "The Sociology of Affect and Emotion." Pp. 118–48 in *Sociological Perspectives of Social Psychology*, edited by Karen Cook, Gary Allen Fine, and James S. House. Boston: Allyn & Bacon.

Spain, Daphne, and Suzanne M. Bianchi. 1996. *Balancing Act: Motherhood, Marriage, and Employment among American Women*. New York: Russell Sage.

Stacey, Judith. 1993. "Good Riddance to 'the Family': A Response to David Popenoe." *Journal of Marriage and the Family* 5:45–47.

Stacey, Judith and Barrie Thorne. 1985. "The Missing Feminist Revolution in Sociology." *Social Problems* 32:301–16.

Sweet, James A. and Larry L. Bumpass. 1996. "The National Survey of Families and Households Waves 1 and 2: Data Description and Documentation." Center for Demography and Ecology, University of Wisconsin, Madison.

Thoits, Peggy A. 1986. "Multiple Identities: Examining Gender and Marital Status Differences in Psychological Distress." *American Sociological Review* 51:259–72.

———. 1989. "The Sociology of Emotions." *Annual Review of Sociology* 15:317–42.

Thompson, Linda, and Alexis J. Walker. 1989. "Gender in Families: Women and Men in Marriage, Work, and Parenthood." *Journal of Marriage and the Family* 51:845–71.

Umberson, Deborah, Meichu D. Chen, James S. House, Kristen Hopkins, and Ellen Slater. 1996. "The Effect of Social Relationships on Psychological Well-Being: Are Men and Women Really So Different?" *American Sociological Review* 61:837–57.

Umberson, Deborah, Camille B. Wortman, and Ronald C. Kessler. 1992. "Widowhood and Depression: Explaining Long-Term Gender Differences in Vulnerability." *Journal of Health and Social Behavior* 33:10–24.

Waite, Linda J. 1995. "Does Marriage Matter?" *Demography* 32:483–507.

Waite, Linda J., and Margie Gallagher. 2000. *The Case for Marriage: Why Married People Are Happier, Healthier and Better Off Financially*. New York: Doubleday.

Warheit, George J., Charles E. Holzer, Roger A. Bell, and Sandra A. Rey. 1976. "Sex, Marital Status and Mental Health: A Reappraisal." *Social Forces* 55:459–70.

West, Candace, and Don Zimmerman. 1987. "Doing Gender." *Gender and Society* 1:125–51.

DISCUSSION

1. Simon includes depression and alcohol abuse as outcomes in her analysis. Why was it important for her to do so? Are there other outcomes that would have been useful for her to include?

2. The data Simon uses are from the early 1990s. Would you expect her results to hold for couples being married today? Why or why not?

Ranae J. Evenson and Robin W. Simon

Clarifying the Relationship Between Parenthood and Depression

Parenthood is an important social role with profound material and symbolic importance. Popular claims about the effects of parenthood on mental health abound but there is little systematic evidence with which to evaluate them. Evenson and Simon take up the question of whether parenthood carries mental health benefits and, in the process, put some popular myths to rest.

Unlike other major adult social roles in the United States, parenthood does not appear to confer a mental health advantage for individuals. Although there is inconsistency in findings across studies, most research either finds that parents do not significantly differ in emotional well-being from nonparents or that parents report significantly more emotional distress than persons who have never had children. These findings have led mental health and family scholars to conclude that persons do not derive the same emotional benefits from parenthood as they do from marriage and employment. However, because research has mainly compared childless persons to either all persons who have ever had children or parents at particular stages of the life course (i.e., "active" and "emptynest" parents), little is known about the mental health of different types of parents relative to nonparents. More importantly, previous research provides limited insight into variation in emotional distress *among* parents. This is an important and timely topic since increases in nonmarital childbearing and cohabitation as well as divorce and remarriage over the second half of the twentieth century have resulted in an increase in certain types of parents—such as single parents, noncustodial parents, stepparents, and cohabiting parents—who are likely to be at higher risk than others for developing depression. In this article, we overcome some of the limitations of prior research and attempt to clarify the relationship between parenthood and current symptoms of depression using data from a nationally representative sample of adults. For reasons that we elaborate upon later, we hypothesize that most types of parents report more depression than nonparents. We also hypothesize that certain types of parenthood are associated with more depression than others.

BACKGROUND

Parental Status Differences in Mental Health

Social status differences in mental health have been the topic of a large body of research. Prompted in large part by women's increased labor force

Evenson, Ranae J. and Robin W. Simon. 2005. "Clarifying the Relationship Between Parenthood and Depression." *Journal of Health and Social Behavior* 46:341–358.

participation during the second half of the 20th century, much of this research has focused on marital and employment status differences in psychological well-being. It is now well documented that marriage and employment are associated with enhanced mental health for men and women since married and employed persons consistently report significantly fewer symptoms of emotional distress than their nonmarried and non-employed counterparts (e.g., Mirowsky & Ross, 2003; Simon, 2002; Thoits, 1983).

Compared to research on marital and employment status differences in emotional well-being, there has been far less research on the relationship between parenthood and mental health, and the research that does exist has been far less conclusive. While some studies report a positive relationship between parenthood and emotional well-being (Aneshensel, Frerichs, & Clark, 1981; Burton, 1998; Kandel, Davies, & Raveis, 1985), others find a negative relationship (Campbell, Converse, & Rogers, 1976; Glenn & McLanahan, 1981; Gove & Geerken, 1977; Hughes, 1989; McLanahan & Adams, 1985; Radloff, 1975). Still others indicate that there is no relationship between parenthood and mental health (Andrews & Withey, 1976; Cleary & Mechanic, 1983; McLanahan & Adams, 1985; Ross, Mirowsky, & Goldsteen, 1990; Umberson & Gove, 1989).

These inconsistencies in findings across studies are attributable, at least in part, to inconsistencies in the parent groups to which nonparents are compared (McLanahan & Adams, 1987, 1989). For example, when nonparents are compared to all persons who have ever had children, parenthood is not associated with psychological well-being (Aneshensel et al., 1981). However, when childless persons are compared to parents residing with minor children, parenthood is negatively associated with mental health (McLanahan & Adams, 1987; Umberson & Gove, 1989). Moreover, when childless adults are compared to emptynest parents, parenthood is positively associated with emotional well-being (Ross & Mirowsky, 1988; Umberson & Gove, 1989). On the basis of these latter two findings, some scholars have speculated that the mental health benefits of parenthood are limited to the stage in the life course when children are grown and independent (Kandel et al., 1985; Umberson & Gove, 1989). Overall, despite some inconsistencies in findings across studies, these observations have led mental health and family scholars to conclude that individuals do not derive as much emotional benefit from parenthood as they do from marriage and employment (Gore & Mangione, 1983; McLanahan & Adams, 1987; Mirowsky & Ross, 2003). That is, unlike other major adult social roles in the United States, parenthood does not appear to confer a mental health advantage for individuals.

Interestingly, both micro- and macro-sociological explanations have been offered to account for why parenthood is not associated with enhanced mental health. Drawing on theories about the psychological consequences of social role involvement, social-psychologically oriented mental health researchers have argued that the emotional benefits associated with parenthood are cancelled out, or exceeded, by the emotional costs associated with the role. According to this argument, parenthood (like other social roles) provides individuals with personal gratification as well as a sense of purpose and meaning in life, both of which promote emotional well-being (Menaghan, 1989; Sieber, 1974; Thoits, 1983). However, the emotional rewards derived from parenthood are often overshadowed by the numerous demands and stressors associated with the role, particularly when children are young, demands which ultimately undermine mental health (Umberson & Gove, 1989).

Focusing instead on the broader social and policy context in which contemporary parenthood takes place, macro-oriented family scholars and family demographers have argued that there has been a decline over the second half of the twentieth century in the cultural significance of parenthood in the United States, a change that has lessened the social value and esteem formerly attached to the role for both women and men (Blake, 1979; Huber, 1980; Preston, 1984, 1986). According to this line of reasoning, a consequence of our cultural indifference to parenthood is that we currently lack institutional supports that would help ease the social and economic burdens and subsequent stressfulness and emotional disadvantages associated with the parental role, especially when children are dependent (also see Hewlett & West, 1998; Hewlett, Rankin, & West, 2002).

However, while these complimentary theoretical arguments are persuasive, research on parental status differences in mental health has focused on *all* persons who have ever had children and parents at *particular stages in the life course;* we therefore know little about the mental health of certain types of parents—such as non-custodial parents—relative to nonparents. Moreover, because parents residing with minor children may include persons living with biological and/or adopted children as well as those living with stepchildren, we know little about the relative mental health of these two different types of parents. Similarly, because emptynest parents may include persons who have their own non-residential adult children as well as those who have nonresidential adult stepchildren, we also know little about the mental health of these different types of emptynest parents compared to childless persons. Nevertheless, on the basis of the research findings and theoretical arguments discussed above, it is likely that most types of parents—especially parents of minor children—report more emotional distress than childless persons.

Variations in Mental Health among Parents

Because most research on the relationship between parenthood and mental health has examined parental status differences in emotional well-being, we also have little information about variations in emotional distress *among* parents. Almost all of the research on this topic has focused on marital status differences in mental health among parents residing with minor children. Not surprisingly, studies show that unmarried persons living with dependent children (i.e., "single" parents) report more mental health problems than their married peers (Andrews & Withey, 1976; Kandel et al., 1985; McLanahan, 1983). Single parents' greater distress appears to be due in large part to the fewer social and economic resources available to them (Brown &

Harris 1978; McLanahan & Adams, 1987; Pearlin & Johnson, 1977). However, while this research is informative, it provides limited insight into distress differences between married relative to single and cohabiting persons residing with young children. This research also offers limited insight into marital status differences in distress among other types of parents, particularly those not residing with children.

There has also been some research on gender differences in mental health among parents residing with young children. While most of these studies find that mothers with dependent children at home report more distress than similar fathers (Aneshensel et al., 1981; Bird & Rogers, 1998; Campbell et al., 1976; Glenn & McLanahan, 1981), some show that under certain conditions (i.e., unemployment) married fathers living with minor children report more distress than similar mothers (Menaghan, 1989; Thoits, 1983). Interestingly, Hughes (1989) finds that single parenthood has particularly negative consequences for the mental health of formerly married men relative to formerly married women. In a more recent study, Simon (1998) shows that both married and unmarried mothers of minor children report more depression than their male counterparts, irrespective of their children's custodial status. However, similar to the studies of marital status differences in distress discussed above, these studies have not investigated gender differences in mental health among parents not residing with minor children, including noncustodial and empty-nest parents, as well as gender differences among stepparents.

In addition to the paucity of research on gender and marital status differences in mental health among parents, there is virtually no research that has systematically assessed differences in distress between different types of parents irrespective of gender and marital status. There is some evidence that parents residing with minor children are more distressed than emptynest parents (Aneshensel et al., 1981; Umberson & Gove, 1989). However, although another assumption underlying work in this area is that parents with dependent children in the household are the most distressed type of parent, it is possible that noncustodial parents are more distressed than parents residing with their own minor children. It is also possible that persons residing with minor stepchildren (and possibly those who have nonresidential adult stepchildren) report more distress than persons living with their own minor children.

Elaborating on sociological theories about the emotional consequences of role involvement discussed earlier, it is reasonable to expect that certain types of parenthood are associated with more depression than others. In fact, we believe that variation in mental health among parents reflects a myriad of factors affecting individuals' experiences as parents, including the demands and normative expectations associated with the role, the quality of their relationships with children, their perceptions of their ability to satisfy role expectations, their self-evaluations as parents, the social and economic resources available to them, the stressfulness of the role, and the emotional gratification and sense of purpose and meaning they derive from parenthood.

For example, the lack of daily contact with one's minor children contradicts the normative expectations of parenthood with dependent offspring, and may negatively affect individuals' relationships with their children as well as their perceptions of their ability to fulfill parental role expectations. Therefore, it is likely that noncustodial parenthood is perceived as stressful and that noncustodial parents report more depression than parents residing with their own dependent children. Similarly, given the absence of cultural norms for stepparents and resentment stepparents and stepchildren of all ages may feel toward one another (Cherlin, 1978; Cherlin & Furstenberg, 1994), it is likely that stepparenthood is perceived as stressful and that stepparents report more depression than parents living with their own minor children. On the other hand, since most of the demands associated with parenting dependent children dissipate as children mature and develop independent lives, it is likely that parenthood involving one's own nonresidential adult children is perceived as less stressful and that these parents report less depression than persons residing with young biological and/or adopted children. In other words, we argue that variation in emotional distress among parents reflects variation in their experiences: Some types of parenthood are associated with more emotional distress than others.

Clarifying the Relationship between Parenthood and Depression

In our article, we address some of the limitations of earlier research and attempt to clarify the relationship between parenthood and current symptoms of depression using data from a nationally representative sample of adults. The following three hypotheses guide our research. First, we hypothesize that unlike other major adult social roles (i.e., marriage and employment), *parenthood is not associated with enhanced emotional well-being*. With the exception of emptynest parents, we expect that most types of parents report more depression than nonparents. However, we also hypothesize that there is considerable *variation in depression among parents* and expect that certain types of parents (e.g., noncustodial and stepparents) report more depression than others (e.g., parents living with their own minor children). We further hypothesize that there are both *gender and marital status differences in the association between parenthood and depression*. Given the female excess of depression in the United States, we expect (1) that most types of mothers report more depression than most types of fathers; and (2) that the association between

SEXUAL ORIENTATION AND MENTAL HEALTH

The previous three selections have assumed that most adult men and women are involved in heterosexual relationships. There is an active line of research concerned with the more general implications of sexual orientation for mental health. One study from that line of research, by Stephen T.

Russell and Kara Joyner, analyzes suicide risk among youth with same-sex as compared to opposite-sex romantic attractions using data from the National Longitudinal Survey of Adolescent Health. The authors find that youth with same-sex romantic attractions are between 1.68 and 2.48 as likely as other youth to express suicidal thoughts and to have attempted suicide, with the risk being slightly higher for girls than for boys. The differences in risk between youth with same-sex and opposite-sex attractions are explained, to a great extent, by the higher levels of victimization, alcohol use, and depression reported by youth with same-sex attractions. These explanatory variables are common predictors of suicide risk among youth, leading the authors to urge attention both to the unique and the common developmental challenges faced by sexual minority youth. Their analysis is an important corrective to the heterosexist bias of mental health research.

Stephen T. Russell and Kara Joyner. 2001. "Adolescent Sexual Orientation and Suicide Risk: Evidence from a National Study." *American Journal of Public Health* 91:1276–1281.

most types of parenthood—especially those involving minor children—and depression is greater for women than for men. Moreover, because research finds that marriage is associated with enhanced mental health for men and women, we further expect that most types of *unmarried* (including single and cohabiting) parents report more depression than their married peers.

In their study of trends in the effects of children on adults' psychological well-being between 1957 and 1976, McLanahan and Adams (1989) showed that different types of parenthood are associated with different levels of distress. Although we focus on different "types" of parents than they did, our study builds on their work and contributes to research on this topic by examining variations in depression among parents with more recent national data. Overall, in addition to clarifying the relationship between parenthood and depression in the United States today, our article attempts to take stock of the meaning of contemporary parenthood and contributes to ongoing theoretical debates about the advantages of social role involvement for individuals' mental health.

METHODS

Data

We conducted our analyses on data from the first wave of the National Survey of Families and Households (NSFH), which was based on a national probability sample of 13,017 adults in the United States. Interviews were administered in 1987–1988 with 9,643 individuals age 19 and older, and an additional 3,374 persons from an oversampling of blacks and Hispanics, cohabiting and recently married persons, and both single and stepparents. The survey's response rate was 74 percent (see Sweet, Bumpass, & Call, 1988 for details). Due to oversampling, the sample includes high proportions of single parents, cohabiting parents, and stepparents. The NSFH is ideal for this study because it contains detailed information about the ages and types of children residing in the respondent's household as well as the ages and types of children living elsewhere.

Measures

Depression. Depression is assessed with 12 items from the Center for Epidemiological Studies Depression CES-D Scale—a measure of depressed mood that has high construct validity and internal consistency (Radloff, 1977). Respondents were asked how many days in the past week: "you were bothered by things that usually don't bother you," "you felt lonely," "you felt you could not shake off the blues, even with the help of your family or friends," "your sleep was restless," "you felt depressed," "you felt that everything you did was an effort," "you felt fearful," "you had trouble keeping your mind on what you were doing," "you talked less than usual," "you did not feel like eating, your appetite was poor," "you felt sad," and "you could not get going?" Item responses (0 to 7 days) were summed; scores on these measures range from 0 to 81 (chronbach's alpha = .93).

In this article, we investigate differences in current levels of depression between childless persons and all parents as well as different types of parents. We also examine variation in symptoms among parents. We therefore created two sets of dummy variables for parental status.

Parental status. Because previous research has examined depression differences between nonparents and all parents, we computed: *"childless adults"* (coded 1), which indicates respondents who have neither given birth to, fathered, adopted, nor had stepchildren; and *"all parents"* (coded 1), which indicates respondents who have either given birth to, fathered, adopted, or had stepchildren. Moreover, because research has investigated depression differences between childless adults and parents at different stages of the life course, we created additional variables: *"fullnest parents"* (coded 1), which indicates persons who *only* have coresidential biological and/or adopted children under the age of 18; and *"emptynest parents"* (coded 1), which indicates persons who *only* have nonresidential biological and/or adopted children 18 years old and over. These four parental status variables are mutually exclusive; respondents who are assigned to these parent status categories are only these types of persons.

Additionally, to assess differences in depression between nonparents and different types of parents (i.e., persons who have different ages and types of children residing in the household and elsewhere) as well as variations in depression among parents, we created six other dummy measures: *"parents with minor children at home"* (coded 1), which indicates persons who have a biological and/or adopted child under 18 in the household; *"parents with minor stepchildren at home"* (coded 1), which indicates people who have a step-child less than 18 in the household; *"noncustodial parents"* (coded 1), which refers to individuals who have a biological and/or adopted child under 18 with whom they are not living; *"parents with adult children at home"* (coded 1), which indicates persons who have a biological and/or adopted child 18 years or older in the household; *"parents with nonresidential adult children"* (coded 1), which refers to persons who have a nonresidential biological and/or adopted child 18 or older; and *"parents with nonresidential adult stepchildren"* (coded 1), which refers to persons who have a nonresidential stepchild 18 years or older. These six parental status variables are not mutually exclusive; respondents who are assigned to each of these parent categories may be more than one type of parent. Throughout the article, we use the term "children" to refer to biological and/or adopted children.

Sociodemographic and status characteristics. In order to hold constant factors that may influence the relationship between parenthood and depression, we include the following sociodemographic and status variables in all of our analyses: respondents' gender (female = 1), race (black = 1; persons from racial backgrounds other than black or white = 1), age (in years), education (in years completed), household income (in dollars), marital status (single = 1; cohabiting = 1), and employment status (employed full-time = 1). We also include a term for age-squared to control for nonlinearity in the associations between age and depression (see Mirowsky & Ross, 1989). Additionally, we assigned a predicted value for household income to respondents who had missing data on this variable, an imputation that was based on their values for gender, race, age, education, marital status, and employment status. A series of interaction terms was created in order to investigate gender differences in the associations between different types of parenthood and symptoms. We also conducted interactional analyses for all of the socio-demographic variables with all of the parental status variables in order to explore whether the associations between different types of parenthood and depression differ by age, race, education, and household income. Although they do not appear in our tables, we report significant interactions in the discussion of our results.

Analysis Sample

The analysis sample comprises of respondents whose parental status is unambiguous and who have complete data on all variables in our models. In the section that follows, we present the results of two main sets of analyses. The first set examines differences in current levels of depression between nonparents and all parents as well as different types of parents ($N = 11{,}473$). The second set of analyses investigates variation in symptoms among parents ($N = 8{,}520$). For the sake of clarity, we discuss the specific plan for each analysis before the presentation of the tables.

Table 1 Selected Sociodemographic Characteristics by Parental Status (N = 11,473)

	Childless Adults[a] (N = 2,953)	All Parents[a] (N = 8,520)	Fullnest Parents[a] (N = 3,703)	Emptynest Parents[a] (N = 2,060)	Parents with Minor Children at Home[b] (N = 4,859)	Parents with Minor Stepchildren at Home[b] (N = 389)	Noncustodial Parents[b] (N = 812)	Parents with Adult Children at Home[b] (N = 838)	Parents with Nonresidential Adult Children[b] (N = 3,467)	Parents with Nonresidential Adult Stepchildren[b] (N = 669)
Gender (%)										
Male	50.5	37.7	30.2	36.7	32.5	76.6	71.2	33.4	37.6	38.3
Female	49.5	62.3	69.8	63.3	67.5	23.4	28.8	66.6	62.4	61.7
Age	36.3	44.3	32.4	63.6	34.5	35.3	37.3	52.3	59.1	52.9
Race (%)										
Black	14.6	18.3	17.7	15.3	18.9	14.4	25.3	22.0	17.8	17.8
White	77.2	72.8	71.0	79.6	70.2	77.6	64.8	67.7	76.0	78.0
Other	8.1	8.9	11.3	5.1	10.9	8.0	10.0	10.4	6.2	4.2
Education	13.1	12.1	12.8	11.1	12.6	12.6	12.2	11.5	11.2	11.7
Household income (in dollars)	25,084	31,517	32,543	26,368	33,199	34,406	28,399	39,465	29,074	34,945
Marital status (%)										
Married	33.0	63.9	69.1	55.7	68.6	77.1	41.4	69.0	59.7	79.1
Cohabiting	8.6	3.9	3.3	1.7	3.7	22.1	12.0	1.1	2.0	1.6
Single	58.5	32.2	27.6	42.6	27.7	0.1	46.7	30.0	38.3	19.3
Full-time employment (%)	77.4	63.0	71.8	37.6	72.1	83.6	81.2	63.6	47.4	59.5
Depression	15.0	15.3	15.6	13.7	15.8	14.4	18.1	15.1	14.6	15.8

Note: Age and education are given in mean years, household income is given in mean dollars, and depression is given in mean CES-D score.
[a]These parental status variables are mutually exclusive.
[b]These parental status variables are not mutually exclusive.

Sociodemographic Characteristics of Childless Adults, All Parents, and Different Types of Parents

Table 1 presents the sociodemographic and status characteristics of nonparents, all parents, and different types of parents. Mean levels of depression for each parental status subgroup are shown as well. Several patterns are evident in this table. First, while this national sample includes a large proportion of parents (74 percent), one-fourth of the respondents are childless. There are several differences between parents and nonparents; parents are older and have less education, but they have higher household incomes than childless persons. Parents are also more likely than nonparents to be female and married and are less likely to be employed full-time. Interestingly, there is no significant difference in the mean level of depression between all parents and nonparents.

Second, while the sample includes several types of parents, the majority (67 percent) are at either the stage in the life course when they are residing with their own minor children or the emptynest stage of parenthood, both of which have been the focus of much prior research on parenthood and mental health. Forty-three percent of the parents are fullnest parents, and another 24 percent are emptynest parents. Not surprisingly, there are sociodemographic and status differences between persons at these different stages of the life course; fullnest parents are younger, have more education and household income, and are more likely to be employed full-time than emptynest parents. Once again, there is no significant difference in the mean level of depression between childless adults and either fullnest or emptynest parents.

There are, however, gender differences across different types of parents. Reflecting contemporary living arrangements in the United States—in which women are more likely to have custody of dependent children upon divorce and remarriage and are more likely to reside with out-of-wedlock offspring—68 percent of parents with minor children at home are female, whereas 77 percent of parents with minor stepchildren at home and 71 percent of noncustodial parents are male. Interestingly, a greater percentage of parents with adult children at home, nonresidential adult children, and nonresidential adult stepchildren are female as well. Mirroring the female excess of depression in the United States, additional analyses (available upon request) indicate that women report significantly higher symptom levels than men among nonparents and all types of parents.

RESULTS

Parental Status Differences in Depression

Table 2 contains the results of dummy variable analyses in which respondents' current level of depression is regressed on their gender, sociodemographic and status characteristics, and parental status. This first set of

Table 2 Unstandardized Coefficients from Regressions of Depression on Childless Adults and Different Types of Parents

Independent Variables	Model 1 (N = 11,473)	Model 2 (N = 8,716)	Model 3 (N = 11,473)
Female (yes = 1)	1.97*** (.33)	2.00*** (.38)	2.19*** (.34)
Age	−.19** (.06)	−.25*** (.07)	−.26*** (.06)
Age-squared	.00 (.01)	.01 (.01)	.01 (.01)
Black[a] (yes = 1)	1.25** (.43)	1.49** (.50)	1.17** (.43)
Other racial background[a] (yes = 1)	−1.22* (.57)	−.91 (.64)	−1.17* (.57)
Education	−.69*** (.06)	−.67*** (.07)	−.66*** (.06)
Household income	−.16*** (.05)	−.13* (.06)	−.17*** (.05)
Cohabiting[b] (yes = 1)	2.35*** (.74)	2.67** (.87)	2.10** (.75)
Single[b] (yes = 1)	4.20*** (.37)	3.83*** (.42)	4.13*** (.37)
Full-time employment (yes = 1)	−3.71*** (.39)	−3.34*** (.44)	−3.78*** (.39)
All parents[c] (yes = 1)	1.36*** (.40)	—	—
Fullnest parents[c] (yes = 1)	—	.87* (.45)	—
Emptynest parents[c] (yes = 1)	—	.26 (.63)	—
Parents with minor children at home[c] (yes = 1)	—	—	.92** (.38)
Parents with minor stepchildren at home[c] (yes = 1)	—	—	.61 (.88)
Noncustodial parents[c] (yes = 1)	—	—	3.04*** (.62)
Parents with adult children at home[c] (yes = 1)	—	—	.145 (.62)
Parents with nonresidential adult children[c] (yes = 1)	—	—	.84 (.48)
Parents with nonresidential adult stepchildren[c] (yes = 1)	—	—	2.47*** (.68)
Constant	29.78	30.33	30.85
Adjusted R^2	.064	.061	.067

*$p < .05$; **$p < .01$; ***$p < .001$ (two-tailed tests)

Note: Numbers in parentheses are standard errors.
[a]White persons are the reference group.
[b]Married persons are the reference group.
[c]Childless persons are the reference group.

analyses examines differences in depressive symptoms between childless adults and all parents (see model 1); childless adults and parents at different stages of the life course, that is, between nonparents and both fullnest and emptynest parents (see model 2); and childless adults and different types of parents (see model 3). Note that childless persons are the reference category in all of these analyses. There are several interesting findings in Table 2.

Consistent with epidemiological research (Mirowsky & Ross, 2003), model 1 indicates that women and younger people, blacks, persons with less education and household income, non-married persons, and those not employed fulltime report significantly higher levels of depression. However, in contrast to some prior research that finds no difference in mental health between childless adults and parents in general (e.g., Aneshensel et al., 1981), we find that as a group parents report significantly *higher* levels of depression than nonparents once sociodemographic and status characteristics are held constant. We suspect that the inconsistency between our and others' findings reflects the relatively high percentage of single, noncustodial, cohabiting, and stepparents in our national sample. Moreover, in contrast to the assumption that the disadvantages of parenthood are greater for women than for men, supplemental interactional analyses (not shown) reveal that there is no gender difference in the association between current depression and being a parent compared to not being a parent.

Additionally, and in accord with earlier work—which shows that persons residing with young children are more distressed than nonparents (Aneshensel et al., 1981; Pearlin & Johnson, 1977; Umberson & Gove, 1989)—model 2 indicates that fullnest parents are significantly more depressed than their childless peers, controlling for sociodemographic and status variables. However, in contrast to some prior studies that find that emptynest parents are less distressed than nonparents (Mirowsky & Ross, 2003; Umberson & Gove, 1989), we find that emptynest parents do not significantly differ from their childless counterparts with respect to depression, even when sociodemographic and status variables are held constant. That is, while parents at the stage of the life course when their children are young and living at home report significantly more depression than nonparents, parents at the stage of the life course when their children are grown and living independently do not enjoy better mental health than persons who never had children. Auxiliary interactional analyses (not shown) also indicate that the association between parenthood (compared to nonparents) and depression at these two different stages of the life course does not significantly differ by gender.

Finally, model 3 shows that persons who have minor children at home, noncustodial children, adult children at home, and nonresidential adult stepchildren all report significantly more symptoms than nonparents when control variables are included. In fact, there is *no* type of parent in this national sample that reports less depression than nonparents. While persons who have minor stepchildren in the household and nonresidential adult children do not significantly differ from persons who have never had children, most types of parents report significantly more depression than childless persons. Once again, additional interactional analyses (not shown) indicate that there are no gender differences in the association of depression and being any of these types of parents compared to not being a parent.

Taken together, this set of analyses provides support for our first hypothesis: Unlike other major adult roles in the United States, parenthood is not associated with lower levels of depressive symptoms. Our results for emptynest parents are interesting and can be interpreted in two ways. On the one hand, they indicate that the emotional disadvantages of parenthood do not apply to persons at the stage of the life course when their own children are grown and independent. On the other hand, they indicate that there are no emotional benefits of emptynest parenthood for current depression. The findings for stepparents, especially those residing with minor stepchildren, are counterintuitive in light of cultural beliefs about the negative consequences of stepparenthood. Although persons who have nonresidential adult stepchildren report more symptoms, persons residing with minor stepchildren do not differ from nonparents with respect to depression. The latter finding may reflect the social selection of persons into this type of stepparenthood on the basis of their mental health status. While stepparenthood may be distressing, it is possible that those who enjoy better mental health and have more coping resources and social support are more likely to become

Table 3 Unstandardized Coefficients from Regressions of Depression on Different Types of Parents

Independent Variables	Model 1[a] (N = 5,763)	Model 2[a] (N = 5,763)	Model 3[b] (N = 8,520)	Model 4[b] (N = 8,520)
Emptynest parents (yes = 1)	.91 (.94)	.75 (1.12)	—	—
Female × emptynest parents	—	.24 (.96)	—	—
Parents with minor stepchildren at home (yes = 1)	—	—	.38 (.91)	−.05 (1.05)
Noncustodial parents (yes = 1)	—	—	2.50*** (.66)	1.68* (.81)
Parents with adult children at home (yes = 1)	—	—	1.59** (.64)	1.62** (.64)
Parents with nonresidential adult children (yes = 1)	—	—	1.51** (.61)	.77 (.79)
Parents with nonresidential adult stepchildren (yes = 1)	—	—	2.68*** (.69)	1.72 (1.10)
Female × parents with minor stepchildren at home	—	—	—	1.86 (2.06)
Female × noncustodial parents	—	—	—	2.28 (1.37)
Female × parents with adult children at home	—	—	—	.54 (.81)
Female × parents with nonresidential adult children	—	—	—	1.38 (.99)
Female × parents with nonresidential adult stepchildren	—	—	—	1.59 (1.41)
Constant	34.73	34.84	35.16	36.07
Adjusted R^2	.073	.073	.076	.077

*$p < .05$; **$p < .01$; ***$p < .001$ (two-tailed tests)

Notes: Numbers in parentheses are standard errors. Each model controls for gender, sociodemographic variables including age, race, education, and household income as well as respondents' marital and employment status.

[a]Fullnest parents are the reference category.

[b]Parents who have at least one minor biological/adopted child at home are the reference category.

stepparents of minor children. Finally, in contrast to the assumption that parenthood is associated with more depression for women than for men, the emotional disadvantages of being a parent relative to not being a parent are not greater for women, and this appears to be the case regardless of the type of parent one is. Having assessed parental status differences in mental health, we next examine variation among parents.

Variation in Depression among Parents

Our second set of analyses investigates (1) whether some types of parents report more depression than others, and (2) whether there are gender differences in the association between parenthood and depression. Table 3 presents the results of dummy variable analyses in which respondents' symptoms are regressed on their gender, sociodemographic and status characteristics, and the type of parent they are. To assess differences in depression between parents at different stages of the life course, model 1 focuses on fullnest and emptynest parents. Model 2 assesses gender differences in the association between symptoms and parenthood at these two different stages of the life course. The reference group for models 1 and 2 is fullnest parents. Recall that an assumption underlying theory and research in this area is that parents who have dependent children in the household are more distressed than most other types of parents. To examine whether this assumption is correct, model 3 focuses on depression differences between parents who have minor children at home and all other types of parents. Model 4 assesses gender differences in the association between symptoms and these different types of parenthood. The reference group for models 3 and 4 is parents who have minor children in the household. Table 3 contains several intriguing results.

In contrast to some previous research indicating that persons at the emptynest stage of parenthood enjoy better mental health than persons at the stage in the life course when they are residing with their minor children (Aneshensel et al., 1981; Kandel et al., 1985; Umberson & Gove, 1989), we find no significant difference in depression between emptynest and fullnest parents (see model 1). Moreover, although some qualitative research suggests that emptynest parenthood is more beneficial for women's mental health than for men's (Rubin, 1979), there is no significant gender difference in the association between emptynest parenthood and symptoms (see model 2). Supplemental analyses (not shown) further reveal that the association between fullnest parenthood and depression does not significantly differ for women and men. This finding is also in contrast to some prior studies showing that residing with young children is more disadvantageous for the well-being of women than of men (Aneshensel et al., 1981; Bird & Rogers, 1998; Glenn & McLanahan, 1981). Differences between our findings for fullnest compared to emptynest parents and those of some other studies may reflect differences in measures across studies; recall that our measure of fullnest parents includes people residing with minor children under the age of 18, whereas some other studies focus only on those living with children under the age of 6.

We do, however, find significant depression differences between parents who have minor children living at home and most other types of parents. Although persons residing with minor stepchildren do not significantly differ from people living with their own minor children, those who have noncustodial children, adult children at home, nonresidential adult children, and nonresidential adult stepchildren all report significantly *higher* symptom levels (see model 3). Interactional analyses reveal no significant gender difference in the associations between any of these different types of parenthood and depression (see model 4). Moreover, supplemental analyses (not shown) show no significant gender difference in the association between being a parent with minor children at home and depression.

On balance, these analyses provide support for our second hypothesis: There is considerable variation in depression among parents. Although fullnest and emptynest parents do not differ as some research suggests, parents residing with their own minor children actually report less (rather than more) depression than most other types of parents. Together, these findings contradict the assumption that parents with minor children in the household are the most distressed type of parent. In light of cultural assumptions about the stressfulness of stepparenthood, we are once again surprised by our findings for stepparents. Our failure to find depression differences between parents residing with their own minor children and those living with minor stepchildren may reflect underlying selection processes. Along similar lines, while noncustodial parenthood is likely to be stressful and depressing, our finding that non-custodial parents report higher symptom levels than custodial parents may reflect the selection of depressed people out of custodial parenthood. We are also surprised to find that having non-residential adult children is associated with more depression than having minor children in the household—a finding for which we do not have a ready explanation. At the same time that these analyses provide support for our hypothesis that there is variation in distress among parents, they provide no support for the hypothesis that there are gender differences in the association between parenthood and depression. Despite the female excess of depression among all types of parents, there is no type of parenthood that is more closely associated with depression for women than for men. This finding contradicts the assumption that parenthood is more consequential for the emotional well-being of women.

Marital Status Variation in the Associations between Parenthood and Depression

We now evaluate our final hypothesis that most types of unmarried parents (including both single and cohabiting parents) report more depression than

Table 4 Unstandardized Coefficients from Regressions of Depression on Different Types of Parents by Marital Status

Independent Variables	Model 1 (N = 4,859)	Model 2 (N = 389)	Model 3 (N = 812)	Model 4 (N = 838)	Model 5 (N = 3,467)	Model 6 (N = 669)
Single parents with minor children at home[a] (yes = 1)	5.15*** (.61)	—	—	—	—	—
Cohabiting parents with minor children at home[a] (yes = 1)	3.83* (1.30)	—	—	—	—	—
Single parents with minor stepchildren at home[a] (yes = 1)	—	21.03* (9.27)	—	—	—	—
Cohabiting parents with minor stepchildren at home[a] (yes = 1)	—	2.52 (2.07)	—	—	—	—
Single noncustodial parents[a] (yes = 1)	—	—	5.56*** (1.41)	—	—	—
Cohabiting noncustodial parents[a] (yes = 1)	—	—	−1.36 (2.08)	—	—	—
Single parents with adult children at home[a] (yes = 1)	—	—	—	4.46** (1.45)	—	—
Cohabiting parents with adult children at home[a] (yes = 1)	—	—	—	9.31 (5.78)	—	—
Single parents with nonresidential adult children[a] (yes = 1)	—	—	—	—	3.91*** (.67)	—
Cohabiting parents with nonresidential adult children[a] (yes = 1)	—	—	—	—	−2.76 (2.10)	—
Single parents with nonresidential adult stepchildren[a] (yes = 1)	—	—	—	—	—	4.27* (1.92)
Cohabiting parents with nonresidential adult stepchildren[a] (yes = 1)	—	—	—	—	—	1.02 (5.63)
Constant	33.16	34.01	52.48	26.47	61.96	23.84
Adjusted R²	.073	.069	.105	.084	.071	.042

*$p < .05$; **$p < .01$; ***$p < .001$ (two-tailed tests)

Notes: Numbers in parentheses are standard errors. Each model controls for gender, sociodemographic variables including age, race, education, and household income as well as respondents' employment status.
[a]Married parents are the reference group.

their married peers. Table 4 presents analyses in which respondents' symptoms are regressed on the same set of variables. However, since the purpose of these analyses is to assess depression differences not only between different types of married and single parents but also between different types of married and cohabiting parents, we included dummy variables for each marital status for each type of parent. The married are the reference category in these analyses.

From an initial glance at Table 4, it is clear that single persons report significantly more symptoms than married persons among all types of parents. However, upon close investigation, Table 4 also reveals that depression differences between cohabiting and married persons are evident only among certain types of parents. Consistent with previous research showing that single persons living with minor children are more distressed than their married counter-parts (Aneshensel et al., 1981; Brown & Harris, 1978; Glenn & McLanahan, 1981; Pearlin & Johnson, 1977), model 1 indicates that both single and cohabiting persons who have minor children at home report significantly more symptoms than their married counterparts. However, while single persons residing with minor stepchildren report significantly more symptoms than their married peers, there is no significant depression difference between married and cohabiting persons living with minor stepchildren (model 2). Although these findings should be interpreted cautiously due to the small number of single persons residing with minor stepchildren, similar results are evident among persons who have noncustodial children (model 3), residential adult children (model 4), nonresidential adult children (model 5), and nonresidential adult stepchildren (model 6). In other words, while single persons who have noncustodial children, adult children at home, nonresidential adult children, and nonresidential adult stepchildren all report more symptoms than similar married persons, there are no differences between these types of married and cohabiting parents.

Overall, Table 4 results provide some support for our final hypothesis regarding marital status differences in the association between parenthood and mental health. However, in contrast to our expectation that most types of unmarried parents report higher levels of depression than their married peers, these analyses reveal depression differences between married and cohabiting persons only among certain types of parents. That is, while all types of single parents report higher symptom levels than all types of married parents, differences between married and cohabiting parents are evident only among those residing with their own minor children. This latter finding strongly suggests that the emotional benefits of marriage relative to cohabitation only apply to persons living with dependent biological and/or adopted children.

CONCLUSIONS AND DISCUSSION

In contrast to some earlier research, our analyses indicate that as a group parents report significantly higher levels of depression than nonparents when sociodemographic and status variables are held constant. We noted that inconsistencies between our and others' findings probably reflect the relatively high percentage of single, noncustodial, cohabiting, and stepparents in this relatively recent national sample. Moreover, and consistent with other research, we found that persons at the stage of the life course when they are residing with their minor children report significantly more depression than their childless peers when sociodemographic and status variables are included in analyses. We concur with other authors (e.g., McLanahan & Adams, 1985; Umberson & Gove, 1989) that the emotional demands of parenthood at this stage of the life course may simply outweigh the emotional rewards of having children. However, we also found that emptynest parents do not significantly differ from persons who have never had children, even when sociodemographic and status characteristics are controlled, which suggests that there are no emotional benefits associated with emptynest parenthood with respect to current depression. While it is inconsistent with some previous studies, our finding for emptynest parents is not too surprising. Although the demands associated with parenthood subside as children age and become independent—freeing parents to reap the rewards of having children—most parents are probably involved in their adult children's lives and continue to be concerned with their well-being, which can also be emotionally costly. In fact, one of our most interesting findings is that there is *no* type of parent that reports less depression than nonparents. Another interesting finding is that the association between all types of parenthood—relative to not being a parent—and depression does *not* significantly differ for women and men. This finding contradicts assumptions about gender differences in the emotional consequences of parenthood—a point to which we will return. Overall, the first set of analyses provides support for our first hypothesis: Unlike other major adult roles in the United States, parenthood is not associated with enhanced emotional well-being.

Subsequent analyses also provide support for our second hypothesis: There is considerable variation in depression among parents, irrespective of gender and marital status. Although there is no depression difference between fullnest and emptynest parents, as some prior research suggests, persons living with minor biological and/or adopted children report *fewer*, rather than more, depressive symptoms than most other types of parents. We noted that this finding contradicts the assumption underlying theory and research that persons residing with minor children are the most distressed type of parent. We also acknowledged that differences between our findings and those of other studies may be due to differences in the measures used for this type of parent.

However, additional analyses failed to support our hypothesis regarding gender differences in the association between parenthood and depression. Despite the female excess of depression among all types of parents (and nonparents) in our national sample, the association between parenthood and symptoms does *not* significantly differ for women and men. These findings are not only inconsistent with some earlier studies, but they are also inconsistent with another assumption of work in this area, which is that parenthood is more consequential for the emotional well-being of women than of men. Although we did not find gender differences in the associations between parenthood and depression, our findings clearly show that certain types of parenthood are predominantly male, whereas other types are predominantly female. These gendered parenting patterns no doubt reflect contemporary custodial arrangements in the United States, where mothers are more likely than fathers to reside with their young biological and/or adopted children in the event of nonmarital childbearing, cohabitation, separation, divorce, and remarriage.

Additional analyses nevertheless revealed marital status differences in the association between parenthood and depression; most types of unmarried parents report more symptoms than most types of married parents. However, depression differences between married and cohabiting persons are evident only among certain types of parents; while all types of single parents report more symptoms than all types of married parents, depression differences between married and cohabiting parents are evident only among persons residing with their own minor children. On the basis of these findings, we suggested that the emotional benefits of marriage relative to cohabitation only apply to persons living with their own dependent children.

Taken as a whole, the results provide support, albeit indirect support, for our argument that variation in mental health among parents reflects a myriad of factors affecting different parenting experiences. While data limitations prevented us from doing so, future research should directly examine whether these social-psychological, sociocultural, and social-structural factors contribute to the emotional costs and rewards associated with parenthood at different stages of the adult life course and different types of parenthood. While we agree with mental health and family scholars that the benefits derived from parenthood may be canceled out or exceeded by the costs associated with the role, definitive conclusions about this argument await further work.

It is equally important for future research to investigate whether individuals select themselves into—and out of—certain types of parenthood on the basis of their mental health status. Although our theoretical framework assumes social causation, we believe that social selection processes operate, especially for certain types of parents. Recall that persons residing with minor stepchildren are no more depressed than persons living with their own children. We suggested that while stepparenthood with residential minor children may be depressing, persons who select themselves into this type of stepparenthood may also enjoy better mental health to begin with. We provided a similar interpretation for our findings for noncustodial parents who report more symptoms than custodial parents. While noncustodial parenthood is also likely to be distressing, depressed persons may be more likely to select themselves out of custodial parenthood for the sake of themselves and their children.

At the same time that our research opens up some new lines of inquiry into the relationship between parenthood and mental health, our findings urge theory and research about the emotional consequences of social role involvement to go beyond simplistic conceptions of adult roles. Building on McLanahan's and Adams's study (1989), we have shown that, although parenthood is currently not associated with enhanced mental health, there are different types of parenthood that appear to be differentially consequential for emotional distress. These different types of parenthood no doubt reflect a diverse range of experiences individuals have as parents. Our analyses clearly indicate that certain types of parenthood—particularly parenthood with minor children in the household—are associated with less depression than other types of parenthood.

References

Andrews, F. M. and S. B. Withey. 1976. *Social Indicators of Well-Being: American's Perceptions of Life Quality*. New York: Plenum.

Aneshensel, Carol S., Ralph R. Frerichs, and Virginia A. Clark. 1981. "Family Roles and Sex Differences in Depression." *Journal of Health and Social Behavior* 22:379–93.

Bird, Chloe E. and Michelle L. Rogers. 1998. "Parenting and Depression: The Impact of the Division of Labor within Couples and Perceptions of Equity." PSTC Working Paper #98–09. Population Studies and Training Center. Brown University Providence, RI.

Blake, Judith. 1979. "Is Zero Preferred? American Attitudes toward Childlessness in the 1970s." *Journal of Marriage and the Family* 41:245–57.

Brown, George W. and Tirril Harris. 1978. *Social Origins of Depression*. New York: Free Press.

Burton, Russell. 1998. "Global Integrative Meaning as a Mediating Factor in the Relationship between Social Roles and Psychological Distress." *Journal of Health and Social Behavior* 39:201–15.

Campbell, Angus, Philip E. Converse, and Willard L. Rogers. 1976. *The Quality of American Life*. New York: Sage.

Cherlin, Andrew. 1978. "Remarriage as an Incomplete Institution." *American Journal of Sociology* 84:634–50.

Cherlin, Andrew and Frank Furstenberg, Jr. 1994. "Step-families in the United States: A Reconsideration." *Annual Review of Sociology* 20:359–81.

Cleary, Paul D. and David Mechanic. 1983. "Sex Differences in Psychological Distress Among Married People." *Journal of Health and Social Behavior* 24:111–21.

Glenn, Norval D. and Sara McLanahan. 1981. "The Effects of Children on the Psychological Well-Being of Older Adults." *Journal of Marriage and the Family* 43:409–21.

Gore, Susan and Thomas W. Mangione. 1983. "Social Roles, Sex Roles, and Psychological Distress." *Journal of Health and Social Behavior* 24:300–312.

Gove, W. R. and M. R. Geerken. 1977. "The Effect of Children and Employment on the Mental Health of Married Men and Women." *Social Forces* 56:66–76.

Hewlett, Sylvia, Nancy Rankin, and Cornel West. 2002. *Taking Parenting Public: The Case for a New Social Movement*. New York: Rowman and Littlefield.

Hewlett, Sylvia Ann and Cornel West. 1998. *The War against Parents*. New York: Houghton Mifflin.

Huber, Joan. 1980. "Will U.S. Fertility Decline toward Zero?" *Sociological Quarterly* 21:481–92.

Hughes, Michael. 1989. "Parenthood and Psychological Well-Being among the Formerly Married: Are Children the Primary Source of Psychological Distress?" *Journal of Family Issues* 10:463–82.

Kandel, Denise B., Mark Davies, and Victoria H. Raveis. 1985. "The Stressfulness of Daily Social Roles for Women." *Journal of Health and Social Behavior* 26:64–78.

McLanahan, Sara. 1983. "Family Structure and Stress: A Longitudinal Comparison of Two-Parent and Female-Headed Families." *Journal of Marriage and the Family* 45:347–57.

McLanahan, Sara and Julia Adams. 1985. "Explaining the Decline in Parents' Psychological Well-Being: The Role of Employment, Marital Disruption and Social Integration." Center for Demography and Ecology, Working Paper No. 85–25, University of Wisconsin, Madison, WI.

———. 1987. "Parenthood and Psychological Well-Being." *Annual Review of Sociology* 13:237–57.

———. 1989. "The Effects of Children on Adult's Psychological Well-Being: 1957–1976." *Social Forces* 68:124–46.

Menaghan, Elizabeth G. 1989. "Role Changes and Psychological Well-Being: Variations in Effects by Gender and Role Repertoire." *Social Forces* 67:59–85.

Mirowsky, John and Catherine E. Ross. 1989. "Age and Depression." *Journal of Health and Social Behavior* 33:187–205.

———. 2003. *Social Causes of Psychological Distress*. 2nd Edition. New York: Aldine de Gruyter.

Pearlin, Leonard I. and Joyce Johnson. 1977. "Marital Status, Life Strains, and Depression." *American Sociological Review* 42:704–15.

Preston, Samuel H. 1984. "Children and the Elderly: Divergent Paths for America's Dependents." *Demography* 21:435–57.

———. 1986. "Changing Values and Falling Birth Rates." *Population and Development Review* (Issue Supplement: "Below-Replacement Fertility in Industrial Societies: Causes, Consequences, Policies") 12:176–95.

Radloff, Lenore S. 1975. "Sex Differences in Depression: The Effects of Occupation and Marital Status." *Sex Roles* 1:249–65.

———. 1977. "The CES-D Scale: A Self-Report Depression Scale for Research in the General Population." *Applied Sociological Measurement* 1:385–401.

Ross, Catherine E. and John Mirowsky. 1988. "Child Care and Emotional Adjustment to Wives' Employment." *Journal of Health and Social Behavior* 29:127–38.

Ross, Catherine E., John Mirowsky, and Karen Goldsteen. 1990. "The Impact of the Family on Health: The Decade in Review." *Annual Review of Sociology* 52:1059–78.

Rubin, Lillian B. 1979. *Women of a Certain Age: The Midlife Search for Self*. New York: Harper and Row.

Sieber, Sam D. 1974. "Toward a Theory of Role Accumulation." *American Sociological Review* 39:567–78.

Simon, Robin. W. 1998. "Assessing Sex Differences in Vulnerability among Employed Parents: The Importance of Marital Status." *Journal of Health and Social Behavior* 39:37–53.

———. 2002. "Revisiting the Relationships among Gender, Marital Status, and Mental Health." *American Journal of Sociology* 4:1065–96.

Sweet, James, Larry Bumpass, and Vaughn Call. 1988. "The Design and Content of the National Survey of Families and Households." Working Paper NSFH-1, Center for Demography and Ecology, University of Wisconsin, Madison, WI.

Thoits, Peggy A. 1983. "Multiple Identities and Psychological Well-Being." *American Sociological Review* 48:174–87.

Umberson, Debra and Walter R. Gove. 1989. "Parenthood and Psychological Well-Being: Theory, Measurement, and Stage in the Family Life Course." *Journal of Family Issues* 10:440–62.

DISCUSSION

1. Ranae Evenson and Robin Simon report that, as a group, no type of parent reports less depression than nonparents. Do you find their results surprising? Are there other factors they did not consider that might identify a subset of parents who are less depressed than nonparents?

2. Would you expect the authors' conclusions to hold in other historical periods? In other countries? Why or why not?

3. When this article was first published, it received a lot of media attention. Headlines such as "Kids are Depressing" and "Feeling the Holiday Blues? Then You Must Have Children" appeared in news outlets worldwide. Most media descriptions of the study were reasonably accurate but some were not. What responsibility do researchers have to make sure that the results of their research are presented fairly and accurately?

Richard A. Miech, Avshalom Caspi, Terrie E. Moffitt, Bradley R. Entner Wright, Phil A. Silva

Low Socioeconomic Status and Mental Disorders: A Longitudinal Study of Selection and Causation during Young Adulthood[†]

When researchers observe that a status or condition is associated with mental health, one important question they must answer is: did the status or condition cause mental health or did mental health cause the status or condition? These two possibilities—known as the social causation and social selection explanations—apply across many statuses and conditions but are invoked most often in the case of socioeconomic status. In the selection that follows, Richard Miech and colleagues analyze the evidence for each explanation and introduce the important point that causation and selection processes may operate differently for different disorders.

Mental disorders are overrepresented in the lower social strata (Dohrenwend et al., 1992; Holzer et al., 1986; Kessler et al., 1994; Link & Dohrenwend, 1989; Neugebauer, Dohrenwend, & Dohrenwend, 1980; Wheaton, 1978). Efforts to

Miech, Richard A., Avshalom Caspi, Terrie E. Moffitt, Bradley R. Entner Wright, and Phil A. Silva. 1999. "Low socioeconomic status and mental disorders: A longitudinal study of selection and causation during young adulthood." *American Journal of Sociology* 104:1096–1131.

distinguish low socioeconomic status (SES) as a cause or consequence of mental disorder address some of the most vexing problems in social demography and medical sociology. On the one hand, mental disorders may play an important role in determining who gets ahead in society, a topic pursued by sociological research in the "selection" tradition that examines the extent to which disorders impair status attainment (Dohrenwend, 1975; Eaton, 1980; Eaton, 1985). On the other hand, adversities linked to low SES may damage the psychological functioning of individuals and play a role in the etiology of mental disorders, a topic pursued by sociological research in the "causation" tradition (Kohn, 1981; Link, Lennon, & Dohrenwend, 1993; Turner, Wheaton, & Lloyd, 1995; Wheaton, 1978). Despite 50 years of research, key theoretical issues regarding the causal direction between low SES and mental disorders still remain unsettled (Dohrenwend et al., 1992; Fox, 1990; Ortega & Corzine, 1990).

In this article, we examine the selection and causation hypotheses by using a panel study to investigate the association between mental disorders and educational attainment, a key component of social status (Sewell, Hauser, & Featherman, 1976). Our prospective study of adolescents as they make the transition to adulthood allows us to evaluate the temporal ordering of mental disorders and educational attainment more directly than past studies. As a consequence, we are able to test whether the relation between educational attainment and nonpsychotic mental disorders results from selection, social causation, or a combination of both processes—three alternative interpretations that have not yet been disentangled with the research designs used in the current literature. The data come from the Dunedin Multidisciplinary Health and Development Study ($N = 1037$), which has followed a group of children from birth to age 21 and includes psychiatric diagnoses for all study members at ages 15 and 21 using criteria from the *Diagnostic and Statistical Manual of Mental Disorders* (the *DSM-III* and *DSM-IIIR*; see APA 1980, 1987).

SELECTION AND CAUSATION

The Hypotheses

Research in the "selection" perspective suggests that mental disorders are overrepresented in the lower socioeconomic strata as a consequence of impaired social mobility. Selection processes operate both within and across generations. Within a generation, mental disorders may cause downward mobility among adults and lead them to "drift" into the lower socioeconomic strata (Eaton, 1980; Jarvis, 1971, 55–56). Across generations, a disorder may be transmitted to offspring, as suggested by recent twin and adoption studies that indicate a role for both genetic and environmental factors in mental disorders (Kendler et al., 1995). A transmitted disorder that impairs status attainment may have cumulative effects across successive generations of a lineage, ultimately leading to the creation of a "residue" of people with mental disorders in the lower socioeconomic strata (Dohrenwend et al., 1992; Gruenberg, 1961). All studies that investigate selection processes are characterized by a causal arrow that points from mental disorders to SES, unlike research in the causation perspective, which points the arrow the other way.

Research on the causation hypothesis suggests a wide array of mechanisms through which SES may affect psychopathology. These mechanisms may either cause illnesses or serve as catalysts to people with genetic predispositions for disorders, and they include stress (Kessler, 1979; Link, Dohrenwend, & Skodol, 1986; Pearlin & Johnson, 1977; Turner et al., 1995), poor social or psychological coping resources (Dohrenwend & Dohrenwend, 1970; Kessler & Cleary, 1980; Kohn, 1981; Liem & Liem, 1978), and lack of occupational direction, control, and planning (Link et al., 1993). While the very different processes of selection and causation might at first appear easily distinguishable, disentangling their effects has proven an elusive goal.

Selection and causation research to date has faced two main obstacles that have prevented a clear test between the interpretations of causation, selection, and combined effects. First, the temporal ordering of mental disorders and low SES has been difficult to establish without longitudinal research designs. Second, the absence of a standardized psychiatric nosology has hindered the ability of researchers to compare findings about social status and mental disorders across different studies that use different measures. In the present study, we address these two limitations by conducting a longitudinal analysis of selection and causation and by examining these processes in relation to multiple, specific mental disorders diagnosed in accordance with a standardized nosology.

The Research Strategies

The study of selection and causation centers on temporal ordering and whether the onset of mental disorders occurs before or after low socioeconomic experience: evidence that it occurs before provides strong support for selection, while evidence that it occurs after is consistent with a social causation interpretation. With temporal ordering in mind, an initial research strategy focused on whether adults with mental disorders came disproportionately from lower-SES family backgrounds. If they did, this evidence suggests that low socioeconomic experience preceded the onset of mental disorder and, consequently, favors a causation interpretation. Yet, while many studies find that the parents of people with mental disorders are concentrated in the lower social strata (see, e.g., Kessler et al., 1994), the interpretation of this finding is more complex than originally expected. For example, an illness such as conduct disorder may impair a person's status attainment and then be passed on to offspring, either through parental socialization or through increased exposure to socioeconomic-based stressors that foster the illness. In this case, the finding that children with conduct disorder are overrepresented among parents with low SES stems both from causation processes that operated on the child, and, in addition, selection processes that operated on the parents (Dohrenwend, 1975). In short, this initial research strategy can suggest preliminary evidence for causation effects, but it is limited because it does not evaluate their size relative to selection effects, nor does it determine whether causation acts to the exclusion of selection.

Subsequent research has pursued two main research strategies to determine the temporal order between mental disorders and SES. The first relies on retrospective reports of study members. Kessler et al. (1995), for example, sought to determine the temporal order between mental disorders and educational dropout by relying on the respondents' ability to recall their mental state before major educational transitions, such as high school completion and college entrance. On average, study members were asked to recall their mental state 15 years before the date of interview. Using these retrospective reports, they find support for the selection perspective to the extent that study members who failed to make major educational transitions reported an overrepresentation of anxiety disorders, mood disorders (including depression), and conduct disorder that predated their educational dropout. Conceivably, this research design could be extended to measure simultaneously the influence of causation processes. It is important to note, however, that conclusions based on analyses using this research design rest on the assumption that retrospective reports of the occurrence and timing of childhood and adolescent mental disorders are valid and reliable, a matter of considerable debate (see Aneshensel et al., 1987; Henry et al., 1994; Holmshaw & Simonoff, 1996; Rogler, Malgady, & Tryon, 1992).

The questionable validity of retrospective reports has led some researchers to forgo them and to pursue a second research strategy instead. This approach does not measure temporal order directly but rather infers it from the insight that ethnic discrimination has distinctly different consequences for selection and causation outcomes (for a detailed discussion see Dohrenwend [1975] and Dohrenwend et al. [1992]). In brief, the selection perspective leads to the expectation that disorders will have smaller, diluted prevalence rates across all SES levels of disadvantaged groups because ethnic discrimination hinders social mobility and keeps greater numbers of healthy members at lower SES levels. In contrast, the causation perspective leads to the competing expectation that disorders will have higher prevalence rates among disadvantaged groups, who presumably experience higher stress levels. Analysis employing this research design supports the presence of causation processes for nonpsychotic mental disorders such as depression and antisocial personality disorder (Dohrenwend et al., 1992) but provides little information regarding the possibility that smaller selection effects are operating at the same time. The design succeeds in evaluating the relative strength of selection and causation, but it fails to provide a test to determine if either process is operating exclusively. This limitation is critical because the assumption of exclusive social causation underpins much of the social stress literature.

A longitudinal research design offers the opportunity to test between selection, causation, and combined-effects interpretations without relying on retrospective information. However, such prospective studies are rare due to the cost and logistics involved in repeated evaluations of large samples. Wheaton (1978) conducted one of the few panel studies of psychological disorder and social status, using occupational prestige to index social status in the adult years. Relying on a general measure of mental illness that combines symptoms of both anxiety and depression (the Langner index, see Langner, 1962), he finds evidence for causation effects and no evidence for selection effects among adults. More recent longitudinal research supporting causation in regard to clinical levels of depression and anxiety comes from the study of Bruce, Takeuchi, and Leaf (1991), based on a six-month follow-up of 5,000 adults ages 18 and over. The existing field of longitudinal research leaves room for advances in at least two ways, however, as we discuss below.

The Transition to Young Adulthood

The transition from adolescence to adulthood has not yet been examined with a longitudinal research design, although adolescence is a strategic time period for the study of both selection and causation. In terms of selection, adolescence is a period when individuals make decisions about their educational attainment and, consequently, their social status. Educational attainment is both itself a primary component of SES indices and also a major predictor of subsequent income and occupational prestige over the life course (Blau & Duncan, 1967; Hauser, 1994; Jencks et al., 1979; Sewell, Hauser, & Featherman, 1976). Indeed, as an initial and powerful step, education is the "key" factor in the status attainment process (Sewell & Hauser, 1976, 13). Through limited educational attainment, adolescents may have already selected themselves into the lower social strata before adulthood, a process that represents selection effects to the extent that it is influenced by adolescent mental illness. In the present study, we investigate this potential process in the framework of a longitudinal study designed to capture the transition from adolescence to adulthood.

In terms of causation, the peak risk period for the emergence of new cases of DSM mental disorders is during the transition from adolescence to young adulthood (Burke et al., 1990; Institute of Medicine, 1994), suggesting that the factors that cause mental disorders are especially influential during this developmental period of the life course. Young adult cohorts have higher *DSM* period-prevalence rates than older cohorts in national cross-sectional studies (Kessler et al., 1994; Robins & Regier, 1991), and the Dunedin cohort analyzed in this study shows a large increase (almost twofold) in the rates of mental disorder between ages 15 and 21 (Newman et al., 1996). Family SES origins appear to play an influential role during this formative period, as the literature on child and adolescent psychopathology documents a significant association between SES and mental disorders (Costello et al., 1997; Rutter et al., 1974; Velez, Johnson, & Cohen, 1989). However, this literature has yet to examine the association in detail and to separate causation from selection effects, and, as such, relatively little is known about the SES-linked factors that are associated with increased risk of mental disorder from adolescence to young adulthood (Institute of Medicine, 1994).

Are Selection and Causation Effects Disorder Specific?

We examine the ways in which selection and causation processes vary across different mental disorders in the transition to adulthood, a topic that has not yet been examined with a longitudinal research design. Current research suggests that different mental disorders are related to social status in different ways (Dohrenwend et al., 1992). Detailing differences across disorders can better inform selection and causation theories, many of which are not disorder specific but have only been evaluated with regard to depression or anxiety (Aneshensel, Rutter, & Lachenbruch, 1991). The standardized *DSM* classification system that we use in this study is well suited for an investigation of disorder-specific relations with socioeconomic status because it provides formal guidelines to distinguish between different mental disorders.

We focus on the internalizing and externalizing disorders, the major mental disorders that afflict adolescents (Achenbach & Edelbrock, 1983). Internalizing disorders involve emotional distress that is turned inward and include anxiety and depression. These are the disorders that have received the most sociological attention in studies of adults, and our study of adolescents serves to complement this literature. The applicability of adult anxiety and depression symptoms to adolescents was once a matter of controversy (Rutter, 1986) but is now generally accepted in the field (Reynolds, 1992).

Externalizing disorders, in contrast, are characterized by "acting out" behavior, such as poorly controlled, impulsive behavior, as well as attention problems and hyperactivity. In adolescence, they are composed mainly of conduct disorder and attention deficit disorder. In adulthood, the antisocial behavior that characterizes conduct disorder may manifest itself as antisocial personality disorder (Lynam, 1996; Moffitt, 1993). We extend our knowledge of selection and causation processes by examining these disorders, which have not yet been formally examined in the sociological literature to date.

In sum, the longitudinal Dunedin study enables us to avoid retrospective reports, extend the selection and causation literature by focusing on the formative transition from adolescence to adulthood, and examine disorder-specific relations with SES. This study both complements the literature on adults and, more generally, adds to the underdeveloped field of adolescent mental health (Institute of Medicine Committee, 1995).

SAMPLE AND METHOD

The Dunedin Study

Subjects for this follow-up study were members of a complete birth cohort that has been studied extensively in the Dunedin Multidisciplinary Health and Development Study since birth. The sample and the history of the study have been described elsewhere (Silva, 1990; Silva & Stanton, 1996). Briefly, the study is a longitudinal investigation of the health, development, and behavior of children born between April 1, 1972, and March 31, 1973, in Dunedin, New Zealand, a city of approximately 120,000. Perinatal data were obtained at delivery. When the children were later traced for follow-up at age 3, 1,037 (52 percent males and 48 percent females, 91 percent of the eligible births) participated in the assessment, forming the base sample for the longitudinal study. Prevalence rates of psychiatric disorders such as major depression and conduct disorder in the Dunedin sample match rates from national U.S. surveys (Costello, 1989; Kessler et al., 1994; Newman et al., 1996).

The Dunedin sample has been assessed with a diverse battery of psychological, medical, and sociological measures at ages 3, 5, 7, 9, 11, 13, 15, 18, and 21. The basic procedure for data collection in the Dunedin study involves bringing each sample member into the research unit within 60 days of his or her birthday for a full day of data collection in which various research topics are presented as standardized modules (e.g., mental health interview, Life History Calendar, physical examination) by different trained examiners in counterbalanced order. Auxiliary data are also collected from parents, teachers, peers, and official records. The present study uses data collected at ages 15 and 21.

Mental Health Measures

Mental health data were collected at ages 15 and 21 using the most current version of the *DSM* available at the time of interview. Age-15 interviews were conducted using the Diagnostic Interview Schedule for Children (DISC-C; Costello et al., 1982), an instrument designed to assess reliably the criteria of the *DSM-III* (APA, 1980). Age-21 interviews were conducted using the Diagnostic Interview Schedule (DIS; Robins et al., 1989), an instrument designed to assess reliably the criteria of the *DSM-IIIR* (APA, 1987). The DISC-C and DIS were used to obtain diagnoses of mental disorders in the 12 months prior to the study member's 15th and 21st birthday interview.

For the current study, we investigated the internalizing disorders of anxiety and depression and the externalizing disorders of conduct disorder, attention deficit disorder, and antisocial personality disorder. At age 15, the anxiety disorder group ($n = 100$) consisted of study members who met criteria for the *DSM-III* anxiety disorders of childhood: overanxious disorder, separation anxiety, simple phobia, social phobia, or any combination of these disorders. At age 21, the anxiety disorder group ($n = 185$) consisted of study members who met the criteria for the *DSM-IIIR* anxiety disorders of adult-hood: generalized anxiety disorder, obsessive-compulsive disorder, panic disorder, agoraphobia, social phobia, simple phobia, or any combination of these disorders. The depression disorder group ($n = 37$ at age 15, $n = 163$ at age 21) consisted of study members who met *DSM-III* criteria for a major depressive episode, dysthymia, or both. The conduct disorder group con-sisted of study members who met *DSM-III* criteria for conduct disorder or oppositional disorder at age 15 ($n = 81$), and our antisocial disorder group ($n = 50$) consisted of study members who met *DSM-IIIR* criteria for either anti-social personality disorder (ASPD) or conduct disorder at age 21. Finally, the attention deficit disorder (ADD) group consisted of study members who met *DSM-III* criteria for ADD at 15 ($n = 20$).

In addition to categorical measures, we created continuous scales by sum-ming the study member's scores on interview symptom items relevant to each disorder (see Krueger et al., 1996). Because symptom counts are highly skewed with a mode of zero, they were transformed by taking the log of the count plus one. This transformation changes their interpretation when used in regression equations so that they reference relative, rather than absolute, changes in mental disorder. For example, when used as an independent var-iable, the beta coefficient refers to the change in Y given a 1 percent change in the disorder scale. When used as a dependent variable, the beta coefficient refers to the percentage change in the disorder scale given a change in the independent variable (Gujarati, 1988).

Social Status Measures

We indexed familial socioeconomic status at age 15 with information obtained directly from parents, using New Zealand–specific measures of parents' occupational socioeconomic status, parents' education, and fam-ily income. Parents' occupational status was measured with the Elley and Irving (1976) scale, a 6-point scale based on the average income and educa-tion levels for 546 occupations of the New Zealand labor force. We assigned scores on the basis of the higher status of either caregiver, whether father or mother. Parents' education was measured with the same scale used by Elley and Irving (1976), which categorizes attainment into three levels on the basis of primary, secondary, and tertiary degrees. As with occupational status, we assigned the score of the higher-ranking parent. Familial income was mea-sured as the combined gross income of both parents from all sources. The SES index was a linear composite of occupational status, educational attain-ment, and familial income, using weights from confirmatory factor analysis (the loadings were 0.80, 0.68, and 0.67, respectively).

Study members' educational attainment by age 21 came from their own self-reports. We broke overall educational attainment by age 21 into three separate transitions because the factors influencing educational dropout may differ across educational levels (Mare, 1980; Mare, 1981). We first exam-ined whether mental disorders influenced study members' performance on the New Zealand school certificate examinations. Almost all students take these national exams by age 16 because they determine promotion in secondary school and technical schools, and passing also helps secure better employment in the labor market (Kennedy, 1981). Of the sample, 87 percent earned a school certificate in at least one subject, and among this subsample we then examined the influence of mental disorders on the study members' ability to earn a sixth form certificate, which is comparable to a high school degree in the United States (Kennedy, 1981). Of those who earned a school certificate, 76 percent also earned a sixth form certificate, and among this subsample we then examined the effects of mental disorders on continuing to tertiary education at a university (37 percent of the study members who earned a sixth form certificate continued to a university education). The variable "Educational Attainment at 21" represents study members' highest educational transition achieved by age 21 (0 = no school certificate, 1 = school certificate, 2 = sixth form certificate, 3 = university attendance).

Four additional measures were used in our analysis to control for confounding influences. We included controls for gender and the study member's ability and motivation to continue education. Intelligence was assessed with the Wechsler Intelligence Scale for Children–Revised (Wechsler, 1974) between ages 7 and 11. Academic ability was assessed with the Burt Word Reading Test (Scottish Council for Research in Education, 1976) when the subjects were 15 years old. School involvement, an important predictor of educational attainment (Kerckhoff, 1993), was measured at age 15.

Analytic Strategy

Our analysis centers on mental disorders during the 12 months prior to the age-15 birthday, the birthday after which the New Zealand adolescents in our study were first legally entitled to leave school and consequently the age at which they were first at risk of "selection" into the lower social strata. We

Table 1 Expected Patterns of Evidence for Selection and Causation Processes

Type of Evidence	Association between Parental SES and Disorder at Age 15	Effect of Disorder at 15 on Subsequent Educational Attainment	Effects of Truncated Education on Increased Disorder between 15 and 21
Exclusive evidence for selection	No	Yes	No
Exclusive evidence for causation	Yes	No	Yes
Evidence for joint effects	Yes	Yes	Yes
Evidence for no effects during early adulthood	No	No	No

employed three empirical tests to examine the influences of selection and causation. First, we examined the association between mental disorders at age 15 and family SES background. Second, we examined the extent to which these mental disorders impaired social mobility by evaluating their influence on subsequent educational attainment, using models that contained traditional status attainment controls such as IQ, family SES background, and gender. Third, we examined the extent to which increases in mental disorder between ages 15 and 21 were associated with early adulthood SES, as indexed by educational attainment at age 21. No test by itself provides enough information to discriminate between the three interpretations of selection, causation, and joint effects, but, taken together, they lead to discerning patterns of expected results, as outlined below.

Table 1 provides a summary of empirical tests and expected patterns of findings. Exclusive evidence for selection would be indicated by the pattern of findings in which, over time, mental disorders impaired the status attainment of study members but were uninfluenced by socioeconomic standing of origin and socioeconomic standing of early adulthood. Exclusive evidence for social causation would be indicated by the contrasting pattern, in which mental disorders were influenced by both SES of origin and SES of early adulthood but exerted no significant influence on status attainment. Evidence for the joint effects of selection and causation processes would be indicated by a pattern in which mental disorders were influenced by SES of origin and impaired status attainment, and additionally were influenced by SES of early adulthood. Finally, evidence for the lack of both causation and selection effects in early adulthood would be indicated by nonsignificant associations across all three tests.

RESULTS

Family SES Background and Adolescent Mental Disorders

The well-documented relationship between SES and mental disorders replicated among the adolescents in our sample. We found that adolescent mental disorders were more likely to be found among youth in families with low SES than would be expected by chance alone.

We limited our methods in this first section to simple bivariate associations because the association between family SES and mental disorders may represent both selection and causation (Dohrenwend, 1975), and we did not know the direction of causality a priori. The results are presented separately for diagnostic categories in Table 2 and symptom scales in Table 3. Overall, adolescents with any *DSM-III* diagnosis were approximately 0.18 of a SD lower in family SES origins than their peers (Table 2, col. 4; $-.07 - .11 = -.18$). Adolescents' total psychiatric symptom scores on the DISC-C schedule were also significantly correlated with their SES background, at a magnitude of 0.16 (Table 3, col. 4).

Table 2 *DSM-III* Diagnoses at Age 15 and Social Class: Mean-Level Comparisons between Disordered and Nondisordered Adolescents[a]

	Parents' Mean Occupational Status	Parents' Mean Education Level	Parents' Mean Income	Parents' Mean Composite SES[b]	N
Mean	4.00	.89	36,070	.03	939
SD	1.25	.63	16,082	.99	939
Range	1–6	0–2	0–80,000	−2.49–2.30	
Any DSM-III disorder	3.78**	.83	35,487	−.11*	207[c]
No disorder	4.06	.90	36,235	.07	732
Internalizing disorders:					
DSM-III anxiety	3.74*	.81	34,338	−.16*	100
No anxiety	4.03	.90	36,276	.05	839
DSM-III depression	3.81	.84	36,383	−.07	37
No depression	4.01	.89	36,057	.04	902
Externalizing disorders: *DSM-III*					
conduct disorder	3.78+	.89	37,292	−.07	81
No conduct disorder	4.02	.84	35,954	.04	858
DSM-III attention deficit disorder	3.45*	.60*	31,275+	−.42*	20
No attention deficit disorder	4.01	.89	36,174	.04	919

[a]Differences between group means are evaluated using *t*-tests for all variables except for parents' education, which is categorical and evaluated using the Mantel-Haenszel chi-square.
[b]The mean composite SES measure has been transformed to z scores.
[c]Due to comorbidity, the number of study members who met *DSM* criteria for "any disorder" is less than the sum of study members who met criteria for individual disorders.
+$P < .10$.
*$P < .05$.
**$P < .01$.

Differences in the relation between SES and mental disorders emerged when mental disorders were considered individually. Among the internalizing disorders, anxiety and depression had different associations with family social status. Whether assessed categorically or continuously, anxiety was disproportionately found in families with lower SES as expected, but depression was not.

Among the externalizing disorders, support for an association between family SES and mental disorders was more robust in analyses of attention deficit disorder than conduct disorder. Based on symptom scales, both disorders showed a significant association with SES (Table 3), but only attention

Table 3 Number of *DSM-III* Mental Disorder Symptoms at Age 15 (Logged) and Social Class: Bivariate Correlations

Types of Symptom	Parents' Occupational Status	Parents' Education	Parents' Income	Parents' Composite SES
Total symptoms	−.16**	−.12**	−.10**	−.16**
Internalizing symptoms:				
Anxiety	−.12**	−.10**	−.07*	−.12**
Depression	.02	.05	.03	.03
Externalizing symptoms:				
Conduct disorder	−.15**	−.11**	−.11**	−.15**
Attention deficit disorder	−.13**	−.12**	−.08*	−.13**

Note: N = 931.
*P < .05.
**P < .01.

deficit disorder showed the expected association when measured categorically (Table 2). The *DSM-III* categorical measure of conduct disorder was not significantly related to overall family SES, but it was negatively associated with parents' occupational status (Table 2, col. 1), providing some evidence for an association with SES.

In general, the relation between mental disorders and social status was more robust using continuous symptom scales rather than categorical classifications of mental disorders. For example, Table 3 shows that the symptom scales for disorders related to the overall SES measure were associated with all three individual components of the SES measure. In contrast, the diagnostic categories in Table 2 were usually associated with only one or two SES components. We suspect that this difference stems more from methodological than substantive reasons and reflects the fact that categorical classifications lose information and statistical power by compressing information on mental disorders into a dichotomous measure (see Mirowsky & Ross, 1989).

Mental Disorders and Subsequent Educational Attainment

We next examined the influence of adolescent mental disorders on educational attainment. We found effects that varied by mental illness: internalizing disorders had no effect on educational attainment, while externalizing disorders exerted a strong negative influence.

We used mental disorders at age 15 as predictor variables in logistic regression equations modeling educational transitions. We present the results separately for the two different measures of mental disorders: Table 4 presents results using categorical diagnoses, and Table 5 presents results using symptom scales. In each table, we analyzed the effects of adolescent mental disorders on three educational transitions: the acquisition of at least one school certificate, completion of the sixth form certificate, and continuation to university training. For each transition, we present two models. The first

Table 4 *DSM* Diagnoses at Age 15 as Predictors of Educational Attainment: Unstandardized Coefficients from Logistic Regression Equations

Variable	Transition 1: Failure To Earn Any School Certificate (N = 939)		Transition 2: Failure to Earn Sixth Form Among School Certificate Recipients (N = 815)		Transition 3: Failure to Enter University among Sixth Form Recipients (N = 617)	
	Model 1	Model 2	Model 1	Model 2	Model 1	Model 2
Internalizing diagnoses:						
Anxiety	-.14	-.23	.26	.28	.29	.25
Depression	.28	.48	-.04	.16	-.62	-.49
Externalizing diagnoses:						
Conduct disorder	1.51**	1.59**	.92**	1.21**	.84	1.04*
Attention deficit disorder	1.72**	.36	1.98**	1.57	...	...
Controls:						
Family SES at 15	-.92**	-.76**	-.57**	-.40*	-.52**	-.32**
Female	...	-.77**	...	-.41**	...	-.08
IQ	...	-.04**	...	-.06**	...	-.04**
Reading ability	...	-.04**	...	-.03**	...	-.04**
School involvement	...	-.49**	...	-.20	...	-.22
Intercept	-2.57**	6.72**	-1.37**	8.22**	.66**	10.01**

Note: The New Zealand sixth form certificate is comparable to a U.S. high school diploma (Kennedy, 1981). Ellipses indicate variable excluded in model 1, and included in model 2.

*P < .05.

**P < .01.

Table 5 Number of *DSM-III* Mental Disorder Symptoms at Age 15 (Logged) as Predictors of Educational Attainment: Unstandardized Coefficients from Logistic Regression Equations

Variable	Transition 1: Failure to Earn Any School Certificate (N = 931)		Transition 2: Failure to Earn Sixth Form among School Certificate Recipients (N = 806)		Transition 3: Failure to Enter University among Sixth Form Recipients (N = 613)	
	Model 1	Model 2	Model 1	Model 2	Model 1	Model 2
Internalizing diagnoses:						
Anxiety	−.14	−.24	−.11	−.25	−.05	−.16
Depression	−.19	.03	−.18	−.07	−.08	−.00
Externalizing diagnoses:						
Conduct disorder	.54**	.47**	.35**	.40**	.29*	.35*
Attention deficit disorder	.90**	.64*	.92**	.74**	.25	.11
Controls:						
Family SES at 15	−.86**	−.70**	−.52**	−.34*	−.49**	−.32**
Female	...	−.59*	...	−.19	...	−.03
IQ	...	−.04**	...	−.06**	...	−.04**
Reading ability	...	−.04**	...	−.03**	...	−.04**
School involvement	...	−.48**	...	−.17	...	−.24
Intercept	−4.47**	4.97**	−3.08**	6.63**	.13	9.24**

Note: The New Zealand sixth form certificate is comparable to a U.S. high school diploma (Kennedy, 1981). Ellipses indicate variable excluded in model 1 and included in model 2.
*$P < .05$.
**$P < .01$.

includes only measures of mental disorders and family SES as predictors of educational achievement. The second includes all the predictors included in the first model and adds status attainment controls to isolate the unique effects of adolescent mental disorders on educational attainment from other factors implicated in the status attainment process.

The internalizing disorders of anxiety and depression did not significantly affect educational attainment in any of the models, whether using *DSM* diagnoses or *DSM* symptom scales. These results suggest that adolescents with internalizing disorders are not "selected" into the lower social strata through truncated education.

In contrast, we found strong evidence for selection processes among adolescents with externalizing disorders. Conduct disorder impaired achievement at every educational transition in this study. Adolescents who met the *DSM* criteria for a diagnosis of conduct disorder were less likely to earn a school certificate by an odds ratio of 4.53, even after controlling for family socioeconomic background and the presence of other comorbid mental disorders (Table 4, model 1 of the first transition; $e^{1.51} = 4.53$). This effect was still strong after status attainment controls were entered into the equation (Table 4, model 2 of the first transition). Adolescents meeting *DSM* criteria for a diagnosis of conduct disorder who earned a school certificate were then significantly less likely to earn a sixth form certificate by an odds ratio of 2.51, after controlling for family socioeconomic background and the presence of other mental disorders (Table 4, model 1 of the second transition; $e^{92} = 2.51$). Again, this effect was still significant after introducing status attainment controls into the equation (Table 4, model 2 of the second transition). In the final educational stage of the analysis, we found evidence that adolescents with conduct disorder who overcame the odds against them and received both a school certificate and a sixth form certificate were later less likely to continue to a university education. Using a *DSM* diagnosis, this effect is significant only in the full model, at the .10 level (Table 4, model 2 of the third transition). When substituting *DSM* symptom counts for diagnoses, however, the effect of conduct disorder on educational attainment is significant for all educational transitions, in both the abbreviated and full models. In sum, by the time adolescents with conduct disorder reach adulthood, they appear to be "selected" into the lower socioeconomic strata through restricted educational attainment.

Attention deficit disorder also impaired educational attainment, although its effects in our models were contingent, in part, on its measurement. Using a *DSM* diagnosis, we found that adolescents with attention deficit disorder (ADD) were less likely to earn a school certificate by an odds ratio of 5.58 (Table 4, model 1 of the first transition; $e^{1.72} = 5.58$), although this effect lost statistical significance after introducing the status attainment controls into the equation (Table 4, model 2 of the first transition). Those adolescents who met *DSM* criteria for ADD that did earn a school certificate were then significantly less likely to earn a sixth form certificate (Table 4, model 1 of the second transition), although, again, this effect was not significant after status attainment controls were introduced into the equation (Table 4, model 2 of the second transition). The effect of ADD on educational attainment past the sixth form was difficult to measure because the sample size became extremely small. Only three (15 percent) adolescents with ADD earned both a school certificate and sixth form certificate, a number too small to enter into our models predicting university attendance.

The results differed in one important way when ADD was measured with a symptom count instead of a dichotomous diagnosis. Namely, the symptom count continued to predict failure at educational transitions, even after the status attainment controls were added to the equation (Table 5, model 2 in transitions 1 and 2). The only models in which ADD did not exert a significant influence were in the equations predicting university attendance (Table 5, models 1 and 2 of the third transition), when the number of sixth form recipients displaying serious ADD symptoms was so small that we believe it precluded us from finding significant effects. In sum, our analysis of ADD indicates strong support for selection effects early in the educational career of adolescents.

Table 6 Educational Attainment as a Predictor of Mental Disorder at Age 21: Unstandardized Coefficients from Regression Equations[a]

Variable	Anxiety at 21		Depression at 21		Antisocial Disorder at 21	
	Model 1	Model 2	Model 1	Model 2	Model 1	Model 2
Educational attainment at 21	−.20[+]	−.15[*]	−.08	−.04	−.72[**]	−.08[**]
Controls:						
Disorder at 15[b]	1.35[**]	.57[**]	1.56[**]	.29[**]	1.27[**]	.24[**]
Family SES at 15	−.18	.01	−.02	−.08	.15	.01
Female	.87[**]	.28[**]	.86[**]	.31[**]	−2.52[**]	−.33[**]
Intercept	−1.70[**]	1.05[**]	−1.93[**]	.87[**]	−1.31[*]	.92[**]
N	903	893	903	896	905	916

[a]Model 1 uses dichotomous DSM diagnoses as measures of mental disorder at ages 15 and 21, and coefficients are from logistic regression equations. Model 2 uses continuous DSM symptom scales (logged) as measures of mental disorders at ages 15 and 21, and coefficients are from OLS equations.
[b]In models predicting age-21 anxiety, depression, and antisocial disorders, control disorders are age-15 anxiety, depression, and conduct disorder, respectively.
[+]$P < .10$.
[*]$P < .05$.
[**]$P < .01$.

Early Adulthood SES and Mental Disorders

In the third part of the analysis, we focused on early adulthood SES, as indexed by educational attainment at age 21, and examined its association with increased disorder between ages 15 and 21. We found that respondents with lower educational attainment were more likely to experience increases in anxiety and antisocial disorders but not depression.

We used logistic and ordinary least squares (OLS) regressions to predict age-21 disorders from educational attainment, statistically controlling the influence of age-15 disorders, gender, and parental SES. For all disorders, model 1 in Table 6 presents results using symptom scales and OLS regression, while model 2 in Table 6 presents results using dichotomous diagnoses and logistic regression.

We found that study members with low educational attainment at age 21 reported significantly higher levels of anxiety, after statistically controlling for age-15 levels of anxiety, parental SES, and gender (Table 6, anxiety models 1 and 2). Slightly higher levels of depression were also found among study members with low educational attainment at age 21. This effect was not significant using either *DSM* diagnoses or symptom scales (Table 6, depression models 1 and 2).

In our final analysis, we focused on antisocial disorders and found that they were overrepresented among respondents with low educational attainment. Because conduct disorder at age 15 may continue as antisocial personality in adulthood (APA, 1987), we used both age-21 conduct disorder and antisocial personality disorder as measures of antisocial disorder in early adulthood. At age 21, study members with low educational attainment were more likely to meet *DSM* criteria for either conduct disorder or antisocial personality disorder, a finding that persists after statistically controlling the influence of conduct disorder at age 15, parental SES, and gender (Table 6, antisocial disorder models 1 and 2).

DISCUSSION

The aim of this study was to examine whether low SES serves as a cause or consequence of mental illness, and we focused our inquiry on a cohort of adolescents as they made the transition to adulthood. Consistent with previous research in this area, we used educational attainment as a proxy for SES in early adulthood, a time period when many young adults have not yet realized their potential in terms of other status measures such as income and occupational prestige. Our analysis was especially well suited to study mental disorders and educational attainment for four reasons. First, we used a prospective longitudinal study that allowed us to test between the three interpretations of selection, causation, and joint effects. Second, we evaluated subjects for a wide array of *DSM-III* disorders, allowing us to examine selection and causation processes across different psychiatric disorders. Third, we studied the sample during the transition from adolescence to young adulthood, a developmental period that includes both the peak onset of psychiatric disorders and the normative educational transitions that constitute a key first step in the status attainment process. Finally, the high response rate of the longitudinal Dunedin study diminished any bias introduced by selective missing data.

We found that the relation between mental disorders and SES is unique for every disorder examined in this study. The main difference centers on selection effects—the extent to which adolescents with mental disorders "select" themselves into the lower social strata through curtailed education. We found no evidence for selection effects among youth with the internalizing disorders of anxiety and depression. In contrast, we found strong evidence for selection effects among youth with the externalizing disorders of conduct disorder and attention deficit disorder.

Conclusion

Different mental health problems are differently related to social status. Each adolescent disorder in this study (anxiety, depression, conduct disorder, and attention deficit disorder) bore a different relation to educational attainment, indicating that differences between disorders extend beyond the simple psychotic/nonpsychotic dichotomy currently recognized in sociological research on social selection and social causation. In terms of methodology, our findings suggest that research on social status and mental health has much to gain by incorporating measures of specific mental illness, rather than relying on the omnibus concept and measure of "psychological distress," which combines symptoms of different disorders. Of course, available interview schedules are expensive to administer—and the methods of diagnoses recommended by different classification systems are imperfect—but the alternative to well-conceived, mental health measurement may be misspecified theories of the relations between social status and mental illness.

In terms of treatment, the finding that different psychiatric diagnoses are differently related to social status suggests that the need for interventions and therapeutic strategies varies by disorder. Our results indicate that anxiety and depression do not significantly impair educational attainment and consequently do not require special intervention programs to counteract their effect on educational attainment. By contrast, conduct disorder and attention deficit disorder uniquely impair educational attainment and thereby damage the future life chances of the persons they afflict. It is particularly important for treatment regimens targeted at these latter adolescent mental health problems to include interventions that improve school performance and curb the initial slide into downward drift.

In terms of theory, our findings highlight the need for disorder-specific explanations of the relations between social status and mental disorders. Our findings about anxiety and antisocial disorders underscore the importance of social-causation processes in the life course; the elevated prevalence rate of these disorders in the lower social strata is partly a product of social inequalities and class-related social conditions. These results thus confirm a role for social structure in the etiology of anxiety and antisocial disorder and highlight the need for research to identify the mechanisms that account for these SES differentials. We also find evidence that conduct disorder and ADD exert strong selection effects, indicating that they disrupt the status attainment process during the transition from adolescence to adulthood. To the extent that these disorders are passed to offspring, either through socialization or biological factors, they play a heretofore overlooked and powerful role in the reproduction of class structure and social inequality. These selection processes violate the assumption of social causation and point to the need for research to identify the mechanisms that lead to their disruptive intra- and intergenerational patterns of influence.

Sociological research offers a unique perspective on the social causes and consequences of mental disorders. While anxiety and depression have captured much of the sociological imagination, our results suggest that other psychiatric conditions—historically neglected in sociology—merit careful scrutiny in order to enable a fuller understanding of how social conditions influence individual lives.

References

Achenbach, Thomas M., and Craig S. Edelbrock. 1983. "Taxonomic Issues in Child Psychopathology." Pp. 65–93 in *Handbook of Child Psychopathology*, edited by T. H. Ollendick and M. Hersen. New York: Plenum Press.

Aneshensel, Carol S., Antonio L. Estrada, Mary Jo Hansell, and Virginia A. Clark. 1987. "Social Psychological Aspects of Reporting Behavior: Lifetime Depressive Episode Reports." *Journal of Health and Social Behavior* 28:232–46.

Aneshensel, Carol S., Carolyn M. Rutter, and Peter A. Lachenbruch. 1991. "Social Structure, Stress, and Mental Health: Competing Conceptual and Analytic Models." *American Sociological Review* 56:166–78.

APA (American Psychiatric Association). 1980. *Diagnostic and Statistical Manual of Mental Disorders,* 3rd ed. Washington DC: APA.

———. 1987. *Diagnostic and Statistical Manual of Mental Disorders: DSM-IIIR.* Washington D.C.: APA.

Blau, Peter, and Otis Dudley Duncan. 1967. *The American Occupational Structure.* New York: Wiley.

Bruce, Martha L., David T. Takeuchi, and Philip J. Leaf. 1991. "Poverty and Psychiatric Status." *Archives of General Psychiatry* 48:470–74.

Burke, Kimberly C., Jack D. Burke, Darrel A. Regier, and Donald S. Rae. 1990. "Age at Onset of Selected Mental Disorders in Five Community Populations." *Archives of General Psychiatry* 47:511–18.

Costello, Anthony, Craig Edelbrock, R. Kalas, Marie Kessler, and S. Klaric. 1982. *Diagnostic Interview Schedule for Children.* Bethesda, Md.: National Institute of Mental Health.

Costello, Elizabeth Jane. 1989. "Developments in Child Psychiatric Epidemiology." *Journal of the American Academy of Child and Adolescent Psychiatry* 28:836–41.

Costello, Elizabeth Jane, Elizabeth M. S. Farmer, Adrian Angold, Barbara J. Burns, and Alaattin Erkanli. 1997. "Psychiatric Disorders among American Indian and White Youth in Appalachia: The Great Smoky Mountains Study." *American Journal of Public Health* 87:827–32.

Dohrenwend, Bruce P. 1975. "Sociocultural and Socio-Psychological Factors in the Genesis of Mental Disorders." *Journal of Health and Social Behavior* 16:365–92.

Dohrenwend, Bruce, and Barbara Dohrenwend. 1970. "Class and Race as Status Related Sources of Stress." Pp. 111–40 in *Social Stress,* edited by S. Levine and N. Scotch. Chicago: Aldine.

Dohrenwend, Bruce P., Itzhak Levav, Patrick Shrout, Sharon Schwartz, Guedalia Naveh, Bruce Link, Andrew Skodol, and Ann Stueve. 1992. "Socioeconomic Status and Psychiatric Disorders: The Causation-Selection Issue." *Science* 255:946–52.

Eaton, William W. 1980. "A Formal Theory of Selection for Schizophrenia." *American Journal of Sociology* 86:149–58.

———. 1985. "Epidemiology of Schizophrenia." *Epidemiologic Reviews* 7:105–26.

Elley, Warwick B., and James C. Irving. 1976. "Revised Socio-Economic Index for New Zealand." *New Zealand Journal of Educational Studies* 11:25–36.

Fox, John W. 1990. "Social Class, Mental Illness, and Social Mobility: The Social Selection-Drift Hypothesis for Serious Mental Illness." *Journal of Health and Social Behavior* 31:344–53.

Gruenberg, Ernest M. 1961. "Comments on 'Social Structures and Mental Disorders: Competing Hypotheses of Explanation' by H. W. Dunham." Pp. 265–70 in *Causes of Mental Disorders: A Review of Epidemiological Knowledge, 1959.* New York: Millbank Memorial Fund.

Gujarati, Damodar N. 1988. *Basic Econometrics.* New York: McGraw-Hill.

Hauser, Robert M. 1994. "Measuring Socioeconomic Status in Studies of Child Development." *Child Development* 65:1541–45.

Henry, Bill, Terrie E. Moffitt, Avshalom Caspi, John Langley, and Phil A. Silva. 1994. "On the 'Remembrance of Things Past': A Longitudinal Evaluation of the Retrospective Method." *Psychological Assessment* 6:92–101.

Holmshaw, Janet, and Emily Simonoff. 1996. "Retrospective Recall of Childhood Psychopathology." *International Journal of Methods in Psychiatric Research* 6:79–88.

Holzer, Charles E., Brent M. Shea, Jeffrey W. Swanson, Philip J. Leaf, Jerome K. Myers, Linda George, Myrna Weissman, Phillip Bednarski. 1986. "The Increased Risk for Specific Psychiatric Disorders among Persons of Low Socioeconomic Status." *American Journal of Social Psychiatry* 6:259–71.

Institute of Medicine, Committee on Prevention of Mental Disorders, Division of Biobehavioral Sciences and Mental Disorders. 1994. *Reducing Risks for Mental Disorders: Frontiers for Preventive Intervention Research*. Washington, D.C. National Academy Press.

Institute of Medicine, Committee for the Study of Research on Child and Adolescent Mental Disorders. 1995. *Report Card on the National Plan for Research on Child and Adolescent Mental Disorders: The Midway Point*. Washington, D.C.: American Academy of Child and Adolescent Psychiatry.

Jarvis, Edward. 1971. *Insanity and Idiocy in Massachusetts: Report of the Commission on Lunacy*. Cambridge, Mass.: Harvard University Press.

Jencks, Christopher, Susan Bartlet, Mary Corcoran, James Crouse, David Eaglesfield, Gregory Jackson, Kent McClelland, Peter Mueser, Michael Olneck, Joseph Schwartz, Sherry Ward, and Jill Williams. 1979. *Who Gets Ahead? The Determinants of Economic Success in America*. New York: Basic Books.

Kendler, Kenneth S., Ellen E. Walters, Michael C. Neale, Ronald C. Kessler, Andrew C. Health, and Lindon J. Eaves. 1995. "The Structure of the Genetic and Environmental Risk Factors for Six Major Psychiatric Disorders in Women: Phobia, Generalized Anxiety Disorder, Panic Disorder, Bulimia, Major Depression, and Alcoholism." *Archives of General Psychiatry* 52:374–83.

Kennedy, Patrick J. 1981. *New Zealand: A Study of the Educational System of New Zealand and a Guide to the Academic Placement of Students in Educational Institutions of the United States*. World Education Series, American Association of Collegiate Registrars and Admissions Officers. ERIC, ED249894.

Kerckhoff, Alan C. 1993. *Diverging Pathways: Social Structure and Career Deflections*. Cambridge: Cambridge University Press.

Kessler, Ronald. 1979. "Stress, Social Status, and Psychological Distress." *Journal of Health and Social Behavior* 20:259–72.

Kessler, Ronald C., and Paul D. Cleary. 1980. "Social Class and Psychological Distress." *American Sociological Review* 45:463–78.

Kessler, Ronald C., Cindy L. Foster, William Saunders, and Paul Stang. 1995. "Social Consequences of Psychiatric Disorders, I: Educational Attainment." *American Journal of Psychiatry* 152:1026–32.

Kessler, Ronald C., Katherine A. McGonagle, Shanyang Zhao, Christopher B. Nelson, Michael Hughes, Suzann Eshleman, Hans-Ulrich Wittchen, and Kenneth S. Kendler. 1994. "Lifetime and 12-Month Prevalence of DSM-III-R Psychiatric Disorders in the United States: Results from the National Comorbidity Study." *Archives of General Psychiatry* 51:8–19.

Kohn, Melvin. 1981. "Social Class and Schizophrenia: A Critical Review and a Reformulation." Pp. 127–43 in *The Sociology of Mental Illness: Basic Studies*, edited by O. Grusky and M. Pollner. New York: Holt, Rinehart & Winston.

Krueger, Robert F., Avshalom Caspi, Terrie E. Moffitt, Phil A. Silva, and Rob McGee. 1996. "Personality Traits Are Differentially Linked to Mental Disorders: A Multitrait-Multidiagnosis Study of an Adolescent Birth Cohort." *Journal of Abnormal Psychology* 105:299–312.

Langner, Thomas S. 1962. "A Twenty-Two Item Screening Score of Psychiatric Symptoms Indicating Impairment." *Journal of Health and Social Behavior* 3:269–76.

Liem, Ramsey, and Joan Liem. 1978. "Social Class and Mental Illness Reconsidered: The Role of Economic Stress and Social Support." *Journal of Health and Social Behavior* 19:139–56.

Link, Bruce G., and Bruce Dohrenwend. 1989. "The Epidemiology of Mental Disorders." Pp. 102–27 in *The Handbook of Medical Sociology,* edited by Howard Freeman and Sol Levine. Englewood Cliffs, N.J.: Prentice-Hall.

Link, Bruce G., Bruce Dohrenwend, and Andrew Skodol. 1986. "Socioeconomic Status and Schizophrenia: Noisome Occupational Characteristics as a Risk Factor." *American Sociological Review* 51:242–58.

Link, Bruce G., Mary Clare Lennon, and Bruce P. Dohrenwend. 1993. "Socioeconomic Status and Depression: The Role of Occupations Involving Direction, Control, and Planning." *American Journal of Sociology* 98:1351–87.

Little, Roderick J., and Donald Rubin. 1987. *Statistical Analysis with Missing Data.* New York: Wiley.

Lynam, Donald R. 1996. "Early Identification of Chronic Offenders: Who Is the Fledgling Psychopath?" *Psychological Bulletin* 120:209–34.

Mare, Robert D. 1980. "Social Background and School Continuation Decisions." *Journal of the American Statistical Association* 75:295–305.

———. 1981. "Change and Stability in Educational Stratification." *American Sociological Review* 46:72–87.

Mirowsky, John and Catherine E. Ross. 1989. "Psychiatric Diagnosis as Reified Measurement." *Journal of Health and Social Behavior* 30:11–25.

Moffitt, Terrie E. 1993. "Adolescence-Limited and Life-Course Persistent Antisocial Behavior: A Developmental Taxonomy." *Psychological Review* 100:674–701.

Neugebauer, Richard, Bruce P. Dohrenwend, and Barbara Dohrenwend. 1980. "Formulation of Hypotheses about the True Prevalence of Functional Psychiatric Disorders among Adults in the United States." Pp. 45–94 in *Mental Illness in the United States: Epidemiological Estimates,* edited by B. P. Dohrenwend et al. New York: Praeger.

Newman, Denise L., Terrie E. Moffitt, Avshalom Caspi, Lynn Magdol, Phil A. Silva, and Warren R. Stanton. 1996. "Psychiatric Disorder in a Birth Cohort of Young Adults: Prevalence, Co-Morbidity, Clinical Significance, and New Case Incidence from Age 11 to 21." *Journal of Consulting and Clinical Psychology* 64:552–62.

Ortega, Suzanne T., and Jay Corzine. 1990. "Socioeconomic Status and Mental Disorders." *Research in Community and Mental Health* 6:149–82.

Pearlin, Leonard I., and Joyce S. Johnson. 1977. "Marital Status, Life-Strains and Depression." *American Sociological Review* 42:704–15.

Reynolds, William M. 1992. "Depression in Children and Adolescents." Pp. 149–253 in *Internalizing Disorders in Children and Adolescents,* edited by W. M. Reynolds. New York: Wiley.

Robins, Lee N., and Darrel A. Regier, eds. 1991. *Psychiatric Disorders in America.* New York: Free Press.

Robins, Lee N., J. E. Helzer, L. Cottler, and E. Goldring. 1989. "Diagnostic Interview Schedule, Version III-R." Unpublished manuscript, Washington University, St. Louis.

Rogler, Lloyd H., Robert G. Malgady, and Warren W. Tryon. 1992. "Evaluation of Mental Health: Issues of Memory in the Diagnostic Interview Schedule." *Journal of Nervous and Mental Disease* 180:215–22.

Rutter, Michael. 1986. "The Developmental Psychopathology of Depression: Issues and Perspectives." Pp. 3–30 in *Depression in Young People: Developmental and Clinical Perspectives*, edited by M. Rutter, C. E. Izard, and P. B. Read. New York: Guilford Press.

Rutter, Michael, Bridget Yule, David Quinton, Olwen Rowlands, William Yule, and Michael Berger. 1974. "Attainment and Adjustment in Two Geographical Areas: III. Some Factors Accounting for Area Differences." *British Journal of Psychiatry* 125:520–33.

Scottish Council for Research in Education. 1976. *The Burt Word Reading Test*. London: Hodder & Stoughton.

Sewell, William H., and Robert Hauser. 1976. "Causes and Consequences of Higher Education: Models of the Status Attainment Process." Pp. 9–27 in *Schooling and Achievement in American Society*, edited by W. Sewell, R. Hauser, and D. Featherman. New York: Academic Press.

Sewell, William H., Robert Hauser, and David Featherman, eds. 1976. *Schooling and Achievement in American Society*. New York: Academic Press.

Silva, Phil A. 1990. "The Dunedin Multidisciplinary Health and Development Study: A Fifteen Year Longitudinal Study." *Pediatric and Perinatal Epidemiology* 4:96–127.

Silva, Phil A., and Warren Stanton, eds. 1996. *From Child to Adult: The Dunedin Multidisciplinary Health and Development Study*. Auckland: Oxford University Press.

Turner, R. Jay, Blair Wheaton, and Donald A. Lloyd. 1995. "The Epidemiology of Social Stress." *American Sociological Review* 60:104–25.

Velez, Carmen N., Jim Johnson, and Patricia Cohen. 1989. "A Longitudinal Analysis of Selected Risk Factors of Childhood Psychopathology." *Journal of the American Academy of Child and Adolescent Psychiatry* 28:861–67.

Wechsler, David. 1974. *Manual of the Wechsler Intelligence Scale for Children—Revised*. New York: Psychological Corporation.

Wheaton, Blair. 1978. "The Sociogenesis of Psychological Disorder: Reexamining the Causal Issues with Longitudinal Data." *American Sociological Review* 43:383–403.

DISCUSSION QUESTIONS

1. Miech and colleagues find that social causation processes operate differently for different disorders. What might explain the differences in results across disorders?

2. What might account for the selection effects the authors observed in the case of conduct disorder and ADHD? Through what processes might symptoms of those disorders affect educational attainment? Why would those same processes not apply in the case of depression and anxiety? Would you expect them to apply to other disorders, such as bipolar disorder or schizophrenia? Why or why not?

3. The data that the authors used were from New Zealand. Would you expect to observe the same patterns in the United States? Why or why not?

Mark Tausig and Rudy Fenwick

Recession and Well-Being

The authors of this selection take a uniquely sociological approach to analyzing the effects of economic conditions on mental health by considering the implications of macroeconomic change for the well-being of the population. The specific change they analyze is the 1974–75 recession—a profound economic change characterized by inflation combined with slow economic growth and rising unemployment. They trace the effects of the recession on population well-being through changes in job characteristics, particularly job demands and pay. Although their analysis is highly technical, it is worth the effort. Students with limited backgrounds in statistics may want to skip Tables 2 and 3 in favor of the summary results in Table 4.

In 1974–75 the United States suffered its worst economic contraction since the "great depression" in the 1930s. Although the economic effects of this recession on Americans have been extensively investigated (e.g., Blumberg, 1980; Bluestone & Harrison, 1982; Cummings, 1987), research into its effects on psychological well-being has been less systematic. Despite separate research literatures on the effects of individual unemployment, plant closings, and even aggregate unemployment rates on measures of well-being, we lack an integrated understanding of how recessions affect the well-being of the population as a whole and what intervening factors can explain those effects. However, available data exist to conduct such a study in the form of the 1973–77 Quality of Employment Panel Study. These data, in fact, document dramatic increases in measures of distress and dissatisfaction among workers during this period. In this paper we relate these changes in well-being to the systematic economic changes that accompanied the 1974–75 recession.

THE 1974–75 RECESSION

The recession that hit the United States in 1974 and 1975 marked a watershed in American economic history—the abrupt end of post-World War II economic growth and U.S. domination of the world economy and the beginning of a long period of deindustrialization and economic stagnation (Bluestone & Harrison, 1982; Cummings, 1987). The early 1970s had been one of the most prosperous periods in U.S. history, with "real" wages and median family income reaching their all-time peaks in 1973 (Blumberg, 1980). However, between the end of 1973 and the middle of 1975 industrial production declined by 14.4 percent and nearly one-third of the nation's productive capacity was

Tausig, Mark, and Rudy Fenwick. 1999. "Recession and Well-Being." *Journal of Health and Social Behavior* 40:1–16.

idled (Cummings, 1987). Unemployment increased from 4.9 percent in 1973 to 8.5 percent by the end of 1975, and was still at 7.0 percent in 1977, a year after the recession had officially ended (U.S. Bureau of the Census, 1978).

Increasing unemployment rates during this period were accompanied by rapid increases in the cost of living. The Consumer Price Index, which had been increasing at an annual rate of 7 percent from 1970 to 1973, jumped to over 12 percent in 1974 (Blumberg, 1980). The resulting "stagflation" (the combination of recession and inflation) compounded the "psychology of recession" with a "psychology of inflation." Concerns about losing one's job were added to concerns about keeping up with the rapidly increasing cost of living and a fear that even having a stable, secure job was no longer enough to maintain one's standard of living. These concerns were reflected in opinion surveys of the time, which reported widespread feelings of helplessness and "mental strain" (i.e., anger, worry, irritation, and depression) in the face of perceived increases in financial pressures and declines in financial well-being and standards of living (Caplovitz, 1979; Blumberg, 1980).

Although these surveys provided snapshots of the public's anguish over economic problems during the mid-1970s, they neither systematically examine the extent to which this anguish was brought on by the problems surrounding the recession (e.g., actual unemployment or fear of losing one's job or job restructuring) or inflation nor whether the popular anguish had increased substantially from the early 1970s. In order to address these issues we turn to theoretical and methodological perspectives on economy and well-being developed in sociological and epidemiological research.

PERSPECTIVES ON THE ECONOMY AND WELL-BEING

Sociology has a long tradition of examining the noneconomic effects of economic events and changes on societies, including the effects on various aggregate measures of well-being. A century ago, Durkheim ([1897] 1951) argued that business crises increase anomie, resulting in higher rates of social pathology, including suicide (Horwitz, 1984). Assessments of the impact of the great depression of the 1930s also focused on the social isolation and mental health problems that resulted from mass unemployment (Bakke, 1940; Komarovsky, 1940). More recently, many researchers have used aggregate time series analyses to uncover relationships between economic indicators, such as unemployment rates, cost of living indices, and a variety of health and well-being indicators like mortality from cardiovascular disease (Brenner, 1973, 1976), suicide rates (Marshall & Hodge, 1981), infant mortality rates (Brenner, 1973), and admissions to mental hospitals (Brenner, 1976).

Reviewing these results, Brenner (1984) and his colleagues (Brenner & Mooney, 1983) have argued that increased unemployment rates negatively affect health and well-being because they reduce personal resources and increase stress based on increasing risk of unemployment and the perceived risk of unemployment (job insecurity), and because attempts to relieve stress may lead to health-risky behaviors like increased consumption of alcohol or drugs. They also speculate that these effects spill over into the ranks of the employed through other mechanisms—restricted mobility, pay reductions, and job restructuring—as well as reduced public resources to deal with health problems (Brenner & Mooney, 1983).

However, these intervening mechanisms have been left largely unmeasured. Thus, the specific connections between aggregate economic processes and well-being have remained speculative rather than resting on a firm conceptual and theoretical base (Catalano & Dooley, 1983). As a consequence, these studies have been criticized for committing the "ecological fallacy" by which associations at the aggregate level are incorrectly assumed to describe actual individual experiences (Dooley & Catalano, 1980; Catalano & Dooley, 1983).

Partly as a result of these criticisms, the focus of this research has shifted from a macrostructural analysis of the general relationship between economic conditions and aggregate well-being to the use of social psychological models that link economic and social processes to individual outcomes. For example, Catalano and Dooley (1983) found that economic contraction (i.e., higher unemployment rates) increased the individual incidence of undesirable job and financial events that in turn increased the incidence of illness and injury, even among employed workers. A later analysis also suggested that higher unemployment rates increased help-seeking among workers because of increased perceptions of employment insecurity (Catalano, Rook, & Dooley, 1986). Using a similar analytic strategy, Fenwick and Tausig (1994) found that increased occupational unemployment rates during the mid-1970s recession often led to restructuring of jobs among employed workers—increasing job demands and decreasing decision latitude—which in turn were related to increased distress and dissatisfaction among these workers. Turner (1995) has shown that the personal effects of unemployment are most significant when regional unemployment rates are high. He argues that poor prospects for reemployment affect the psychological reaction to personal unemployment. Still other studies have minimized the economic context in favor of examining the individual-level relationship between personal unemployment and well-being (Cobb & Kasl, 1977; Jahoda, 1982; Liem & Rayman, 1982).

EARLY RESEARCH ON THE ECONOMY AND MENTAL ILLNESS

One of the first examples of research linking the economy to mental illness was M. Harvey Brenner's analysis of the association between the

New York State employment index (for manufacturing industries) and mental hospital admissions from 1910–60. Brenner found that mental hospital admissions rose during periods of low employment, especially for men and for "functional psychoses" (schizophrenia, bipolar disorder). (See figures below.) He concluded that, "the level of psychiatric symptomatology is frequently increased by precipitating sociocultural stresses, among which economic factors loom large in the sequence of causation (Brenner, 1967, 187–88). Brenner was later criticized for drawing conclusions about the experiences of individuals based on data from the population, a problematic form of inference sometimes referred to as the ecological fallacy. His data do not tell us, for example, whether

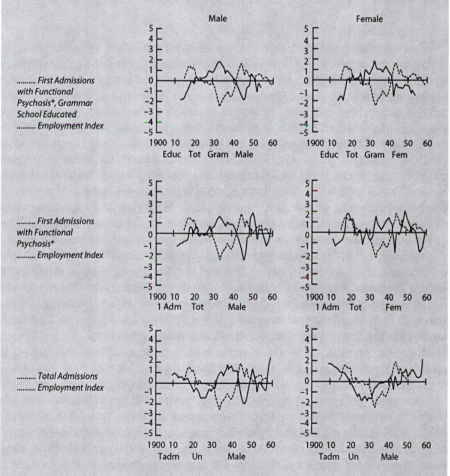

Figure 1 Admissions to Civil State Mental Hospitals Compared with the Employment Index *New York State, 1910–1960* Linearly Detrended Data (Least-Squares Technique), in Standard Deviations

the people who were most affected by periods of low employment were most likely to be admitted to mental hospitals. More generally, they cannot tell us whether adverse economic circumstances contribute to mental illness or whether they lead to lower tolerance and support of people with mental health problems in the community. Despite the problems with Brenner's study, it remains a classic in the field because it alerted mental health scholars to the possible mental health implications of economic downturns.

Brenner, M. Harvey. 1967. "Economic Change and Mental Hospitalization: New York State, 1910–1960." *Social Psychiatry* 2:180–88.

These studies have been able to shed light on pathways by which macroeconomic processes affect individual well-being by explaining differences in individual outcomes and changes in these outcomes (e.g., which individuals become more or less distressed and why). Although important, this is not the same issue that was of concern in much of the earlier research from Durkheim to Brenner. Rather, their interest was in explaining the magnitude of aggregate change in a population's distress level that may occur because of these economic processes. The distinction is important since aggregate changes can occur without changing the distribution of individual outcomes. This is especially likely to happen when change is experienced extensively throughout a population (Susser, 1994). For example, in a widespread economic recession all workers might experience increased distress. The aggregate (mean) distress level for the labor force would increase, but the distribution of distress among individual workers would remain relatively unchanged (e.g., workers having the highest (or lowest) levels of distress before the recession would continue to have the highest (or lowest) levels during or after the recession). An exclusive concern with explaining differences in individual outcomes would show little or no change at this level while missing the change that occurred at the aggregate level.

However, even if all workers experienced increased distress during a recession, as in this example, they may have done so for different reasons—some because of the personal experience of unemployment, others because of increased job insecurity, reduced pay, restricted opportunities for job mobility, or job restructuring (e.g., as discussed above in Brenner & Mooney, 1983). And, in the case of the 1974–75 recession, increased distress for some may have resulted from rapid increases in the cost of living. Still others may have experienced increased distress for reasons unrelated to the recession, such as divorce or widowhood. Since some or all of these experiences could account for some or all of the aggregate increase in distress, we need to be able to measure the contribution each type of experience makes toward the total aggregate change.

In the analysis and discussion that follows, we demonstrate a technique that allows us to measure the contributions made by different types of experiences to aggregate changes in well-being. It does so by decomposing measured changes in well-being into their various components, taking into account both the degree of association between relevant experiences and well-being and the amount of changes in these variables (Mirowsky, 1998). Using this technique we will measure how much various types of sociodemographic, labor market, and job experiences and changes (e.g., marriage/divorce, unemployment, job restructuring) contributed to aggregate changes in measures of well-being (e.g., distress and dissatisfaction) in the U.S. labor force before and after the mid-1970s recession.

DATA AND MEASURES

Data for the analysis come from the 1973–77 Quality of Employment Panel Study (QES). The QES is one of the few national longitudinal studies of the U.S. labor force and provides comprehensive information on workers, their job structures, and distress and dissatisfaction during the period of interest—the mid-1970s. Indeed, because of the timing of the two waves of interviews—the first was conducted in 1973, shortly before the onset of the recession, and the second wave in 1977, shortly after the end of the recession—the panel, in effect, represents pre-and post-tests of the effects of the recession on workers in the labor force.

The first wave of the QES was a national probability sample of 1,455 full-time workers (i.e., 20 hours or more per week) in the U.S. labor force, 16 years of age or older. Of the time-one respondents, 1,086 were reinterviewed in the second wave in 1977, and of these 830 reported still working full-time. Because only full-time respondents were asked in-depth questions on variables important to this study, such as job structures and distress and dissatisfaction, the analysis is limited to these 830.

Variables and Measurement

To provide a comprehensive analysis of the effects of the mid-1970s recession on changes in levels of distress and dissatisfaction of the U.S. labor force, we include several types of variables: sociodemographic determinants of occupational position and sociodemographic change; occupational and labor market position and change; job characteristics and changes in these characteristics; distress; dissatisfaction; and change. Because the analysis which follows is concerned with explaining how much of the aggregate changes in distress and dissatisfaction can be accounted for by changes in sociodemographic statuses, labor market positions, and job characteristics (restructuring), many of these variables have been recoded so that higher scores suggest higher distress or dissatisfaction (with the exception of variables whose coding direction is nonarbitrary: age, years of education, and organizational size).

Sociodemographic characteristics include: *age* (in years), *gender, race* (white versus non-white), *marital status* (married versus not married, i.e., single, divorced, or widowed), *number of children* (age 15 and under who were living at home), and the *number of years of education.* Age, gender, and race are measured only at time-one (1973), while marital status, children, and education are measured in both 1973 and 1977. These variables are included not only because of their known effects on occupational position but also because of their effects on distress and dissatisfaction levels. To reflect higher levels of distress, females and non-whites are coded 1, while males and whites are coded 0.

Occupational and labor market positions measured here are *workplace size, union versus nonunion, economic sector* (core versus periphery), and *occupational unemployment rates.* These variables, which are measured at both time-one and time-two, reflect the relative vulnerability of workers to economic changes, such as recessions. Larger firms, unions, and firms in the core tend to produce more stable and secure job structures, such as job ladders and internal labor markets, that offer workers some protection from the recession (Lincoln & Kalleberg, 1985). However, firm size also tends to increase worker isolation, powerlessness, and dissatisfaction due, paradoxically, to these same bureaucratic job structures (Blauner, 1964; Spenner, 1983; Hodson, 1984). Size is measured as the natural log of the number of employees working at the respondents' work sites. The natural log is used instead of the absolute number because the effects of organizational size on structure, attitudes, and behavior generally has been found to best fit the log function (Stolzenberg, 1978). Union versus nonunion is measured by whether or not the respondent was a member of a labor union or employee association at the times of the interviews. The distinction between core and peripheral economic sectors was measured according to the Census Bureau's 1970 industry codes. Core industries tend to have a high concentration of capital resources that enable them to produce for oligopolistic markets, thus providing more secure job structures for their workers. In contrast, industries in the periphery have fewer capital resources and produce for markets in which there is a high degree of competition among firms; therefore, there is greater vulnerability of both these firms and their workers to market forces (Lincoln & Kalleberg, 1985). To reflect the greater vulnerability of nonunion and peripheral workers to recession and resultant distress, these respondents were coded 1, while union members and core workers were coded 0.

Occupational unemployment rates are the most direct measure of the relative vulnerability of workers to economic recession, as well as the most commonly used in the literature on the health effects of recession (e.g., Brenner, 1976; Catalano & Dooley, 1977, 1979; Dooley &Catalano, 1980). In this study, unemployment rates are measured in each of ten broad occupational categories used by the U.S. Census Bureau: (1) professional and technical; (2) managers and administrators; (3) sales workers; (4) clerical; (5) craft and kindred; (6) operatives, except transport; (7) transport equipment operators; (8) nonfarm laborers; (9) service workers; and (10) farm workers (U.S. Bureau of the Census, 1978). Each respondent was assigned the rate of unemployment for his or her occupational category that had existed two years prior to the times of the surveys—1971 rates for the 1973 survey and 1975 rates for the 1977 survey. This was done to account for the lagged effects of unemployment rates on stress-related outcomes that have been found in prior research, with two years appearing to be about the optimal lag time (Brenner, 1987, 1995).

In addition, we include measures of the *personal employment history* of workers by assessing whether *respondents had been unemployed* (i.e., "out of work for a month or more") and whether they *changed jobs* between 1973 and 1977. The job change measure combines both those who changed employers and those who changed jobs within their old firms (versus those working in the same jobs in the same firms). Both personal unemployment and job change were measured dichotomously at time two. Those who experienced unemployment were coded 1; those who did not were coded 0. However, to be consistent with Brenner and Mooney's (1983) argument that restricted mobility is one of the ways in which recessions are experienced as stressful, we have coded 1 respondents who remained in the same jobs over the four year period and 0 those who changed.

Five *job characteristics* are included in the analysis and measured at both times one and two. Three of the measures tap extrinsic characteristics of work and are recoded so that higher scores reflect more distress: *job insecurity, lack of opportunities for promotions,* and *poor pay.* Each is measured by a single item asking respondent to evaluate that aspect of their current jobs: "not true at all" (1) to "very true" (4).

Two multiple-item variables measure intrinsic job characteristics: *decision constraints* and *job demands.* These measures are derived from the job demands-control model developed by Karasek (1979). Decision constraints is the reverse of Karasek's (1979) concept of "decision latitude," which is defined as the "working individual's potential control over tasks and conduct during the working day" (289–90). It is constructed by computing the mean of respondents' scores on eight items that reflect evaluations of various aspects of the respondent's job, such as the degree to which they feel the job requires high levels of skill, learning new things, nonrepetitious and creative work, as well as the degree to which the job allows for freedom and ability to have input about how the job is done. As with the above extrinsic characteristics, we have recoded these items so that higher scores suggest greater distress (greater constraints on decision-making rather than latitude). Job demands measures "the psychological stressors involved in accomplishing workload" (291) and is constructed by computing respondents' mean scores on seven items evaluating how much their jobs require working hard and fast, whether they are allowed time to finish the tasks, and whether or not they are subject to conflicting job demands.

Our dependent variables, *distress* and *dissatisfaction,* are measures of psychological (mental health) functioning in 1973 and 1977. Distress measures the psycho-physiological symptoms of distress, and is computed by taking respondents' mean scores on nine items that reflect physiological conditions associated with depression and anxiety, such as sweating palms, pounding heart, and sleep difficulties (Mirowsky & Ross, 1989). Dissatisfaction measures respondents' general feelings about their present (at the time of the interview) lives and reflects lack of well-being (Campbell et al., 1976). It is computed by taking respondents' mean scores on eight recoded items that probe feelings that one's life is neither interesting, enjoyable, full nor worthwhile.

Means and standard deviations for these variables are presented in Table 1, along with the results of t-tests for differences in means between 1973 and 1977. Comparing variable means in 1977 with those in 1973 we can see the overall amount of aggregate changes that occurred during this period. With the exceptions of increasing years of education, relative growth of core sector employment, and decreasing decision constraints, changes in the variables show declining labor market positions and job characteristics and higher levels of distress and dissatisfaction indicative of recessionary periods.

Occupational unemployment rates increased by almost 50 percent between 1973 to 1977, from 4.42 percent to 6.48 percent, while 14 percent of respondents reported having been out of work at some time during this period. Slightly more than half (53 percent) of the respondents were in the same jobs in 1977 as they had been in 1973. There was also a significant shift from

Table 1 Means and Standard Deviations for Demographic, Socioeconomic, Job, and Mental Health Variables

| | 1973 | | 1977 | | |
	$\bar{x}$	SD	$\bar{x}$	SD	T-Value
Age[a]	37.59	12.03	—	—	—
Female[ab]	.29	.46	—	—	—
Nonwhite[ab]	.10	.30	—	—	—
Married[b]	.78	.41	.78	.41	−.30
Children	1.21	1.35	1.21	1.38	.07
Education	12.48	2.96	12.61	3.01	2.84**
Size	4.29	2.11	4.34	2.06	.68
Nonunion[b]	.68	.87	.72	.95	2.93**
Periphery[b]	.29	.45	.24	.43	−3.07**
Unemployment Rate (1971, 1975)	4.42	2.70	6.48	3.90	15.45***
Unemployed[ab]	—	—	.14	.28	—
Same Job[ab]	—	—	.53	.50	—
Demands	2.71	.52	2.88	.51	8.22***
Decision Constraints	2.09	.64	2.05	.57	−1.73
Insecurity	1.72	.94	1.81	.90	2.42*
Lack of Promotions	1.63	.89	2.69	.93	25.03***
Poor Pay	1.46	.67	2.04	.90	15.20***
Distress	1.52	.47	1.72	.49	12.40***
Dissatisfaction	2.11	.97	2.33	.98	6.28***

*$p \le .05$; **$p \le .01$; ***$p \le .001$
[a]Variable measured only at one time.
[b]Mean represents percentage of respondents in the particular category.

union to nonunion employment. Aside from decision constraints, measures of job characteristics showed significant shifts in the direction of more stressful jobs: job demands increased by one-third of a standard deviation, lack of promotional opportunities increased by over one standard deviation, and inadequate pay increased by almost one standard deviation. The increase in job insecurity, although smaller, was nonetheless significant.

The shift to more stressful jobs was indeed borne out by significant increases in distress and dissatisfaction. Distress increased by almost half a standard deviation, and dissatisfaction increased by a quarter of a standard deviation.

ANALYSIS

How much of these large aggregate changes in distress and dissatisfaction were due to the equally large changes in labor market and job characteristics as well as the smaller sociodemographic changes? To answer this question we will use a statistical model that allows us to analyze the amount of aggregate change in distress and dissatisfaction that can be explained by the aggregate changes in each of the sociodemographic, occupational, labor market, and job characteristics in Table 1. The model was developed by John Mirowsky to enable the decomposition of aggregate change (Mirowsky, 1998). Mirowsky's model takes the form of the following equation:

$$\Delta Y = a_0 + a_1 y_1 + a_2 x_1 + \Delta X + e, \tag{1}$$

where Y is distress or dissatisfaction and X is an attribute of the individual's occupation, job characteristic, or sociodemographic status. In this equation, Y and X are measured as deviations from their respective time 1 means; $y_i = Y_i - \bar{Y}_i$ and $x_i = X_i - \bar{X}_i$ are measured for continuous variables. For nominal variables measured at time 1, such as race and gender, the deviation score $d_i = \bar{D}_i - D_i = D_i - P_{Di}$, where P_{Di}, is the proportion of the sample in the category (coded 1). Change scores (ΔY and ΔX) are measured as the difference between the raw score at time 2 and the raw score at time 1: $\Delta Y = Y_2 - Y_1$ and $\Delta X = X_2 - X_1$. The logic of change score measurement can also be adapted to include variables that refer to events that occurred (or not) between times 1 and 2, such as unemployment (or staying in the same job). Since the events occurred after time 1, the raw score for the these variables at time 1 would be zero; thus, the change score would equal the raw score at time 2: $\Delta X = X_2 - X_1 = X_2 - 0 = X_2$.

The intercept a_0 in equation 1 equals the expected change in Y for the average person in the sample (for whom $y_1 = x_1 = 0$) in the absence of any change in X ($\Delta X = 0$). Thus, the t-test associated with the intercept tests the proposition that the aggregate change in Y would have been zero if the aggregate change in X had been zero. Coefficients a_1 and a_2 measure the effects of the initial (time 1) measures of distress or dissatisfaction (Y_1) and sociodemographic, occupational, and job variables (X_1), respectively, on the expected changes in psychological functioning: ΔY. Coefficient a_3 measures the effect of a unit increase in X on the expected change in Y. Its t-value tests the proposition that changes in X predict corresponding changes in Y.

As discussed above, sociodemographic, occupational and job variables (X) have been coded or recoded so that an increase in X predicts an increase in Y (distress and dissatisfaction). This enables us to find the percentage of the aggregate change in Y that is attributable to the aggregate change in X by taking expected values in equation 1:

$$\Delta \bar{Y} = a_0 + a_1 \bar{Y}_1 + a_2 \bar{X}_2 + a_3 \Delta \bar{X} + \bar{e} \tag{2}$$

Since Y and X are measured as deviations from their respective means, these terms drop out; thus:

$$\Delta \bar{Y} = a_0 + a_1(0) + a_2(0) + a_3 \Delta \bar{X} + (0) \tag{3}$$

$$\Delta \bar{Y} = a_0 + a_3 \Delta \bar{X}. \tag{4}$$

The percentage of change in Y attributable to any X is:

$$\text{Attributable percentage} = 100 \times a_3 \Delta \bar{X}_i / \Delta Y. \tag{5}$$

The values for ΔX and ΔY can be obtained from Table 1. To obtain the values for a_3 we next regress changes in distress and dissatisfaction on changes in sociodemographic, labor market, and job characteristics, along with their initial (time 1) deviation scores. By entering similar groups of X variables (sociodemographic, labor market, job) into regression equations in progressive stages we can determine how the aggregate change in each Y (distress and dissatisfaction) relates to changes in each group of X variables, which group of variables accounts for the most aggregate change in Y, and which groups mediate the effects of initial status on subsequent changes in Y. This progressive adjustment begins by regressing the change in Y on initial (time 1) sociodemographic, occupational, and job characteristics as well as initial level of distress or dissatisfaction. The intercept for this equation should equal $\Delta \bar{Y} = Y_2 - Y_1$. Sociodemographic changes between 1973 and 1977 (married, unmarried, number of children, and years of education) are added in the second stage equation. Personal employment history—unemployment experience and staying in the same job—are entered in the third equation; occupational and labor market changes (size, nonunion, periphery, and unemployment rates) are added in the fourth; and job characteristics (decision constraint, demands, insecurity, lack of promotions, and poor pay) are added in the fifth. The intercept for each of these equations represents the change in distress or dissatisfaction (Y) expected in the absence of any change in these groups of X variables. And since the intercept in the first equation is equal to $\Delta \bar{Y}$, or $\bar{Y}_2 - \bar{Y}_1$, we can determine the percentage of this change attributable to a group of X variables by comparing the intercepts in equations two through five with the intercepts in the preceding equations. The percentage of change attributable to each X change variable can then be determined by plugging the respective regression coefficient into formula 5.

Results of this progressive adjustment procedure on changes in distress are presented in Table 2. The first equation shows the effects on initial socio-demographic, occupational, and job characteristics and initial levels of distress on changes in distress. As expected, the intercept (a_0 = .202) was equal, within rounding, to the mean difference in distress between 1973 and 1977 ($\Delta \bar{Y}$ = .20). Together, these time-1 variables accounted for almost a quarter of the variance in changes in distress (R^2 = .231), but only one—initial (i.e., 1973) distress—had significant effect on changes in distress. Typical of regression to the mean, this effect was negative: The higher the initial level of distress, the less the subsequent increase.

Sociodemographic changes are introduced in the second equation. Although they accounted for six percent of the aggregate change in distress (as indicated by the reduction of the intercept), none had a significant effect on changes in distress. Labor market experiences and changes are included in the next two stages. The inclusion of personal employment history in equation three accounted for another 18 percent of the change in distress, with those experiencing unemployment between 1973 and 1977 having significantly greater increases in distress than those who did not undergo this experience. Another 6 percent of the aggregate change in distress is attributable to changes in occupational structures (equation four). Increased occupational unemployment rates and movement to the periphery are significantly related to increased distress. However, changes in job characteristics appear to have had the most impact on increasing levels of distress, accounting for 20 percent of the aggregate change (equation five). Measures of intrinsic change were particularly significant as changes in distress were positively related to changes in both job demands and decision constraints. These variables also mediated the effects of changes in occupational structures. When all measures of changes in sociodemographic status, employment history, occupational structures, and job characteristics are included, the model accounts for over a quarter of the variance in the change in distress R^2 = .288) and over half (51 percent) of its aggregate increase between 1973 and 1977.

Table 3 presents the results for change in dissatisfaction, with equation one again showing the effects of initial characteristics on this change. The intercept (a_0 = .217) was again equal, within rounding, to the mean difference between 1973 and 1977 dissatisfaction ($\Delta \bar{Y}$ = .22), while the initial variables accounted for slightly more than a quarter of the variance in change in dissatisfaction (R^2 = .279). As with distress, there was a significant negative relationship between the level of dissatisfaction in 1973 and subsequent changes in dissatisfaction. However, unlike distress, there were other time-1 variables that were related to changes in dissatisfaction. Increases in dissatisfaction were greater among younger workers, those working in the periphery, and those lacking promotional opportunities in 1973.

Table 2 Metric Coefficients from the Regression of Aggregate Change in Distress Adjusting Sequentially for Baseline Sociodemographics, Job Characteristics, Distress (1), Sociodemographic Changes (2), Personal Employment Experience (3), Labor Market Changes (4), and Changes in Job Characteristics (5), 1973–77

Independent Variables	Equation				
	1	2	3	4	5
Age	−.002 (.001)	−.001 (.001)	−.001 (.001)	−.001 (.001)	.000 (.001)
Female	.050 (.035)	.050 (.035)	.050 (.035)	.061 (.035)	.053 (.035)
Nonwhite	−.080 (.050)	−.083 (.051)	−.077 (.051)	−.078 (.051)	−.088 (.050)
Married 1973	−.014 (.039)	.009 (.045)	.008 (.045)	.007 (.045)	.004 (.044)
Children 1973	.015 (.011)	.015 (.013)	.015 (.013)	.017 (.018)	.014 (.012)
Education 1973	−.008 (.006)	−.007 (.006)	−.007 (.006)	−.004 (.006)	−.007 (.006)
Size 1973	.000 (.008)	.001 (.008)	.000 (.007)	−.003 (.008)	−.003 (.008)
Nonunion 1973	−.032 (.033)	−.029 (.033)	−.025 (.033)	−.023 (.038)	−.016 (.038)
Periphery 1973	.062 (.035)	.060 (.035)	.065 (.035)	.098* (.040)	.077* (.039)
Unemployment Rate 1971	.002 (.007)	.003 (.007)	.002 (.007)	.007 (.007)	.005 (.007)
Demands 1973	.009 (.030)	.006 (.030)	.006 (.030)	.004 (.030)	.115** (.037)
Decision Constraints 1973	.024 (.028)	.023 (.028)	.022 (.028)	.016 (.028)	.066 (.036)
Insecurity 1973	.012 (.017)	.013 (.017)	.011 (.017)	.011 (.017)	.020 (.022)
Lack of Promotions 1973	.005 (.018)	.004 (.018)	.002 (.018)	.000 (.018)	−.007 (.023)
Poor Pay 1973	.005 (.023)	.003 (.023)	.004 (.023)	.006 (.023)	.023 (.028)
Distress 1973	−.492*** (.032)	−.493*** (.032)	.494*** (.032)	−.493*** (.032)	−.506*** (.032)
Got Married 1973–77		.118 (.071)	.119 (.071)	.119 (.071)	.111 (.069)
Unmarried 1973–77		.098 (.063)	.093 (.063)	.100 (.063)	.096 (.064)
ΔChildren 1973–77		.001 (.017)	.003 (.017)	.000 (.017)	.003 (.017)
ΔEducation 1973–77		−.003 (.015)	−.003 (.015)	.002 (.015)	.000 (.015)
Same Job 1973–77			.029 (.031)	.028 (.031)	.027 (.031)
Unemployment 1973–77			.158** (.051)	.155** (.051)	.154** (.051)
ΔSize 1973–77				−.004 (.010)	−.008 (.010)
ΔNonunion 1973–77				−.001 (.044)	−.005 (.043)
ΔPeriphery 1973–77				.091* (.044)	.076 (.043)
ΔUnemployment Rates 1971–75				.008* (.004)	.007 (.004)
ΔDemands 1973–77					.156*** (.031)
ΔDecision Constraints 1973–77					.086** (.033)
ΔInsecurity 1973–19					.012 (.018)
ΔLack of Promotions 1973–77					.008 (.017)
ΔPoor Pay 1973–77					.019 (.018)
Intercept (a)	.202*** (.014)	.189*** (.016)	.152*** (.024)	.140*** (.026)	.117*** (.031)
R²	.231***	.236***	.246***	.253***	.288***
ΔR²		.005	.010**	.007	.035***
%ΔIntercept		.064	.247	.307	.510

*p ≤ .05; **p ≤ .01; ***p ≤ .001
Note: Numbers in parentheses are standard errors; N = 860.

Table 3 Metric Coefficients From the Regression of Aggregate Change in Dissatisfaction Adjusting Sequentially for Baseline Sociodemographics, Job Characteristics, Dissatisfaction (1), Sociodemographic Changes (2), Personal Employment Experience (3), Labor Market Changes (4), and Changes in Job Characteristics (5), 1973–77

Independent Variables	Equation				
	1	2	3	4	5
Age	−.009 (.003)	−.009** (.003)	−.009** (.003)	−.008** (.003)	−.008** (.003)
Female	−.015 (.071)	−.011 (.071)	−.011 (.071)	−.010 (.072)	−.073 (.071)
Nonwhite	−.091 (.104)	−.125 (.103)	−.120 (.104)	−.145 (.104)	−.207* (.101)
Married 1973	.114 (.080)	.054 (.093)	.052 (.093)	.036 (.093)	.030 (.090)
Children 1973	.009 (.024)	−.001 (.026)	−.000 (.026)	−.001 (.026)	−.003 (.025)
Education 1973	−.015 (.012)	−.014 (.013)	−.014 (.013)	−.006 (.013)	−.008 (.013)
Size 1973	.012 (.015)	.014 (.015)	.013 (.015)	.018 (.017)	.021 (.017)
Nonunion 1973	.021 (.069)	.030 (.068)	.033 (.068)	.085 (.079)	.099 (.077)
Periphery 1973	.141* (.072)	.146* (.072)	.151* (.072)	.109 (.083)	.076 (.080)
Unemployment Rate 1971	−.021 (.013)	−.020 (.014)	−.021 (.014)	−.003 (.015)	−.017 (.015)
Demands 1973	−.019 (.062)	−.028 (.061)	−.029 (.061)	−.022 (.061)	.095 (.076)
Decision Constraints 1973	.080 (.059)	.071 (.059)	.072 (.059)	.057 (.059)	.250*** (.074)
Insecurity 1973	.013 (.034)	.022 (.034)	.022 (.034)	.012 (.034)	.052 (.044)
Lack of Promotions 1973	.090* (.036)	.083* (.036)	.081* (.036)	.082* (.036)	.107* (.047)
Poor Pay 1973	.010 (.048)	.014 (.048)	.016 (.048)	.019 (.048)	.111* (.057)
Dissatisfaction 1973	−.526*** (.032)	−.536*** (.032)	−.536*** (.032)	−.535*** (.032)	−.566*** (.032)
Got Married 1973–77		−.091 (.145)	−.089 (.145)	−.122 (.145)	−.139 (.141)
Unmarried 1973–77		.413** (.129)	.412** (.129)	.400** (.128)	.390** (.125)
ΔChildren 1973–77		−.037 (.035)	−.035 (.035)	−.041 (.035)	−.033 (.034)
ΔEducation 1973–77		.014 (.031)	.014 (.031)	.021 (.031)	.021 (.030)
Same Job 1973–77			.040 (.064)	.037 (.064)	.046 (.063)
Unemployed 1973–77			.116 (.105)	.106 (.105)	.121 (.102)
ΔSize 1973–77				.028 (.020)	.022 (.020)
ΔNonunion 1973–77				.050 (.090)	.045 (.088)
ΔPeriphery 1973–77				−.040 (.091)	−.076 (.088)
ΔUnemployment Rates 1971–75				.023** (.008)	.014 (.009)
ΔDemands 1973–77					.176** (.064)
ΔDecision Constraints 1973–77					.314*** (.069)
ΔInsecurity 1973–77					.058 (.036)
ΔLack of Promotions 1973–77					.026 (.034)
ΔPoor Pay 1973–77					.098** (.036)
Intercept (a)	.217*** (.034)	.194*** (.032)	.157** (.049)	.109* (.053)	.017 (.064)
R²	.279***	.292***	.293***	.301***	.347***
ΔR²		.013	.001	.008*	.046***
%ΔIntercept		.106	.276	.498	.922

*p ≤ .05; **p ≤ .01; ***p ≤ .001
Note: Numbers in parentheses are standard errors; N = 860.

Sociodemographic changes between 1973 and 1977 accounted for almost 11 percent of the aggregate change in dissatisfaction, as shown in the second equation. In particular, increased dissatisfaction was related to changes in marital status from married to unmarried (divorced, separated, or widowed). Another 17 percent of the aggregate increase in dissatisfaction was attributable to personal employment history from 1973 to 1977, although neither of these variables had a significant effect on change in distress. Occupational structure changes (equation four) accounted for an additional 22 percent of the aggregate increase, although only one—increased unemployment rates—was significantly related to increased dissatisfaction. However, as with distress, the greatest amount of aggregate change in dissatisfaction was attributable to changes in job characteristics presented in the fifth equation—over 42 percent by these variables alone. Changes in intrinsic characteristics—job demands and decision constraints—were again positively related to changes in dissatisfaction, as was one extrinsic change: increasingly poor pay. Changes in job characteristics mediated the effects of occupational structure changes but also uncovered some significant effects of time 1 variables. Dissatisfaction increased more among nonwhites than whites and was related to high initial levels of decision constraints and poor pay. Overall, while the model accounted for a third of the variance in changes in dissatisfaction ($R = .347$), the changes in sociodemographic statuses, personal employment history, occupational structures, and job characteristics together accounted for nearly all (92 percent) of the aggregate increase in labor force dissatisfaction between 1973 and 1977.

We now apply formula (5) to determine the percentage of change in distress and dissatisfaction attributable to change in each independent variable. Table 4 presents the results of this procedure using the regression coefficients from the full structural (fifth) equations in Tables 2 and 3. Results for distress are presented in the first column; those for dissatisfaction in the second. The total percentages shown at the bottom of the columns are calculated by adding together the percentages attributable to the individual variables in the respective columns. Note that these total percentages are, within rounding, equal to the total percentages calculated from differences in intercepts in Tables 2 and 3.

Results in Table 4 are generally consistent with those in Tables 2 and 3 in that variables accounting for the greatest percentages of change in distress and dissatisfaction were those that had significant regression effects. Most of the largest changes in these measures of well-being were attributable to changes in job structures. The greatest amount of the increase in distress was due to increased job demands (13.26 percent), followed by personal unemployment experience (10.78 percent). Increasingly inadequate or poor pay accounted for the greatest increase in dissatisfaction—indeed, a quarter (25.84 percent) of the total. This was followed by increased job demands (13.60 percent) and changes in marital status from married to unmarried (11.34 percent).

Table 4 Percent Aggregate (Mean) Change in Distress and Dissatisfaction Accounted for by Aggregate Changes in Sociodemographic, Occupational, and Job Characteristics, 1973–77

	Distress	Dissatisfaction
Got Married 1973–77	3.33%	−3.79%
Unmarried 1973–77	3.07	11.34
ΔChildren 1973–77	.00	.00
ΔEducation 1973–77	.00	1.24
Same Job 1973–77	7.16	11.08
Unemployed 1973–77	10.78	7.70
ΔSize 1973–77	−.20	.50
ΔNonunion 1973–77	−.10	.82
ΔPeriphery 1973–77	−1.90	1.73
ΔUnemployment Rates 1971–75	7.21	13.11
ΔDemands 1973–77	13.26	13.60
ΔDecision Constraints 1973–77	−1.72	−5.70
ΔInsecurity 1973–77	.54	2.27
ΔLack of Promotions 1973–77	4.24	12.53
ΔPoor Pay 1973–77	5.51	25.84
Total % Δ $\bar{y}$ 1973–77	51.18	92.37

Some variables having only modest regression effects nonetheless accounted for relatively large changes in the measures of well-being due to the size of their means or mean changes. This was particularly true for change in dissatisfaction, where decreasing opportunities for promotion (12.53 percent), increased unemployment rates (13.11 percent), and remaining in the same job (11.08 percent), each accounted for over a tenth of the total change despite insignificant regression effects. In contrast, because of the relatively small mean change in decision constraints, it accounted for a relatively small percentages of the changes in distress (−1.72 percent) and dissatisfaction (−5.70 percent), despite its significant regression effects. Moreover, because the mean change was toward less constraint, the percentages accounted for were negative. Had this change not occurred, in other words, the aggregate increases in distress and dissatisfaction between 1973 and 1977 would have been slightly larger than what was observed.

Although seemingly paradoxical, these results regarding changes in decision constraints clearly point out the difference between explaining individual outcomes and accounting for aggregate changes. Decision constraints (or, conversely, "latitude") has consistently been found to be related to various measures of individual well-being (Karasek, 1979). And changes in the level of constraints has been found to be one of the most significant variables affecting change in individual's well-being among this panel: Those whose jobs became more constrained (or had less latitude) became more distressed and dissatisfied relative to other individuals whose jobs did not become more constrained, and vice versa (Fenwick & Tausig, 1994). However, because its overall (mean) level in the labor force changed little, changes in decision constraints accounted for little of the aggregate changes in the measures of well-being.

DISCUSSION AND CONCLUSIONS

In this paper we have addressed two related questions: how much do recessions affect the well-being of a population, and by what means? With respect to the effects of the 1974–75 recession on full-time workers in the U.S. labor force, the answer to the first question is "considerable." Mean distress scores increased by almost one-half a standard deviation, and mean dissatisfaction levels increased by one-fourth of a standard deviation during the period from 1973 to 1977. Overall, our model explained just over 50 percent of the aggregate increase in distress and 92 percent of the aggregate increase in dissatisfaction. Subtracting the amount of this change due to changes in non-economic demographic statuses, such as marriage and having children (6 percent and 11 percent, respectively), this still means that nearly half of the change in distress and over 80 percent of the aggregate change in dissatisfaction is due to labor market experiences and changes in job characteristics during this period that straddles the recession.

As to the second question, results clearly point to the importance of changing job characteristics—job restructuring—as accounting for the greatest amounts of change in distress and dissatisfaction: About 20 percent of the increase in distress and 42 percent of the increase in dissatisfaction is accounted for by the model. Of particular importance were the increases in job demands and perceptions of increasingly inadequate pay, which alone accounted for a quarter of the increase in dissatisfaction.

These results are in contrast with the usual emphasis given to the effects of unemployment on well-being during economic downturns. Actual unemployment experiences, even during recessions, are, in fact, limited to a relatively small percentage of workers: Only 14 percent of the sample reported having been unemployed at any time between 1973 and 1977. In contrast, job restructuring could hypothetically be experienced by all workers. However, it has been noted that the effects of unemployment extend beyond the unemployed (Brenner & Mooney, 1983) and that job restructuring is related to high and increasing unemployment rates (Fenwick & Tausig, 1994). Both appear to be the case here. Increasing occupational unemployment rates accounted for almost as much increase in distress as personal unemployment experiences (7 percent versus 10 percent) and almost twice as much of the increase in dissatisfaction (13 percent versus 7 percent). Increasing unemployment rates also had indirect effects through changing job characteristics (Tables 2 and 3). When these job measures are omitted from the model, increased unemployment rates accounted for 8 percent of the increase in distress and 21 percent of the increase in dissatisfaction (data not shown; based on applying formula (5) to the fourth equation in Tables 2 and 3).

The impact of unemployment may also have been somewhat limited by the nature of the sample. Because the QES panel consisted only of full-time workers in both 1973 and 1977, it excluded more marginal groups, such as younger, minority, and less educated workers who would have been more vulnerable to unemployment. Still, although the impact of unemployment (direct and indirect) was not inconsequential, job restructuring was the most substantial cause of declining well-being for these full-time workers.

Much of the recent research describing the effects of economic change on the psychological well-being of individuals uses a social psychological model in which the recession is seen as an "event generator" that increases *individual risk* of distress through exposure to stressors. These studies are important for understanding how macroeconomic changes affect individuals, but they do not explain why aggregate levels of distress and dissatisfaction rose following the 1970s recession. By contrast, the method of analysis used in this paper emphasizes the importance of structural or *systematic risk*. Systematic risk underscores both the widespread consequences of recession (e.g., unemployment and job restructuring) and the fact that groups of workers are differentially vulnerable to these consequences based on positions in social and labor market structures. In this sense, systematic risk represents a highly appropriate way to investigate the relationship between social and economic organization and health. Systematic risk emphasizes the idea that well-being levels change because contextual conditions change and not simply because individuals are exposed to negative experiences. Individuals neither choose to become unemployed nor to have levels of job demands increase. Rather, they become unemployed because firms lay them off in response to the effects of the recession on the firm's economic well-being, and firms increase job demands for the same reason. Individual risk does not convey the influence of structural change on population well-being. The approach that we have developed here seems to capture such a process.

Finally, we need to consider the generalizability of our findings with respect to the psychological health effects of recessions. The 1974–75 recession was distinguished by a simultaneous rise in unemployment and inflation. It is quite possible that the importance of perceptions of inadequate pay for predicting dissatisfaction, for example, is related to the inflationary aspect of this particular recession. Nevertheless, there is reason to believe that the central findings would apply to the analysis of the health effects of other recessions. We tend to think of recessions solely in terms of increased unemployment, but, in fact, such unemployment affects relatively few workers. By contrast, firms' attempts to adjust to more demanding economic conditions by changing job conditions has the potential to affect every worker. Thus, our conclusion that restructuring accounts for the greatest amount of change in distress and dissatisfaction levels is consistent with both theory and the data. A recession represents a macrostructural change in economic and social relationships and should, thereby, widely affect well-being. The specifics of each recession may differ (e.g., the 1991–92 recession took place during long-term efforts to downsize firms and reduce reliance on permanent employees). However, increases in unemployment rates and productivity declines are defining characteristics of recessions so that the effects of unemployment and productivity-related job restructuring are also fundamental to understanding any consequent changes in emotional well-being.

References

Bakke, Edward Wight. 1940. *Citizens Without Work: A Study of the Task of Making a Living Without a Job.* New Haven: Yale University Press.

Blauner, Robert. 1964. *Alienation and Freedom: The Factory Worker and His Industry.* Chicago: University of Chicago Press.

Bluestone, Barry and Bennett Harrison. 1982. *The Deindustrialization of America.* New York: Basic Books.

Blumberg, Paul. 1980. *Inequality in an Age of Decline.* Oxford: Oxford University Press.

Brenner, M. Harvey. 1973. *Mental Illness and the Economy.* Cambridge, MA: Harvard University Press.

———. 1976. *Estimating the Social Costs of Economic Policy: Implications for Mental and Physical Health, and Criminal Aggression.* Congressional Research Service of the Library of Congress Joint Economic Committee of Congress. Washington, DC: Government Printing Office.

———. 1984. *Estimating the Effect of Economic Change on National Mental Health and Social Well-Being.* Subcommittee on Economic Goals and Intergovernmental Policy of the Joint Economic Committee, U.S. Congress. Washington, DC: Government Printing Office.

———. 1987. "Relation of Economic Change to Swedish Health and Social Well-Being, 1950–1980." *Social Science and Medicine* 25:183–95.

———. 1995. "Political Economy and Health." Pp. 21–246 in *Society and Health,* edited by B. C. Amick, S. Levine, A. R. Tarlov, and D. C. Walsh. New York: Oxford University Press.

Brenner, M. Harvey and Anne Mooney. 1983. "Unemployment and Health in the Context of Economic Change." *Social Science and Medicine* 17(16):1125–38.

Campbell, Angus, Philip E. Converse, W. Ward, and L. Rogers. 1976. *The Quality of American Life.* New York: Russell Sage.

Caplovitz, David. 1979. *Making Ends Meet.* Beverly Hills, CA: Sage.

Catalano, Ralph and David Dooley. 1977. "Economic Predictors of Depressed Mood and Stressful Live Events." *Journal of Health and Social Behavior* 18:292–307.

———. 1979. "The Economy as Stressor: A Sectoral Analysis." *Review of Social Economy* 37:175–87.

———. 1983. "Health Effects of Economic Instability: A Test of Economic Stress Hypothesis." *Journal of Health and Social Behavior* 24:46–60.

Catalano, Ralph, Karen Rook, and David Dooley. 1986. "Labor Markets and Help-Seeking: A Test of the Employment Security Hypothesis." *Journal of Health and Social Behavior* 27:277–87.

Cobb, Sidney and Stanislav V. Kasl. 1977. *Termination: The Consequences of Job Loss.* Cincinnati: National Institute for Occupational Safety and Health.

Cummings, Scott. 1987. "Vulnerability to the Effects of Recession: Minority and Female Workers." *Social Forces* 65:834–57.

Dooley, David and Ralph Catalano. 1980. "Economic Change as a Cause of Behavioral Disorder." *Psychological Bulletin* 87:450–68.

Durkheim, Emile. [1897]1951. *Suicide: A Study in Sociology.* Translated by John A. Spalding and George Simpson. New York: Free Press.

Fenwick, Rudy and Mark Tausig. 1994. "The Macroeconomic Context of Job Stress." *Journal of Health and Social Behavior* 35:266–82.

Hodson, Randy D. 1984. "Corporate Structure and Job Satisfaction: A Focus on Employer Characteristics." *Sociology and Social Research* 69:22–49.

Horwitz, Allan. 1984. "The Economy and Social Pathology." *Annual Review of Sociology* 10: 95–119.

Jahoda, Marie. 1982. *Employment and Unemployment: A Social Psychological Analysis.* New York: Cambridge University Press.

Karasek, Robert A. 1979. "Job Demands, Job Decision Latitude, and Mental Strain: Implications for Job Redesign." *Administrative Science Quarterly* 24:285–306.

Komarovsky, Mira. 1940. *The Unemployed Man and His Family.* New York: Dryden.

Liem, Ramsay and Paula Rayman. 1982. "Health and Social Costs of Unemployment Research and Policy Considerations." *American Psychologist* 37:1116–23.

Lincoln, James R. and Arne L. Kalleberg. 1985. "Work Organization and Work Commitment: A Study of Plants and Employees in the US and Japan." *American Sociological Review* 50:738–60.

Marshall, James R. and Hodge, R. W. 1981. "Durkheim and Pierce on Suicide and Economic Change." *Social Science Research* 10:101–14.

Mirowsky, John. 1998. Personal Communication, January 23.

Mirowsky, John and Catherine E. Ross. 1989. *Social Causes of Psychological Distress.* New York: Aldine.

Spenner, Kenneth. 1983. "Deciphering Prometheus: Temporal Change in the Skill Level of Work." *American Sociological Review* 48:824–37.

Stolzenberg, Ross M. 1978. "Bringing the Boss Back In: Employer Size, Employee Schooling and Socioeconomic Achievement." *American Sociological Review* 43:813–28.

Susser, Mervyn. 1994. "The Logic in Ecological: II. The Logic of Design." *American Journal of Public Health* 84:830–35.

Turner, Blake. 1995. "Employment Context and the Health Effects of Unemployment." *Journal of Health and Social Behavior* 36:213–29.

U.S. Bureau of the Census. 1978. *Statistical Abstracts of the United States.* Washington, DC: Government Printing Office.

DISCUSSION

1. Tausig and Fenwick introduce the concept of systematic risk as distinct from individual risk. What are the differences between the two concepts? How does the concept of systematic risk add to our understanding of the effects of macroeconomic change on the well-being of the population?

2. Do you think that Tausig and Fenwick's results would generalize to other recessions? Why or why not?

3. In contrast to Evenson and Simon's study, which received a great deal of media attention, Tausig and Fenwick's study received almost none. Why might the media have been less interested in Tausig and Fenwick's study? What angle might you take to generate media interest in this kind of research?

David R. Williams, Yan Yu, James S. Jackson, and Norman B. Anderson

Racial Differences in Physical and Mental Health: Socioeconomic Status, Stress, and Discrimination

In this selection, David R. Williams and colleagues take up the important question of what accounts for racial differences in physical and mental health. Specifically, they evaluate the ability of socioeconomic status, perceived discrimination, and general measures of stress to explain the poorer physical and mental health outcomes observed among African Americans as compared to whites in the United States. Their analysis provides answers and also raises new questions about the complex mechanisms through which racism, in all of its forms, damages health.

One of the most firmly established and frequently reported patterns in the distribution of health status in the United States is that African Americans (or blacks) have higher rates of death, disease, and disability than whites have. This pattern has been documented for over 150 years (Krieger, 1987) and in 1990 blacks had higher rates than whites for 13 of the 15 leading causes of death in the United States (National Center for Health Statistics, 1994). Although the findings are not uniform, studies of mental health status also generally find that, compared to whites, blacks have higher levels of psychological distress (nonspecific emotional symptoms) and lower levels of subjective well-being (Vega & Rumbaut, 1991). Recent data reveal that for some indicators of health status, such as infant mortality and low birth weight, the relative gap between blacks and whites has widened in recent decades, while for other indicators, such as life expectancy and sexually transmitted diseases, there has been an absolute decline in the health of the African American population in some recent years (Williams & Collins, 1995).

Despite decades of research, our understanding of the factors responsible for racial differences in health is still limited. Historically, research on racial differences in health has been premised on the notion that blacks and whites were biologically distinct groups and that observed disparities could be traced to biological differences between the races (Krieger, 1987). Much of this research was blatantly racist and explicitly attempted to provide a scientific rationale for policies of racial inequality. Blatant racial bias is rare in current research in the medical sciences, but there is a persistent tendency, even in the face of scientific evidence to the contrary, to define race in terms of underlying genetic homogeneity and to understand racial differences in health in terms of innate biological differences (Williams, Lavizzo-Mourey, & Warren, 1994; Witzig, 1996). In contrast, anthropologists (Gould, 1977; Lewontin, 1972) and

Williams, David R., Yan Yu, James S. Jackson, and Norman B. Anderson. 1997. "Racial differences in physical and mental health: Socio-economic status, stress and discrimination." *Journal of Health Psychology* 2:335–351.

health researchers (Cooper & David, 1986; Krieger, Rowley, Herman, Avery, & Phillips, 1993; Williams, in press) emphasize the scientific information that indicates that race is a gross indicator of distinctive social and individual histories and not a measure of biological distinctiveness. Races are socially constructed categories that have emerged in the context of social and economic oppression and have been used to perpetuate economic, cultural, ideological, political, and legal systems of inequality (Omi & Winant, 1986). This view of race does not deny that there may be biological aspects to race. However, genetic or biologic factors are not the central defining characteristics of race and are unlikely to be the primary sources of racial differences in health. Although racial differences in biological processes have been found (e.g., in sodium secretion), these processes may be influenced by psychosocial factors (Anderson, McNeilly, & Myers, 1991). Moreover, not only can social conditions produce physiological differences between races, they may also interact with any innate biological differences to affect health.

RACE, SES, AND HEALTH

The worsening health status of African Americans must be understood within the larger context of the increasing polarization of income and wealth in the United States. In recent years much of the past gains in economic status of blacks relative to whites has been arrested. For some economic indicators blacks have experienced a decline relative to whites, while others reveal an absolute decline in the economic situation of African Americans (Karoly, 1992; Smith & Welch, 1989). The United States is not unique. There is growing income inequality in other western industrialized countries (Danziger & Gottschalk, 1993), and a commensurate widening in socio-economic status (SES) differences in health (Williams & Collins, 1995).

Given the strong relationship between race and systems of inequality, social and behavioral scientists have emphasized that differences between the races in socio-economic circumstances are centrally responsible for racial variations in health. There are large racial differences in SES. The 1990 Census, for example, indicated that compared to whites, African Americans have a median family income that is 63 percent less, are more than twice as likely to be unemployed, three times as likely to be poor and twice as likely not to have graduated from college (National Center for Health Statistics, 1993). Accordingly, studies of racial differences in health routinely control for SES and it is generally found that adjustment for SES substantially reduces and sometimes eliminates racial disparities in health (Krieger et al., 1993; Lillie-Blanton, Parsons, Gayle, & Dievler, 1996).

Although racial differences are markedly reduced, it is frequently found that they persist even after adjustment for SES (Lillie-Blanton et al., 1996). Moreover, for some indicators of SES, racial differences increase as SES increases (Krieger et al., 1993). Accordingly, several recent critiques have emphasized that the current paradigm of an almost exclusive focus on differences in SES as responsible for racial differences in health is inadequate (Cooper & David, 1986; Hummer, 1996; Krieger et al., 1993; Williams et al., 1994). First, SES measures are not equivalent across racial groups. That is, there are racial differences in income returns for a given level of education, the quality of education, the level of wealth associated with a given level of income, the purchasing power of income, the stability of employment and the health risks associated with working in particular occupations (Williams & Collins, 1995). Thus, even when race differences in health are "explained" by SES, group differences in the very nature of SES make the interpretation of such findings difficult.

Second, it has been emphasized that SES is not just a confounder of the relationship between race and health, but part of the causal pathway by which race affects health (Cooper & David, 1986). That is, race is an antecedent and determinant of SES, and SES differences between blacks and whites reflect, in part, the impact of economic discrimination as produced by large-scale societal structures. Racial residential segregation is a prime example of a societal structure that importantly restricts socio-economic opportunity and mobility for blacks (Massey & Denton, 1993). Third, the conceptualization and measurement of SES is limited. SES is too often used in a static, routine and atheoretical manner. Finally, the persistence of racial differences after adjustment for SES emphasizes that race is more than SES and that additional research attention is required to understand the ways in which unique experiences linked to race, such as non-economic forms of racial discrimination can adversely affect health.

At the present time it is unclear whether the failure of SES to account completely for racial differences in health reflects limitations of the measures of SES or the failure of researchers to consider race-related risk factors such as racial discrimination. Enhancing our understanding of the ways in which race and SES combine to affect health will require research initiatives in two directions. First, we need more comprehensive and theoretically informed measures of socio-economic position. Second, we need more concerted attention to conceptualize and measure the effects of racism on health.

IMPROVED MEASUREMENT OF SOCIAL POSITION

Much prior research on the role of socio-economic status in racial differences in health has used only one indicator of SES in a given study. Currently, the extent to which limitations in the measurement of SES accounts for the failure of SES to account completely for racial differences in health is not known. In particular, the contribution of multiple indicators of SES to racial differences in health is unclear. In addition, health researchers have recently emphasized the importance of including in epidemiologic studies theoretically driven measures of social class to characterize fully the relationship between social stratification and health (Krieger et al., 1993; Krieger, Williams, & Moss, 1997). Current measures give greater emphasis to Weberian notions of social stratification than to the Marxist emphasis on relationship to the system of production. The Marxist view of class emphasizes that social classes are collectivities defined in relationship to other social classes on the basis of opposing interests. The distribution of power and resources vary across social classes but social classes are not primarily gradational in the extent to which they possess particular attributes. Wright (1985) indicates that social classes in contemporary society are rooted in the complex intersection of exploitation based on the ownership of capital assets, organizational assets, and the possession of skill or credential assets. From a comprehensive battery of survey items to measure social class, Wright (1997) has recently identified a smaller subset of items that capture most of the variation in the concept.

THE EXPERIENCE OF RACIAL BIAS AND HEALTH

A growing number of researchers have emphasized that racism is a neglected but central societal force that adversely affects the health of racial and ethnic minority populations (Cooper, 1993; Cooper, Steinhauer, Miller, David, & Shatzkin, 1981; King & Williams, 1995; Krieger et al., 1993; Williams, 1996a; Williams et al., 1994). The term *racism* includes an ideology of superiority that categorizes and ranks various groups, negative attitudes and beliefs about outgroups and differential treatment of outgroups by individuals and societal institutions. The most profound impact of racism is at the level of societal institutions in shaping the socio-economic opportunities, mobility and life chances of racialized groups. The quality and quantity of a broad range of health-enhancing resources, including medical care, are differentially distributed by societal institutions, to members of discriminated against racial groups. Much of the observed racial differences in SES reflects the results of these processes.

In addition to discrimination at the societal level, stressful life experiences linked to race can also adversely impact the health of minority populations. Stress can affect racial differences in health in at least two ways. First, stress is not randomly distributed in the population. It is linked to social structure, and social status and social roles determine both the types and quantities of stress to which an individual is exposed (Pearlin, 1989; Williams & House, 1991). The structural location of blacks in society would lead them to have higher levels of stress than whites. Second, the experience of specific incidents of racial bias can generate psychic distress and lead to alterations in physiological processes that can adversely affect health. There is growing attention to the pervasiveness and persistence of racial discrimination for African Americans (Cose, 1993; Essed, 1991; Feagin, 1991).

Descriptions of these experiences suggest that they capture important elements of stressful experiences that are known to be predictive of adverse changes in health. Critiques of the stress literature have also emphasized that the current approaches to the assessment of stress are not comprehensive and do not capture some of the stressful life experiences of poor populations in general and racial minority populations in particular (Aneshensel, 1992; Thoits, 1983). Several studies indicate that experiences of discrimination based on race or ethnicity can adversely affect physical and mental health (Amaro, Russo, & Johnson, 1987; Jackson et al., 1996; James, La Croix, Kleinbaum, & Strogatz, 1984; Krieger, 1990; Salgado de Snyder, 1987; Williams & Chung, in press). And one recent study found that racial discrimination not only is associated with systolic and diastolic blood pressure but accounts for a part of the association between race and blood pressure (Krieger & Sidney, 1996).

Studies of the relationship between racial discrimination and health are still in their infancy and are subject to several limitations. First, although experiences of racial bias are complex and multidimensional (McNeilly et al., 1996), the conceptualization of discrimination has been limited in many of the studies to date such that the phenomenon has not been comprehensively assessed. Some studies, for example, have utilized only a single-item global measure of discrimination. Second, studies have typically focused only on major experiences of discrimination. In contrast, Essed (1991) emphasizes that discrimination is a structured part of everyday experiences and includes not only major stressful life experiences but recurrent indignities and irritations in everyday situations.

Third, limited attention has been given to experiences of unfair treatment for the white population. It has been emphasized that the major forces affecting the health of minority populations are important societal factors that affect the health of the larger society on a smaller scale and in less intensive a manner (Cooper et al., 1981; Jackson & Inglehart, 1995). Consistent with this perspective some evidence indicates that the experience of unfair treatment, irrespective of race or ethnicity, may have negative consequences for health (Harburg et al., 1973). It is likely that African Americans will have more frequent and more intense experiences of unfair treatment than will whites, but perceived racial or ethnic bias, including perceptions of reverse discrimination, could also adversely affect the health of whites (Jackson, Williams, & Torres, in press). Thus, studying the impact of experiences of unfair treatment on the health of black and white adults can highlight the extent to which patterns observed among blacks are unique.

This article analyses probability sample data from a large metropolitan area in the United States to examine the extent to which multiple measures of social stratification combine with race-related stressful experiences and more general measures of stress to affect health and explain racial/ethnic variations in health status. Prior research has tended to test these major classes of explanatory factors in isolation or in pairs. We have multiple measures within each class of factors and can examine how each class performs in relation to the others. This model of competing explanations has rarely been tested in the literature with the breadth and range of measures in this article.

The goals of this study are to assess the extent to which: (1) levels of general stress and race-related stress vary by race; (2) indicators of socio-economic status and social class, considered singly and in combination, can account for black-white differences in physical and mental health; and (3) race-related stressors and general measures of stress can account for racial differences in health. We hypothesize that multiple measures of SES will account for a large part of racial differences in health. We also hypothesize that the comprehensive assessment of stress, both race-related and general sources of stress, will play incremental roles in accounting for reported racial differences in health.

METHODS

Sample

The data for our analyses come from the 1995 Detroit Area Study (DAS). The DAS is a multistage area probability sample consisting of 1139 adult respondents, 18 years of age and older, residing in Wayne, Oakland and Macomb counties in Michigan, including the city of Detroit. Face-to-face interviews were completed between April and October 1995 by University of Michigan graduate students in a research-training practicum in survey research and professional interviewers from the Survey Research Center. The response rate was 70 percent. Race was measured by respondent self-identification Blacks were oversampled and the final sample included 520 whites; 586 blacks; and 33 Asians, Native Americans, and Hispanics. All of the analyses reported in this article use only the black and white respondents.

Measures and Analyses

All intervally scaled measures were coded in the direction of the variable name so that a high score reflected a high value of the variable name. Four measures of health status are used as dependent variables in the analyses. Self-rated ill health is a widely used general indicator of health status that is strongly related to mortality and other objective measures of health. It captures a respondent's overall assessment of health as "excellent, very good, good, fair, or poor." Psychological distress sums the frequency with which respondents felt sad, nervous, restless or fidgety, hopeless, worthless, and that everything was an effort in the past 30 days. Bed-days, a measure of physical incapacitation, is a count of the number of days in the last month that the respondent was totally unable to work or carry out normal activities because of both physical health problems and emotional distress. Measures of psychological well-being attempt to assess an individual's overall perception of the quality of life. Our well-being measure combines each respondent's assessment of overall life satisfaction on a 5-point scale ranging from "completely satisfied" to "not at all satisfied" with the respondent's agreement with the statement: "My life is full of joy and satisfaction" on a 4-point agree–disagree scale.

RACIAL BIAS IN RESEARCH ON MENTAL ILLNESS

Race and mental health have been entangled since the early days of U.S. history. Krieger (1987) describes an early scholarly article on mulattoes that deliberately falsified data on rates of mental illness from the 1840 U.S. Census to make it appear as if persons of mixed white-black heritage had higher rates of mental illness than either "pure" whites or blacks. In the 1850s, many physicians considered blacks constitutionally suited for slavery, so much so that blacks who tried to escape slavery were designated as suffering from "drapetomania," a mental disorder. Tony Brown (2003) contends that racial biases still exist in contemporary research on mental health. Specifically, he believes that racial stratification results in unique mental health problems for both blacks and whites that are not captured in traditional diagnostic classifications. These include nihilistic tendencies (tendencies to destroy oneself), anti-self issues (internalization of negative stereotypes and estrangement from one's racial identity), and suppressed anger, all of which are common among blacks, delusional denial, which occurs among both blacks and whites, and extreme racial paranoia (extreme fear of interacting with blacks), which occurs among whites. By failing to include these kinds of mental health problems in our studies, we may mischaracterize racial differences in mental health. Together, these authors' writings suggest that any attempt to document racial and ethnic differences in mental health must first address complex arguments about the nature and measurement of mental illness.

Krieger, Nancy. 1987. "Shades of Difference: Theoretical Underpinnings of the Medical Controversy on Black/White Differences in the United States: 1830–1870." *International Journal of Health Services* 17:259–278.

Brown, Tony N. 2003. "Critical Race Theory Speaks to the Sociology of Mental Health: Mental Health Problems Produced by Racial Stratification." *Journal of Health and Social Behavior* 44:292–301.

Age (in years) and gender (1 = female, 0 = male) are sociodemographic control variables used in the analyses. Race was assessed by respondent self-report. It was coded as a dummy variable in the regression analyses (1 = blacks, 0 = whites). Income and education are two measures of socio-economic status. Our income measure captures total household income in the previous year. Since income is a highly skewed variable, we used its logarithm. Because the meaning of a given level of income is related to the number of persons in the analyses, household size is included in the analyses whenever we analyse income. Household size is a count of the number of persons living in the household ranging from 1 to 6 or more. Education is divided into four categories that capture meaningful differences in educational credentials: 0–11 years, 12 years, 13–15 years, and 16 or more years.

Education is used as a set of dummy variables in the regression analyses with 16 years or more as an omitted category.

Following Wright (1997) we classified respondents into social classes based on their pattern of responses to three questions:

1. "Do you hold a managerial position at your place of employment?"
2. "As an official part of your job, do you supervise the work of other employees, have responsibility for or tell other employees what work to do?"
3. "At your work place, do you participate in making decisions about such things as the products or services offered, the total number of people employed, budgets, and so forth?"

Respondents who gave an affirmative response to all three questions were categorized as Managers, while respondents who answered "no" to all three questions were categorized as Workers. Those who answered "yes" or "no" to the managerial question, "yes" to the supervisory question and "no" to the decision-making question are Supervisors. Manager was treated as the omitted category in our regression analyses.

Two measures of race-related stress were utilized: discrimination and everyday discrimination. Unlike prior research, both of them were framed in the context of unfairness instead of in the context of race. Discrimination, a measure of major experiences of unfair treatment, is a count of three items:

1. "Do you think you have ever been *unfairly* fired or denied promotion?"
2. "For *unfair* reasons, do you think you have ever not been hired for a job?"
3. "Do you think you have ever been *unfairly* stopped, searched, questioned, physically threatened or abused by the police?"

Our second measure, everyday discrimination, attempts to measure more chronic, routine, and relatively minor experiences of unfair treatment (Essed, 1991). It sums nine items that capture the frequency of the following experiences in the day-to-day lives of respondents: being treated with less courtesy than others; less respect than others; receiving poorer service than others in restaurants or stores; people acting as if you are not smart; they are better than you; they are afraid of you; they think you are dishonest; being called names or insulted; and being threatened or harassed.

Three general indicators of stress were also utilized. Chronic stress is a count of problems in the last month or so, with aging parents, spouse or partner, children, hassles at work, and balancing work and family demands. Financial stress is measured by the respondent's assessment of the difficulty of meeting the family's monthly payments on a 5-point scale ranging from extremely difficult to not difficult at all. Life events is a count of nine possible experiences in the year prior to the interview. These include serious illness or injury, physical attack or assault, robbery or burglary, involuntary retirement, unemployment, a move to a worse residence or neighborhood, serious financial problems, interracial arguments or conflicts and death of a loved one.

The data were weighted to take into account differential probabilities of selection and to adjust the demographics of the sample to that of the area from which it was drawn. Simple descriptive analyses are used to present racial differences in the distribution of responses on SES, social class, and stress. Ordinary least squares regression is used to estimate the size and statistical significance of the associations between our independent variables and health status.

RESULTS

Racial differences in SES and stress

Table 1 presents the distributions of SES, social class, and stress by race. Racial differences for all of the variables are significant at $p \leq .05$. Blacks have significantly higher scores than have whites on all variables in Table 1 except the measure of chronic stress, where the mean for whites exceeds that for blacks. Levels of educational attainment vary by race, with the racial gap being especially pronounced at both ends of the educational distribution. Blacks are 1.6 times more likely than whites to have completed less than 12 years of education. There are no racial differences in the middle of the educational distribution (high-school graduation, some college), but whites are almost twice as likely as African Americans to have graduated from college. A similar pattern is evident for income. Blacks are almost four times as likely as whites to have a total annual income of less than $10,000 (21 percent vs 6 percent) and are 1.4 times more likely than whites to be in the $10,000–$29,999 range. Equivalent percentages of blacks and whites are in the middle-income category ($30,000–$59,999), but whites are 2.5 times more likely than blacks to have incomes over $60,000 (41 percent vs 16 percent). The lower average income of blacks provides for households that on average are significantly larger than those of whites. The racial distribution by social class follows the familiar pattern noted for education and income. Blacks are more likely than whites to be in the worker category (61 percent vs 51 percent), equivalent numbers of blacks and whites are supervisors, but whites are almost twice as likely as blacks to be managers (24 percent vs 13 percent).

Table 1 also shows differences between the races for the stress measures. Blacks are more likely than whites to report major experiences of discrimination in employment and in contact with the police. Only slightly more African Americans than whites (29 percent vs 25 percent) report one discriminatory event, but blacks are twice as likely to report two discriminatory experiences and seven times more likely to report three experiences. Blacks also have significantly higher scores on the chronic ongoing indicators of everyday discrimination, although the magnitude of the racial gap is not as large as for the major experiences of discrimination. There is a significant

Table 1 Race Differences in the Distribution of SES, Social Class, and Stress, Means and Percentages (P)

	Blacks	Whites
Socioeconomic status		
1. Education (P)		
a. 0–11 yrs	19.5	11.8
b. 12 yrs	31.9	30.4
c. 13–15 yrs	33.0	28.4
d. 16+ yrs	15.5	29.4
2. Household income (P)		
a. $0–9,999	21.0	5.7
b. $10,000–$29,999	32.4	23.4
c. $30,000–$59,999	30.3	29.7
d. $60,000+	16.3	41.2
3. Household Size	3.098	2.88
Social Class		
4. Social class (P)		
a. Worker	60.6	50.8
b. Supervisor	26.5	25.5
c. Manager	12.9	23.7
Race-related stress		
5. Discrimination (P)		
a. None	37.7	63.8
b. One event	28.7	24.8
c. Two events	22.1	9.8
d. Three events	11.5	1.6
6. Everyday discrimination	2.099	1.71
General stress		
7. Chronic stress	0.90	1.07
8. Financial stress	1.996	1.65
9. Life events	1.561	0.85

racial difference on chronic stress, with whites having higher levels of chronic stress than blacks. Levels of financial stress are significantly higher for blacks than for whites and the average score on the life-events scale for blacks is almost twice that of whites.

Race, SES, and Health

Table 2 presents the findings for the association among race, SES and social class, with self-reported ill health and bed-days. Five regression models are presented for each of the health outcomes. The first model shows the association between race and health, adjusted for the demographic variables (age and gender). The next three models consider the impact of education, income and occupation, considered singly, while the final model enters the three measures of social position simultaneously. As expected, Table 2 shows that blacks report higher levels of poor health than do whites. This difference is

Table 2 Unstandardized Regression Coefficients for the Association of Race, SES, and Social Class to Self-Reported Ill Health and Bed-Days for Blacks and Whites, Detroit Area Study (DAS)

	Self-reported ill health					Bed-days				
	I	II	III	IV	V	I	II	III	IV	V
1. Race (black)	.315**	.241**	.140*	.303**	.131†	.194**	.170**	.087†	.186**	.086†
2. Age	.018**	.018**	.019**	.019**	.018**	.005**	.004**	.004**	.005**	.004**
3. Sex (female)	.061	.030	−.012	.046	−.014	.034	.029	−.013	.025	−.008
4. Education										
a. 0–11 yrs		.682**			.485**		.257**			.099
b. 12 yrs		.386**			.286**		.123*			.027
c. 13–15 yrs		.315**			.266**		.048			−.011
d. 16+ yrs (omitted)										
5. Household income (log)			−.630**		−.503**			−.394**		−.365**
6. Household size			.048		.037			.010		.006
7. Social Class										
a. Worker				.117	−.083				.093	−.002
b. Supervisor				.029	−.138				.077	.036
c. Manager (omitted)										
Constant	1.494	1.252	4.285	1.433	3.614	−.070	−.125	1.761	−.130	1.627
R^2	.118	.149	.170	.120	.189	.028	.041	.072	.030	.075

†= $p \le .10$; *= $p \le .05$; **= $p \le .01$

significant, after adjusted for age and gender and is reduced by almost 25 percent when adjusted for education. The race effect is dramatically reduced when economic status is considered but it remains significant. Controlling for income reduced the coefficient for race by 56 percent from the first model. Social class is unrelated to variations in self-reported health and makes no contribution to explaining racial differences in health. When all three measures of social position are considered in Model V, the racial difference is reduced by more than half, to marginal significance. When considered simultaneously, the association of both education and income with health is reduced from the earlier models, but they both remain significant predictors of variations in self-reported ill health.

A similar pattern is evident for bed-days. Blacks report higher levels of bed-days than do whites. People with a high-school education or less report higher levels of bed-days than do college graduates. However, adjusting for education only minimally reduces the racial difference on this health income. Income is inversely related to bed-days and adjustment for income reduces the coefficient for race by 55 percent, to marginal significance. Similar to the pattern observed for self-reported ill health, social class is unrelated to bed-days and plays no role in accounting for racial differences. The final model

Table 3 Unstandardized Regression Coefficients for the Association of Race, SES, and Social Class to Well-Being and Psychological Distress for Blacks and Whites, Detroit Area Study (DAS)

	Well-being					Psychological distress				
	I	II	III	IV	V	I	II	III	IV	V
1. Race (black)	−.331**	−.262**	−.083	−.320**	−.083	.493	.244	−.117	.467	−.114
2. Age	.003	.004†	.003	.003	.003	−.014†	−.020*	−.007	−.014†	−.013
3. Sex (female)	.115	.139†	.210*	.130	.202*	.828**	.776**	.579†	.809**	.684*
4. Education										
a. 0–11 yrs		−.654**			−.355*		2.608**			1.944**
b. 12 yrs		−.441**			−.277*		1.282**			.817*
c. 13–15 yrs		−.228*			−.144		.335			.075
d. 16+yrs (omitted)										
5. Household income (log)			.879**		.782**			−.2169**		−1.666**
6. Household size			−.076*		−.067*			.398**		.334**
7. Social class										
a. Worker				−.117	.109				.201	−.473
b. Supervisor				−.007	.183				.980*	.479
c. Manager (omitted)										
Constant	5.782	6.006	1.919	5.838	2.382	6.840	6.314	15.474	6.476	13.166
R^2	.014	.039	.071	.016	.079	.012	.043	.046	.018	.067

†$= p \le .10$; *$= p \le .05$; **$= p \le .01$

indicates that the racial difference in bed-days remains marginally significant when adjusted for education, income, and social class. Instructively, unlike the pattern observed for self-reported ill health, educational differences disappear when adjusted for income. Thus, income emerges as the strongest predictor of variations in bed-days.

Table 3 presents similar models for the two measures of mental health status—psychological well-being and psychological distress. The table shows that although levels of psychological well-being are unrelated to age and gender, African Americans report lower levels of well-being than whites do. Education is positively related to well-being. College graduates enjoy higher levels of psychological well-being than do people with less education. Moreover, the education–well-being association fits the pattern of a linear graded relationship. Persons in each educational category report lower levels of well-being than do the category just above them. The consideration of education reduces racial differences in well-being by more than 20 percent. The third model reveals that there is also a strong positive relationship between income and well-being and an inverse relationship between well-being and household size. Moreover, consideration of economic status reduces racial differences in well-being by 75 percent to non-significance. Similar to the pattern observed earlier, social class is unrelated to variations in well-being. The fifth model shows that when income and education are considered simultaneously, the association of each with well-being is reduced, but both of them remain significantly related to the health outcome.

The findings for psychological distress are also presented in Table 3. Although the coefficient for race is in the direction of higher levels of psychological distress for blacks vs whites, the coefficient is not significant in the first model that also includes the demographic variables. As expected, women report higher levels of psychological distress than men do. However, education is related to psychological distress, with persons with 12 years of education or less having higher levels of distress than college graduates had. Income and household size are also related to psychological distress. Distress decreases with increasing levels of income, but increases with the number of persons in the household. Social class is related to psychological distress, with supervisors reporting higher levels of distress than managers did. This relationship between social class and distress is reduced to non-significance when adjusted for income and education in the fifth model; however, both of these variables are somewhat reduced but remain significantly related to distress in this final model that considers the three social status measures together.

Race, SES, Stress, and Health

Table 4 shows the incremental contribution of stress to understanding variations in levels of self-reported ill health and bed-days. Three hierarchical regression models are presented for each outcome. The first shows the relationship between race and health, adjusted for the demographic factors, as well as, education, income, and social class. The second model considers race-related stressors and the third adds general measures of stress. While major experiences of discrimination are unrelated to self-assessed ill health, everyday discrimination is positively related to ill health. There is a small but significant increase in the explained variance from Model I to Model II. Moreover, the adjustment for the discrimination measures reduces the race coefficient by almost 40 percent, to nonsignificance. Thus, race-related stressors make a small incremental contribution to accounting for SES differences in self-reported ill health. The third model adds the three general indicators of stress and consideration of these variables produces a significant increase in the R^2. Chronic stress is unrelated to self-reported ill health, but both financial stress and major life events are positively related to ill health. That is, higher levels of stress are generally related with poorer health status. The coefficient for everyday discrimination is no longer associated with ill health once adjusted for the other measures of stress. For self-reported health, educational differentials are virtually unchanged when adjusted for stress. In contrast, adjustment for general measures of stress reduces the association between income and self-reported health by 30 percent.

Table 4 Unstandardized Regression Coefficients for the Association of Race, SES, Social Class, Race-Related Stress and General Stress to Self-Reported Ill Health and Bed-Days for Blacks and Whites, Detroit Area Study (DAS)[1]

	Self-reported ill health			Bed-days		
	I	II	III	I	II	III
1. Race (black)	.131[†]	.080	.063	.086[†]	.037	.004
2. Education						
a. 0–11 yrs	.485**	.488**	.445**	.099	.104	.054
b. 12 yrs	.286**	.280**	.287**	.027	.022	.022
c. 13–15 yrs	.266**	.257**	.236**	−.011	−.017	−.043
d. 16 + yrs (omitted)						
3. Household income (log)	−.503**	−.501**	−.353**	−.365**	−.361**	−.276**
4. Household size	.037	.039†	.012	.006	.008	−.009
Race-related stress						
5. Discrimination		.022	−.030		.014	−.029
6. Everyday discrimination		.108*	.047		.118**	.079*
General stress						
7. Chronic stress			.014			.011
8. Financial stress			.099**			.031
9. Life events			.125**			.126**
Constant	3.614	3.307	2.533	1.627	1.297	.850
R^2	.189	.194	.226	.075	.086	.131
Net R^2	—	.005*	.030**	—	.011**	.041**

[†] $= p \le .10$; * $= p \le .05$; ** $= p \le .01$
[1] Adjusted for age, gender, and social class

Similar to the findings for self-reported ill-health major experiences of discrimination are unrelated to bed-days, while everyday discrimination is positively related. Adjustment for race-related stress also reduces the marginally significant relationship between race and bed-days by almost 60 percent to non-significance. The relationship between everyday discrimination and bed-days is reduced by over 30 percent but remains significant when controlled for general indicators of stress. Of the three general indicators, only life events is positively related to bed-days. Both classes of stress variables produce a significant increase in the explained variance with the general stress variables having a larger impact. Similar to the pattern observed for self-reported ill health, consideration of stress, especially general measures of stress, reduces the association between income and bed-days by almost 25 percent from the first model. In sum, for both of the outcomes in Table 4, the consideration of stress makes an incremental contribution and, in combination with SES, completely accounts for racial differences in these health outcomes.

Table 5 shows the relationship among race, SES, and stress for psychological well-being and psychological distress. It was noted earlier that racial differences in well-being were completely accounted for when adjusted for income,

Table 5 Unstandardized Regression Coefficients for the Association of Race, SES, Social Class, Race-Related Stress and General Stress to Well-Being and Psychological Distress for Blacks and Whites, Detroit Area Study (DAS)[1]

	Well-being			Psychological distress		
	I	II	III	I	II	III
1. Race (black)	−.083	.199†	.141	−.114	−1.083**	−.830*
2. Education						
a. 0–11 yrs	−.355*	−.368*	−.374**	1.944**	2.021**	2.154**
b. 12 yrs	−.277*	−.248*	−.322**	.817*	.659†	.967*
c. 13–15 yrs	−.144	−.096	−.101	.075	−.044	.021
d. 16+ yrs (omitted)						
3. Household income (log)	.782**	.762**	.575**	−1.666**	−.550**	−1.085**
4. Household size	−.067*	−.080*	−.003	.334**	.355**	.090
Race-related stress						
5. Discrimination		−.150**	−.066		−.046	−.331†
6. Everyday discrimination		−.550**	−.391**		2.818**	2.215**
General stress						
7. Chronic stress			−.181**			.805**
8. Financial stress			−.213**			.557**
9. Life events			−.094*			.304*
Constant	2.382	4.027	5.016	13.166	5.699	3.323
R^2	.079	.157	.213	.067	.185	.241
Net R^2	—	.078**	.055**	—	.118**	.056**

† = $p \leq .10$; * = $p \leq .05$; ** = $p \leq .01$

[1]Adjusted for age, gender, and social class

while race was unrelated to psychological distress. At the same time, it was of interest to note the relationship between stress and these indicators of mental health status. Models similar to those in Table 4 are presented for each of the mental health outcomes in Table 5. Both of the measures of race-related stress are inversely related to psychological well-being. Persons who report higher levels of major experiences of discrimination and everyday discrimination report lower levels of psychological well-being. Consideration of race-related stress produces a substantial increase in the explained variance.

Interestingly, when the two measures of race-related stress are included in the model, the association between race and psychological well-being becomes positive and marginally significant. That is, there is a tendency for blacks to report higher levels of psychological well-being when race-related stressors are taken into account. This marginally significant positive association between race and psychological well-being in Model II is reduced by one-third to non-significance when adjusted for the general measures of stress in Model III. Chronic stress, financial stress, and life events are all inversely related to psychological well-being and this set of stress measures significantly increases the variance explained in well-being, When controlled for the general measures of stress, the coefficient for everyday discrimination is reduced by almost one-third, but remains significant, while the coefficient for major experiences of discrimination is reduced to non-significance.

The findings for psychological distress are similar to those observed for well-being. There is a strong positive relationship between everyday discrimination and psychological distress. Persons who report that they frequently experienced everyday discrimination also report higher levels of psychological distress. Major experiences of discrimination are unrelated to psychological distress, but consideration of race-related stress makes an incremental contribution of 12 percent to the explained variance. Importantly, once the coefficients for race-related stress are included in the model the relationship between race and psychological distress become significant. That is, when experiences of unfairness are controlled for blacks and whites, blacks report significantly *lower* levels of psychological distress than whites do.

DISCUSSION

This study has several limitations. First, the data are cross-sectional and provide no basis for causal directionality. At the same time, the findings are consistent with a large body of work that suggests that social conditions are important determinants of variations in health. High levels of stress and low socio-economic status are two important social factors that have been identified in prior research as pathogenic. Second, the measures of discrimination utilized in this study are based on respondent self-report. This criticism is frequently raised about the measurement of racial discrimination, although it applies to much of the measurement of stress more generally. Considerable evidence suggests that discrimination is ubiquitous in U.S. society (Cose, 1993; Feagin, 1991; Gardner, 1995). The stressfulness of a life experience is determined, in part, by the meaning it has for the individual, which is importantly linked to that individual's personal and social history. Thus, a respondent's perception and appraisal of a life experience is a critical component of the experience of stress. Nonetheless, strategies that have been developed to improve the measurement of stress (Cohen, Kessler, & Gordon, 1995), also apply to the assessment of discrimination.

MENTAL HEALTH AMONG AMERICAN INDIANS

The research of Spero Manson and his colleagues at the American Indian and Alaskan Natives Program at the University of Colorado Health Sciences Center adds depth to our understanding of the role of race and ethnicity in mental health. In a study conducted with members of one southwest and two northern plains tribes, they assessed 16 types of trauma including being a victim of a disaster (e.g., flood, fire), interpersonal trauma (e.g., rape, molestation, physical abuse), and witnessing trauma, among others. They summarize their results as follows: "Male northern plains tribal members were most likely to have experienced noninterpersonal trauma, and female southwest tribal members were least likely. Female tribal members were more likely than male tribal members to have experienced interpersonal trauma. Specifically, they were more likely to report physical abuse, particularly by a spouse, which demonstrated the highest prevalence. Witnessed traumas were common in all groups. Female members of the northern plains tribe were more likely than men of the southwest tribe to have witnessed family violence. A third of the sample reported that someone close to them had experienced a trauma. Finally, lifetime experience of any trauma was high across both populations and genders, ranging from 62.4 % for male southwest tribe members to 69.8% for female northern plains tribe members (p. 852)." These rates can be compared to national estimates of 51.2 percent and 60.7 percent for men and women, respectively. Trauma was more common among people with higher levels of education and less common among people living in poverty. Compared to national estimates, American Indians also have higher rates of alcohol dependence and posttraumatic stress disorder, controlling for education, marital status, and poverty status. These findings highlight the unique mental health disadvantages of the American Indian population in the United States.

Manson, Spero M., Janette Beals, Suzell A. Klein, Calvin D. Croy, and AI-SUPERPFP Team. 2005. "Social Epidemiology of Trauma Among 2 American Indian Reservation Populations." *American Journal of Public Health* 95:851–859.

Beals, Janette, Douglas K. Novins, Nancy R. Whitesell, Paul Spicer, Christina M. Mitchell, and Spero M. Manson. 1005. "Prevalence of Mental Disorders and Utilization of Mental Health Services in Two American Indian Reservation Populations: Mental Health Disparities in a National Context." *American Journal of Psychiatry* 162:1723–1732.

Finally, this study focused only on blacks and whites. There is considerably more racial and ethnic variation in the United States that is also importantly linked to variations in SES and health (Williams, 1996b). Recent studies find that other minority groups, such as Asians (Kim & Lewis, 1994) and Hispanics (Telles & Murgia, 1990) also experience discrimination. Future research must explore the health consequences of discrimination for the various groups that make up the racial and ethnic diversity of the U.S. population.

At the same time, this study provides important additional evidence of the importance of the social environment in understanding racial variations in health. We found racial differences in the expected direction for three of the four health outcomes considered. African Americans reported lower levels of psychological well-being; higher rates of self-reported ill health; and more bed-days than whites did. Education and especially income were importantly related to all of the health outcomes examined and played a major role in explaining racial differences in health. Social class, as measured in this study, was generally unrelated to health and played no role in racial differences in disease. Our analyses also found that race-related stress, as well as general measures of stress, are generally adversely related to health and make an incremental contribution to explaining racial differences in health. Race-related stress was more strongly related to our indicators of mental health than it was to physical health.

For both measures of mental health status, the mental health of blacks tended to exceed that of whites once we adjusted for race-related stress. This pattern is consistent with the notion that these stressful experiences may affect the health of whites more adversely than that of blacks. A recent review noted that for a number of child and infant health outcomes, although blacks are more exposed to adverse risk factors, these factors have a larger impact on the health status of whites than that of blacks (Williams & Collins, 1995). Kessler (1979) documented a similar pattern for the relationship between stressful life events and psychological distress for nonwhites (mainly blacks) and low SES persons. Both of these economically disadvantaged groups were more exposed to stress. However, compared to nonwhites and low SES individuals, comparable stressful events more adversely affected the mental health of whites and high SES persons, respectively. Kessler (1979) suggested some possible reasons for this relative advantage.

First, due to earlier exposure and/or more frequent exposure to adversity, African Americans could become more accustomed to dealing with stress, such that a new stressful experience has less of an impact. Second, compared to whites, African Americans may respond to stress with greater emotional flexibility (that is, emotional expression), which may facilitate recovery. In addition, African Americans may have greater access than that of whites to other coping resources, such as religious involvement, that some have argued may importantly reduce the negative effects of stress (Williams, 1994).

The hypothesis that blacks cope better with stress than whites do could shed light on an important paradox in the literature. Compared to whites, African Americans have higher rates of disease and death for virtually all measures of physical health (U.S. Department of Health and Human Services, 1985), but they also have equivalent or lower rates of psychiatric illness (Kessler et al., 1994; Robins & Regier, 1991) and lower rates of suicide (Griffith & Bell, 1989). If blacks cope better with stress, there may be a consequential trade-off. Although effective coping may shield African Americans from the psychological sequelae of stress, the cumulative effects of high exposure to stress may take a heavy physical toll and leave them more vulnerable to a broad range of physical ailments (cf. Geronimus, 1992). This issue deserves careful research attention.

Our analyses also emphasize that understanding racial differences in health importantly requires an appropriate theoretical framework. Because we conceptualized race as not reflecting biological distinctiveness, we examined other factors (socio-economic status and stress) that are linked to the social situation of racial groups. A different understanding of race could have led to a search for genetic and biological differences. At the same time, our findings document that the associations among race, racism, SES, and health are complex. Racism is a part of the structure of society and arguably the most profound health impact of racism is at the level of societal institutions (Williams, 1996a). Racial differences in SES reflect some of the economic manifestations of racial discrimination. Cooper and David (1986) argue that since SES is an intermediate variable in the causal pathway between race and health, adjusting racial differences for SES is a form of overcontrol and should not be used in health studies. Although we agree that SES is not technically a confounder of racial differences in health, it is an important intermediate factor. Our approach suggests that analytic control can be usefully employed for non-confounders. We control for these intermediate factors, not to eliminate bias but to facilitate an understanding of the processes that link race (a marker of social privilege or economic disadvantage) to health.

In an era of waning public support and government commitment to making the needed investment to improve the social and economic conditions of the most vulnerable populations in the USA, our analyses document that race matters a lot in terms of health. Moreover, the sources of racial disparities are not unknown, individual, or obscure. They can be traced to inequalities that have been created and maintained by the economic, legal, and political structures of society. These systems, and not individual beliefs and behavior, are the fundamental causes of racial and socio-economic inequalities in health (Williams, 1990; Williams, in press). Eliminating these health disparities will thus require changes in the fundamental social systems in society.

References

Amaro, H., Russo, N. F., & Johnson, J. (1987). Family and work predictors of psychological wellbeing among Hispanic women professionals. *Psychology of Women Quarterly, 11*, 505–521.

Anderson, N. B., McNeilly, M., & Myers, H. (1991). Autonomic reactivity and hypertension in blacks: A review and proposed model. *Ethnicity and Disease, 1*, 154–170.

Aneshensel, C. S. (1992). Social stress: Theory and research. *American Sociological Review, 18*, 15–38.

Cohen, S., Kessler, R. C., & Gordon, L. U. (1995). *Measuring stress: A guide for health and social scientists.* New York: Oxford University Press.

Cooper, R. S. (1993). Health and the social status of blacks in the United States. *Annals of Epidemiology, 3*, 137–144.

Cooper, R. S., & David, R. (1986). The biological concept of race and its application to public health and epidemiology. *Journal of Health and Politics, Policy and Law, 11*, 97–116.

Cooper, R. S., Steinhauer, M., Miller, W., David, R., & Schatzkin, A. (1981). Racism, society, and disease: An exploration of the social and biological mechanisms of differential mortality. *International Journal of Health Services, 11*(3), 389–414.

Cose, E. (1993). *The rage of a privileged class.* New York: HarperCollins.

Danziger, S., & Gottschalk, P. (Eds.) (1993). *Uneven tides: Rising inequality in America.* New York: Russell Sage.

Essed, P. (1991). *Understanding everyday racism.* Newbury Park, CA: Sage.

Feagin, J. R. (1991). The continuing significance of race: Antiblack discrimination in public places. *American Sociological Review, 56,* 101–116.

Gardner, C. B. (1995). *Passing by: Gender and public harassment.* Berkeley: University of California Press.

Geronimus, A. T. (1992). The weathering hypothesis and the health of African-American women and infants. *Ethnicity and Disease, 2,* 207–221.

Gould, S. J. (1977). Why we should not name human races: A biological view. In S. J. Gould (Ed.), *Ever since Darwin* (pp. 231–236). New York: Norton.

Griffith, E., & Bell, C. (1989). Recent trends in suicide and homicide among blacks. *Journal of the American Medical Association, 262,* 2265–2269.

Harburg, E., Erfurt, J., Chape, C., Havenstein, L., Schull, W., & Schork, M. A. (1973). Socioecological stressor areas and black–white blood pressure: Detroit. *Journal of Chronic Disease, 26,* 595–611.

Hummer, R. A. (1996). Black–white differences in health and mortality: A review and conceptual model. *Sociological Quarterly, 37*(1), 105–125.

Jackson, J. S., Brown, T. N., Williams, D. R., Torres, M., Sellers, S. L., & Brown, K. (1996). Racism and the physical and mental health status of African Americans: A thirteen year national panel study. *Ethnicity and Disease, 6*(1,2), 132–147.

Jackson, J. S., & Inglehart, M. R. (1995). Reverberation theory: Stress and racism in hierarchically structured communities. In S. E. Hobfoll & M. DeVries (Eds.), *Extreme stress and communities: Impact and interventions* (pp. 353–373). Dordrecht: Kluwer Academic.

Jackson, J. S., Williams, D. R., & Torres, M. (in press). *Racial discrimination, stress, action orientation and physical and psychological health.* National Institute of Mental Health.

James, S. A., LaCroix, A. Z., Kleinbaum, D. G., & Strogatz, D. S. (1984). John Henryism and blood pressure differences among black men. II. The role of occupational stressors. *Journal of Behavioral Medicine, 7,* 259–275.

Karoly, L. A. (1992). *The trend in inequality among families, individuals, and workers in the United States: A twenty-five year perspective.* Santa Monica, CA: Rand.

Kessler, R. C. (1979). Stress, social status, and psychological distress. *Journal of Health and Social Behavior, 20,* 259–273.

Kessler, R. C., McGonagle, K. A., Zhao, S., Nelson, C. B., Hughers, M., Eshleman, S., Wittchen, H., & Kendler, K. S. (1994). Lifetime and 12-month prevalence of DSM-III-R psychiatric disorders in the United States. *Archives of General Psychiatry, 51,* 8–19.

Kim, P. S., & Lewis, G. B. (1994). Americans in the public service: Success, diversity, and discrimination. *Public Administration Review, 54,* 285–290.

King, G., & Williams, D. R. (1995). Race and health: A multi-dimensional approach to African American Health. In B. C. Amick, S. Levine, D. C. Walsh, & A. Tarlov (Eds.), *Society and health* (pp. 93–130). New York: Oxford University Press.

Krieger, N. (1987). Shades of difference: Theoretical underpinnings of the medical controversy on black/white differences in the United States, 1830–1870. *International Journal of Health Services, 17,* 259–278.

Krieger, N. (1990). Racial and gender discrimination: Risk factors for high blood pressure? *Social Science and Medicine, 30*(12), 1273–1281.

Krieger, N., Rowley, D. L., Herman, A. A., Avery, B., & Phillips, M. T. (1993). Racism, sexism, and social class: Implications for studies of health, disease, and well-being. *American Journal of Preventive Medicine, 9* (Suppl. 6), 82–122.

Krieger, N., & Sidney, S. (1996). Racial discrimination and blood pressure: the CARDIA study of young black and white women and men. *American Journal of Public Health, 86*(10), 1370–1378.

Krieger, N., Williams, D. R., & Moss, N. E. (1997). Measuring social class in U.S. public health research: Concepts, methodologies, and guidelines. *Annual Review of Public Health, 18,* 341–378.

Lewontin, R. C. (1972). The apportionment of human diversity. In Th. Dobzhansky, M. K. Hecht, & W. C. Steere (Eds.), *Evolutionary biology* (Vol. 6, pp. 381–386). New York: Appleton-Century-Crofts.

Lillie-Blanton, M., Parsons, P. E., Gayle, H., & Dievler, A. (1996). Racial differences in health: Not just black and white, but shades of gray. *Annual Review of Public Health, 17,* 411–448.

Massey, D. S., & Denton, N. A. (1993). *American apartheid: Segregation and the making of the underclass.* Cambridge, MA: Harvard University Press.

McNeilly, M. D., Anderson, N. B., Armstead, C. A., Clark, R., Corbett, M., Robinson, E. L., Pieper, C. F., & Lepisto, E. M. (1996). The perceived racism scale: A multidimensional assessment of the experience of white racism among African Americans. *Ethnicity and Disease, 6*(1,2), 154–166.

National Center for Health Statistics (1993). *Health, United States, 1992 and healthy people review.* Washington, DC: U.S. Government Printing Office.

National Center for Health Statistics (1994). *Vital statistics of the United States, 1990. Vol. II, Mortality Part A.* Hyattsville, MD: Public Health Service.

Omi, M., & Winant, H. (1986). *Racial formation in the United States: From the 1960s to the 1980s.* New York: Routledge.

Pearlin, L. I. (1989). The sociological study of stress. *Journal of Health and Social Behavior, 30*(3), 241–256.

Robins, L. N., & Regier, D. A. (1991). *Psychiatric disorders in America: The epidemiologic catchment area study.* New York: Free Press.

Salgado de Snyder, V. N. (1987). Factors associated with acculturative stress and depressive symptomatology among married Mexican immigrant women. *Psychology of Women Quarterly, 11,* 475–488.

Smith, J. P., & Welch, F. R. (1989). Black economic progress after Myrdal. *Journal of Economic Literature, 27,* 519–564.

Telles, E. E., & Murgia, E. (1990). Phenotypic discrimination and income differences among Mexican Americans. *Social Science Quarterly, 71,* 682–697.

Thoits, P. A. (1983). Dimensions of life events that influence psychological distress: An evaluation and synthesis of the literature. In H. B. Kaplan (Ed.), *Psychosocial research: Trends in theory and research* (pp. 33–103). New York: Academic.

U.S. Department of Health and Human Services (1985). *Report of the Secretary's task force on black and minority health.* Washington, DC: U.S Government Printing Office.

Vega, W. A., & Rumbaut, R. G. (1991). Ethnic minorities and mental health. *Annual Review of Sociology, 71,* 351–383.

Williams, D. R. (1990). Socioeconomic differential in health: A review and redirection. *Social Psychology Quarterly, 3,* 81–99.

Williams, D. R. (1994). The measurement of religion in epidemiologic studies: Problems and prospect. In J. S. Levin (Ed.), *Religion in aging and health: Theoretical foundations and methodological frontiers* (pp. 125–148). Thousand Oaks, CA: Sage.

Williams, D. R. (1996a). Racism and health: A research agenda. *Ethnicity and Disease, 6,* 1–6.

Williams, D. R. (1996b). Race, ethnicity, and socioeconomic status: Measurement and methodological issues. *International Journal of Health Services, 26*(3), 483–505.

Williams, D. R. (in press). Race and health: Basic questions, emerging directions. *Annals of Epidemiology.*

Williams, D. R., & Chung, A-M. (in press). Racism and health. In R. Gibson & J. S. Jackson (Eds.), *Health in black America*. Thousand Oaks, CA: Sage.

Williams, D. R., & Collins, C. (1995). Socioeconomic and racial differences in health. *Annual Review of Sociology, 21,* 349–386.

Williams, D. R., & House, J. S. (1991). Stress, social support, control and coping: A social epidemiologic view. In B. Badura & I. Kickbusch (Eds.), *Health promotion research: Towards a new social epidemiology*. Copenhagen: World Health Organization.

Williams, D. R., Lavizzo-Mourey, R., & Warren, R. C. (1994). The concept of race and health status in America. *Public Health Reports, 109,* 26–41.

Witzig, R. (1996). The medicalization of race: Scientific legitimization of a flawed social construct. *Annals of Internal Medicine, 125,* 675–679.

Wright, E. O. (1985). *Classes*. London: Verso.

Wright, E. O. (1997). *Class counts: Comparative studies in class analysis*. New York: Cambridge University Press.

DISCUSSION

1. The authors assert that socioeconomic status (SES) is more than a confounder of the race-health relationship (i.e., something that is related to race and that has to be controlled in order to accurately estimate the effect of race) but, rather, that it is an important causal mechanism through which race affects health. What do they mean by that?

2. The effects of race on well-being and psychological distress were generally weaker than the effects of race on physical health in this study. Develop two or three hypotheses to explain the difference. What information would you need to test those hypotheses?

3. Take the role of a staff member to a U.S. senator who works on health-related policies. What policy recommendations would you present based on the results of this study?

Jane D. McLeod

Childhood Parental Loss and Adult Depression

This selection is an early example of research that applies the life course perspective to the study of mental health. The life course perspective is an orienting framework that directs our attention to the connections among developmental

McLeod, Jane D. 1991. "Childhood Parental Loss and Adult Depression." *Journal of Health and Social Behavior* 32:205–220.

processes, institutionalized life paths (e.g., the transition from schooling to work), and ongoing changes in society. Two important principles of the life course perspective are that human development is a lifelong process and that lives are lived interdependently—the things that happen to significant others have implications for our own lives as well. These principles are evident in this analysis, which evaluates the effects of childhood parental death and divorce for the life course of children.

A growing body of evidence supports the contention that parental deaths and parental divorces that occur during childhood have implications for adult well-being. Early studies documented significantly higher rates of depressive disorders among persons who lost a parent as compared to those who did not in clinical samples (e.g., Brown, 1961; Forrest, Fraser, & Priest, 1965). More recently, those findings have been extended to the general population (Brown, Harris, & Copeland, 1977; Hallstrom, 1987; Harris, Brown, & Bifulco, 1986), although with somewhat less consistency (e.g., Tennant, Bebbington, & Hurry, 1982). Furthermore, parental divorce has implications for well-being defined more broadly. Adults from divorced backgrounds achieve relatively low levels of education (Greenberg & Wolf, 1982; Keith & Amato, 1990; Keith & Finlay, 1988), marry at younger ages (McLanahan & Bumpass, 1988), and are more likely to divorce themselves (McLanahan & Bumpass, 1988; Pope & Mueller, 1976) than their counterparts from intact homes, even after corrections for socioeconomic background are introduced. Although many of the relationships between loss and these outcomes are modest in size, their consistency and pervasiveness argue for their substantive importance.

While the bivariate relationships between parental loss and these indicators of adult well-being have received substantial attention, the interconnections among the processes implied by these relationships have not. Specifically, we know little about whether the socioeconomic and marital outcomes of parental loss are implicated in the observed higher levels of depression. Depression, defined variously by diagnostic criteria or by the presence of high levels of depressed mood, represents the most commonly studied mental health outcome of parental loss, in part because of the proposed centrality of loss in some theories of the etiology of depression. Psychosocial epidemiological research supports the plausibility of the interconnections among parental loss, socioeconomic and marital outcomes, and depression. Persons with low levels of education report higher levels of psychological distress than persons with high levels of education (Dohrenwend & Dohrenwend, 1969). Furthermore, the quality of the marital relationship is a key correlate of depression (Brown & Harris, 1978). In this analysis, I integrate these two areas of research by examining the extent to which the socioeconomic and marital outcomes of parental loss mediate and/or modify their relationship to depression among married men and women.

DIVERGENT TRADITIONS IN PREVIOUS RESEARCH

The failure of previous research to link the socioeconomic and marital outcomes of parental loss to depression results in part from the divergent theoretical and empirical traditions out of which each relevant literature grew. A consideration of these traditions sheds light on the ways in which they complement one another, and on potential specifications of the relationships between loss and life course outcomes by the type of loss (death v. divorce) and by gender.

Research on the relationship between parental loss and depression developed out of a general epidemiological concern with the origins of depressive disorders in adulthood. In the context of this type of investigation, Brown, Harris, and their colleagues at Bedford New College identified maternal loss before age 11 as one background social condition with demonstrable relationships to adult depression (Brown & Harris, 1978; Brown, Harris, & Bifulco, 1986; Brown, Harris, & Copeland, 1977). They reported odds-ratios of 1.5 to 2.4 for the development of adult depression following an early maternal loss among samples of working-class and middle-class women in boroughs of London and the Outer Hebrides. Significant relationships between losses, losses at ages 11 to 17, and adult depression have been documented in other general population samples (e.g., Barnes & Prosen, 1985).

In trying to understand the origins of these patterns, depression researchers have typically relied on intrapsychic explanations, such as Freudian psychoanalytic theory (Abraham, 1924; Freud, 1917) and Bowlby's attachment theory (Bowlby, 1969, 1980). While these explanations vary in the specific intrapsychic processes they propose, they share a common focus on the primacy of deep-seated personality and cognitive deficits as the ultimate causes of the adult depression which results from childhood parental loss.

This focus on intrapsychic deficits accounts, in part, for the lack of attention traditionally given by depression researchers to the distinctions among parental death, parental divorce, and other parental losses in theoretical and empirical analyses. Although these losses may differ in their implications for the structure of the child's subsequent life experience, because they may all have intrapsychic ramifications, they are all thought to be potential precipitants of depression. Thus, evidence about the relative importance of these different losses in predicting depression is lacking.

Furthermore, most researchers interested in the childhood origins of adult depression have also failed to give adequate attention to the variety of life course outcomes which may mediate the loss-depression relationship, such as educational attainment and age at marriage. Presumably, their lack of attention to other outcomes can be traced to the proposed primacy of psychological continuities as determinative of adult mental health.

In contrast to depression research which favors intrapsychic explanations, research on the socioeconomic and marital outcomes of loss has favored structural explanations. In particular, much of this research has been grounded in a sociological life course perspective which focuses on the ways in which interdependencies among structured events and transitions shape current and future life outcomes (Elder, 1985). This perspective argues for the importance of distinguishing losses by their cause, and for the simultaneous consideration of multiple outcomes in analyses of depression. To the extent that parental death and parental divorce initiate different sequences of events, we might expect their relationships with depression to differ as well.

Demographic research documents different life course experiences for persons from homes broken by divorce and death. Persons from divorced homes report lower levels of life satisfaction, health (Glenn & Kramer, 1985), economic well-being (Greenberg & Wolf, 1982), and marital stability (Bumpass & Sweet, 1972; McLanahan & Bumpass, 1988; Pope & Mueller, 1976) than others in nationally representative samples. In addition, several characteristics of intact marriages appear to covary in predictable ways with parental divorce, including the presence of conflict, the use of conflictual problem-solving strategies, and positive feelings toward one's spouse (Pond, Ryle, & Hamilton, 1963). Most comparisons of these relationships with comparable relationships for parental death indicate that the latter are much weaker and rarely achieve significance (Glenn & Kramer, 1985, 1987; Pope & Mueller, 1976). Demographers have attributed these differences to the lower levels of economic deprivation and parental conflict in homes broken by death versus divorce. What demographers have not done is to take the additional step to link these outcomes with the development of depression in adulthood.

While I have focused on the failure of previous research to examine the interconnections among the different life course outcomes of parental loss, there is a second limitation of that work which motivates the present study. Neither depression research nor demographic research has examined gender differences in the relationships between parental loss and adult outcomes consistently, despite some empirical evidence for the existence of such differences (Glenn & Kramer, 1985, 1987). Theoretical considerations support the hypothesis that parental losses will have stronger relationships with adult marital and depression outcomes among women as compared to men. Carol Gilligan (1982) and others (including Chodorow, 1978) proposed that girls more than boys define their identities through intimate relationships and through their ability to maintain those relationships. If this were true, disruptions in parental relationships would influence girls more strongly, both in terms of their sense of self-worth and in terms of their perceptions of future relationships. Furthermore, one could posit that parental losses would also lead to greater socioeconomic disadvantage among girls than among boys, as families coping with economic deprivation would be more likely to deprive their daughters of educational opportunities (Elder, 1974).

This analysis uses data from a sample of married men and women to consider the interconnections among the various outcomes of childhood parental death and divorce, and to examine differences in those processes by gender. Specifically, I propose three hypotheses.

1. The relationships between parental loss and adult depressive, socioeconomic, and marital outcomes are stronger for parental divorce than for

parental death. Furthermore, these relationships are stronger among women than among men.

2. Observed relationships between parental loss and adult depression can be explained by socioeconomic and marital disadvantages experienced by persons who lost a parent.

This hypothesis emphasizes a mediational model whereby parental losses create socioeconomic and relational disadvantages which, in turn, lead to the development of depression. One could make an equally strong argument for the importance of interactive relationships between parental losses and their socioeconomic and marital outcomes in predicting depression. Achieving a high level of education or income, despite having lost a parent, may protect the individual from the mental health outcomes of loss through the sense of competence it promotes (Kessler & Cleary, 1980). In addition, attachment theory argues that the relationship between parental loss and disrupted adult attachments is not inevitable, but can be tempered through the establishment of a secure relationship with another adult (Bowlby, 1980). Both of these processes are interactive rather than additive.

Thus, I propose a third hypothesis:

3. The relationship between parental loss and adult depression is stronger among persons who achieve low levels of socioeconomic status, who marry at younger ages, and who experience poor marital quality than among others.

DATA AND METHODS

Data

The data for the analysis are from the 1985 Detroit Area Study, an annual survey of general population respondents sponsored by the Department of Sociology at the University of Michigan. That year, the topic of the survey was stressful life experiences and related psychopathology among married couples. The sample included white married couples living together in suburban Detroit, in which at least one member of the couple was between the ages of 18 and 64. We obtained completed interviews with one or both members of the married couple in 73 percent of the eligible households, yielding a total of 1,755 respondents. Our decision to interview only whites was based on the low rate of intact marriages among nonwhites in the Detroit metropolitan area. Most analyses suggest that the relationships between parental losses and later life outcomes are weaker among blacks than whites (e.g., Glenn & Kramer, 1987; Keith & Amato, 1990).

My decision to pursue this analysis using a data set of married couples deserves special comment as it has implications for the interpretation of these results. By focusing on married couples, I leave open the possibility that the results of this analysis are biased by the nature of the sample. Men and women with the most conflictual marriages may have already selected themselves out. Given the higher rate of marital disruption among persons from divorced homes (Glenn & Kramer, 1987), this type of selection would lead to underestimates of the relationship between parental divorce and marital quality, assuming that persons from divorced backgrounds are equally or more likely to pursue divorce as a means of resolving marital conflict.

Given this disadvantage, it is important to emphasize the gains that can be achieved by focusing on married couples. As noted above, previous research suggests that both the probability of being married and marital quality are influenced by childhood parental loss. The former finding is much more well-established than the latter because most analyses of the effect of parental divorce on marital functioning focus on marital dissolution. By doing so, however, those analyses fail to acknowledge evidence that marital dissolution and marital quality may result from very different processes (Lewis & Spanier, 1979) which require different analytic strategies. A thorough examination of the predictors of marital quality requires a sample of ever-married persons and their ratings of marital quality for at least one of their marriages. As noted above, because this sample includes only currently married couples instead of ever-married persons, the estimates of the relationships between parental divorce and marital quality are likely to be biased downwards.

The five types of variables included in the analysis are childhood parental loss, depression, socioeconomic status, marital transition behaviors, and marital quality.

Childhood parental loss. Respondents to the survey were asked whether or not they lived with both of their natural parents up through the age of 16. If they did not, they were asked what happened, how old they were at the time, and with whom they lived afterward. Of the 1,755 respondents, 157 (8.9 percent) reported a childhood parental death, 171 (9.7 percent) reported a childhood parental divorce, and 35 (2.0 percent) reported not living with their parents up through age 16 for some other reason. The latter 35 respondents were excluded from the analysis because the reasons for their losses were so diverse.

Depression. I included two indicators of depression in the analysis: a categorical, diagnostic measure and a symptom scale. These indicators represent the two main alternative operationalizations of depression used in epidemiological research. Categorical indicators are generally thought to measure the presence of a discrete, clinically-relevant depressive disorder while symptom scales measure continuous variations in depressed mood, which may or may not manifest as a clinical disorder. They may be thought of as representing more or less serious depression experiences, respectively.

The categorical indicator is a dummy variable for the experience of recent depressive episodes, based on the stem question from the Diagnostic Interview Schedule depression section (Robins et al., 1981). Respondents who responded affirmatively to that question (experiencing an episode lasting at least two weeks during the past six months) are identified as depressed according to this indicator. This outcome measure approximates a diagnostic approach to defining depression, but reflects more inclusive criteria than traditional diagnoses. Of the 1,661 respondents with complete data on the analysis variables, 317 met this criteria.

The second indicator is a depression index created from a 10-item subset of the depression subscale of the SCL-90-R, the revised version of the Hopkins Symptom Checklist (Derogatis, 1977). The 10 items were chosen from the original 13 items based on high reported factor loadings. The items collectively assess the frequency of occurrences of a variety of depressive symptoms in the 30 days before the interview, including dysphoric mood, loss of energy, feelings of hopelessness, and withdrawal from activities (Derogatis, Lipman, & Covi, 1973). While the SCL-90-R depression index is best thought of as a measure of depressed mood, its score has been shown to discriminate normal populations and psychiatric outpatients, suggesting its validity as a measure of depression among the general population. In creating the depression index, each item score was standardized, the item scores were summed, and the final index score was standardized.

Socioeconomic Status. The respondent's socioeconomic status was measured in three ways: number of years of education; a dummy variable for whether or not the respondent had pursued some education beyond high school; and reported total family income for 1984. Respondents reported their incomes in 16 categories, for which the midpoints were coded. Previous research documents significant relationships between parental divorce and these outcomes among men (Greenberg & Wolf, 1982; Wadsworth & Maclean, 1986).

Marital Transition Behaviors. Transitions into and out of marriage were also represented by three variables: age at the respondent's first marriage; whether or not the respondent was married before age 18; and whether or not the respondent had been married previously. As noted earlier, parental divorce has been shown to predict an earlier age at marriage and higher probability of marital dissolution in previous research (Glenn & Kramer, 1987; McLanahan & Bumpass, 1988).

Marital Quality. I used five indicators of perceived marital quality: presence of recent (12-month) serious marital problems; frequency of disagreements with spouse; use of calm problem-solving strategies (e.g., discuss differences calmly); use of conflictual problem-solving strategies (e.g., say cruel and angry things); and marital trust (items listed in Appendix A). Use of calm and conflictual problem-solving strategies and marital trust are multi-item indices. The correlations among these indicators range in absolute value from .29 to .53 with the highest correlations observed for the three indices. The presence of conflict, styles of conflict resolution, and positive feelings toward one's spouse comprise the indicators of marital adjustment that have been related to childhood experiences in previous research (Pond et al., 1963).

Background controls. I controlled for current age and for parental socioeconomic status throughout the analysis. Both variables are related to the likelihood of childhood parental loss (Glick, 1979) and to adult mental health (Langner & Michael, 1963; Veroff, Douvan, & Kulka, 1981). Failure to control for them could lead to inaccurate estimates of the relationship between loss and mental health. Parental socioeconomic status was operationalized with two indicators: years of education and the occupational status of the reported "major financial support" of the respondent's childhood household. Occupational status was coded as an eight-category prestige index, with the lowest category representing professional and technical workers.

Statistical Methods

I used ordinary least squares regression to examine the relationship between childhood parental loss and adult mental health. The baseline regression equation in the analysis was $D = b_0 + b_1\text{Death} + b_2\text{Divorce} + b_3C$, where D represents an indicator of depression, Death and Divorce represent dummy variables for parental death or parental divorce, and C represents control variables. Similar equations were used to estimate the relationships among parental loss experiences, socioeconomic status, marital transitions, and marital quality. Because the depression diagnosis and several of the socio-economic and marital variables are dichotomous, ordinary least squares regression is not technically the most appropriate statistical technique. I present results using OLS for ease of interpretation (the coefficients can be interpreted in terms of adjusted differences in probabilities), but confirmed the significance (or nonsignificance) of the observed relationships with these outcomes using logistic regression. All models presented in this paper included the control variables but those coefficients are excluded from the tables for clarity of presentation. Estimated effects with significance levels of .05 and below (two-tailed tests) are considered statistically significant.

RESULTS

Depressive Outcomes

The first concern of this analysis was whether childhood parental losses are significantly related to adult depression among married men and women, and whether gender specifies those relationships. According to these data, parental losses have different life course implications for married men and women. Table 1 lists the coefficients from the initial regressions of depression on childhood parental death and parental divorce among men and women separately. Women who lost a parent reported higher levels of depressed mood than women who did not. The coefficients for these effects are comparable in size to those observed for the effects of recent losses on psychological distress (Kessler & McLeod, 1984) suggesting that these relationships are not trivial, and are of approximately equal size for both types of loss experiences. Despite this clear pattern with respect to depressed mood, the relationships between parental losses and depression are not significant for the indicator of depressive episodes. Parental losses are more highly predictive of mood variations than of discrete episodes in this sample. Furthermore, in contrast

Table 1 Coefficients (and Standard Errors) from the Regressions of Depression on Parental Loss for Women and Men Separately

Depression	Women (n = 884)		Men (n = 777)	
	Death	Divorce	Death	Divorce
Mood	.26*	.31*	−.01	.11
	(.12)	(.11)	(.11)	(.11)
Episode	.08	.03	.06	−.03
	(.05)	(.05)	(.04)	(.05)

*p < .05; **p < .01.

to the results among women, neither type of parental loss is significantly related to either indicator of depression among men. These results are consistent with previous research (Harris & Brown, 1985) in documenting small relationships between parental loss and mental health among men.

It is worth noting that the nonsignificance of these relationships among men does not appear to be solely an artifact of my decision to focus on depressive outcomes. Clearly, one could make a strong case for the expectation that other types of outcomes, such as alcohol use, physical health problems, or antisocial behavior, might capture the distress reactions of men more effectively (Dohrenwend & Dohrenwend, 1976). If parental loss had strong relationships to other indicators of mental health among men, the observed gender difference for depression would reflect a difference in the *style* of response to adversity rather than in the *degree* of response. I estimated the strengths of the relationships between parental losses and three additional variables in order to assess this possibility: a count of days of high alcohol or drug use; a count of physical health problems; and a diagnostic measure of antisocial behavior (available for only a subset of study participants). The only significant relationships with these outcomes existed among women (results not shown but available from the author). Therefore, while I cannot eliminate the possibility that there would be consistent, significant relationships between parental loss and other outcomes among men, these results render that interpretation less plausible, and suggest a more general gender difference in the relationships between parental loss and adult well-being.

Socioeconomic Status, Marital Transitions, and Marital Quality

The estimated regressions of socioeconomic status, marital transition behaviors, and marital quality on parental death and parental divorce further support that conclusion. Table 2 presents the coefficients from those regressions. Two patterns are immediately evident: many more of these relationships are significant for women than for men and the relationships are stronger for parental divorce than for parental death. Women whose parents divorced achieved over two-thirds of one year less education and over $5,000 per year less income on average than women who did not lose a parent. They were

Table 2 Coefficients (and Standard Errors) from the Regressions of Other Adult Outcomes on Parental Loss, for Women and Men Separately

Outcome	Women (n = 884)			Men (n = 777)		
	Death	Divorce	R^2	Death	Divorce	R^2
Socioeconomic Status						
Education	−.20	−.68**	.23	−.35	−.78*	.19
	(.23)	(.21)		(.30)	(.31)	
Ed > High School	.03	−.20**	.17	−.07	−.09	.13
	(.05)	(.05)		(.06)	(.06)	
1984 Income	−1.14	−5.48**	.09	.54	−.51	.05
	(2.31)	(2.11)		(.50)	(2.56)	
Marital Transitions						
Age at Marriage	−.20	−.94*	.05	−1.13*	−.69	.06
	(.45)	(.41)		(.50)	(.51)	
Age < 18	.08	.15**	.06	.00	.06*	.01
	(.04)	(.04)		(.02)	(.02)	
Previously Married	.02	.09*	.02	.02	.08	.02
	(.04)	(.04)		(.05)	(.05)	
Marital Quality						
Disagreements	−.07	−.30	.03	.16	−.07	.04
	(.11)	(.10)		(.12)	(.12)	
Serious Problems	.09*	.10*	.02	−.02	−.05	.02
	(.04)	(.04)		(.04)	(.04)	
Trust	−.04	−.34**	.03	−.03	.02	.00
	(.13)	(.12)		(.10)	(.10)	
Calm Problem-Solving	.07	−.25*	.02	.15	−.12	.01
	(.12)	(.11)		(.12)	(.12)	
Conflictual Problem-Solving	−.01	.25*	.02	.13	.07	.00
	(.12)	(.11)		(.12)	(.12)	

*p < .05; **p < .01

also more likely to marry at young ages, to be previously married, and to report more conflictual, and less supportive, marital relationships.

The estimated effects of parental divorce on socioeconomic and marital outcomes are much weaker among men. In fact, out of the 11 outcomes, only 2 show significant relationships with parental divorce: education in years and being married before age 18. Income levels, rates of previous marriage, and self-reported marital quality do not differ between men from divorced and intact backgrounds. The gender difference documented for depressive outcomes appears to extend to more general indictors of well-being.

The second pattern noted above is that parental divorce has much stronger relationships with socioeconomic and marital outcomes than parental death for both men and women. Consistent with the findings of demographic research (Wadsworth & Maclean, 1986) parental death is not related to adult socioeconomic levels, nor does it predict significant differences in marital quality among intact marriages. The two exceptions to this pattern—for the experience of serious marital problems among women, and for age at marriage among men—may represent true relationships worthy of further attention. However, it is equally plausible that we would observe one significant relationship among 11 outcomes for each gender just by chance. Thus, I hesitate to accord these relationships much importance.

Although the relationships of parental divorce to adult outcomes appear to be much stronger among women than men according to the gender-specific analyses, it is important to note that most of the gender differences are not significant for depression, socioeconomic status, and marital transitions. In contrast, the gender differences with respect to marital quality are both clear and pervasive. Parental divorce is much more strongly related to marital quality among women as compared to men. One of the more important differences between men and women from divorced backgrounds appears to be the differences in their perceptions of the quality of their marriages.

Relationships Among Outcomes of Parental Loss

The core issue in this analysis is the extent to which the socioeconomic and marital outcomes of parental death and parental divorce mediate or condition the observed relationships between parental losses and adult depression. In deciding how to examine the interrelationships among the varied outcomes of parental death and parental divorce, one could posit a number of different causal mechanisms. For example, parental losses could lead to decreased socioeconomic attainment which, in turn, predicts higher levels of depressed mood, or parental loss could manifest itself in higher levels of depressed mood, which lead to lower levels of attainment at school and in the labor market. In the first instance, socioeconomic status is viewed as an intervening variable in the loss-depression relationship, akin to social causation arguments. In the latter, depressed mood takes that role, changing the argument to one of social selection. One could make comparable arguments for marital outcomes: parental loss (especially divorce) leads to poor marital outcomes, which create high levels of depressed mood; or parental loss creates distress, which leads to a diminishment in marital functioning. For the purposes of this analysis, I assume that socioeconomic status and marital outcomes act as mediators of the relationship between parental death or divorce and adult depression. While the alternative models have obvious plausibility, the processes that they imply have tended to receive somewhat less support than causation arguments, particularly for nonpathological levels of depressive symptomatology (see, for example, Wheaton, 1978).

Table 3 displays the coefficients from regressions models that added socioeconomic, marital transition, and marital quality variables to the baseline models predicting depressed mood from parental death and parental divorce among women. I estimated the explanatory power of each group of variables separately in order to assess their relative importance for understanding loss-depression relationships. The relationships between parental

Table 3 Coefficients (and Standard Errors) from the Regression of Depressed Mood on Parental Loss Controlling for Mediating Variables, for Women

	Women			
	I	II	III	IV
Loss				
Death	.26* (.12)	.25* (.12)	.26* (.12)	.25** (.11)
Divorce	.31** (.11)	.30** (.11)	.31** (.11)	.15 (.10)
Socioeconomic Outcomes		.08 (.08)		
Ed > High Schoolc				
1984 Income		−.01** (.00)		
Marital Transitions				
Age < 18			−.08 (.10)	
Previously Married			.19 (.10)	
Marital Quality				
Disagreements				.15** (.04)
Serious Problems				.27** (.10)
Trust				−.13** (.04)
Calm Problem-Solving				−.19** (.04)
Conflictual Problem-Solving				.00 (.04)
R^2	.02	.03	.03	.18

*$p < .05$; **$p < .01$.

Note: I: baseline model
II: mediating effects of socioeconomic outcomes
III: mediating effects of marital transition behaviors
IV: mediating effects of perceived marital quality

loss and depressive episodes were not significant in either group, so I do not present explanatory models for that outcome.

The addition of indicators of socioeconomic status to the baseline equation for the loss-depression relationship did not change the death or divorce coefficients substantially among women. (The table lists results with education greater than high school as the indicator of education; the results were virtually the same when the continuous version of education was used instead.) Marital transition behaviors are equally ineffective as mediators. In contrast, perceived marital quality is strongly implicated in the relationship between parental divorce and depressed mood. Controlling for the five indicators of perceived marital quality reduced the coefficient for parental divorce by over 50 percent, and made that coefficient nonsignificant. Thus, marital quality appears to offer potential in explicating the process linking parental divorce and depressed mood. The relationship between parental death and depressed mood is not explained by any of these intervening conditions. Although the mental health implications of parental death and parental divorce appear similar, the processes behind those relationships may be quite different.

The models listed in Table 3 may misrepresent the processes linking the socioeconomic, marital, and depressive outcomes of parental losses if those processes are interactive rather than additive. For example, the relationship between parental divorce and adult depression may be conditioned by the degree of socioeconomic success experienced by those individuals, with more successful individuals being less affected by early experiences. Alternatively, the relationship may be stronger among persons whose current marriages are conflictual than among persons who enjoy conflict-free, satisfying marital relationships.

The results from this analysis do not support those hypotheses. I estimated the multiplicative interactions among parental death, parental divorce, and each socioeconomic and marital variable in predicting depressed mood and the experience of depressive episodes for women. Only three achieved significance, well within the realm of chance. Furthermore, each variable had an approximately equal number of positive and negative interactions, suggesting a total lack of patterns. The only consistent patterns of interaction for individual variables, judged so by the sign of the interaction, are not consistent across variables. For example, the relationships of parental death and parental divorce with depressive episodes are stronger both among women who experienced serious marital problems and among those who reported high levels of marital trust. Thus, this analysis provides virtually no support for the existence of interactions between childhood parental losses and other adult life outcomes in predicting adult depression.

DISCUSSION

The results of this analysis generally support my expectations. Parental divorce was more strongly related to most adult life outcomes than parental death. These relationships were also stronger among women than men. Furthermore, adult life outcomes were able to explain a substantial amount of the relationship between parental divorce and depressed mood. The one expectation for which there was little support was the existence of interactions between parental loss and adult outcomes in predicting depression.

Despite the general consistency between expectations and results, this analysis also revealed several exceptions and/or specifications of the interconnections among parental losses and their varied adult outcomes. Perceived marital quality played a much stronger role in the relationship between parental divorce and depression than did socioeconomic status or marital transition behaviors. This finding implies that intimate relationships are key in understanding the higher levels of depressed mood observed among women whose parents divorced. Variations of this finding have been obtained in a number of other studies of the long-term effects of childhood experiences. Brown and his colleagues (1986) found that women who lost a mother during childhood were more likely than women who did not to marry men who offered little intimacy or support. Furthermore, these differences were instrumental in explaining the higher rate of clinical depression observed among the former group. Quinton, Rutter, and Liddle (1984) reported a similar finding in a comparison of women who had and had not been raised in institutions. Women with institutional backgrounds were much more likely than others to experience poor mental health, as indicated by high levels of psychiatric disorder and criminality. The authors were able to explain this difference almost entirely by the lack of marital support experienced among women with institutional backgrounds. Thus, the patterns of relationship observed in this sample do not appear to be idiosyncratic. Rather, they become part of a larger pattern of relationship between disruptive childhood experiences, lack of success in intimate relationships, and poor mental health.

Given the pervasiveness of this pattern in previous research, it may seem puzzling that my analysis provided no evidence of a similar pattern for parental death. Parental death and divorce have approximately equivalent relationships with depressed mood, but perceived marital quality plays a much less significant mediating role in the case of the former than of the latter. Empirically, this can be explained by the smaller observed relationships between parental death and most adult outcomes. Given that parental death and marital quality are only weakly related, it is not surprising to discover that marital quality cannot explain the relationship between death and depression. Furthermore, the weaker relationships between parental death and most adult outcomes were, in fact, predicted, based on the lower levels of family disruption and conflict experienced by bereaved as compared to divorced families.

What remains unclear, however, is why parental death should have a significant relationship with depressed mood in the absence of a relationship with marital quality. A sociological life course perspective implies that the interconnections among events over the life course determine current functioning. Two obvious possibilities for my failure to observe these interconnections exist. First, the relationships between parental death and adult depression may be explained by other adult life outcomes which I did not include in the analysis. In other words, I may have failed to identify the relevant life events for persons from homes broken by death. A second possibility is that parental death may have a stronger influence on unobservable, intrapsychic processes than parental divorce, while parental divorce has a stronger influence on observable life experience. In that case, the death-depression relationship would be explained with reference to the unconscious conflicts or negative self-perceptions caused by the death—explanations favored by psychoanalytic and attachment theorists. I cannot offer additional evidence with which to evaluate these alternatives. The variation in the results for death and divorce awaits further replication and consideration.

Finally, consistent with expectation, this analysis documented stronger relationships between parental loss and adult outcomes among women as compared to men. I advanced this expectation based primarily on arguments about the relative importance of interpersonal disruptions in girls' and boys' development. However, there are alternative interpretations for the findings. Girls may be more likely than boys to model the post-divorce attitudes of their custodial parent (usually the mother), leaving them less confident of their potential to have successful interpersonal relationships (Glenn & Kramer, 1987). Or, girls may delay their efforts to cope with the divorce while boys resolve their unhappiness more quickly. Research on children of divorce indicates that parents are more likely to fight in front of boys than girls (Emery, 1982; Hetherington, 1979), and that they offer less consistent discipline to boys than girls following the divorce (Emery, 1982). As a result, boys may be forced to cope with the implications of divorce at the time while girls are not. Consistent with this interpretation, research on short-term reactions to divorce typically documents more negative outcomes among boys than girls (Emery, 1982). Wallerstein and Blakeslee (1989) speculated that the implications of parental divorce for girls' well-being may become visible only as they enter into intimate relationships themselves. This alternative suggests that it is not the greater reliance on interpersonal relationships that places girls at risk, but the fact that they delay their coping efforts until a later time. Although it is not possible for me to choose among these alternatives, each suggests greater long-term implications of parental loss for women than for men.

The conclusions I have drawn from this analysis are necessarily tentative. No analysis which focuses on cross-sectional or retrospective data can provide definitive evidence in favor of particular longitudinal processes. While this analysis provides strong suggestive evidence of the interconnections between the relational and mental health implications of parental divorces, alternative interpretations of the results remain plausible. For example, these results might be spurious due to the influence of childhood and adolescent depression. Kandel and Davies (1986) reported that adolescent girls who experienced high levels of depressed mood reported more problems in their adult marriages and also experienced problems with depression in adulthood. The data which I used in this analysis are not adequate for addressing these types of complexities.

In addition, the sample composition clearly limits the generalizability of these findings. A sample of married persons who experienced a loss may not be representative of the total loss population. One might expect, for example, that the mean difference in age at first marriage between women whose parents got divorced and women with no loss would be larger in a general population sample than it was here because women who get married at younger ages are more likely to get divorced (Glenn & Supancic, 1984; Glick & Norton, 1979). Similarly, early age at marriage might be more strongly implicated in the divorce-depression relationship in a sample that included ever-married persons.

Despite these limitations, this analysis serves as a reminder that understanding why some people experience high levels of depressed mood and others do not requires a consideration of the interconnections among a variety of experiences and responses over the life course. Childhood parental losses appear to begin a chain of events which result in life conditions conducive to the development of poor mental health. Our understanding of the complexities of this chain would be greatly enhanced by prospective studies of development over the life course.

APPENDIX A. DESCRIPTION OF MARITAL QUALITY INDICES

Frequency of disagreements
How often do you and your husband have an unpleasant disagreement?
> 5 = Once a week or more
> 4 = 2 or 3 times a month
> 3 = About once each month
> 2 = Less often
> 1 = Never

Marital problems
In the past 12 months have you:
Had serious marital problems or difficulties? Separated from spouse? Relations with spouse got much worse?
> 1 = Yes to at least one
> 0 = No to all three

Marital trust
How often would you say your husband understands the way you feel about things?
How much can you depend on him to be there when you really need him?
How much concern does he show for your feelings and problems?
How much can you trust him to keep his promises to you?
> 1 = Not at all
> 2 = A little
> 3 = Some
> 4 = A lot

Calm problem-solving strategies
When the two of you disagree…
How often do you discuss your differences calmly?
How often do you try to appreciate your husband's point of view?
How often do you work things out so that both of you are satisfied?
> 5 = Always
> 4 = Usually
> 3 = Sometimes
> 2 = Hardly Ever
> 1 = Never

Conflictual problem-solving strategies
How often do things become tense and unpleasant?
How often does your husband say cruel and angry things to you?
How often do you both refuse to compromise?
(see Calm Problem-Solving)

References

Abraham, Karl. 1924. "A Short Study on the Development of the Libido Viewed in the Light of Mental Disorders." Pp. 418–501 In *Selected Papers of Karl Abraham* (1927). London: Hogarth.

Barnes, Gordon E. and Harry Prosen. 1985. "Parental Death and Depression." *Journal of Abnormal Psychology* 94:64–69.

Bowlby, John. 1969. *Attachment and Loss. Volume I: Attachment.* London: Hogarth Press.

———. 1980. *Attachment and Loss. Volume III: Loss.* New York: Basic Books.

Brown, Felix. 1961. "Depression and Childhood Bereavement." *Journal of Mental Science* 107:74–77.

Brown, George W. and Tirrill O. Harris. 1978. *The Social Origins of Depression: A Study of Psychiatric Disorder in Women.* New York: Free Press.

Brown, George W., Tirril O. Harris, and Antonia Bifulco. 1986. "Long-term Effects of Early Loss of Parent." Pp. 251–96 in *Depression in Young People,* edited by M. Rutter, G. E. Izard, and P. B. Read. New York: Guilford.

Brown, George W., Tirrill O. Harris, and John R. Copeland. 1977. "Depression and Loss." *British Journal of Psychiatry* 130:1–18.

Bumpass, Larry L. and James A. Sweet. 1972. "Differentials in Marital Instability: 1970." *American Sociological Review* 37:754–66.

Chodorow, Nancy. 1978. *The Reproduction of Mothering.* Berkeley, CA: University of California Press.

Derogatis, Leonard I. 1977. *SCL-90: Administration, Scoring & Procedures Manual—I for the Revised Version.* Baltimore: Johns Hopkins School of Medicine.

Derogatis, Leonard I., Ronald S. Lipman, and Lino Covi. 1973. "SCL-90: An Outpatient Psychiatric Rating Scale—Preliminary Report." *Psychopharmacology Bulletin* 9:13–27.

Dohrenwend, Bruce P. and Barbara Snell Dohrenwend. 1969. *Social Status and Psychological Disorder: A Causal Inquiry.* New York: Wiley.

———. 1976. "Sex Differences and Psychiatric Disorders." *American Journal of Sociology* 81:1447–54.

Elder, Glen H., Jr. 1974. *Children of the Great Depression.* Chicago: University of Chicago Press.

———. 1985. "Perspectives on the Life Course." Pp. 23–49 in *Life Course Dynamics,* edited by G. H. Elder, Jr. Ithaca, NY: Cornell University Press.

Emery, Robert E. 1982. "Interparental Conflict and the Children of Discord and Divorce." *Psychological Bulletin* 92:310–30.

Forrest, A.D., R.H. Fraser, and R.G. Priest. 1965. "Environmental Factors in Depressive Illness." *British Journal of Psychiatry* 111:243–53.

Freud, Sigmund. 1917. "Mourning and Melancholia." In *Complete Psychological Works, Volume 14* (1957). London: Hogarth.

Gilligan, Carol. 1982. *In a Different Voice.* Cambridge, MA: Harvard University Press.

Glenn, Norval D. and Kathryn B. Kramer. 1985. "The Psychological Well-being of Adult Children of Divorce." *Journal of Marriage and the Family* 47:905–12.

———. 1987. "The Marriages and Divorces of the Children of Divorce." *Journal of Marriage and the Family* 49:811–25.

Glenn, Norval D. and Michael Supanic. 1984. "The Social and Demographic Correlates of Divorce and Separation in the United States: An Update and Reconsideration." *Journal of Marriage and the Family* 46:563–75.

Glick, Paul C. 1979. "Children of Divorced Parents in Demographic Perspective." *Journal of Social Issues* 35:170–82.

Glick, Paul C. and Arthur J. Norton. 1979. "Marrying, Divorcing, and Living Together in the U.S. Today." *Population Bulletin* 32:3–41.

Greenberg, David and Douglas Wolf. 1982. "The Economic Consequences of Experiencing Parental Marital Disruption." *Child and Youth Services Review* 4:141–62.

Hallstrom, T. 1987. "The Relationships of Childhood Socio-demographic Factors and Early Parental Loss to Major Depression in Adult Life." *Acta Psychiatrica Scandinavica* 75:212–16.

Harris, Tirril O. and George W. Brown. 1985. "Interpreting Data in Aetiological Studies of Affective Disorder: Some Pitfalls and Ambiguities." *British Journal of Psychiatry* 147:5–15.

Harris, Tirrill O., George W. Brown, and Antonia Bifulco. 1986. "Loss of Parent in Childhood and Adult Psychiatric Disorder: The Role of Lack of Adequate Parental Care." *Psychological Medicine* 16:641–59.

Hetherington, E. Mavis. 1979. "Divorce: A Child's Perspective." *American Psychologist* 34:851–58.

Kandel, Denise B. and Mark Davies. 1986. "Adult Sequelae of Adolescent Depressive Symptoms." *Archives of General Psychiatry* 43:255–62.

Keith, Bruce and Paul R. Amato. 1990. "Consequences of Childhood Family Disruptions on Subsequent Adult Well-being." Paper presented at the Midwest Sociological Society Conference, Chicago, IL.

Keith, Verna M. and Barbara Finlay. 1988. "The Impact of Parental Divorce on Children's Educational Attainment, Marital Timing, and Likelihood of Divorce." *Journal of Marriage and the Family* 50:797–809.

Kessler, Ronald C. and Paul D. Cleary. 1980. "Social Class and Psychological Distress." *American Sociological Review* 45:463–78.

Kessler, Ronald C. and Jane D. McLeod. 1984. "Sex Differences in Vulnerability to Undesirable Life Events." *American Sociological Review* 49:620–31.

Langner, Thomas S. and Stanley T. Michael. 1963. *Life Stress and Mental Health*. New York: Free Press.

Lewis, Robert A. and Graham B. Spanier. 1979. "Theorizing About the Quality and Stability of Marriage." Pp. 268–94 in *Contemporary Theories About the Family (Vol. 1)*, edited by W.R. Burr, R. Hill, F.I. Nye, and I.L. Reiss. New York: Free Press.

McLanahan, Sara and Larry Bumpass. 1988. "Intergenerational Consequences of Family Disruption." *American Journal of Sociology* 94:130–52.

Pond, D.A., A. Ryle, and Madge Hamilton. 1963. "Marriage and Neurosis in a Working-class Population." *British Journal of Psychiatry* 109:592–98.

Pope, Hallowell and Charles W. Mueller. 1976. "The Intergenerational Transmission of Marital Instability: Comparisons by Sex and Race." *Journal of Social Issues* 32:49–66.

Quinton, David, Michael Rutter, and Christine Liddle. 1984. "Institutional Rearing, Parenting Difficulties and Marital Support." *Psychological Medicine* 14:107–24.

Robins, Lee N., John E. Helzer, Jack Croughan, and Kathryn L. Ratcliff. 1981. "National Institute of Mental Health Diagnostic Interview Schedule: Its History, Characteristics and Validity." *Archives of General Psychiatry* 38:381–89.

Tennant, Christopher, Paul Bebbington, and Jane Hurry. 1982. "Social Experiences in Childhood and Adult Psychiatric Morbidity: A Multiple Regression Analysis." *Psychological Medicine* 12:321–27.

Veroff, Joseph, Elizabeth Douvan, and Richard Kulka. 1981. *The Inner American: A Self-Portrait from 1957 to 1976.* New York: Basic Books.

Wadsworth, M.E.J. and M. Maclean. 1986. "Parents' Divorce and Children's Life Chances." *Children and Youth Services Review* 8:145–59.

Wallerstein, Judith S. and Sandra Blakeslee. 1989. *Second Chances.* New York: Ticknor & Fields.

Wheaton, Blair. 1978. "The Sociogenesis of Psychological Disorder: Reexamining the Causal Issues with Longitudinal Data." *American Sociological Review* 43:383–403.

DISCUSSION

1. In what ways are the principles of human development as a lifelong process and of interdependent lives evident in McLeod's research?

2. The life course perspective also emphasizes the importance of the historical context in shaping the effects of specific life experiences on individuals. Do you think McLeod's results would generalize to people who grew up during other historical periods? Why or why not?

Scott Schieman, Karen van Gundy, and John Taylor

Status, Role, and Resource Explanations for Age Patterns in Psychological Distress

Schieman and colleagues focus on an important sociodemographic pattern in research on psychological distress: the U-shaped association with age. The explanations they offer for the association link to previous selections on socioeconomic status, roles, and the stress process model. In addition to its substantive contributions, this selection introduces the concept of a suppressor variable—a variable whose presence in an analysis reveals a previously null association. In this case, the greater satisfaction with finances and fewer religious doubts associated with increasing age mask the upturn in distress among older Americans. Suppressor effects are omnipresent in research on mental health but are often ignored.

Are there age patterns in psychological distress? Turner and Lloyd (1999) assert that age is among several core social characteristics that have "reliably defined variations in risk for depression" (p. 391). However, Newmann (1989) argues, "we are left with many unanswered questions about the aging process" (p. 162) and its relationship to mental health. A number of studies

Schieman, Scott, Karen van Gundy, and John Taylor. 2001. "Status, Role, and Resource Explanations for Age Patterns in Psychological Distress." *Journal of Health and Social Behavior* 42:80–96.

document a U-shaped age pattern in depression or distress (Kessler et al., 1992; Mirowsky & Reynolds, 2000; Mirowsky & Ross, 1992, 1999a; Wade & Cairney, 1997). However, others fail to detect a substantial old-age upturn in psychological distress (Feinson, 1985; Newmann, 1989; Turner, Noh, & Levin, 1985). While several of the studies cited above examine mediating effects, only one that we are aware of considers conditions that suppress the old-age upturn in depression (see Wade & Cairney, 2000). Thus, our study has three aims: (1) to replicate the U-shaped cross section in two recent U.S. data sets, (2) to confirm and elaborate the mediators of the age-distress relationship, and (3) to explore further an array of potential suppression effects. We examine data from two U.S. samples—the 1996 and 1998 General Social Surveys—to explore the relationships among age, age-linked personal and social qualities, and two different measures of psychological distress: depressive symptoms (1996) and generalized psychological distress (1998).

STRAINS, RESOURCES, AND AGE PATTERNS IN DISTRESS

Recent calls for an "alliance" between stress and life course research (see Pearlin & Skaff, 1996) guide our ideas about age-correlated factors that may *explain* or *suppress* parts of the age-distress association. Specifically, we organize our paper around three general themes: (1) possible "status strains," measured by low education, financial dissatisfaction, and poor health; (2) potential "role strains," assessed by retirement and widowhood statuses, dissatisfaction with family, time demands, and shameful emotional experiences; and (3) personal "resources" related to the sense of control, religious participation and confidence, optimism about human nature, and the sense of forgiveness for past regrets and offenses (see Figure 1). We focus on age variations in the structural *and* subjective organization of lives and propose that less dissatisfaction with finances and family, fewer time demands, greater religious participation and confidence, a more optimistic viewpoint, less shame, and a sense of forgiveness may provide an emotional counterbalance to potential threats to well-being in later life, such as retirement, widowhood, poor health, and a lower sense of control.

Status Strains

Age patterns in education, financial dissatisfaction, and poor health may contribute to age differences in psychological distress. Health and financial difficulties are status strains that often vary across the life course (Pearlin & Skaff, 1996). Along with those strains, we include low educational attainment. As a resource and a source of human capital, education ripens personal qualities such as persistence, effectiveness (Becker, 1993), and a sense of control (Mirowsky & Ross 1998). However, historical trends in economic patterns and labor market needs may produce a negative correlation between age and education—which, in turn, may partly contribute to higher depression in the

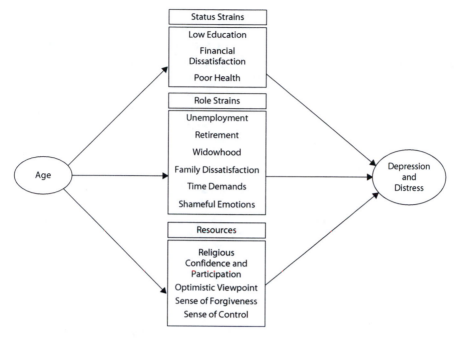

Figure 1 Conceptual Model

latter part of the life span (Mirowsky & Ross, 1992; Wade & Cairney, 1997). Moreover, the effect of low education may occur through the greater risk of unemployment, poorer finances, and health, and a lower sense of personal control (Ross & Van Willigen, 1997).

Economic quandaries can incite daily stress for people at any age (Pearlin & Skaff, 1996). Financial strains may obstruct goals and increase a sense of powerlessness, which, in turn, can threaten mental health (Ross & Huber, 1985). During young adulthood, many individuals embark on careers and the accumulation of pecuniary assets. In midlife, occupational achievements tend to consolidate and furnish an overall sense of financial worth and stability. In later life, having fewer young dependents and greater governmental assistance with medical expenses may ease fiscal burdens. Indeed, some studies demonstrate that average levels of economic hardship (Mirowsky & Ross, 1999b) and dissatisfaction with finances (Schieman, 1999) *decrease* among older age groups. Dissatisfaction's positive association with distress and its negative association with age may contribute to better mental health among older adults. Although research documents the effect of objective income measures (Mirowsky & Ross, 1992), to our knowledge no studies test the effect of subjective accounts of financial satisfaction *and* income comparisons to "average families" on the age-psychological distress relationship.

Poor health and physical impairment is a prevalent strain in later life (Pearlin & Skaff, 1996) and may be related to mental health (Gatz & Zarit,

1999). Age-linked physiological processes can increase impairment and pain, and erode subjective health (Johnson & Wolinsky, 1993). In addition, age-related decline in sensory, motor, and cognitive abilities may impede role performance and generate a sense of powerlessness (Rodin, 1986). Unlike objective measures, subjective indicators of health reflect one's overall condition relative to social reference-based expectations. In sum, as a "status strain," we suspect that declining health during midlife and beyond contributes to poorer mental health during those periods. Additionally, low education and financial dissatisfaction represent status strains that are related positively to distress. However, based on previous studies, older adults tend to report less education and poorer health—patterns that predict *more* psychological distress in later life. In contrast, despite reporting less income, older people tend to report less financial dissatisfaction—a pattern that may suppress levels of psychological distress among older adults. We test both possibilities.

Role Strains

Pearlin and Skaff (1996) identify potential emotional consequences of "the social warp and weave of aging, especially transitions into and out of social roles..." (p. 239). For example, work and family roles often breed challenges that can elevate the risk of emotions (Pearlin, 1983; Schieman, 1999, 2000). Role sets influence self-structures, which, in turn, organize emotional experiences (Labouvie-Vief, 1999). In addition, the full-time employee role can cultivate personal qualities, such as the sense of control, that protect against distress (Ross & Mirowsky, 1995). However, many people also struggle to balance the time pressures caused by competing full-time work and family roles (Hochschild, 1997). Moreover, problematic aspects of work and family may produce feelings of inequity, unfairness, dissatisfaction, and negative affect (Ross & Van Willigen, 1996). Additionally, social exchanges within core role domains often reflect emotional ties in which opinions are shared and are highly esteemed. In such domains, where the propensity for failure and disappointment is greater, the risk of experiencing shameful emotions may be higher (Scheff, 2000). Moreover, feelings of embarrassment may be strongly related to social judgments that threaten identity. Although some research shows the relevance of shame for emotions like anger (Scheff, 2000; Schieman, 1999), less is known about the role and significance of age patterns in shame for the relationship between age and psychological distress.

We suspect that role strains related to time demands, dissatisfaction with family life, and shameful emotional experiences are associated positively with psychological distress. Strains associated with multiple role commitments may be more prevalent during the young adulthood years. Additionally, social-emotional selectivity theory proposes that older people are more proficient at conserving their emotions, are less acutely affected by others, and show greater restraint, tolerance, and an ability to express affection, even in conflictual situations (Carstensen, 1993; Labouvie-Vief, 1999). Some research shows that older people tend to report fewer conflictual relationships relative to younger adults (Schieman & Van Gundy, 2000)—relationships that may threaten emotional well-being. The view of age as *maturity* suggests, "with growing insight and skill, social and psychological traits and tendencies merge into an increasingly harmonious whole" (Mirowsky & Ross, 1992, 188). A sense of others and a "know-how" may accrue with time and experience to help people manage discordant social appraisals. By extension, older people may report fewer emotions that entail disapproving self- and social-evaluations such as embarrassment and shame. A lower risk of shameful emotions among older adults may suppress an old-age upturn in distress. A previous study documents that older people tend to report fewer time demands, less dissatisfaction with family, and fewer shameful emotions, and those patterns contribute to less *anger* among older people (Schieman, 1999). In the present study, we examine if those same patterns also suppress psychological distress during midlife and old age.

In contrast to maturity reflected in a "good old age," stressful challenges related to role losses may offset the personal growth associated with maturity. For instance, retirement may reduce involvement in activities, the sense of purpose, and control (Ross & Drentea, 1998). Additionally, many older adults often confront extraordinary ordeals related to the loss of a spouse (Pitcher & Larson, 1989). Widowhood eliminates a source of companionship and can undercut a sense of purpose and meaning. Moreover, it may force individuals to confront death, which, in turn, may wear down an individual's sense of control and optimism about life (Ferraro, 1989). Diminished financial resources further compound isolation and other forms of distress among widowers (Umberson, Wortman, & Kessler, 1992). Thus, a higher probability of retirement and widowhood during the later years may contribute to higher levels of depression in old age.

Personal Resources

The stress process model identifies personal qualities, such as a high sense of control, that promote coping and bolster resilience to adversity (Pearlin, 1999). Conversely, low control implies a sense of powerlessness and a belief that life chances are ruled by fate (Mirowsky & Ross, 1991). Empirical and theoretical observations provide grounds for expecting age patterns in control. For example, theories of the life cycle describe midlife as a time of increased power and control (Mirowsky & Ross, 1992). In general, many cross-sectional studies show a curvilinear association such that average levels of control increase through early adulthood, peak during middle age, and then are lower among older adults (Gecas, 1989), although the evidence is still inconclusive (see Clark-Plaskie & Lachman, 1999). However, recent international (Sastry & Ross, 1998), U.S. (Mirowsky, 1995), and Canadian (Schieman & Turner, 1998) surveys show that older people tend to report less control. Greater personal control in young adulthood through midlife predicts less distress during that period; conversely, lower levels of control in later life predict more distress among older adults.

Religion is another potential resource that may affect individual emotionality. Research shows that religious behavior can enhance coping resources and well-being for older adults (Krause et al., 1999b; Levin & Chatters, 1998; Musick, Blazer, & Hays, 2000). Religious principles often provide meaning and guidance, enhance the emotional lives of the faithful (Krause et al., 1999a), and foster one's capacity to reconcile past grievances. In contrast, people who view the world in terms of pain, evil, and suffering may have reservations about their faith and be disinclined to pardon the self and others for bygone faults and offenses. Additionally, having a pessimistic outlook and misgivings about faith may foster cognitive dissonance (Festinger, 1957) and leave individuals feeling unsettled, conflicted, and ashamed (Krause et al., 1999a). Conversely, greater confidence and participation in religious activities may provide a sense of emotional calm and a crucial source of social support.

Are there age patterns in religious participation and confidence, optimistic viewpoint, and the sense of forgiveness? Role losses can motivate older people to seek alternative sources of purpose, meaning, and integration in later life (Payne, 1988). Although inconclusive, studies generally show a high salience of religion, spirituality, church affiliation, and devotion to religious attendance among older adults (Koenig, 1995; Krause et al., 1999b). Theoretical views of age as maturity imply that over the life span individuals attain insight, practice, and experience. Age affords time for individuals to solidify their faith, acquire a sense of absolution of the self and others for shortcomings and earlier transgressions, and to come to terms with feelings of anger and resentment. Additionally, an outlook marked by the capacity for "forgiveness" may be associated with "optimal aging" (Labouvie-Vief, 1999). Thus, we suspect that greater religious participation and confidence, an optimistic viewpoint, and a greater sense of forgiveness among older adults suppress an old-age upturn in depression and distress.

Summary of Hypotheses

Based on the majority of existing research we suspect a parabolic relationship between age and psychological distress such that young adults (under age 30) and adults in later life (over age 70) have higher levels of distress compared to adults in midlife. Lower levels of education and poorer self-rated health among successively older age groups may suppress a decline in distress and explain part of an old-age upturn. Conversely, greater financial satisfaction among older age groups may contribute to a downward slope and suppress part of an old-age upturn in distress. In addition, strains related to retirement and widowhood may contribute to an upward age curve in distress. However, there may be suppression effects that counter threats to well-being among the oldest-old: Fewer time demands, greater family satisfaction, greater religious confidence, and participation, fewer shameful emotions, greater optimism, and a sense of forgiveness among older age groups may counteract challenges to emotional well-being in late life.

DATA AND METHODS

Samples

We use data from the 1996 and 1998 General Social Surveys (see Davis & Smith, 1999). The General Social Survey is a probability sample of English speaking adults living in households in the United States. The 1996 survey had a response rate of about 76 percent (2,904 out of 3,814 cases). In 1996, a subset of 1,460 respondents was asked questions about emotions. Our analyses are based on 1,408 individuals who had complete responses to depression items. The 1998 survey had a response rate of about 76 percent (2,832 out of 3,745 cases). In 1998, a subset of 1,445 respondents was asked questions about generalized psychological distress. Our analyses are based on 1,409 individuals who had complete responses to distress items. In both samples, the age range is 18 to 89, with a mean around 45 years. About 55 percent are female. About 80 percent are white.

Measures

Dependent variables. The 1996 and 1998 surveys use different measures to assess respondents' levels of psychological distress. The 1996 depression index uses items similar to the Center for Epidemiological Studies' Depression Scale (CES-D) (Radloff, 1977). Seven items ask, "On how many days in the *past 7 days* have you felt:" "sad," "lonely," "happy," "anxious and tense," "fearful about something that might happen to you," "you couldn't shake the blues," and "so restless that you couldn't sit long in a chair?" We reversed the "happy" item and averaged responses such that higher scores reflect greater depression.

In contrast, the six items in the 1998 survey assess one-month prevalence rates of generalized distress (Wade & Cairney, 1997). The items ask, "In the *past 30 days,* how often did you feel:" "so sad nothing could cheer you up," "nervous," "restless or fidgety," "hopeless," "that everything was an effort," and "worthless?" The response categories range from "all of the time" (1) to "none of the time" (5). We reversed coding so that higher scores reflect greater generalized distress.

Independent variables. Age is measured in years. Although peripheral to our hypotheses, we also adjust for ascribed statuses of sex and race. Gender is coded 1 for females. Minority status is coded 1 if respondents are non-white. In both surveys, education is measured in years of schooling. Available in both the 1996 and 1998 General Social Surveys, "never married," "divorced or separated," and "widowed" roles are each coded 1 in a series of dummy variables, with "married" as the omitted contrast category. "Full-time," "part-time," "school," "homemaker," and "retired" roles are each coded 1, with "unemployed" as the contrast category. In both surveys, an item that measures subjective global health asks, "Would you say your own health, in general, is excellent (4), good (3), fair (2), or poor (1)?" Higher scores reflect better health.

In both surveys, two items assess satisfaction with financial circumstances. One asks, "So far as you and your family are concerned, would you say that you are (1) pretty well satisfied with your present financial situation, (2) more or less satisfied, or (3) not satisfied at all?" We reverse the codes such that higher scores reflect greater satisfaction. The second asks, "Compared with American families in general, would you say your family income is far below average (1), below average (2), average (3), above average (4), or far above average (5)?" We standardized and averaged the items to create the index. The items reflect the subjective account of financial conditions relative to social comparisons with the respondent's image of the "average American family."

Questions about the perceptions about time demands, satisfaction with family life, and the experience of shameful emotional experiences are only available in the 1996 General Social Survey. One item that measures perceptions about time demands asks, "In general, how do you feel about your time—would you say that you (1) never feel rushed even to do things you have to do, (2) only sometimes feel rushed, or (3) almost always feel rushed?" Also, a satisfaction with family life item asks, "How successful do you feel in your family life?" Choices range from "not at all successful" (1) to "very successful" (5). Additionally, several questions ask respondents about the experience of shameful emotions: "On how many days in the past 7 days have you" (1) "felt ashamed of something you'd done" and (2) "felt embarrassed about something?" These two items are summed to form a composite measure in which higher scores reflect more shame.

In 1996, sense of control items ask respondents the extent they agree or disagree with four statements: (1) "There is no sense in planning a lot—if something good is going to happen, it will;" (2) "Most of my problems are due to bad breaks;" (3) "The really good things that happen to me are mostly luck;" and (4) "I have little control over the bad things that happen to me" (Mirowsky &Ross, 1991). Choices range from "strongly agree" (1) to "strongly disagree" (5). We summed items; higher scores reflect greater control.

In both 1996 and 1998 surveys, a religious attendance item asks, "how often do you attend religious services?" Response choices range from "never" (0) to "several times a week" (8). Measures of religious doubt, optimistic viewpoint, and the sense of forgiveness are available only in the 1998 survey. Items that measure an individual's religious doubt ask, "How often have these problems caused doubts about your religious faith?" Items include "evil in the world" and "personal suffering." Response choices are "often" (1), "sometimes" (2), and "never" (3). We reversed the codes such that higher scores reflect more religious doubt; we summed and averaged the items.

Several items measure optimistic viewpoint with the following statements:

People have different views of the world and human nature. We'd like to know the kinds of images you have. Where would you place your image of the world?

The items are: (1) "The world is basically filled with evil and sin...there is much goodness in the world which hints at God's goodness" and (2) "Human nature is basically good...human nature is fundamentally perverse and corrupt." Items are coded on a 7-point scale. We reversed the second item and averaged the two items. Higher scores indicate a more optimistic viewpoint.

Items that measure a sense of forgiveness asks respondents, "Because of your religious or spiritual beliefs have you always, almost always, often, seldom, or never felt the following ways:" (1) "I have forgiven myself for things that I have done wrong" and (2) "I have forgiven those who hurt me." Response choices range from 1 to 4; we reversed codes and averaged the items such that higher scores indicate a greater sense of forgiveness.

Analytic Strategy

To obtain an overall age profile, we examine crude mean levels of distress across 10-year age categories. To what extent are these patterns attributable to age-correlated patterns in our independent variables? We estimate a model with ordinary least squares regression to establish the total association without adjustments. Next, we adjust for sex, race, and education to establish the total effect of age on depression. Education is a factor that tends to stabilize early in the life course and changes little over time (Mirowsky & Ross, 1992). Then, to assess their unique contribution to age patterns in depression, we adjust for sets of variables such as marital and work statuses, religious attitudes and participation, role strains, health status (in both surveys), and the sense of control (in the 1996 survey only). In each step we examine change in the age coefficients. An *increase* in the age coefficient indicates a suppressor effect; a *decrease* could indicate a link from age through that set of variables. We add some of the variables from Figure 1 simultaneously because we suspect that taken together they explain a downward age pattern and suppress an old-age upturn.

RESULTS

The 1996 Sample

The top panel of Figure 2 shows that average levels of depression tend to decrease from young adulthood through midlife and are higher among the oldest age groups in the 1996 sample. In particular, the 60-year-old age group has the lowest average depression. To model the falling and rising means, we regress depression on age and age squared. Additionally, we adjust for age-correlated independent variables shown in Table 1.

Equation 1 of Table 2 reports the negative linear and positive quadratic age coefficients, which reflect the patterns shown in the top panel of Figure 2. Line 1 of Figure 3 represents the linear and quadratic age coefficients shown in equation 1. Next, we compare age and age^2 coefficients from equation 1

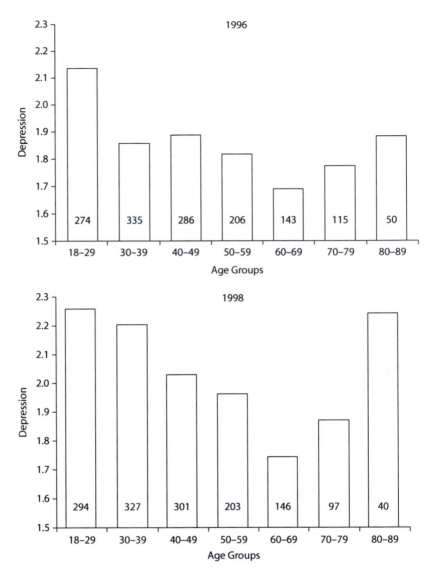

Figure 2 Average Levels of Depression in 1996 (upper) and Generalized Distress in 1998 (lower) across Age Groups.

Note: The numbers of cases are shown inside the bars.

with those obtained in adjustment of the hypothesized mediating variables (equations 2 through 6).

Equation 2 of Table 2 shows that women report more depression, but race has no effect. Adjustment for sex and race influences the age-depression association by a trivial amount. Equation 3 shows that education is associated negatively with depression. In addition Table 1 shows that average levels of

Table 1 Average Levels of Independent Variables across Age Groups (1996 Survey)

Age Group	Years of Education	Financial Satisfaction	Family Satisfaction	Time Demands	Shameful Emotions	Religious Attendance	Sense of Control	Global Health
18–29	13.435	−.054	3.493	2.180	1.231	3.071	13.346	3.204
	(2.273)	(.840)	(.811)	(.599)	(2.037)	(2.430)	(3.157)	(.695)
30–39	13.639	−.073	3.419	2.284	1.168	3.550	13.961	3.196
	(2.552)	(.780)	(.849)	(.618)	(2.045)	(2.579)	(3.061)	(.677)
40–49	14.247	−.024	3.559	2.279	1.169	3.425	14.314	3.093
	(2.714)	(.770)	(.868)	(.633)	(2.143)	(2.599)	(3.190)	(.768)
50–59	13.790	.046	3.685	2.147	.813	3.778	14.865	2.951
	(2.976)	(.871)	(.800)	(.673)	(1.808)	(2.549)	(2.914)	(.877)
60–69	12.610	.135	3.767	1.773	.794	4.458	14.183	2.822
	(3.592)	(.862)	(.830)	(.651)	(1.922)	(2.494)	(3.001)	(.828)
70–79	11.804	.160	3.733	1.659	.969	4.835	13.047	2.793
	(2.988)	(.828)	(.880)	(.690)	(1.911)	(2.675)	(3.191)	(.802)
80 and older	11.400	.069	3.642	1.450	.750	4.675	13.098	2.800
	(3.045)	(.743)	(.883)	(.677)	(2.227)	(2.711)	(2.676)	(.882)

Note: Standard deviations shown in parentheses.

Table 2 Regression of Depression on Age (1); Ascribed Statuses (2); Education (3); Roles (4); Satisfactions, Time Demands, Shame, and Religious Attendance (5); and the Sense of Control and Global Health Status (6) (1996 Survey, N =1,408)

Variables	1	2	3	4	5	6
$(Age)10^{-4}$	−.103***	−.106***	−.112***	−.133***	−.052**	−.079**
	(−5.277)	(−5.430)	(−5.735)	(−5.173)	(−2.872)	(−3.414)
$(Age^2)10^{-3}$	.215*	.207*	.106	.013	.234**	.100
	(2.227)	(2.140)	(1.090)	(.115)	(2.608)	(.946)
Women = 1		.171**	.165**	.110	.179**	.139*
		(2.948)	(2.867)	(1.804)	(3.426)	(2.556)
Nonwhite = 1		−.088	−.128	−.172*	−.088	−.183**
		(−1.181)	(−1.727)	(−2.298)	(−1.286)	(−2.671)
Education			−.051***	−.042***	−.036***	−.001
			(−4.932)	(−3.969)	(−3.806)	(−.163)
Full-time[a]				−.334**		−.195
				(−2.888)		(−1.869)
Part-time[a]				−.353*		−.234
				(−2.500)		(−1.867)
In School[a]				−.328		−.136
				(−1.640)		(−.765)
Homemaker[a]				−.183		−.090
				(−1.289)		(−.718)
Retired[a]				−.224		−.089
				(−1.392)		(−.626)
Never Married[b]				.171*		.082
				(2.020)		(1.074)
Divorced[b]				.295***		.146*
				(3.888)		(2.100)
Widowed[b]				.470***		.356***
				(4.136)		(3.531)
Financial Satisfaction					−.194***	−.132***
					(−5.850)	(−3.969)
Family Satisfaction					−.068*	−.022
					(−2.159)	(−.709)
Time Demands					.194***	.214***
					(4.759)	(5.235)
Shameful Emotions					.188***	.183***
					(14.671)	(14.683)
Religious Attendance					−.045***	−.039***
					(−4.398)	(−3.952)
Sense of Control						−.055***
						(−6.068)
Global Health						−.161***
						(−4.556)
Constant	2.015	1.937	2.666	2.745	2.214	2.947
R^2	.019	.026	.042	.067	.230	.277

[e]p <.10; *p <.05; **p <.01; ***p <.001 (two-tailed test)
Note: Unstandardized regression coefficients with t-statistics in parentheses.
[a]Compared to unemployed.
[b]Compared to married.

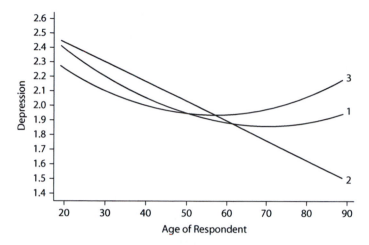

Figure 3 Age and Depression (1996 Survey)

Note: Regression line 1 reflects the unadjusted age and age-squared coefficients from equation 1 of Table 2; line 2 reflects the slope adjusted for sex, race, education, and social roles in equation 4 of Table 2; line 3 reflects the slope adjusted for financial satisfaction, family satisfaction, time demands, shameful emotions, and religious attendance in equation 5 of Table 2.

education tend to increase through young adulthood into midlife, and older people report the fewest years of education. Adjustment for those patterns suppresses the age coefficient by 5.6 percent and reduces the age² coefficient from .207 to .106, or by 48.7 percent, to statistical insignificance ($t = 1.090$).

Equation 4 shows that, compared to unemployed individuals, people employed full- and part-time report significantly less depression. Compared to married individuals, people who are never married, divorced, or widowed report significantly more depression. Adjustment for statuses increases the age term from −.112 to −.133, or by 18.7 percent, and reduces the age² coefficient from .106 to .013, or by 87.7 percent. Separate analyses (not shown here) comparing the effects of employment versus marital status reveal that widowhood has a larger influence. That is, higher rates of widowhood among older people accounts for part of the positive component of the age curve. Conversely, higher rates of marriage among middle-aged people account for some of the negative age slope. However, the greater probability of being never married, divorced, or separated during young adulthood and early midlife offsets marriage's beneficial effect, suppressing the downward pattern by 19 percent. Line 2 in Figure 3 shows the effect of those adjustments.

Equation 5 shows that financial satisfaction and religious attendance are associated negatively with depression, and means of those factors tend to increase from young adulthood through midlife (see Table 1). In addition, shame and time demands are associated positively with depression, and means of those factors tend to decrease from young adulthood through midlife. Thus, adjustment for those age patterns decrease the age term from .112 to .052, or by about 53.5 percent. However, the negative age term remains statistically significant. Additionally, the age^2 term increases by 120 percent with adjustment for satisfaction with family (5 percent) and finances (42 percent), time demands (100 percent), shame (1 percent), and religious attendance (12 percent). Time demands and satisfaction with finances have the largest suppression effect on the old-age upturn. That is, older people would report even higher depression were it not for their greater financial satisfaction and fewer time demands.

Equation 6 shows that the sense of control and self-rated health are associated negatively with depression. In addition, age differences in the sense of control have an inverted u-shape that is almost the mirror opposite of age patterns in depression (see Table 1). In separate analyses (not shown here), we adjust for the sense of control and exclude health. That decreases the age term by 16 percent and decreases the age^2 term by about 72 percent. We also adjust for self-rated health and exclude the sense of control. That increases the age coefficient by 19 percent and increases the age^2 coefficient by 24 percent. Those increases may be due to the fact that average self-rated health declines until about age 60 and then stabilizes in later life (see Table 1). Comparing equations 3 and 6 in Table 2, the inclusion of both control and health in the full model reduces the age coefficient from −.112 to −.079, or by 30 percent, and has little effect on the age^2 coefficient (.106 to .100).

The 1998 Sample

The bottom panel of Figure 2 shows that average levels of generalized distress tend to decrease across young adulthood through midlife and are higher among the oldest age group in the 1998 sample. Similar to the 1996 sample, the 60-year-old age group has the lowest average distress. We expect that age-correlated personal and social conditions shown in Table 3 contribute to age differences in distress.

Equation 1 of Table 4 presents the total association between age and distress, controlling for ascribed statuses. The negative age and positive age^2 coefficients indicate a significant parabolic association between age and distress (see line 1 of Figure 4). In equation 2, the sex and race effects are not significant and, therefore, cannot mediate any of age's association with distress. Equation 3 shows that education is associated negatively with distress. Average education increases through young adulthood into midlife, but older people report less education (see Table 3). Adjustment for education increases the age coefficient from −.086 to −.092 or by 7 percent, and reduces the age^2 coefficient from .272 to .183, or by 32.7 percent.

Equation 4 of Table 4 shows that, compared to the unemployed, individuals who are employed full-time, part-time, or are retired report less distress. Compared to married respondents, the never married and divorced report more distress. Adjustment for marital and work status reduces the age term from −.092 to −.081, or by 12 percent, and it reduces the age^2 coefficient from .183 to .146, or by 20.2 percent. Higher rates of retirement contribute to the upward age curve; conversely, higher rates of marriage and full-time

Table 3 Average Levels of Independent Variables across Age Groups (1998 Survey)

Age Group	Years of Education	Financial Satisfaction	Religious Doubts	Sense of Forgiveness	Optimistic Viewpoint	Religious Attendance	Global Health
18–29	13.179	–.286	1.664	3.075	4.324	2.849	3.178
	(2.288)	(.806)	(.613)	(.764)	(1.277)	(2.430)	(.736)
30–39	13.722	–.015	1.573	3.239	4.569	3.691	3.247
	(2.435)	(.817)	(.604)	(.691)	(1.350)	(2.683)	(.697)
40–49	13.553	–.051	1.555	3.258	4.690	3.638	3.052
	(2.904)	(.858)	(.607)	(.683)	(1.343)	(2.740)	(.816)
50–59	13.740	.294	1.529	3.307	4.814	3.720	3.000
	(3.083)	(.881)	(.620)	(.668)	(1.454)	(2.809)	(.921)
60–69	12.741	.107	1.510	3.326	4.749	3.679	2.825
	(3.364)	(.736)	(.573)	(.709)	(1.391)	(2.929)	(.858)
70–79	12.217	.121	1.478	3.243	5.082	4.434	2.730
	(3.407)	(.858)	(.571)	(.779)	(1.143)	(2.938)	(.911)
80 and older	10.240	.172	1.350	3.405	5.209	4.420	2.400
	(3.217)	(.662)	(.573)	(.726)	(1.465)	(2.983)	(.903)

Note: Standard deviations shown in parentheses.

Table 4 Regression of Generalized Distress on Age (1); Ascribed Statuses (2); Education (3); Roles (4); Financial Satisfaction, Religious Doubt and Attendance, Optimism and Forgiveness (5); and Global Health (6) (1998 Survey $N = 1,409$)

Variables	1	2	3	4	5	6
$(Age)10^{-1}$	−.088***	−.086***	−.092***	−.081***	−.053***	−.075***
	(−6.892)	(−6.665)	(−7.171)	(−4.726)	(−4.264)	(−4.645)
$(Age^2)10^{-3}$	.275***	.272***	.183**	.146ᵠ	.175**	.203**
	(4.332)	(4.261)	(2.850)	(1.884)	(2.888)	(2.831)
Women = 1		.015	.016	−.028	.008	−.018
		(.383)	(.436)	(−.688)	(.242)	(−.475)
Nonwhite = 1		.049	.002	−.012	−.035	−.057
		(1.019)	(.052)	(−.251)	(−.755)	(−1.276)
Education			−.044***	−.036***	−.027***	−.013*
			(−6.498)	(−5.164)	(−3.082)	(−2.053)
Full-timeª				−.394***		−.184*
				(−4.572)		(−2.266)
Part-timeª				−345**		−159.
				(−3.347)		(−1.656)
In Schoolª				−.291ᵠ		−.116
				(−1.896)		(−.817)
Homemakerª				−.114		−.001
				(−1.122)		(−.013)
Retiredª				−.322**		−.246*
				(−3.012)		(−2.484)
Never Marriedᵇ				.159**		.029
				(2.865)		(.567)
Divorcedᵇ				.204***		.083ᵠ
				(3.819)		(1.644)
Widowedᵇ				.039		−.009
				(.498)		(−.130)
Financial Satisfaction					−.174***	−.110***
					(−7.511)	(−4.711)
Religious Doubts					.255***	.238***
					(8.388)	(8.066)
Sense of Forgiveness					−.106***	−.108***
					(−3.979)	(−4.199)
Optimistic Viewpoint					−.031*	−.018
					(−2.272)	(−1.381)
Religious Attendance					−.007	.000
					(−1.081)	(.097)
Global Health						−.218***
						(−9.140)
Constant	1.812	1.795	2.424	2.592	2.324	2.906
R^2	.034	.034	.063	.095	.171	.235

ᵠ$p < .10$; *$p < .05$; **$p < .01$; ***$p < .001$ (two-tailed test)
Note: Unstandardized regression coefficients with t-statistics in parentheses.
ªCompared to unemployed.
ᵇCompared to married.

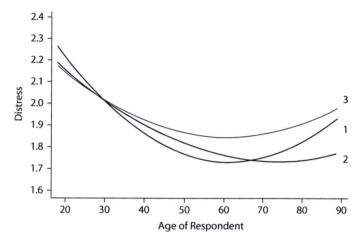

Figure 4 Age and Generalized Psychological Distress (1998 Survey)

Note: Regression line 1 reflects the unadjusted age and age-squared coefficients from equation 1 of Table 4; line 2 reflects the slope adjusted for sex, race, education, and social roles in equation 4 of Table 4; line 3 reflects the slope adjusted for financial satisfaction, religious doubts, forgiveness, optimistic viewpoint, and religious attendance in equation 5 of Table 4.

employment contribute to the downward age pattern. Line 2 in Figure 4 shows the association with those adjustments.

Age is generally associated positively with financial satisfaction, the sense of forgiveness, optimistic viewpoint, and religious attendance; conversely, it is associated negatively with religious doubts (see Table 3). People with greater satisfaction with finances, fewer religious doubts, a greater sense of forgiveness, and a more optimistic viewpoint report less distress (see equation 5 of Table 4). The age term decreases by 42.4 percent with adjustment for satisfaction with finances (23 percent), religious doubts (12 percent), forgiveness (8 percent), optimism (7 percent), and religious attendance (7 percent). In addition, the age^2 coefficient decreases with adjustment for satisfaction with finances (23 percent) and forgiveness (6 percent), and it increases with adjustment for religious doubts (6 percent). Line 3 of Figure 4 illustrates the association with those adjustments.

Equation 6 in Table 4 adjusts for subjective health status. Health is associated negatively with distress, and average levels of health decrease across age groups (see Table 3). A separate analysis that adjusts for self-rated health alone increases the age term by 30 percent.

Those patterns indicate that declining subjective health *suppresses* the downward age curve in distress by 30 percent. However, adjustment for subjective health in the full model shows that the age term decreases from −.092 to −.075, or by 18.5 percent (comparing equations 3 and 6 in Table 4). In addition, adjustment for self-rated health in the full model increases the age^2 coefficient from .183 to .203, or by 11.5 percent.

To sum, in the 1996 sample, less education, lower control, and widowhood contribute to higher depression in later life. However, fewer time demands and greater financial satisfaction suppress the upward age pattern in depression. Greater control, fewer demands, less shame, and greater religious attendance explain part of the lower depression from the young adulthood through midlife years. Conversely, declining health among adults in midlife suppresses the size of the negative age coefficient. Comparing equations 3 and 6 in Table 2, the lack of an effect on the age^2 coefficient is attributable to competing influences of age-linked personal and social conditions. In the 1998 survey, greater satisfaction with finances and fewer religious doubts contribute to the downward age pattern in distress. However, declining levels of health suppress the downturn. Conversely, less education and retired status account for some of the old-age upturn. We did not detect substantial suppression effects of personal and social conditions on the age^2 term in the 1998 data.

DISCUSSION

We examined age differences in psychological distress and the conditions that contribute to those differences. In the 1996 General Social Survey, average levels of depression decrease across young adulthood through middle age and increase among the oldest age groups. Similar patterns exist for generalized distress in the 1998 survey. We document statistically significant linear and quadratic age coefficients, results that generally reinforce previous findings of an overall u-shaped age pattern in depression (Kessler et al., 1992; Mirowsky & Ross, 1992, 1999a; Wade & Cairney, 1997, 2000). In addition, we document a significant old-age upturn in depression and distress, with a steeper increase in the 1998 survey. That pattern may be related to the different measures: The 1996 items measure short-term and transient symptoms of depression in the *past seven days*. The 1998 measure, which has better reliability, taps psychological distress over the *past 30 days*. The measure for the longer time period may capture a more accurate profile of emotional experience. In addition, the "nervous" and "restless or fidgety" items reflect anxiety more than depression. Some researchers observe that older people report low levels of anxiety (Mirowsky & Ross, 1999a). However, our results show similar age patterns across the six items; in contrast, we find that older people report somewhat higher means on the "anxiety items."

Previously, some scholars speculated about the distressing features of midlife (Reid & Willis, 1999). Like others, our results refute the "midlife emotional crisis" (Keyes & Ryff, 1999). Surveys in the 1980s and early 1990s show that individuals aged 40 to 50 have the lowest levels of depression (Kessler, et al., 1992; Mirowsky & Ross, 1992). However, our findings show an "optimum age" around age 63—a finding consistent with others (Wade & Cairney, 1997). What causes cross-study variation in the "optimum age?" During the 1980s and early 1990s, the economic outlook was less promising. Older workers may have had less optimism about work prospects, perhaps worrying about downsizing or corporate restructuring during those recession periods. In contrast, the 1996 and 1998 surveys occurred during prosperous times. The recent stronger economy may have alleviated fears about layoffs for adults in midlife and contributed to greater contentment during early and late midlife. Future studies should elaborate on age patterns in economic and occupational *insecurity* and determine if they contribute to age variation in depression and distress.

Some researchers cite "historical trend" explanations for age differences in depression (Mirowsky & Ross, 1992). Age-linked education patterns represent historical trends. For instance, young and middle aged adults have higher levels of education than older adults do, and those patterns contribute to the upward age pattern in depression and distress. Current trends, however, indicate that older cohorts are increasingly reporting more education. Specifically, in 1980 roughly 9 million adults over age 55 reported some college; in 1998 that number increased to almost 20 million (U.S. Bureau of the Census, 1998). In addition racial differences in emotions, and their link to educational attainment, have received little attention. Therefore, future work should examine the emotional effect of age trends in education, and race-linked differentials in education, as they impact emotionality across the life course.

Additionally, the view of age as "maturity" predicts better emotional health among adults in midlife and later life. Midlife is often a period in which adults reach peaks in career and family roles, and achieve a sense of full maturity (Erikson, 1982). The research focus on losses neglects more "favorable" indicators that peak during midlife, such as the sense of control, satisfaction with family and finances, fewer time demands, greater religious participation and confidence, and an optimistic worldview. These factors contribute to the *downward* age pattern in distress across the midlife years. In contrast, however, self-rated health is associated negatively with depression, and average levels of health decrease across age. Thus, were it not for declining levels of self-rated health, the decline in depression and distress would be even steeper. Our results are similar to recent studies that uncover suppression effects with adjustment for self-rated health, health status, and physical impairment (Mirowsky & Reynolds, 2000; Wade & Cairney, 2000).

In our study, older people tend to both report *below average* economic standing and *more satisfaction* with finances, and that suppresses an upturn in depression and distress among older adults. Future research should consider the way economic and social policy changes cause financial circumstances to shift across age groups. In addition, our findings reinforce others that show that lower control contributes to the old-age upturn in depression (Mirowsky & Ross, 1992). Some of that lower control may be due specifically to economic uncertainties associated with declining health of health care coverage. However, if policymakers enact reforms that cover prescription drugs then elders may report less economic hardship and greater satisfaction with financial circumstances. These ideas reflect the potential for period effects on the age-distress relationship.

Over a lifetime, the congruence between aspirations and achievements may nurture self-actualization, satisfaction, and growth (Erikson, 1982). In some cases, emotions have a *function*, such as sadness inspiring a person to disengage from a loss (Kubzansky & Kawachi, 2000). Additionally, theories of age propose that opposing objective and subjective factors determine the emotional status of older adults (Gatz & Zarit, 1999; Schulz, 1985). For example, older people report fewer time demands, religious doubts, and shameful emotions—patterns that suppress an old-age upturn in depression. Those patterns may also reflect facets of maturity that equalize distressing losses. However, panel designs are needed to address temporal ordering and reciprocal associations within the complex processes related to "maturity." Roles may shift feelings of control and family satisfaction. A pessimistic worldview could fuel marital problems, while the exit from a difficult relationship could spark a sense of optimism. Retirement can reduce time demands—but those demands may have reflected a salient identity. Taken together the functions of emotions within roles represent a challenging direction for future research in aging and mental health.

Additionally, elders who are available for surveys may have high levels of vigor, energy, and commitment for interviews and may over-represent the fewer cases among the oldest-old (Newmann, 1989). The depressed may be more likely to die young, leaving a pool of "optimal agers." Survival bias can underestimate depression among elders (Mirowsky & Ross, 1992), but we can describe individuals who survive and are able to respond to surveys (Whitbourne, 1996). Some researchers, however, assuage those concerns by reporting evidence that "cohort and survivor bias of the cross-sectional age curve is replaced by the far more difficult attrition bias of the panel survey" (see Mirowsky & Reynolds, 2000, 502).

In conclusion, life course and stress research can identify the transitions, events, and historical patterns that contribute to age patterns in well-being. However, cross-sectional analyses seems unable to truly inform us about the way that historical changes impact generations, nor are they able to inform us about the way societal-level readjustments influence the social distribution of status strains, role strains, and personal resources. The age-linked factors that explain or suppress age patterns in mental health will undoubtedly shift in the coming years. As social, cultural, and economic institutions adjust to demographic shifts, the study of well-being of young, middle-aged, and older adults will require a deeper accounting of the interplay among demography, social structure, aging related policy and individual's well-being.

References

Becker, Gary S. 1993. *Human Capital.* 3d ed. New York: Columbia University Press.
Carstensen, Laura L. 1993. "Motivation for Social Contact across the Life Span: A Theory of Socioemotional Selectivity." Pp. 209–54 in *Nebraska Symposium on Motivation,* edited by J. E. Jacobs. Lincoln: Nebraska University Press.

Clark-Plaskie, Margaret and Margie E. Lachman. 1999. "The Sense of Control in Midlife." Pp. 181–208 in *Life in the Middle: Psychosocial and Social Development in Middle Age*, edited by Sherry L. Lewis and James D. Reid. San Diego, CA: Academic Press.

Davis, James and Tom Smith. 1999. *General Social Surveys, 1972–1998: Cumulative Codebook and Data File*. Chicago, IL: National Opinion Research Center and the University of Chicago.

Erikson, Erik H. 1982. *The Life Cycle Completed*. New York: Norton.

Feinson, Marjorie Chary. 1985. "Aging and Mental Health: Distinguishing Myth from Reality." *Research on Aging* 7:155–74.

Ferraro, Kenneth F. 1989. "Widowhood and Health." Pp. 69–89 in *Aging, Stress, and Health*, edited by Kyriakos S. Markides and Cary L. Cooper. Chichester, UK: John Wiley & Sons.

Festinger, Leon. 1957. *A Theory of Cognitive Dissonance*. Stanford, CA: Stanford University Press.

Gatz, Margaret and Steven H. Zarit. 1999. "A Good Old Age: Paradox or Possibility." Pp. 396–416 in *Handbook of Theories of Aging*, edited by Vern L. Bengtson and K. Warner Schaie. New York: Springer.

Gecas, Viktor. 1989. "The Social Psychology of Self-efficacy." *Annual Review of Sociology* 15:291–316.

Hochschild, Arlie R. 1997. *The Time Bind: When Work Becomes Home and Home Becomes Work*. New York: Henry Holt and Company.

Johnson, Robert and Fredric Wolinsky. 1993. "The Structure of Health Status among Older Adults: Disease, Disability, Functional Limitations, and Perceived Health." *Journal of Health and Social Behavior* 34:105–21.

Kessler, Ronald C., Cindy Foster, Pamela S. Webster, and James S. House. 1992. "The Relationship between Age and Depressive Symptoms in Two National Surveys." *Psychology and Aging* 7:119–26.

Keyes, Corey Lee M. and Carol D. Ryff. 1999. "Psychological Well-being in Midlife." Pp. 161–80 in *Life in the Middle: Psychological and Social Development in Middle Age*, edited by Sherry Willis and James Reid. San Diego: Academic Press.

Koenig, Harold G. 1995. "Religion and Health in Later Life." Pp. 9–29 in *Aging, Spirituality, and Religion: A Handbook*, edited by Melvin A. Kimble, Susan H. McFadden, James W. Ellor, and James J. Seeber. Minneapolis, MN: Fortress Press.

Krause, Neal, Berit Ingersoll-Dayton, Christopher G. Ellison, and Keith M. Wulff. 1999a. "Aging, Religious Doubt, and Psychological Well-being." *The Gerontologist* 39:525–33.

Krause, Neal, Berit Ingersoll-Dayton, Jersey Liang, and Hidehiro Sugisawa. 1999b. "Religion, Social Support, and Health among the Japanese Elderly." *Journal of Health and Social Behavior* 40:405–21.

Kubzansky, Laura D. and Ichiro Kawachi. 2000. "Affective States and Health." Pp. 213–41 in *Social Epidemiology*, edited by Lisa F. Berkman and Ichiro Kawachi. Oxford, UK: University Press.

Labouvie-Vief, Gisela. 1999. "Emotions in Adulthood." Pp. 253–67 in *Handbook of Theories of Aging*, edited by Vern L. Bengtson and K. Warner Schaie. New York: Springer.

Levin, Jeffrey S. and Linda M. Chatters. 1998. "Religion, Health, and Psychological Well-being in Older Adults." *Journal of Health and Aging* 10:504–31.

Mirowsky, John. 1995. "Age and the Sense of Control." *Social Psychology Quarterly* 58:31–43.

Mirowsky, John and John R. Reynolds. 2000. "Age, Depression, and Attrition in the National Survey of Families and Households." *Sociological Methods and Research* 28:476–504.

Mirowsky, John and Catherine E. Ross. 1991. "Eliminating Defense and Agreement Bias from Measures of the Sense of Control Index: A 2 × 2 Index." *Social Psychology Quarterly* 54:127–45.

————. 1992. "Age and Depression." *Journal of Health and Social Behavior* 33:187–205.

————. 1998. "Education, Personal Control, Lifestyle and Health." *Research on Aging* 20:415–49.

————. 1999a. "Well-being across the Life Course." Pp. 328–47 in *Handbook for the Study of Mental Health: Social Contexts, Theories, and Systems*, edited by Allan V Horwitz and Teresa L. Scheid. Cambridge, UK: Cambridge University Press.

————. 1999b. "Economic Hardship across the Life Course." *American Sociological Review* 64:548–69.

Musick, Marc A., Blazer, D., and Judith C. Hays. 2000. "Religious Activity, Alcohol Use, and Depression in a Sample of Elderly Baptists." *Research on Aging* 22:91–116.

Newmann, Joy Perkins. 1989. "Aging and Depression." *Psychology and Aging* 4:150–65.

Payne, Barbara. 1988. "Religious Patterns and Participation of Older Adults: A Sociological Perspective." *Educational Gerontology* 14:255–67.

Pearlin, Leonard I. 1983. "Role strains and personal stress." Pp. 3–32 in *Psychosocial Stress: Trends in Theory and Research* edited by H. Kaplan. New York: Academic Press.

————. 1999. "Stress and Mental Health: A Conceptual Overview." Pp. 161–75 in *Handbook for the Study of Mental Health: Social Contexts, Theories, and Systems*, edited by Allan V. Horwitz and Teresa L. Scheid. Cambridge, UK: Cambridge University Press.

Pearlin, Leonard I. and Marilyn M. Skaff. 1996. "Stress and the Life Course: A Paradigmatic Alliance." *The Gerontologist* 36:239–47.

Pitcher, P. B. and D. C. Larson. 1989. "Elderly Widowhood." Pp. 59–82 in *Aging and the Family*, edited by S. Bahr and E. Peterson. New York: Lexington.

Radloff, Lenore S. 1977. "The CES-D Scale: A New Self-report Depression Scale for Research in the General Population." *Applied Psychological Measurement* 1:385–401.

Reid, James D. and Sherry L. Willis. 1999. "Middle Age: New Thoughts, New Directions." Pp. 275–80 in *Life in the Middle: Psychological and Social Development in Middle Age*, edited by Sherry L. Willis and James D. Reid. San Diego, CA: Academic Press.

Rodin, Judith. 1986. "Aging and Health: Effects of the Sense of Control." *Science* 233: 1271–76.

Ross, Catherine E. and Patricia Drentea. 1998. "Consequences of Retirement Activities for Distress and the Sense of Personal Control." *Journal of Health and Social Behavior* 39:317–34.

Ross, Catherine E. and Joan Huber. 1985. "Hardship and Depression." *Journal of Health and Social Behavior* 26:312–27.

Ross, Catherine E. and John Mirowsky. 1995. "Does Employment Affect Health?" *Journal of Health and Social Behavior* 36:230–43.

Ross, Catherine E. and Marieke Van Willigen. 1996. "Gender, Parenthood, and Anger." *Journal of Marriage and the Family* 58:572–84.

———. 1997. "Education and the Subjective Quality of Life." *Journal of Health and Social Behavior* 38:275–97.

Sastry, Jaya and Catherine E. Ross. 1998. "Asian Ethnicity and the Sense of Control." *Social Psychology Quarterly* 61:101–20.

Scheff, Thomas J. 2000. "Shame and the Social Bond: A Sociological Theory." *Sociological Theory* 18:84–99.

Schieman, Scott. 1999. "Age and Anger." *Journal of Health and Social Behavior* 40:273–89.

———. 2000. "Education and the Activation, Course, and Management of Anger." *Journal of Health and Social Behavior* 41:20–39.

Schieman, Scott and Heather A. Turner. 1998. "Age, Disability, and the Sense of Mastery." *Journal of Health and Social Behavior* 39:169–86.

Schieman, Scott and Karen Van Gundy. 2000. "The Personal and Social Links between Age and Self-reported Empathy." *Social Psychology Quarterly* 63:152–74.

Schulz, Richard. 1985. "Emotion and Affect." Pp. 531–43 in *Handbook of the Psychology of Aging.* 2d ed., edited by James E. Birren and K. Warner Schaie. New York: Van Nostrand Reinhold Company.

Turner, R. Jay and Donald A. Lloyd. 1999. "The Stress Process and the Social Distribution of Depression." *Journal of Health and Social Behavior* 40:374–404.

Turner, R. Jay, Samuel Noh, and D. Levin. 1985. "Depression across the Life Course: The Significance of Psychosocial Factors among the Disabled." Pp. 32–59 in *Depression: A Multidisciplinary Perspective,* edited by L. Dean. New York: Bruner/Mazel Press.

Umberson, Debra, Camille B. Wortman, and Ronald C. Kessler. 1992. "Widowhood and Depression: Explaining Long-term Gender Differences in Vulnerability." *Journal of Health and Social Behavior* 33:10–24.

U.S. Bureau of the Census. 1998. "Years of School Completed by People 25 Years Old and Over, by Age and Sex: Selected Years 1940 to 1998." Retrieved August 29, 2000 (http://www.census.gov/population/socdemo/education/tablea-01.txt).

Wade, Terrance J. and John Cairney. 1997. "Age and Depression in a Nationally Representative Sample of Canadians: A Preliminary Look at the National Population Health Survey." *Canadian Journal of Public Health* 88:297–302.

———. 2000. "The Effect of Sociodemographics, Social Stressors, Health Status and Psychosocial Resources on the Age-Depression Relationship." *Canadian Journal of Public Health* 91:307–12.

Whitbourne, Susan K. 1996. "Psychosocial Perspectives on Emotions: The Role of Identity in the Aging Process." Pp. 83–98 in *Handbook of Emotion, Adult Development, and Aging,* edited by Carol Magai and Susan H. McFadden. San Diego, CA: Academic Press.

DISCUSSION

1. Draw a visual representation that depicts the associations among age, the proposed mediators and suppressor variables, and distress. What experiences contribute to the decline in distress in middle age? To the increase in distress in older age? What experiences suppress those patterns?

2. Trace the frameworks presented by Aneshensel, Pearlin, and Thoits through this analysis. Where are these earlier frameworks evident in the

research of Schieman and colleagues? How do these frameworks make their analysis sociological?

3. What does this analysis suggest about how public policies might be used to improve the well-being of older Americans?

Benedict Carey

The Struggle to Gauge a War's Psychological Cost

New York Times writer Benedict Carey describes the toll that combat service in Iraq has taken on the soldiers as well as the military's efforts to offer assistance. The experience of solders in combat, the expectable nature of their distress, and the changing nature of responses to combat, link the material on the social origins of mental illness with the social constructionist arguments with which we opened the reader.

It was hardly a traditional therapist's office. The mortar fire was relentless, head-splitting, so close that it raised layers of rubble high off the floor of the bombed-out room.

Capt. William Nash, a Navy psychiatrist, sat on an overturned box of ready-made meals for the troops. He was in Iraq to try to short-circuit combat stress on the spot, before it became disabling, as part of the military's most determined effort yet to bring therapy to the front lines.

His clients, about a dozen young men desperate for help after weeks of living and fighting in Falluja, sat opposite him and told their stories.

One had been spattered with his best friend's blood and blamed himself for the death.

Another was also filled with guilt. He had hesitated while scouting an alley and had seen the man in front of him shot to death.

"They were so young," Captain Nash recalled.

At first, when they talked, he simply listened. Then he did his job, telling them that soldiers always blame themselves when someone is killed, in any war, always.

Grief, he told them, can make us forget how random war is, how much we have done to protect those we are fighting with.

"You try to help them tell a coherent story about what is happening, to make sense of it, so they feel less guilt and shame over protecting others, which is so common," said Captain Nash, who counseled the marines last November as part of the military's increased efforts to defuse psychological troubles.

Carey, Benedict. 2005. "The Struggle to Gauge a War's Psychological Cost." New York Times, November 26.

He added, "You have to help them reconstruct the things they used to believe in that don't make sense anymore, like the basic goodness of humanity."

Military psychiatry has always been close to a contradiction in terms. Psychiatry aims to keep people sane; service in wartime makes demands that seem insane.

This war in particular presents profound mental stresses: unknown and often unseen enemies, suicide bombers, a hostile land with virtually no safe zone, no real front or rear. A 360-degree war, some call it, an asymmetrical battle space that threatens to injure troops' minds as well as their bodies.

But just how deep those mental wounds are, and how many will be disabled by them, are matters of controversy. Some experts suspect that the legacy of Iraq could echo that of Vietnam, when almost a third of returning military personnel reported significant, often chronic, psychological problems.

Others say the mental casualties will be much lower, given the resilience of today's troops and the sophistication of the military's psychological corps, which place therapists like Captain Nash into combat zones.

The numbers so far tell a mixed story. The suicide rate among soldiers was high in 2003 but fell significantly in 2004, according to two Army surveys among more than 2,000 soldiers and mental health support providers in Iraq. Morale rose in the same period, but 54 percent of the troops say morale is low or very low, the report found.

A continuing study of combat units that served in Iraq has found that about 17 percent of the personnel have shown serious symptoms of depression, anxiety or post-traumatic stress disorder—characterized by intrusive thoughts, sleep loss, and hyper-alertness, among other symptoms—in the first few months after returning from Iraq, a higher rate than in Afghanistan but thought to be lower than after Vietnam.

In interviews, many members of the armed services and psychologists who had completed extended tours in Iraq said they had battled feelings of profound grief, anger, and moral ambiguity about the effect of their presence on Iraqi civilians.

And at bases back home, there have been violent outbursts among those who have completed tours. A marine from Camp Pendleton, Calif., has been convicted of murdering his girlfriend. And three members of a special forces unit based at Fort Carson, in Colorado Springs, have committed suicide.

Yet for returning service members, experts say, the question of whether their difficulties are ultimately diagnosed as mental illness may depend not only on the mental health services available, but also on the politics of military psychiatry itself, the definition of what a normal reaction to combat is and the story the nation tells itself about the purpose and value of soldiers' service.

"We must not ever diminish the pain and anguish many soldiers will feel; this kind of experience never leaves you," said David H. Marlowe, a former chief of military psychiatry at the Walter Reed Army Institute of Research.

"But at the same time we have to be careful not to create an attachment to that pain and anguish by pathologizing it."

The legacy of Iraq, Dr. Marlowe said, will depend as much on how service members are received and understood by the society they return to as on their exposure to the trauma of war.

MEMORIES STILL HAUNT

The blood and fury of combat exhilarate some people and mentally scar others, for reasons no one understands.

On an October night in 2003, mortar shells fell on a base camp near Baquba, Iraq, where Specialist Abbie Pickett, then 21, was serving as a combat lifesaver, caring for the wounded. Specialist Pickett continued working all night by the dim blue light of a flashlight, "plugging and chugging" bleeding troops to a makeshift medical tent, she said.

At first, she did not notice that one of the medics who was working with her was bleeding heavily and near death; then, frantically, she treated his wounds and moved him to a medical station not knowing if he would survive.

He did survive, Specialist Pickett later learned. But the horror of that night is still vivid, and the memory stalks her even now, more than a year after she returned home.

"I would say that on a weekly basis I wish I would have died during that attack," said Specialist Pickett, who served with the Wisconsin Army National Guard and whose condition has been diagnosed as post-traumatic stress disorder. "You never want family to hear that, and it's a selfish thing to say. But I'm not a typical 23-year-old, and it's hard being a combat vet and a woman and figuring out where you fit in."

Each war produces its own traumatic syndrome. The trench warfare of World War I produced the shaking and partial paralysis known as shell shock. The long tours and heavy fighting of World War II induced in many young men the numbed exhaustion that was called combat fatigue.

But it is post-traumatic stress disorder, a diagnosis some psychiatrists intended to characterize the mental struggles of Vietnam veterans, that now dominates the study and description of war trauma.

The diagnosis has always been controversial. Few experts doubt that close combat can cause a lingering hair-trigger alertness and play on a person's conscience for a lifetime. But no one knows what level of trauma is necessary to produce a disabling condition or who will become disabled.

The largest study of Vietnam veterans found that about 30 percent of them had post-traumatic stress disorder in the 20 years after the war but that only a fraction of those service members had had combat roles. Another study of Vietnam veterans, done around the same time, found that the lifetime rate of the syndrome was half as high, 15 percent.

And since Vietnam, therapists have diagnosed the disorder in crime victims, disaster victims, people who have witnessed disasters, even those who have seen upsetting events on television. The disorder varies widely depending on the individual and the nature of the trauma, psychiatrists say, but they cannot yet predict how.

Yet the very pervasiveness of post-traumatic stress disorder as a concept shapes not only how researchers study war trauma but also how many soldiers describe their reactions to combat.

Specialist Pickett, for example, has struggled with the intrusive memories typical of post-traumatic stress and with symptoms of depression and a seething resentment over her service, partly because of what she describes as irresponsible leaders and a poorly defined mission. Her memories make good bar stories, she said, but they also follow her back to her apartment, where the combination of anxiety and uncertainty about the value of her service has at times made her feel as if she were losing her mind.

Richard J. McNally, a psychologist at Harvard, said, "It's very difficult to know whether a new kind of syndrome will emerge from this war for the simple reason that the instrument used to assess soldiers presupposes that it will look like P.T.S.D. from Vietnam."

A more thorough assessment, Dr. McNally said, "might ask not only about guilt, shame and the killing of noncombatants, but about camaraderie, leadership, devotion to the mission, about what is meaningful and worthwhile, as well as the negative things."

Sitting amid the broken furniture in his Falluja "office," Captain Nash represents the military's best effort to handle stress on the ground, before it becomes upsetting, and keep service members on the job with the others in their platoon or team, who provide powerful emotional support.

While the military deployed mental health experts in Vietnam, most stayed behind the lines. In part because of that war's difficult legacy, the military has increased the proportion of field therapists and put them closer to the action than ever before.

The Army says it has about 200 mental health workers for a force of about 150,000, including combat stress units that travel to combat zones when called on. The Marines are experimenting with a program in which the therapists stationed at a base are deployed with battalions in the field.

"The idea is simple," said Lt. Cmdr. Gary Hoyt, a Navy psychologist and colleague of Captain Nash in the Marine program. "You have a lot more credibility if you've been there, and soldiers and marines are more likely to talk to you."

Commander Hoyt has struggled with irritability and heightened alertness since returning from Iraq in September 2004.

Psychologists and psychiatrists on the ground have to break through the mental toughness that not only keeps troops fighting but also prevents them from seeking psychological help, which is viewed as a sign of weakness. And they have been among the first to identify the mental reactions particular to this war.

One of them, these experts say, is profound, unreleased anger. Unlike in Vietnam, where service members served shorter tours and were rotated in and out of the country individually, troops in Iraq have deployed as units and tend to have trained together as full-time military or in the Reserves or the National Guard. Group cohesion is strong, and the bonds only deepen in the hostile desert terrain of Iraq.

For these tight-knit groups, certain kinds of ambushes—roadside bombs, for instance—can be mentally devastating, for a variety of reasons.

"These guys go out in convoys, and boom: the first vehicle gets hit, their best friend dies, and now they're seeing life flash before them and get a surge of adrenaline and want to do something," said Lt. Col. Alan Peterson, an Air Force psychologist who completed a tour in Iraq last year. "But often there's nothing they can do. There's no enemy there."

Many, Colonel Peterson said, become deeply frustrated because "they wish they could act out on this adrenaline rush and do what they were trained to do but can't."

Some soldiers and marines describe foot patrols as "drawing fire," and gunmen so often disappear into crowds that many have the feeling that they are fighting ghosts. In roadside ambushes, service men and women may never see the enemy.

Sgt. Benjamin Flanders, 27, a graduate student in math who went to Iraq with the New Hampshire National Guard, recalled: "It was kind of a joke: if you got to shoot back at the enemy, people were jealous. It was a stress reliever, a great release, because usually these guys disappear."

Another powerful factor is ambiguity about the purpose of the mission, and about Iraqi civilians' perception of the American presence.

On a Sunday in April 2004, Commander Hoyt received orders to visit Marine units that had been trapped in a firefight in a town near the Syrian border and that had lost five men. The Americans had been handing out candy to children and helping residents fix their houses the day before the ambush, and they felt they had been set up, he said.

The entire unit, he said, was coursing with rage, asking: "What are we doing here? Why aren't the Iraqis helping us?"

Commander Hoyt added, "There was a breakdown, and some wanted to know how come they couldn't hit mosques" or other off-limits targets where insurgents were suspected of hiding.

In group sessions, the psychologist emphasized to the marines that they could not know for sure whether the civilians they had helped had supported the insurgents. Insurgent fighters scare many Iraqis more than the Americans do, he reminded them, and that fear creates a deep ambivalence, even among those who most welcome the American presence. And following the rules of engagement, he told them, was crucial to setting an example.

Commander Hoyt also reminded the group of some of its successes, in rebuilding houses, for example, and restoring electricity in the area. He also told them it was better to fight in Iraq than back home.

"Having someone killed in World War II, you could say, 'Well, we won this battle to save the world,'" he said. "In this terrorist war, it is much less tangible how to anchor your losses."

SUICIDE RATE FOR SOLDIERS ROSE IN '07

By THE ASSOCIATED PRESS

WASHINGTON (AP)—At least 115 soldiers killed themselves in 2007, up from 102 the previous year, the Army said Thursday.

Nearly one-third of them died at the battlefront, 32 in *Iraq* and 4 in *Afghanistan*. But 26 percent had never been sent to either conflict.

"We see a lot of things that are going on in the war which do contribute," said Col. Elspeth Ritchie, psychiatric consultant to the Army surgeon general.

"Mainly the longtime and multiple deployments away from home, exposure to really terrifying and horrifying things, the easy availability of loaded weapons and a force that's very, very busy right now. And so all of those together we think are part of what may contribute, especially if somebody's having difficulties already," Colonel Ritchie said at a news conference.

Some common factors among those who took their own lives were trouble with relationships, work problems, and legal and financial difficulties, officials said.

The 115 confirmed suicides among active-duty soldiers and National Guard and Reserve troops who had been activated amounted to a rate of 18.8 per 100,000 troops — the highest since the Army began keeping records in 1980.

Ninety-three of the 115 suicides were active-duty troops; 22 were members of the Army National Guard or Reserve who had been mobilized. There were also 166 attempted suicides among troops in Iraq and Afghanistan and 935 in the whole Army. As of Monday, there had been 38 confirmed suicides in 2008 and 12 more deaths that were suspected of being suicides but were still under investigation, said Lt. Col. Thomas E. Languirand, head of command policies and programs.

HELP IN ADJUSTING TO LIFE AT HOME

No one has shown definitively that on-the-spot group or individual therapy in combat lowers the risk of psychological problems later. But military psychiatrists know from earlier wars that separating an individual from his or her unit can significantly worsen feelings of guilt and depression.

About 8 service members per every 1,000 in Iraq have developed psychiatric problems severe enough to require evacuation, according to Defense Department statistics, while the rate of serious psychiatric diagnoses in Vietnam from 1965 to 1969 was more than 10 per 1,000, although improvements in treatment, as well as differences in the conflicts and diagnostic criteria, make a direct comparison very rough.

At the same time, Captain Nash and Commander Hoyt say that psychological consultations by returning marines at Camp Pendleton have been increasing significantly since the war began.

One who comes for regular counseling is Sgt. Robert Willis, who earned a Bronze Star for leading an assault through a graveyard near Najaf in 2004.

Irritable since his return home in February, shaken by loud noises, leery of malls, or other areas that are not well-lighted at night—classic signs of posttraumatic stress—Sergeant Willis has been seeing Commander Hoyt to help adjust to life at home.

"It's been hard," Sergeant Willis said in a telephone interview. "I have been boisterous, overbearing—my family notices it."

He said he had learned to manage his moods rather than react impulsively, after learning to monitor his thoughts and attend more closely to the reactions of others.

"The turning point, I think, was when Dr. Hoyt told me to simply accept that I was going to be different because of this," but not mentally ill, Sergeant Willis said.

The increase in consultations at Camp Pendleton may reflect increasingly taxing conditions, or delayed reactions, experts said. But it may also be evidence that men and women who have fought with ready access to a psychologist or psychiatrist are less constrained by the tough-it-out military ethos and are more comfortable seeking that person's advice when they get back.

"Seeing someone you remember from real time in combat absolutely could help in treatment," as well as help overcome the stigma of seeking counseling, said Rachel Yehuda, director of the post-traumatic stress disorder program at the Veterans Affairs Medical Center in the Bronx. "If this is what is happening, I think it's brilliant."

TRACKING SERIOUS SYMPTOMS

In the coming months, researchers who are following combat units after they return home are expected to report that the number of personnel with serious mental symptoms has increased slightly, up from the 17 percent reported last year.

In an editorial last year in *The New England Journal of Medicine*, Dr. Matthew J. Friedman, executive director of the National Center for Post-Traumatic

Stress Disorder for the Department of Veterans Affairs, wrote that studies suggested that the rates of post-traumatic stress disorder, in particular, "may increase considerably during the two years after veterans return from combat duty."

And on the basis of previous studies, Dr. Friedman wrote, "it is possible that psychiatric disorders will increase now that the conduct of the war has shifted from a campaign for liberation to an ongoing armed conflict with dissident combatants."

But others say that the rates of the disorder are just as likely to diminish in the next year, as studies show they do for disaster victims.

Col. Elspeth Cameron Ritchie, psychiatry consultant to the Army surgeon general, said that given the stresses of this war, it was worth noting that five out of six service members who had seen combat did not show serious signs of mental illness.

The emotional casualties, Colonel Ritchie said, are "not just an Army medical problem, but a problem that the V.A. system, the civilian system and the society as a whole must work to solve."

That is the one thing all seem to agree on. Some veterans, like Sergeant Flanders and Sergeant Willis, have reconnected with other men in their units to help with their psychological adjustment to home life. Sergeant Willis has been transferred to noncombat duty at Camp Pendleton, in an environment he knows and enjoys, and he can see Commander Hoyt when he needs to. Sergeant Flanders is studying to be an officer.

But others, particularly reservists and National Guard troops, have landed right back in civilian society with no one close to them who has shared their experience.

Specialist Pickett, since her return, has felt especially cut off from the company she trained and served with. She has struggled at school, and with the Veterans Affairs system to get counseling, and no one near her has had an experience remotely like hers. She has tried antidepressants, which have helped reduce her suicidal thinking. She has also joined Operation Truth, a nonprofit organization that represents Iraq veterans, which has given her some comfort.

Finally, she said, she has been searching her memory and conscience for reasons to justify the pain of her experience: no one, Specialist Pickett said, looks harder for justification than a soldier.

Dr. Marlowe, the former chief of psychiatry at Walter Reed, knows from studying other wars that this is so.

"The great change among American troops in Germany during the Second World War was when they discovered the concentration camps," Dr. Marlowe said. "That immediately and forever changed the moral appreciation for why we were there."

As soldiers return from Iraq, he said, "it will be enormously important for those who feel psychologically disaffected to find something which justifies the killing, and the death of their friends."

DISCUSSION

1. Apply the concepts from the stress process model to understanding the experiences of soldiers in combat. How would you describe their experiences using the concepts from that model? What structural contexts (in Pearlin's terms) contribute to the stresses they experience? How do soldiers' bonds with their units ameliorate and exacerbate the stresses of combat?

2. How has the nature of soldiers' responses to combat changed over time? What might account for those changes? What would we need to know to decide whether post-traumatic stress disorder is a new condition or a new label for an older condition?

3. Carey hints at a controversy over whether to consider soldiers' responses to combat pathological or normal reactions to difficult circumstances. Which interpretation do you favor and why?

STIGMA AND THE SOCIAL DIMENSIONS OF THE EXPERIENCE OF MENTAL ILLNESS

L abeling theory remains one of the most controversial theories in the sociology of mental health. First applied to mental illness by Thomas Scheff, it identifies important social contingencies in the processes through which people are labeled mentally ill and in the progression of mental illness. Despite the intuitive appeal of the theory, early critics, most notably Walter Gove, charged that empirical research failed to support many of its specific propositions. In part because of this criticism, Link and his colleagues proposed a modified version of the theory that recasts the labeling process with reference to stigma: a distinction that carries negative stereotypes. Their recasting shifted research attention toward the relevance of stigma for the lives of people with mental illness. The first four selections in this section trace the history of debate regarding the importance of mental illness labels from Scheff's original theoretical statement through recent research on mental illness stigma. The final four selections look more in-depth to the ways that stigma can influence the lives and self-concepts of people with mental illness. Central to these latter studies is the concept of the "illness career" and how both societal stigma and other contingencies organize the "careers" of those labeled as having a stigmatizing mental illness.

Labeling

Thomas J. Scheff

The Role of the Mentally Ill and the Dynamics of Mental Disorder: A Research Framework[†]

In this classic statement, Scheff introduces the nine key propositions of labeling theory. These propositions concern the effects of mental illness labels on the future course of mental illness. Following those propositions, he briefly outlines contingencies in the labeling process itself: the characteristics of the deviant and the labeler that determine whether and when labels will be applied. This statement represents the opening salvo in the continuing debate about labeling theory.

One frequently noted deficiency in psychiatric formulations is the failure to incorporate social processes into the dynamics of mental disorder. Although the importance of these processes is increasingly recognized by psychiatrists, the conceptual models used in formulating research questions are basically concerned with individual rather than social systems. Genetic, biochemical, and psychological investigations seek different causal agents, but utilize similar models: dynamic systems which are located within the individual. In these investigations, social processes tend to be relegated to a subsidiary role, because the model focuses attention on individual differences, rather than on the social system in which the individuals are involved.

Recently a number of writers have sought to develop an approach which would give more emphasis to social processes. Lemert, Erikson, Goffman, and Szasz have notably contributed to this approach.[1] Lemert, particularly, by rejecting the more conventional concern with the origins of mental deviance, and stressing instead the potential importance of the societal reaction

---

Scheff, Thomas. 1963. "The Role of the Mentally Ill and the Dynamics of Mental Disorder." *Sociometry* 26:436–453.

[1] Edwin M. Lemert, *Social Pathology*, New York: McGraw-Hill, 1951; Kal T. Erikson, "Patient Role and Social Uncertainty—A Dilemma of the Mentally Ill," *Psychiatry*, 20 (August, 1957), pp. 263–274; Erving Goffman, *Asylums*, New York: Doubleday-Anchor, 1961; Thomas S. Szasz, *The Myth of Mental Illness*, New York: Hoeber-Harper, 1961.

in stabilizing deviance, focuses primarily on mechanisms of social control. The work of all of these authors suggests research avenues which are analytically separable from questions of individual systems and point, therefore, to a theory which would incorporate social processes.

The purpose of the present paper is to contribute to the formulation of such a theory by stating a set of nine propositions which make up basic assumptions for a social system model of mental disorder. This set is largely derived from the work of the authors listed above, all but two of the propositions (#4 and #5) being suggested, with varying degrees of explicitness, in the cited references. This paper also delineates three problems which are crucial for a sociological theory of mental disorder: what are the conditions in a culture under which diverse kinds of deviance become stable and uniform; to what extent, in different phases of careers of mental patients, are symptoms of mental illness the result of conforming behavior; is there a general set of contingencies which lead to the definition of deviant behavior as a manifestation of mental illness? Finally, this paper attempts to formulate special conceptual tools to deal with these problems, which are directly linked to sociological theory. The social institution of insanity, residual deviance, the social role of the mentally ill, and the bifurcation of the societal reaction into the alternative reactions of denial and labeling, are examples of such conceptual tools.

These conceptual tools are utilized to construct a theory of mental disorder in which psychiatric symptoms are considered to be violations of social norms, and stable "mental illness" to be a social role. The validity of this theory depends upon verification of the nine propositions listed below in future studies, and should, therefore, be applied with caution, and with appreciation for its limitations. One such limitation is that the theory attempts to account for a much narrower class of phenomena than is usually found under the rubric of mental disorder; the discussion that follows will be focused exclusively on stable or recurring mental disorder, and does not explain the causes of single deviant episodes. A second major limitation is that the theory probably distorts the phenomena under discussion. Just as the individual system models under-stress social processes, the model presented here probably exaggerates their importance. The social system model "holds constant" individual differences, in order to articulate the relationship between society and mental disorder. Ultimately, a framework which encompassed both individual and social systems would be desirable. Given the present state of knowledge, however, this framework may prove useful by providing an explicit contrast to the more conventional medical and psychological approaches, and thus assisting in the formulation of sociological studies of mental disorder.

THE SYMPTOMS OF "MENTAL ILLNESS" AS RESIDUALLY DEVIANT BEHAVIOR

One source of immediate embarrassment to any social theory of "mental illness" is that the terms used in referring to these phenomena in our society prejudge the issue. The medical metaphor "mental illness" suggests a deter-minate process which occurs within the individual: the unfolding and devel-opment of disease. It is convenient, therefore, to drop terms derived from the disease metaphor in favor of a standard sociological concept, deviant behav-ior, which signifies behavior that violates a social norm in a given society.

If the symptoms of mental illness are to be construed as violations of social norms, it is necessary to specify the type of norms involved. Most norm violations do not cause the violator to be labeled as mentally ill, but as ill-mannered, ignorant, sinful, criminal, or perhaps just harried, depending on the type of norm involved. There are innumerable norms, however, over which consensus is so complete that the members of a group appear to take them for granted. A host of such norms surround even the simplest conver-sation: a person engaged in conversation is expected to face toward his part-ner, rather than directly away from him; if his gaze is toward the partner, he is expected to look toward his eyes, rather than, say, toward his forehead; to stand at a proper conversational distance, neither one inch away not across the room, and so on. A person who regularly violated these expectations probably would not be thought to be merely ill-bred, but as strange, bizarre, and frightening, because his behavior violates the assumptive world of the group, the world that is construed to be the only one that is natural, decent, and possible.

The culture of the group provides a vocabulary of terms for categorizing many norm violations: crime, perversion, drunkenness, and bad manners are familiar examples. Each of these terms is derived from the type of norm broken, and ultimately, from the type of behavior involved. After exhausting these categories, however, there is always a residue of the most diverse kinds of violations, for which the culture provides no explicit label. For example, although there is great cultural variation in what is defined as decent or real, each culture tends to reify its definition of decency and reality, and so pro-vide no way of handling violations of its expectations in these areas. The typical norm governing decency or reality, therefore, literally "goes without saying" and its violation is unthinkable for most of its members. For the con-venience of the society in construing these instances of unnamable deviance which are called to its attention, these violations may be lumped together into a residual category: witchcraft, spirit possession, or, in our own society, mental illness. In this paper, the diverse kinds of deviation for which our society provides no explicit label, and which, therefore, sometimes lead to the labeling of the violator as mentally ill, will be considered to be techni-cally *residual deviance.*

THE ORIGINS, PREVALENCE AND COURSE OF RESIDUAL DEVIANCE

The first proposition concerns the origins of residual deviance. **1. Residual deviance arises from fundamentally diverse sources.** It has been demonstrated that some types of mental disorder are the result of organic causes. It appears likely, therefore, that there are genetic, biochemical or physiological origins for residual deviance. It also appears that residual deviance can arise from individual psychological peculiarities and from differences in upbringing and training. Residual deviance can also probably be produced by various kinds of external stress: the sustained fear and hardship of combat, and deprivation of food, sleep, and even sensory experience.[2] Residual deviance, finally, can be a volitional act of innovation or defiance. The kinds of behavior deemed typical of mental illness, such as hallucinations, delusions, depression, and mania, can all arise from these diverse sources.

The second proposition concerns the prevalence of residual deviance which is analogous to the "total" or "true" prevalence of mental disorder (in contrast to the "treated" prevalence). **2. Relative to the rate of treated mental illness, the rate of unrecorded residual deviance is extremely high.** There is evidence that grossly deviant behavior is often not noticed or, if it is noticed, it is rationalized as eccentricity. Apparently, many persons who are extremely withdrawn, or who "fly off the handle" for extended periods of time, who imagine fantastic events, or who hear voices or see visions, are not labeled as insane either by themselves or others.[3] Their deviance, rather, is unrecognized, ignored, or rationalized. This pattern of inattention and rationalization will be called "denial."[4]

In addition to the kind of evidence cited above there are a number of epidemiological studies of total prevalence. A convenient summary of findings is presented in Plunkett and Gordon.[5] This source compares the methods and populations used in 11 field studies, and lists rates of total prevalence (in percentages) as 1.7, 3.6, 4.5, 4.7, 5.3, 6.1, 10.9, 13.8, 23.2, 23.3, and 33.3.

How do these total rates compare with the rates of treated mental disorder? One of the studies cited by Plunkett and Gordon, the Baltimore study reported by Pasamanick, is useful in this regard since it includes both treated and untreated rates.[6] As compared with the untreated rate of 10.9 per cent, the rate of treatment in state, VA, and private hospitals of Baltimore residents

---

[2] Philip Solomon, *et al.* (eds.), *Sensory Deprivation,* Cambridge: Harvard, 1961; E. L. Bliss, et al., "Studies of Sleep Deprivation—Relationship to Schizophrenia," *A.M.A. Archives of Neurology and Psychiatry,* 81 (March, 1959), pp. 348–359.

[3] See, for example, John A. Clausen and Marian R. Yarrow, "Paths to the Mental Hospital," *Journal of Social Issues,* 11 (December, 1955), pp. 25–32; August B. Hollingshead and Frederick C. Redlich, *Social Class and Mental Illness,* New York: Wiley, 1958, pp. 172–176; Elaine Cumming and John Cumming, *Closed Ranks,* Cambridge: Harvard, 1957, pp. 92–103.

[4] The term "denial" is used in the same sense as in Cumming and Cumming, *ibid.,* Chap. VII.

[5] Richard J. Plunkett and John E. Gordon, *Epidemiology and Mental Illness,* New York: Basic Books, 1960.

[6] Benjamin Pasamanick, "A Survey of Mental Disease in an Urban Population, IV, An Approach to Total Prevalence Rates," *Archives of General Psychiatry,* 5 (August, 1961), pp. 151–155.

was .5 per cent.[7] That is, for every mental patient there were approximately 20 untreated cases located by the survey. It is possible that the treated rate is too low, however, since patients treated by private physicians were not included. Judging from another study, the New Haven study of treated prevalence, the number of patients treated in private practice is small compared to those hospitalized: over 70 percent of the patients located in that study were hospitalized even though extensive case-finding techniques were employed. The overall treated prevalence in the New Haven study was reported as .8 percent, which is in good agreement with my estimate of .7 percent for the Baltimore study.[8] If we accept .8 percent as an estimate of the upper limit of treated prevalence for the Pasamanick study, the ratio of treated to untreated cases is 1/14. That is, for every treated patient we should expect to find 14 untreated cases in the community.

One interpretation of this finding is that the untreated patients in the community represent those cases with less severe disorders, while those patients with severe impairments all fall into the treated group. Some of the findings in the Pasamanick study point in this direction. Of the untreated patients, about half are classified as psychoneurotic. Of the psychoneurotics, in turn, about half again are classified as suffering from minimal impairment. At least a fourth of the untreated group, then, involved very mild disorders.[9]

The evidence from the group diagnosed as psychotic does not support this interpretation, however. Almost all of the cases diagnosed as psychotic were judged to involve severe impairment, yet half of the diagnoses of psychosis occurred in the untreated group. In other words, according to this study there were as many untreated as treated cases of psychoses.[10]

On the basis of the high total prevalence rates cited above and other evidence, it seems plausible that residual deviant behavior is usually transitory, which is the substance of the third proposition. **3. Most residual deviance is "denied" and is transitory.** The high rates of total prevalence suggest that most residual deviancy is unrecognized or rationalized away. For this type of deviance, which is amorphous and uncrystallized, Lemert uses the term "primary deviation."[11]

If residual deviance is highly prevalent among ostensibly "normal" persons and is usually transitory, as suggested by the last two propositions, what accounts for the small percentage of residual deviants who go on to deviant careers? To put the question another way, under what conditions is residual deviance stabilized? The conventional hypothesis is that the answer lies in the deviant himself. The hypothesis suggested here is that the most important single factor (but not the only factor) in the stabilization of residual deviance is the societal reaction. Residual deviance may be stabilized if

---

[7] *Ibid.*, p. 153.
[8] Hollingshead and Redlich, *op. cit.*, p. 199.
[9] Pasamanick, *op. cit.*, pp. 153–154.
[10] *Ibid.*
[11] Lemert, *op. cit.*, Chap. 4.

it is defined to be evidence of mental illness, and/or the deviant is placed in a deviant status, and begins to play the role of the mentally ill. In order to avoid the implication that mental disorder is merely role-playing and pretence, it is first necessary to discuss the social institution of insanity.

SOCIAL CONTROL: INDIVIDUAL AND SOCIAL SYSTEMS OF BEHAVIOR

In *The Myth of Mental Illness,* Szasz proposes that mental disorder be viewed within the framework of "the game-playing model of human behavior." He then describes hysteria, schizophrenia, and other mental disorders as the "impersonation" of sick persons by those whose "real" problem concerns "problems of living." Although Szasz states that role-playing by mental patients may not be completely or even mostly voluntary, the implication is that mental disorder be viewed as a strategy chosen by the individual as a way of obtaining help from others. Thus, the term "impersonation" suggests calculated and deliberate shamming by the patient. In his comparisons of hysteria, malingering, and cheating, although he notes differences between these behavior patterns, he suggests that these differences may be mostly a matter of whose point of view is taken in describing the behavior.

The present paper also uses the role-playing model to analyze mental disorder, but places more emphasis on the involuntary aspects of role-playing than Szasz, who tends to treat role-playing as an individual system of behavior. In many social psychological discussions, however, role-playing is considered as a part of a social system. The individual plays his role by articulating his behavior with the cues and actions of other persons involved in the transaction. The proper performance of a role is dependent on having a cooperative audience. This proposition may also be reversed: having an audience which acts toward the individual in a uniform way may lead the actor to play the expected role even if he is not particularly interested in doing so. The "baby of the family" may come to find this role obnoxious, but the uniform pattern of cues and actions which confronts him in the family may lock in with his own vocabulary of responses so that it is inconvenient and difficult for him not to play the part expected of him. To the degree that alternative roles are closed off, the proffered role may come to be the only way the individual can cope with the situation.

This discussion suggests that a stable role performance may arise when the actor's role imagery locks in with the type of "deference" which he regularly receives. An extreme example of this process may be taken from anthropological and medical reports concerning the "dead role," as in deaths attributed to "bone-pointing." Death from bone-pointing appears to arise from the conjunction of two fundamental processes which characterize all social behavior. First, all individuals continually orient themselves by means of responses which are perceived in social interaction: the individual's identity and continuity of experience are dependent on these cues.[12] Secondly, the individual has his own vocabulary of expectations, which may in a particular situation either agree with or be in conflict with the sanctions to which he is exposed. Entry into a role may be complete when this role is part of the individual's expectations, and when these expectations are reaffirmed in social interaction. In the following pages this principle will be applied to the problem of the causation of mental disorder.

What are the beliefs and practices that constitute the social institution of insanity?[13] And how do they figure in the development of mental disorder? Two propositions concerning beliefs about mental disorder in the general public will now be considered.

4. Stereotyped imagery of mental disorder is learned in early childhood. Although there are no substantiating studies in this area, scattered observations lead the author to conclude that children learn a considerable amount of imagery concerning deviance very early, and that much of the imagery comes from their peers rather than from adults. The literal meaning of "crazy," a term now used in a wide variety of contexts, is probably grasped by children during the first years of elementary school. Since adults are often vague and evasive in their responses to questions in this area, an aura of mystery surrounds it. In this socialization the grossest stereotypes which are heir to childhood fears, e.g., of the "boogie man," survive. These conclusions are quite speculative, of course, and need to be investigated systematically, possibly with techniques similar to those used in studies of the early learning of racial stereotypes.

---

[12] Generalizing from experimental findings, Blake and Mouton make this statement about the processes of conformity, resistance to influence, and conversion to a new role:

> ...an individual requires a stable framework, including salient and firm reference points, in order to orient himself and to regulate his interactions with others. This framework consists of external and internal anchorages available to the individual whether he is aware of them or not. With an acceptable framework he can resist giving or accepting information that is inconsistent with that framework or that requires him to relinquish it. In the absence of a stable framework he actively seeks to establish one through his own strivings by making use of significant and relevant information provided within the context of interaction. *By controlling the amount and kind of information available for orientation, he can be led to embrace conforming attitudes which are entirely foreign to his earlier ways of thinking.*

Robert R. Blake and Jane S. Mouton, "Conformity, Resistance and Conversion," in *Conformity and Deviation*, Irwin A. Berg and Bernard M. Bass (eds.), New York: Harper, 1961, pp. 1–2. For a recent and striking demonstration of the effect on social communication in defining internal stimuli, see Stanley Schachter and Jerome E. Singer, "Cognitive, Social, and Physiological Determinants of Emotional State," *Psychological Review*, 69 (September, 1962), pp. 379–399.

[13] The Cummings describe the social institution of insanity (the "patterned response" to deviance) in terms of denial, isolation, and insulation. Cumming and Cumming, *loc. cit.*

Assuming, however, that this hypothesis is sound, what effect does early learning have on the shared conceptions of insanity held in the community? There is much fallacious material learned in early childhood which is later discarded when more adequate information replaces it. This question leads to hypothesis No. 5. **5. The stereotypes of insanity are continually reaffirmed, inadvertently, in ordinary social interaction.**

Although many adults become acquainted with medical concepts of mental illness, the traditional stereotypes are not discarded, but continue to exist alongside the medical conceptions, because the stereotypes receive almost continual support from the mass media and in ordinary social discourse. In newspapers, it is a common practice to mention that a rapist or a murderer was once a mental patient. This negative information, however, is seldom offset by positive reports. An item like the following is almost inconceivable:

> Mrs. Ralph Jones, an ex-mental patient, was elected president of the Fair-view Home and Garden Society in their meeting last Thursday.

Because of highly biased reporting, the reader is free to make the unwarranted inference that murder and rape occur more frequently among ex-mental patients than among the population at large. Actually, it has been demonstrated that the incidence of crimes of violence, or of any crime, is much lower among ex-mental patients than among the general population.[14] Yet, this is not the picture presented to the public.

Reaffirmation of the stereotype of insanity occurs not only in the mass media, but also in ordinary conversation, in jokes, anecdotes, and even in conventional phrases. Such phrases as "Are you crazy?", or "It would be a madhouse," "It's driving me out of my mind," or "It's driving me distracted," and hundred of others occur frequently in informal conversations. In this usage insanity itself is seldom the topic of conversation; the phrases are so much a part of ordinary language that only the person who considers each word carefully can eliminate them from his speech. Through verbal usages the stereotypes of insanity are a relatively permanent part of the social structure.

DENIAL AND LABELING

According to the analysis presented here, the traditional stereotypes of mental disorder are solidly entrenched in the population because they are learned early in childhood and are continuously reaffirmed in the mass media and in everyday conversation. How do these beliefs function in the

---

[14] Henry Brill and Benjamin Malzberg, "Statistical Report Based on the Arrest Record of 5354 Male Ex-patients Released from New York State Mental Hospitals During the Period 1946–48," mimeographed document available from the authors; L. H. Cohen and H. Freeman, "How Dangerous to the Community are State Hospital Patients?", *Connecticut State Medical Journal*, 9 (September, 1945), pp. 697–701.

processes leading to mental disorder? This question will be considered by first referring to the earlier discussion of the societal reaction to residual deviance.

It was stated that the usual reaction to residual deviance is denial, and that in these cases most residual deviance is transitory. The societal reaction to deviance is not always denial, however. In a small proportion of cases the reaction goes the other way, exaggerating and at times distorting the extent and degree of deviation. This pattern of exaggeration, which we will call "labeling," has been noted by Garfinkel in his discussion of the "degradation" of officially recognized criminals.[15] Goffman makes a similar point in his description of the "discrediting" of mental patients.[16] Apparently under some conditions the societal reaction to deviance is to seek out signs of abnormality in the deviant's history to show that he was always essentially a deviant.

The contrasting social reactions of denial and labeling provide a means of answering two fundamental questions. If deviance arises from diverse sources—physical, psychological, and situational—how does the uniformity of behavior that is associated with insanity develop? Secondly, if deviance is usually transitory, how does it become stabilized in those patients who became chronically deviant? To summarize, what are the sources of uniformity and stability of deviant behavior?

In the approach taken here the answer to this question is based on hypotheses Nos. 4 and 5, that the role imagery of insanity is learned early in childhood, and is reaffirmed in social interaction. In a crisis, when the deviance of an individual becomes a public issue, the traditional stereotype of insanity becomes the guiding imagery for action, both for those reacting to the deviant and, at times, for the deviant himself. When societal agents and persons around the deviant react to him uniformly in terms of the traditional stereotypes of insanity, his amorphous and unstructured deviant behavior tends to crystallize in conformity to these expectations, thus becoming similar to the behavior of other deviants classified as mentally ill, and stable over time. The process of becoming uniform and stable is completed when the traditional imagery becomes a part of the deviant's orientation for guiding his own behavior.

ACCEPTANCE OF THE DEVIANT ROLE

From this point of view, then, most mental disorder can be considered to be a social role. This social role complements and reflects the status of the insane in the social structure. It is through the social processes which maintain the status of the insane that the varied deviancies from which mental disorder

---

[15] Harold Garfinkel, "Conditions of Successful Degradation Ceremonies," *American Journal of Sociology,* 61 (March, 1956), pp. 420–424.

[16] Goffman, "The Moral Career of the Mental Patient," in *Asylums, op. cit.,* pp. 125–171.

arises are made uniform and stable. The stabilization and uniformization of residual deviance are completed when the deviant accepts the role of the insane as the framework within which he organizes his own behavior. Three hypotheses are stated below which suggest some of the processes which cause the deviant to accept such a stigmatized role.

6. Labeled deviants may be rewarded for playing the stereotyped deviant role. Ordinarily patients who display "insight" are rewarded by psychiatrists and other personnel. That is, patients who manage to find evidence of "their illness" in their past and present behavior, confirming the medical and societal diagnosis, receive benefits. This pattern of behavior is a special case of a more general pattern that has been called the "apostolic function" by Balint, in which the physician and others inadvertently cause the patient to display symptoms of the illness the physician thinks the patient has.[17] Not only physicians but other hospital personnel and even other patients, reward the deviant for conforming to the stereotypes.[18]

7. Labeled deviants are punished when they attempt the return to conventional roles. The second process operative is the systematic blockage of entry to nondeviant roles once the label has been publicly applied. Thus the ex-mental patient, although he is urged to rehabilitate himself in the community, usually finds himself discriminated against in seeking to return to his old status, and on trying to find a new one in the occupational, marital, social, and other spheres.[19] Thus, to a degree, the labeled deviant is rewarded for deviating, and punished for attempting to conform.

8. In the crisis occurring when a primary deviant is publicly labeled, the deviant is highly suggestible, and may accept the proffered role of the insane as the only alternative. When gross deviancy is publicly recognized and made an issue, the primary deviant may be profoundly confused, anxious, and ashamed. In this crisis it seems reasonable to assume that the deviant will be suggestible to the cues that he gets from the reactions of others toward him.[20] But those around him are also in a crisis; the incomprehensible nature of the deviance, and the seeming need for immediate action lead them to take collective action against the deviant on the basis of the attitude which all share—the traditional stereotypes of insanity. The deviant is sensitive to the cues provided by these others and begins to think of himself in terms of the stereotyped role of insanity, which is part of his own role vocabulary also, since he, like those reacting to him, learned it early in childhood.

---

17 Balint, *op. cit.,* pp. 215–239; Cf. Thomas J. Scheff, "Decision Rules, Types of Error and Their Consequences in Medical Diagnosis," *Behavioral Science,* 8 (April, 1963), pp. 97–107.

18 William Caudill, F. C. Redlich, H. R. Gilmore, and E. B. Brody, "Social Structure and the Interaction Processes on a Psychiatric Ward," *American Journal of Orthopsychiatry,* 22 (April, 1952), pp. 314–334.

19 Lemert, *op. cit.,* provides an extensive discussion of this process under the heading of "Limitation of Participation," pp. 434–440.

20 This proposition receives support from Erikson's observations: Kai T. Erikson, *loc. cit.*

In this situation his behavior may begin to follow the pattern suggested by his own stereotypes and the reactions of others. That is, when a primary deviant organizes his behavior within the framework of mental disorder, and when his organization is validated by others, particularly prestigeful others such as physicians, he is "hooked" and will proceed on a career of chronic deviance.

The last three propositions suggest that once a person has been placed in a deviant status there are rewards for conforming to the deviant role, and punishments for not conforming to the deviant role. This is not to imply, however, that the symptomatic behavior of persons occupying a deviant status is always a manifestation of conforming behavior. To explain this point, some discussion of the process of self-control in "normals" is necessary.

In a recent discussion of the process of self-control, Shibutani notes that self-control is not automatic, but is an intricate and delicately balanced process, sustainable only under propitious circumstances.[21] He points out that fatigue, the reaction to narcotics, excessive excitement or tension (such as is generated in mobs), or a number of other conditions interfere with self-control; conversely, conditions which produce normal bodily states, and deliberative processes such as symbolization and imaginative rehearsal before action, facilitate it.

One might argue that a crucially important aspect of imaginative rehearsal is the image of himself that the actor projects into his future action. Certainly in American society, the cultural image of the "normal" adult is that of a person endowed with self-control ("will-power," "back-bone," "strength of character," etc.). For the person who sees himself as endowed with the trait of self-control, self-control is facilitated, since he can imagine himself enduring stress during his imaginative rehearsal, and also while under actual stress.

For a person who has acquired an image of himself as lacking the ability to control his own actions, the process of self-control is likely to break down under stress. Such a person may feel that he has reached his "breaking-point" under circumstances which would be endured by a person with a "normal" self-conception. This is to say, a greater lack of self-control than can be explained by stress tends to appear in those roles for which the culture transmits imagery which emphasizes lack of self-control. In American society such imagery is transmitted for the roles of the very young and very old, drunkards and drug addicts, gamblers, and the mentally ill.

Thus, the social role of the mentally ill has a different significance at different phases of residual deviance. When labeling first occurs, it merely gives a name to primary deviation which has other roots. When (and if) the primary deviance becomes an issue, and is not ignored or rationalized away, labeling may create a social type, a pattern of "symptomatic" behavior in

---

[21] T. Shibutani, *Society and Personality*, Englewood Cliffs, N. J.: Prentice-Hall, 1961, Chapter 6, "Consciousness and Voluntary Conduct."

conformity with the stereotyped expectations of others. Finally, to the extent that the deviant role becomes a part of the deviant's self-conception, his ability to control his own behavior may be impaired under stress, resulting in episodes of compulsive behavior.

The preceding eight hypotheses form the basis for the final causal hypothesis.

9. Among residual deviants, labeling is the single most important cause of careers of residual deviance. This hypothesis assumes that most residual deviance, if it does not become the basis for entry into the sick role, will not lead to a deviant career. Most deviant careers, according to this point of view, arise out of career contingencies, and are therefore not directly connected with the origins of the initial deviance.[22] Although there are a wide variety of contingencies which lead to labeling rather than denial, these contingencies can be usefully classified in terms of the nature of the deviant behavior, the person who commits the deviant acts, and the community in which the deviance occurs. Other things being equal, the severity of the societal reaction to deviance is a function of, first, the degree, amount, and visibility of the deviant behavior; second, the power of the deviant, and the social distance between the deviant and the agents of social control; and finally, the tolerance level of the community, and the availability in the culture of the community of alternative nondeviant roles.[23] Particularly crucial for future research is the importance of the first two contingencies (the amount and degree of deviance), which are characteristics of the deviant, relative to the remaining five contingencies, which are characteristics of the social system.[24] To the extent that these five factors are found empirically to be independent determinants of labeling and denial, the status of the mental patient can be considered a partly ascribed rather than a completely achieved status. The

---

[22] It should be noted, however, that these contingencies are causal only because they become part of a dynamic system: the reciprocal and cumulative inter-relation between the deviant's behavior and the societal reaction. For example, the more the deviant enters the role of the mentally ill, the more he is defined by others as mentally ill; but the more he is defined as mentally ill, the more fully he enters the role, and so on. By representing this theory in the form of a flow chart, Walter Buckley pointed out that there are numerous such feedback loops implied here. For an explicit treatment of feedback, see Edwin M. Lemert, "Paranoia and the Dynamics of Exclusion," *Sociometry*, 25 (March, 1962), pp. 2–20.

[23] *Cf.* Lemert, *op. cit.*, pp. 51–53, 55–68; Goffman, "The Moral Career of the Mental Patient," in *Asylums, op. cit.*, pp. 134–135; David Mechanic, "Some Factors in Identifying and Defining Mental Illness," *Mental Hygiene*, 46 (January, 1962), pp. 66–74; for a list of similar factors in the reaction to physical illness, see Earl L. Koos, *The Health of Regionville*, New York: Columbia University Press, 1954, pp. 30–38.

[24] *Cf.* Thomas J. Scheff, "Psychiatric and Social Contingencies in the Release of Mental Patients in a Midwestern State," forthcoming; Simon Dinitz, Mark Lefton, Shirley Angrist, and Benjamin Pasamanick, "Psychiatric and Social Attributes as Predictors of Case Outcome in Mental Hospitalization," *Social Problems*, 8 (Spring, 1961), pp. 322–328.

dynamics of treated mental illness could then be profitably studied quite apart from the individual dynamics of mental disorder.

CONCLUSION

This paper has presented a sociological theory of the causation of stable mental disorder. Since the evidence advanced in support of the theory was scattered and fragmentary, it can only be suggested as a stimulus to further discussion and research. Among the areas pointed out for further investigation are field studies of the prevalence and duration of residual deviance; investigations of stereotypes of mental disorder in children, the mass media, and adult conversations; studies of the rewarding of stereotyped deviation, blockage of return to conventional roles, and of the suggestibility of primary deviants in crises. The final causal hypothesis suggests studies of the conditions under which denial and labeling of residual deviation occur. The variables which might effect the societal reaction concern the nature of the deviance, the deviant himself, and the community in which the deviation occurs. Although many of the hypotheses suggested are largely unverified, they suggest avenues for investigating mental disorder different than those that are usually followed, and the rudiments of a general theory of deviant behavior.

DISCUSSION

1. Scheff proposes that mental illness is a social role. What does he mean by that? How do people learn to "play the role"? Is he suggesting that mental illness is just an act?

2. Theories provide insight into how the world works but are most useful when validated empirically. How would you test Scheff's propositions? What observations would be consistent with his predictions? What observations would be inconsistent with his predictions?

3. Some people are forced into treatment by others and some enter treatment voluntarily. How would Scheff's theory account for voluntary treatment-seeking?

Walter R. Gove

Societal Reaction as an Explanation of Mental Illness: An Evaluation[†]

Walter Gove is one of Thomas Scheff's most ardent critics. In this early critique of labeling theory, he presents evidence against the theory's key propositions. By so doing, he challenges the notion that mental illness labels are applied capriciously and that they have damaging consequences for the individual. Notably, he also challenges the assertion that stigma plays a major role in the lives of people with mental illness—a challenge that Link and his colleagues take up in the selection that follows.

During the 1960s the societal reaction perspective, sometimes referred to as "labeling theory," has been one of the most pervasive and influential sociological approaches to deviance. However, this perspective has received little systematic evaluation. In this paper I will attempt to assess the empirical validity of the explanation of mental illness provided by the societal reaction theorists.

THE SOCIETAL REACTION PERSPECTIVE

One of the most fundamental distinctions made by the societal reaction theorists is between primary deviance, which may cause someone to be labeled as a deviant, and secondary deviance, which is the behavior produced by being placed in a deviant role. Regarding primary and secondary deviance, Lemert (1967, 17) says: "Primary deviation is assumed to arise in a wide variety of social, cultural, and psychological contexts, and at best has only marginal implication for the psychic structure of the individual; it does not lead to symbolic reorganization at the level of self-regarding attitudes and social roles. Secondary deviation is deviant behavior, or social roles based upon it, which becomes a means of defense, attack or adaptation to the overt and covert problems created by the societal reaction to primary deviation."

The societal reaction theorists do not appear to attach significance to an act of primary deviance except insofar as others react toward the commission of the act. To them deviance is not a quality of an act, but instead deviance is produced in the interaction between a person who commits an act and those who respond to it (Becker, 1963, 14).

According to this approach, usually the most crucial step in the development of a stable pattern of deviant behavior is the experience of being

---

Gove, Walter R. 1970. "Societal Reaction as an Explanation of Mental Illness: An Evaluation." *American Sociological Review* 35:873–884.

caught and publicly labeled deviant. Whether or not this happens to a person "depends not so much on what he does as on what other people do" (Becker, 1963, 31). Erikson (1964, 16), writing about the public labeling process, states: "The community's decision to bring deviant sanctions against the individual...is a sharp rite of transition at once moving him out of his normal position in society and transferring him into a distinctive deviant role. The ceremonies which accomplish this change of status, ordinarily, have three related phases. They provide a formal confrontation between the deviant suspect and representatives of his community (as in the criminal trial or psychiatric case conference); they announce some judgment about the nature of his deviancy (a verdict or diagnosis for example), and they perform an act of social placement, assigning him to a special role (like that of a prisoner or patient) which redefines his position in society."

Erikson (1964, 16) goes on to state: "An important feature of these ceremonies in our own culture is that they are almost irreversible." Why might this be the case? According to the societal reaction theorists, the status of deviant is a master status which overrides all other statuses in determining how others will act towards one (Becker, 1963, 33). Once a person is stigmatized by being labeled a deviant, a self-fulfilling prophecy is initiated with others perceiving and responding to the person as a deviant (Becker, 1963, 34; Erikson, 1964, 16). Furthermore, once persons are publicly processed as deviants, they are typically forced into a deviant group (usually by being placed in an institution). As Becker notes (1963, 38), such groups have one thing in common, their deviance. They have a common fate, they face the same problems and because of this they develop a deviant subculture. This subculture combines a perspective on the world with a set of routine activities. According to Becker (1963, 38), "membership in such a group solidifies a deviant identity" and leads to rationalization of their position.

In the view of the societal reaction theorists, once this has occurred it is extremely difficult for the person to break out of his deviant status. As Lemert (1967, 55) states, "Once deviance becomes a way of life the personal issue often becomes the cost of making a change rather than the higher status to be gained through rehabilitation or reform. Such costs are calculated in terms of the time, energy and distress seen as necessary for change." The deviant has learned to carry on his deviant activities with a minimum of trouble (Becker, 1963, 39). He has already failed in the normal world, suggesting to himself and others an inability to make it even when things are relatively normal; now he faces the world as a stigmatized person. If he is in an institution, such as a mental hospital, to become a candidate for reinstatement in society he must, as Lemert (1967, 45) notes, give allegiance to an often anomalous conception of himself and the world. Denial of the organizational ideology may lead to the judgment that the deviant is "unreformed" or still "sick." Even if he is returned to the community, he presumably will face an audience which anticipates the worst and will take steps to protect himself, steps which make it difficult for the person to succeed. Furthermore, in the community he may be on a form of probation which forces him to live by extremely rigorous rules, the violations of which are grounds for reinstitutionalization.

In summary, the argument of the societal reaction theorists is that persons who have passed through a degradation ceremony and have been forced to become members of a deviant group have experienced a profound and frequently irreversible socialization process. They have acquired an inferiority status and have developed a deviant world view and the knowledge and skill that go with it. And perhaps equally important, they have developed a deviant self-image based upon the image of themselves they receive through the actions of others. Although the societal reaction perspective of deviance has been very much in vogue during the 1960s, most of the work based on this perspective has been intuitive and/or theoretical, and there has been very little systematic evaluation and testing of the perspective. What follows in this paper is an attempt to meet this lack of critical evaluation by examining the evidence in a particular area of deviance—that of mental illness.

ENTRANCE INTO THE MENTALLY ILL ROLE

The Theoretical Explanation. A fairly explicit statement of how the societal reaction perspective may be used to explain how a person becomes mentally ill has been provided by Scheff (1966). Scheff views mental illness as an ascribed status, entry into which is primarily dependent upon conditions external to the individual. His formulation is (1) that virtually everyone at sometime commits acts that correspond to the public stereotype of mental illness; (2) if, by some happenstance, these acts become public knowledge, the individual may, depending upon various (unspecified) contingencies, be referred to the appropriate officials; and (3) once this happens the person will be routinely processed as mentally ill and placed in a mental institution. This is an original formulation which very neatly gets around a potentially troublesome aspect of the societal reaction perspective, namely, why does the person commit an act of primary deviance? In most cases it would be very difficult to argue that the person publicly presents psychiatric symptoms for personal gain or because he belongs to a subculture with values in conflict with the dominant group. Instead, Scheff argues that psychiatric symptoms are a common phenomenon, that their presentation is unintended, and only rarely and fortuitously do they cause someone to be labeled mentally ill. The question we must now confront is whether or not this formulation is consistent with available evidence.

The Empirical Evidence. A number of investigations (Star, 1961; Nunnally, 1961; Cumming & Cumming, 1957) have been made of the public's image of mental illness. These studies indicate that the public lacks accurate knowledge about mental disorder, distorting and exaggerating the amount and type of disturbance. In addition, "the mentally ill are regarded with fear, distrust and dislike" (Nunnally, 1961, 46). In the public conception, mental illness appears to involve unpredictable and potentially dangerous behavior.

Furthermore, there is a halo effect: once a person is perceived as mentally ill, he is not only thought to be unpredictable and dangerous but also "dirty, unintelligent, insincere and worthless" (Nunnally, 1961, 233). These investigations clearly indicate that the public has a negative, highly stereotyped image of mental illness and suggest that the public generally views mental illness as a master status that overrides other characteristics of the individual. The question, however, is whether people are treated as mentally ill because they inadvertently perform an act that activates the stereotype of mental illness. The evidence from field surveys and from studies of the path to the mental hospital indicates that this is not the case.

In a pioneering study, Yarrow et al. (1955) investigated how wives came to define their husbands as mentally ill. The research demonstrated that the wives utilized strong defenses to avoid seeing their husbands' behavior as deviant. The wives would make every effort to interpret their husbands' behavior as normal. If that failed, they would minimize the importance of the behavior and balance it off against more normal behavior. Only when the husband's behavior became impossible to deal with would the wife take action to have her husband hospitalized. Even at this time the husband was not always viewed as mentally ill. This pattern appears to be consistent with the findings of other investigators (Schwartz, 1957, 290; Hollingshead & Redlich, 1958; Sampson et al., 1964; also see Jaco, 1960, 18). Furthermore, investigations have indicated that rehospitalization does not typically occur because of the expectations of others but because of the manifestation of severe psychiatric symptoms which have become impossible to handle in the community (Freeman & Simmons, 1963; Angrist et al., 1968).

The results of field surveys also bear upon how people identify the mentally ill. When people are presented with descriptions of persons with various types of mental disorder, the disturbed behavior is not regarded as an indication of mental illness except when the person is presented as dangerous (Cumming & Cumming, 1957; Star, 1961). Phillips (1963), using the same case materials, has shown that rejection of the mentally ill is not related to their behavior but to their being labeled as mentally ill by being in treatment. In sum, the evidence strongly suggests that persons, typically, are hospitalized because they have an active psychiatric disorder which is extremely difficult for themselves and/or others to handle. It would appear that the public's stereotype of mental illness does not lead to persons being inappropriately labeled mentally ill through an inadvertent act of residual rule-breaking. Instead, the evidence suggests that the gross exaggeration of the degree and type of disorder in the stereotype fosters the denial of mental illness, since the disturbed person's behavior does not usually correspond to the stereotype.

Once a person is brought to the attention of public officials as mentally ill, do the officials, as Scheff suggests, act on the assumption of illness and routinely route him to a mental hospital? We might first look at persons who voluntarily seek hospitalization. Mechanic (1962) and Brown (1961, 60) feel that public mental hospitals accept virtually all such patients, but they present no data. To my knowledge there are only two studies that have systematically evaluated hospital acceptance of voluntary mental patients. Mishler and Wexler (1963) found that the public mental hospital they studied accepted for admission only 39 percent ($n = 246$) of the applicants, and the private mental hospital accepted 58 percent ($n = 137$) of the applicants. Similarly, Mandel and Rapport (1969) found that the public mental hospital they studied accepted for admission 41 percent ($n = 269$) of the applicants. Both studies thus found that the public mental hospitals only admitted approximately 40 percent of the voluntary applicants. Although there probably are hospitals that routinely assume illness and admit virtually all voluntary mental patients, it is clearly inappropriate to assume this is always or even usually the case.

Let us turn to involuntary patients. Such persons may be thought of as going through three stages in their contact with public officials: (1) a screening stage where the police or some other screening agency makes the decision to hold or not to hold the person for examination and possible commitment, (2) an examination by a court psychiatrist or other duly qualified board, and (3) the court hearing where the official decision is made to release the person or to commit him to a mental hospital.

First, let us examine the limited data available on the screening stage. A recent study of police discretion in the apprehension of the mentally ill by Bittner (1967, 280) found that the police "like everyone else avail themselves of various forms of denial when it comes to doing something about it (mental illness)." Furthermore, it is Bittner's impression that "except for cases of suicide attempts, the decision to take someone to the hospital is based upon overwhelmingly conclusive evidence of illness" (Bittner, 1967, 285). He goes on to note that the police regularly assist persons in the community whom they and others recognize as having a serious mental disturbance while making no effort to have them hospitalized. There is, to my knowledge, only one study (Wilde, 1968) of a psychiatric screening agency that presents the agency's response to requests to initiate commitment proceedings. In this study when a nonpsychiatrist made a request to initiate commitment proceedings, the screening agency approved the request in only 33 percent of the cases ($n = 6000$). In contrast, when a psychiatrist made a request, the request was apparently routinely approved—the approval rate for hospital psychiatrists being 98 percent ($n = 2000$), and for court psychiatrists 100 percent ($n = 250$)—presumably on the assumption that the psychiatrist had carefully and expertly evaluated the need for hospitalization. Support for this assumption is provided by the fact that the court psychiatrists examined approximately 1,000 suspected mental cases sent by the jails but only requested commitment proceedings on 250 (Wilde, 1968, 216). These studies clearly suggest that during the initial screening stage officials do not assume illness but in fact proceed rather cautiously, screening out a substantial number of persons.

Let us shift to the outcomes of the psychiatric examination of persons held for commitment. Scheff in his study of these examinations found them to be unsystematic, arbitrary, and prejudicial. He felt that "except in very unusual cases, the psychiatric examiner's recommendation to retain the patient is virtually automatic" (Scheff, 1968, 287). Nonetheless, in each of the studies reviewed, release was recommended for at least some persons. Generally, such recommendations were relatively rare; however, in the largest study (Haney & Michielutte, 1968) only 50 percent of the persons under 65 were found to be incompetent.

When we look at the outcome to the court hearing, we find a similar pattern with most, but usually not all, persons being committed. The description of commitment proceedings (Miller & Schwartz, 1966; Scheff, 1967; Wenger & Fletcher, 1969) indicate that they are very rapid, that there is rarely any real exploration of the facts surrounding the case, and that proper legal procedures are not closely observed. From their experience Miller and Schwartz (1966, 34) guess that "the judgment about mental illness had already been made earlier in the commitment process and that the hearing was a rubber stamp to an earlier decision." From the rates presented by Wilde (1968), it would appear that those persons who are released are exclusively those for whom the psychiatrists had recommended such action. Wenger and Fletcher (1969, 68) explicitly state this to be the case in their study. Miller and Schwartz (1966, 34), however, found that "the judge reversed the medical recommendation for commitment...in nearly one-fourth of the cases."

In summary, the available evidence on how people enter the mentally ill role indicates that the societal reaction formulation, at least as stated by Scheff, is false. The evidence is that the vast majority of persons who become patients have a serious disturbance, and it is only when the situation becomes untenable that action is taken. The public officials who perform the major screening role do not simply process all of the persons who come before them as mentally ill but instead screen out a large portion. If the person passes this initial screening, he will probably be committed, and there is reason to assume the process at this point frequently becomes somewhat ritualized. But even here a number of persons are released either through the psychiatric examination or the court hearing.

CONSEQUENCES OF HOSPITALIZATION

Let us now turn to what happens to a person who enters a mental hospital. As noted in the introductory section, the societal reaction theorists feel that once a person has gone through a public hearing, and has been certified as a deviant and placed in an institution, it is extremely difficult for the person to break out of his deviant status. For a number of reasons, the impact of this process is held to be especially pronounced for the mental patient (see Goffman, 1961). First, the mental patient may have been misled, lied to, jailed and testified against by those he trusted; and by the time he arrives at the hospital, he is presumed to feel deserted, betrayed, and estranged from his family and friends, a condition that should promote the acceptance of the mentally ill role. Second, in the hospital the patient is surrounded by severe restrictions and deprivations which are presented as "intended parts of his treatment, part of his need at the time, and therefore an expression of the state his self has fallen to." (Goffman, 1961, 149). Third, the events recorded in the patient's case history are selected in such a manner that they are almost uniformly defamatory and discrediting. These events tend to be public knowledge, and they may be used to keep the patient in his place and to validate his mental illness.

Unfortunately, the research in the societal reaction tradition dealing with the effects of hospitalization has focused almost exclusively on what goes on in the hospital. Such studies have probably focused primarily on long-term patients who make up the bulk of the resident population; they tend to ignore the majority of psychiatric patients whose hospitalization is relatively brief. For this reason much of this research may present an unrepresentative picture. Let us agree, however, that mental hospitals may, in many ways, be debilitating places where patients *may* come to accept the preferred role of the insane and *may*, over time, develop skills and a world view adapted to the institutional setting and gradually lose their roles and even interest in the community.

Restitutive Processes. The fact that debilitating processes may be present does not mean that restitutive processes are not also in operation. One such process may of course be treatment, but that is not the only one. An important study by Sampson et al. (1961, 1964), which looked at the patient before, during, and after hospitalization, found that hospitalization initiated major restitutive processes, most of which were not consciously guided by hospital personnel. Let us outline these processes. It was found that hospitalization interrupted a situation which was experienced as untenable and, by doing so, it blocked actions which threatened irremediable damage to family life. This interruption was "legitimated by the act of hospitalization which ratified the wife as ill and in need of special isolation and treatment" (Sampson et al., 1961, 144). This ratification of illness was decisive in blunting and redefining the negative implications of the interruption. The acts leading to the hospital were not viewed as alienative, "but as actions of an involuntary nature required by and serving the present and future interests of the patient and her family" (Sampson et al., 1961, 144). Furthermore, through moral and legal obstacles the husband was forced to defer a sometimes planned divorce allowing other solutions to marital difficulties to be considered and attempted.

Hospitalization was also found to have initiated processes which served in a positive way to move the family toward reintegration. In some cases the removal of the patient and the conflict situation promoted a revival of positive ties and feelings. In many other cases the dislocation in family life produced by the wife's absence caused considerable problems and "at the first sign of improvement the husband often began to pleasurably anticipate his wife's return and resumption of responsibilities" (Sampson et al., 1961, 152). Furthermore, the hospital, by treating the husband as responsible for his wife and eager for her recovery, put him into a role which frequently reinstituted a relationship of concern and improved marital communication.

A major issue is whether the processes just presented generally have a major impact on the patient or if they are overshadowed by the processes pointed to by the societal reaction theorists. Before the era of the tranquil-izers and the open door policy, the average patient was probably heavily influenced by the deadening institutional procedures of the traditional men-tal hospital. Now, however, the vast majority of mental patients receive fairly rapid and intensive treatment. In such cases the restitutive factors of hospi-talization may well dominate; and, in any case, with a brief hospitalization the impact of many of the processes outlined by the societal reaction theo-rists should be minimal.

Stigma. There is, of course, the possibility that the patient is so stigmatized by having been labeled mentally ill that when he returns to the community he is not *allowed* to resume his previous interpersonal and instrumental roles. In an attempt to evaluate the question of whether or not the stigma of having been a patient in a mental hospital necessarily leads to the chronic occupancy of the mentally ill role, let us turn to a detailed study of 287 women after treatment conducted by Angrist et al. (1968). Their sample of women tended to be severely disturbed but to have an acute rather than chronic illness (for example, only one-third of their sample had been hospitalized previously). Their patients had received fairly intensive treatment and on the average had been in the hospital 52 days. The study was concerned with those patients who had been returned to the community and who were able to remain there for 15 days.

One of the first things to be noted is that the ex-patients were not like their neighbors, or like a random sample of females in the community, the ex-patients being atypical in their lack of education, their singleness, and their household living arrangements. These factors apparently predated their hos-pitalization and could not be considered a consequence of being publicly labeled mentally ill. Once the former mental patients and their neighbors were matched on these characteristics, the groups were extremely similar "in the areas of instrumental role performance, role expectations and toler-ance of deviant behavior" (Angrist et al., 1968, 161). The ex-patients, however, manifested significantly more psychiatric handicaps. The authors also found that "as performance (or the ability to perform) degenerates, the expectations of family members are corroded, so that they become accustomed to expect less of their relative" (Angrist et al. 1968, 171). This suggests that expecta-tions for poor performance may be determined more by ineffectual behavior than the reverse, a conclusion that appears to be consistent with the work of Freeman and Simmons (1963).

For former patients, probably the most important indicator of continued occupancy of the mentally ill role is rehospitalization. Of the patients in this study 15 percent had been rehospitalized after six months; 24 percent after two years; and 32 percent after seven years (Angrist et al., 1968, *passim*). Thus, over two-thirds of these patients had not been rehospitalized after seven years, and probably a significant proportion of these never will.

What caused rehospitalization? The evidence indicated that following the initial hospitalization, the readmitted patients had exhibited more deviant behavior and more psychiatric symptoms (particularly extreme and acutely disordered symptoms) than ex-patients who avoided rehospitalization.

Furthermore, the data showed that in spite of the fact that ex-patients had previously been labeled as mentally ill, the relatives viewed "readmission as a last resort for behavior which cannot be handled without medical help" (Angrist et al., 1968, 100). In conclusion, the authors (Angrist et al., 1968, 176) state that "the fact that the returnees were decidedly sicker than community patients indicates that intrinsic features of the illness are of greater consequence in precipitating readmission than are the variations in the way significant others perceive, evaluate or tolerate such illness."

Although this study clearly suggests that the stigma attached to a former mental patient does not generally have serious consequences, it does not specifically deal with the question of stigma. Unfortunately, very little work has focused directly on this issue. A study of psychiatric patients by Jones et al. (1963) found that patients, typically, felt that the lay public would not view a person as undesirable because he had been in a mental hospital, Cumming and Cumming (1965) found, in a study of 22 former mental patients, that 41 percent felt stigmatized, 4 expressing shame and 5 having a generalized expectation of discrimination. They suggest that with the passage of time, or with the occupancy of normal roles, feelings of stigma will disappear. Freeman and Simmons (1961) in a study of feelings of stigma by relatives of ex-mental patients found that only 24 percent of the families ($n = 394$) felt stigmatized. Furthermore, their findings indicate that feelings of stigma are associated with the perception that the patient is acting in an abnormal fashion and with a fear that persons in the community will discriminate against the family because of the patient's current bizarre behavior. In general, the evidence on stigma, although far from conclusive, suggests that stigma is not a serious problem for most ex-mental patients and that, when stigma is a problem, it is more directly related to the person's current psychiatric status, or general ineffectiveness, than it is to having been in a mental hospital.

DISCUSSION

The societal reaction perspective does not view the deviant as someone who is suffering from an intra-personal disorder but instead as someone who, through a set of circumstances, becomes publicly labeled a deviant and who is forced by the societal reaction into a deviant role. In essence, they view the deviant as someone who is victimized (see Gouldner, 1968). The available evidence, however, indicates that the societal reaction formulation of how a person becomes mentally ill is substantially incorrect. There is very little systematic evidence of victimization. The evidence shows that a substantial majority of the persons who are hospitalized have a serious psychiatric disturbance quite apart from any secondary deviance that may be associated with the mentally ill role. Furthermore, persons in the community do not view someone as mentally ill if he happens to act in a bizarre fashion. On the contrary, they persist in denying mental illness until the situation becomes intolerable. Once prospective patients come into contact with public officials, a substantial screening still occurs, presumably sorting out persons who are being railroaded or who are less disturbed. It is only in the last stages of the commitment process that some ritualization appears to occur, and even here a noticeable proportion of persons are sorted out.

The evidence also indicates that the societal reaction theorists have overstated the degree to which secondary deviance is associated with mental hospitalization. (1) There appear to be many restitutive processes associated with hospitalization even apart from the question of therapy. (2) Patients treated in a modern psychiatric hospital typically do not spend enough time in the hospital to become truly institutionalized. (3) In most cases the stigma of having been a former mental patient does not appear to affect greatly one's performance in the community following discharge. In summary, the studies reviewed, while in no way denying the existence of the processes outlined by the societal reaction theorists, suggest that mental hospitalization does not necessarily or even typically lead to a prolonged occupancy of the mentally ill role. Furthermore, the available evidence indicates that when former patients continue to have difficulty, these difficulties are generally due to the person's confronting a troubled situation or to some psychiatric disorder, and not to the social expectations of others.

The evidence reviewed suggests that a person's behavior determines the expectations of others to a much greater degree than the reverse. This relationship between behavior and expectations is probably generally true in the short run; it certainly appears that it is the person's disturbed behavior that generally leads to the mentally ill role. In the long run, however, the expectations of others may play an important role in determining the behavior of a person, and such expectations should be taken into account in a general theory of mental illness. Unfortunately, the societal reaction theorists have generally treated their framework as a sufficient explanatory system. In doing so they have underemphasized the importance of acts of primary deviance and overemphasized the importance of the forces promoting secondary deviance. Future attempts at explaining mental illness will have to redress the balance.

References

Angrist, Shirley, Mark Lefton, Simon Dinitz and Benjamin Pasamanick. 1968. Women After Treatment. New York: Appleton-Century-Crofts.

Becker, Howard. 1963. Outsiders: Studies in the Sociology of Deviance. New York: The Free Press.

Bittner, Egon. 1967. "Police discretion in apprehending the mentally ill." Social Problems 14 (Winter): 278–292.

Brown, E. L. 1961. Newer Dimensions of Patient Care. New York: Russell Sage Foundation.

Cumming, Elaine and John Cumming. 1957. Closed Ranks. Cambridge: Harvard University Press.

Cumming, John and Elaine Cumming. 1965. "On the stigma of mental illness." Community Mental Health Journal 1:135–143.

Erikson, Kai. 1964. "Notes on the sociology of deviance." Pp. 9–21 in Howard Becker (ed.), The Other Side. New York: The Free Press.

Freeman, Howard and Ozzie Simmons. 1961. "Feelings of stigma among relatives of former mental patients." Social Problems 8:32–321.

Freeman, Howard and Ozzie Simmons. 1963. The Mental Patient Comes Home. New York: Wiley.

Goffman, Erving. 1961. Asylums: Essays on the Social Situation of Mental Patients and Other Inmates. Garden City, N.Y.: Anchor Books.

Gouldner, Alvin. 1968. "The sociologist as partisan: Sociology and the welfare state." The American Sociologist. 3 (May):103–116.

Haney, C. Allen and Robert Michelutte. 1968. "Selective factors operating in the adjudication of incompetency." Journal of Health and Social Behavior 9 (September):233–242.

Hollingshead, August and Fredrick Redlich. 1958. Social Class and Mental Illness. New York: Wiley.

Jaco, E. Gartly. 1960. The Social Epidemiology of Mental Disorders. New York: Russell Sage Foundation.

Jones, Nelson, Marvin Kahn and John MacDonald. 1963. "Psychiatric patients' view of mental illness, hospitalization and treatment." Journal of Nervous and Mental Disease 136:82–87.

Lemert, Edwin. 1967. Human Deviance, Social Problems and Social Control. Engelwood Cliffs, New Jersey: Prentice Hall.

Mechanic, David. 1962. "Some factors in identifying and defining mental illness." Mental Hygiene 46 (January): 66–74.

Mendel, Werner and Samuel Rapport. 1969. "Determinants of the decision for psychiatric hospitalization." Archives of General Psychistry 20 (March):321–328.

Miller, Dorothy and Michael Schwartz. 1966. "County lunacy commission hearings: Some observations of commitments to a state mental hospital." Social Problems 14 (Summer):26–35.

Mishler, Elliott and Nancy Wexler. 1963. "Decision processes in psychiatric hospitalization." American Sociological Review 28:576–587.

Nunnally, Jim 1961 Popular Conceptions of Mental Health. New York: Holt, Rinehart and Winston.

Phillips, Derek. 1963. "Rejection: A possible consequence of seeking help for mental disorders." American Sociological Review 28:963–972.

Sampson, Harold, Sheldon Messinger and Robert Towne. 1961. "The mental hospital and marital family ties." Social Problems 9 (Fall):141–155.

Sampson, Harold, Sheldon Messinger and Robert Towne. 1964. Schizoprenhic Women: Studies in Marital Crisis. New York: Atherton.

Scheff, Thomas. 1966. Being Mentally Ill. Chicago: Aldine.

Scheff, Thomas. 1967. "Social conditions for rationality: How urban and rural courts deal with the mentally ill." Pp. 109–118 in Thomas Scheff (ed.), Mental Illness and Social Progress. New York: Harper and Row.

Scheff, Thomas. 1968. "The societal reaction to deviance: Ascriptive elements in the psychiatric screening of mental patients in a Midwestern state." Pp. 276–290 in Stephen Spitzer and Norman Denzin (eds.), The Mental Patient. New York: McGraw-Hill.

Schwartz, Charlotte. 1957. "Perspectives on deviance—Wives' definitions of their husbands' mental illness." Psychiatry 20:275–291.

Star, Shirley. 1961. The Dilemmas of Mental Illness Citied in the Joint Commission on Mental Illness and Health. Action for Mental Health. Pp. 74–76. New York: Science Editions.

Wenger, Denis and C. Richard Fletcher. 1969. "The effect of legal counsel on admissions to a state mental hospital: A confrontation of professions." Journal of Health and Social Behavior 10 (March): 66–72.

Wilde, William. 1968. "Decision-making in a psychiatric screening agency." Journal of Health and Social Behavior 9 (September):215–221.

Yarrow, Marion, Charlotte Schwartz, Harriet Murphy and Leila Deasy. 1955. "The psychological meaning of mental illness in the family." The Journal of Social Issues XI, (No. 4): 12–24.

DISCUSSION

1. What are the key points of Gove's critique? What evidence does he present in favor of his points? How persuaded are you by the evidence he presents?

2. Based on your knowledge and experience, do you agree with Gove that there is little stigma associated with mental illness?

Bruce G. Link, Francis T. Cullen, Elmer Struening, Patrick E. Shrout, and Bruce P. Dohrenwend

A Modified Labeling Theory Approach to Mental Disorders: An Empirical Assessment[†]

Link and his colleagues propose a "middle ground" theory of labeling—a theory that neither accepts the validity of Scheff's specific propositions nor rejects the independent power of mental illness labels. In this selection, they evaluate the evidence for their theory using data from a community sample as well as from a sample of psychiatric patients. When it was first published, their work motivated a redirection of research away from strict tests of labeling theory and toward an understanding of mental illness stigma.

In recent years, labeling theory propositions that directly link the emergence of mental illness to societal reaction (Scheff, 1966) have received sustained and severe criticism (e.g., Gove, 1970, 1980, 1982; Lehman, Joy, Kreisman, & Simmens, 1976; Weinstein, 1983). More than simply refuting the extreme claim that "labeling causes most career deviance," critics also downplay the

Link, Bruce G., Francis T. Cullen, Elmer Struening, Patrick E. Shrout, and Bruce P. Dohrenwend. 1989. "A Modified Labeling Theory Approach to Mental Disorders: An Empirical Assessment." *American Sociological Review* 54:400–423.

salience of social factors such as stigma and stereotyping and assert that for the "vast majority of mental patients stigma appears to be transitory and does not appear to pose a severe problem" (Gove, 1982, 280). We argue that such an assessment is over pessimistic and misguided in suggesting that stigma is unimportant. Our argument draws on Scheff's (1966) labeling theory but qualifies and extends it to arrive at a "modified labeling approach." In this paper we derive predictions from this approach and test them empirically. Specifically, we examine whether stigmatization affects the social support networks of patients officially labeled by contact with a mental health clinic or hospital.

To begin, we note that critics rely on several types of data to dismiss the stigma of mental disorder as unimportant. Often they point to findings which seem to show that the public does not harbor negative feelings toward the mentally ill. For example, Crocetti, Spiro, and Siassi (1971) found that a sample of automobile workers typically expressed a willingness to work on the same job with, rent a room to, or even to fall in love with a former mental patient. Other critics argue that even if negative attitudes toward patients exist, they do not result in rejecting behavior. As noted by Huffine and Clausen (1979, 1057) and by Gove and Fain (1973, 496–97), present and former patients rarely are able to report concrete instances of rejection. Similarly, Weinstein's (1979, 1983) literature reviews prompted him to conclude that many patients do not feel stigmatized and view favorably their treatment by mental health professionals. Further, a growing body of research concludes that any rejection patients experience is far more likely to occur because of their deviant behavior than because of the label "mental patient." A seemingly convincing approach along these lines involves experimental manipulation of "labeling" and "behavior," and shows that behavior determines peoples' reactions more strongly than does labeling (for a review see Link, Cullen, Frank, & Wozniak, 1987).

Yet recent studies challenge these conclusions. First, with respect to the idea that public attitudes are benign, Link and Cullen (1983) used a vignette experiment to show that although respondents know that the "ideal" response to the mentally ill is one of acceptance, their perception of how "most people" respond is far less positive. Thus it may be that studies based on accepting responses to straight forward social distance items, like Crocetti et al.'s (1971), measure socially desirable attitudes—the ideal response—but overlook more latent and unfavorable views.

Second, studies that compare a wide variety of stigmatized conditions provide little evidence of benign attitudes toward the mentally ill. Albrecht, Walker, and Levy (1982; see also Tringo, 1970) show that "mental illness" is one of the most highly rejected status conditions, clustering with drug addiction, prostitution, ex-convict status, and alcoholism rather than with cancer, diabetes, and heart disease.

Third, the notion that labeled persons are rejected only insofar as they behave inappropriately has been rebutted both in experimental work (Link et al., 1987) and in nonexperimental work (Link. 1982, 1987; Palamara, Cullen,

& Gersten, 1986). Link et al.'s (1987) study is particularly relevant because it shows how tests of labeling need to be conducted in the context of a more fully elaborated model of labeling processes. They presented data illustrating that previous experimental studies may have reached erroneous conclusions on the salience of labeling and may have overestimated the importance of behavior, because the studies' designs failed to explore the meaning of a "mental patient" label for respondents. Thus Link et al. found that among community respondents who perceived the mentally ill as dangerous, the label of "former mental patient" elicited strong expressions of social distance.

To summarize, we believe that it is premature to dismiss labeling and stigma as unimportant in the lives of mental patients. On close examination we find less than convincing much of the evidence that the critics of labeling theory offer to support their position. Though such studies rightly question some of the strongest claims of labeling theory, typically they do not address the more complex ways in which labeling and stigma may be important in the lives of psychiatric patients. Building on this observation, we offer a model for understanding how the stigmatization of the mental patient status can have harmful consequences. Since this framework extends Scheff's (1966) path-breaking theorizing, we refer to our model as a "modified labeling approach."

A MODIFIED LABELING APPROACH

Statement of the Approach

Scheff's model. As a prelude to our approach, we specify central elements of Scheff's labeling model (1966, 1984). Because we focus on the consequences of labeling rather than on factors that lead to it (see Cullen & Cullen, 1978; Thoits, 1985), we do not consider Scheff's entire approach but summarize his main points on the consequences of labeling (see Figure 1A). Once labeled, an individual is subjected to uniform responses from others. Behavior crystallizes in conformity to these expectations and is stabilized by a system of rewards and punishments that constrain the labeled individual to the role of a "mentally ill person." When the individual internalizes this role, incorporating it as a central identity, the process is complete and chronic mental illness is the consequence (Scheff, 1966, especially 82).

Step 1: Beliefs about devaluation and discrimination. A modified labeling perspective (Figure 1B), like Scheff's (1966), relies heavily on the idea that individuals internalize societal conceptions of what it means to be labeled mentally ill. As Mead (1934) observed, during socialization individuals learn the attitude of the community toward many behaviors, objects, and attributes, and internalize these in the form of what he called the "generalized other." Following Mead we note that the attitude of the community toward the mentally ill can be formed by a variety of mechanisms and thereby can function as part of the generalized other. Scheff (1966), for example, emphasizes how jokes, cartoons,

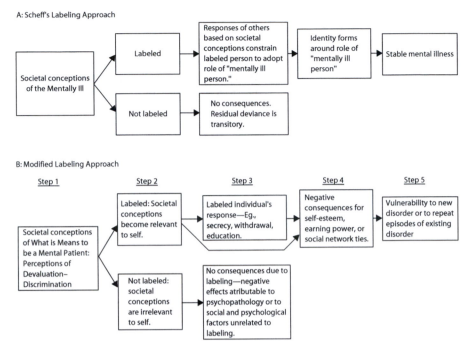

A: Scheff's Labeling Approach

B: Modified Labeling Approach

Figure 1 Diagramatic Representation of Scheff's Labeling Model and the Modified Labeling Approach

and the media's reporting of mental patient status can influence views of what it means to be mentally ill. Drawing on sources like these, all members of society—those who will become psychiatric patients as well as those who will not—form conceptions of what it means to acquire that status.

These conceptions include two important components: the extent to which people believe that mental patients will be devalued and the extent to which they believe that patients will be discriminated against. "Devaluation" comes from Cumming and Cumming's (1965) notion of stigma as "loss of status" and from Goffman's (1963) ideas about the "discrediting" nature of stigmatized statuses. "Discrimination" is suggested by the extensive "social distance" tradition as it applies to mental patients (Link et al., 1987). Our interest in devaluation-discrimination is in the extent to which individuals believe that "most people" (the community at large) will devalue and discriminate against a mental patient. Following Scheff (1966), we expect that community residents believe that most people view the status of mental patient negatively. However, since numerous factors are likely to produce such beliefs, people will almost certainly vary in this regard.

An important implication of this reasoning is that patients' expectations of rejection are an outcome of socialization and the cultural context rather than a pathological state associated with their psychiatric condition (see Crocetti et al., 1974, 130, for an example of the latter view). Thus, patients and nonpatients should share the belief that most people devalue and discriminate against mental patients.

Step 2: Official labeling through treatment contact. An official label is important because it brings personal relevance to a labeled person's views about the attitude of the community toward mental patients (beliefs about devaluation-discrimination). A seemingly innocuous array of beliefs becomes applicable to oneself; it now matters whether one believes that people will devalue and discriminate against a person who is in treatment for mental illness.

Step 3: Patients' responses to their stigmatizing status. We consider three possible responses to labeling and argue that a tendency to endorse them indicates that patients see stigmatization by others as a threat. In the first, *secrecy*, patients may choose to conceal their treatment history from employers, relatives, or potential lovers to avoid rejection (Goffman, 1963). Second is *withdrawal*, or limiting social interaction to those who know about and tend to accept one's stigmatized condition. Goffman (1963) notes that this group tends to consist of persons he calls the "own" (those similarly stigmatized) and the "wise" (those who know about and accept the stigma). When patients adopt this response, they are protected from the rejection that might ensue if they ventured out to seek friends, jobs, and the like in the wider social environment. Third is the attempt at *educating* others ("preventive telling") in hopes of enlightening them so as to ward off negative attitudes (Schneider & Conrad, 1980).[1] Education, with its emphasis on changing others' views, does not connote passive acceptance of others' attitudes toward a label as secrecy and withdrawal might. Still, their need to educate suggests that patients consider stigmatization likely, a possibility that critics of labeling theory deny. Moreover, as Schneider and Conrad (1980) observe, educating implies disclosure and this risks direct discrimination.

Step 4: Consequences of the stigma process on patients' lives. Negative outcomes may arise directly from one's beliefs about community attitudes toward the status of mental patient (see Step 1), or they may follow from attempts to protect oneself by withdrawing (see Step 3). If people believe that others will discriminate against them or devalue them because of a status they possess, powerful and unfortunate consequences can ensue. They may feel shame (Scheff, 1984) or believe that they are set off from others and thus are very different. In addition, beliefs about others' views of a stigmatized status have

---

[1] The nature of the relationships between these adaptive strategies and devaluation-discrimination (Step 1) may be complex because patients can adopt a mixture of responses. A patient who chooses withdrawal or secrecy, for example, may cope simultaneously by denying that mental patients face discrimination. Similarly, a patient may endorse the strategy of education even though he or she feels that most people are accepting of patients and that education is necessary for the minority who are likely to be rejecting. Therefore, we do not predict that beliefs about devaluation-discrimination will be related to these coping strategies in one-to-one, linear fashion.

been shown to negatively affect social interaction (Farina, Gliha, Boudreau, Allen, & Sherman, 1971) and self-esteem (Link, 1987).

The responses of secrecy, withdrawal, and education may also produce negative consequences. While adoption of these responses may protect patients from some negative aspects of labeling, they also may limit their life chances. For example, withdrawal may lead to more constricted social networks and fewer attempts at seeking more satisfying, higher-paying jobs. If present, this effect is consistent with the classical labeling theory idea of secondary deviance with its emphasis on "defense, attack, or adaptation" to factors brought on by labeling (Lemert, 1967, 17).

Step 5: Vulnerability to future disorder. If the processes outlined in Steps 1 through 4 operate, many patients will lack self-esteem, social network ties, and employment as a consequence of their own and others' reactions to labeling. These deficits are regarded as major social and psychological risk factors for the development of psychopathology (Dohrenwend & Dohrenwend, 1981; Turner, 1981). Thus, for some patients, labeling and stigma may induce a state of vulnerability that increases their likelihood of experiencing repeated episodes of disorder.

Comparisons to Scheff's model. The differences between our approach and Scheff's are a matter of emphasis. First, although we agree with Scheff that people will perceive community attitudes toward mental illness as strongly negative (Step 1), we emphasize more than Scheff the importance of variability in these beliefs. Some people believe that mental patients are vilified while others believe that society's conception is far more temperate. Second, although Scheff observes that labeled persons have internalized the same cultural views as the public, he tends to emphasize the responses of others. In contrast, we highlight the labeled individual's response on the basis of his or her beliefs about how others will react unless he or she does something to avoid their reactions. Finally, our approach does not assign to labeling the power to create mental illness directly. Instead, we view labeling and stigma as possible causes of negative outcomes that may place mental patients at risk for the recurrence or prolongation of disorders that resulted from other causes.

Assessing the Modified Labeling Approach

One previous study provided a partial assessment of the modified labeling approach. In keeping with Step 1, Link's study (1987) showed that current patients, former patients, and community residents tended to share the belief that mental patients will be devalued and discriminated against by most people. Moreover, in keeping with Steps 2 and 4, official labeling made these beliefs personally relevant. Specifically, Link found that even when diagnosis and relevant demographic variables were constant, the more strongly the labeled cases feared rejection the more likely they were to (1) feel demoralized, (2) earn less income, and (3) be unemployed. This suggested one reason why untreated cases of disorder tended to function better than patients; they were unaffected by labeling-activated expectations of rejection. The present study extends Link's work in two major ways. First, it adds an analysis about the coping orientations outlines in Step 3 and examines their impact. Second, it extends the test of modified labeling to another set of outcome variables by studying the social support networks of labeled and unlabeled respondents.

Unfortunately our cross-sectional study cannot test the fifth and final step of the approach concerning stabilization in a "career" of mental disorder, and therefore cannot provide definitive evidence on this provocative labeling hypothesis.

We test our hypotheses by comparing data on five groups: (1) psychiatric patients experiencing their first treatment contact, (2) current psychiatric patients with repeated treatment contacts, (3) community residents who report having been in treatment but who are not currently in treatment, (4) community residents who are classified as untreated cases on the basis of systematic evaluations of their symptomatology, and (5) "well" community residents who show no evidence of severe pathology and have no history of treatment.

As Table 1 shows, the five groups vary in three major ways. First, they vary in levels of psychopathology. Untreated community cases, first-treatment contact patients, and repeat-treatment contact patients all experience high levels of psychopathology. Community residents, who were once in treatment, constitute a mixed group: some are well, whereas others still qualify as cases. The remaining community residents show no evidence of psychopathology and have never been in treatment. Second, untreated cases and "well" respondents have not been labeled, whereas first-treatment contact patients, repeat-treatment contact patients, and community residents who were in treatment at one time have been labeled. Third, each treated group has had a different experience with labeling. First-treatment contact patients have been exposed only recently. As a result, their pretreatment support networks cannot have been affected by labeling. Thus, we predict no association between stigma and network support for this group. Repeat-contact patients differ because they have had a history of being labeled, so their network ties may have been affected by stigma. In addition, because repeat-contact patients are currently in treatment, they differ from community respondents who were in treatment at one time but are not in treatment now.

Table 1 summarizes the labeling predictions that we will test. Most of these are derived from Figure 1, but additional theoretical specification is required to test Step 4 and our predictions about social support networks. Specifically we asked our respondents whether each individual named in the network was a relative or a household member. With this information, we constructed network support measures of three kinds: (1) relatives outside the household, (2) nonrelatives outside the household, and (3) household members, including both relatives and nonrelatives. We make different predictions about the effects of stigma processes on these three types of supporters.

Underlying our predictions is a theoretical perspective on stigmatizing conditions developed by Jones, Farina, Hastorf, Markus, Miller, and Scott

Table 1 Summary of Modified Labeling Theory Predictions in Five Groups That Differ in Their Experience with Labeling and in Levels of Psychopathology

	First-Treatment Contact Patients	Repeat-Treatment Contact Patients	Formerly Treated Community Respondents	Community Untreated Cases	Community Respondents without Pathology
Distinguishing Features					
Currently in treatment?	yes	yes	no	no	no
Previous treatment?	no	yes	yes	no	no
Level of psychopathology?	high	high	mixed	high	low
Modified Labeling Theory Predictions					
Step 1					
Level of belief that mental patients will be devalued and discriminated against	high[a]	high[a]	high[a]	high[a]	high[a]
Step 3					
Patients' level of endorsement of protective strategies	high[a]	high[a]	no data	not applicable	not applicable
Steps 2 and 4					
Effect of devaluation-discrimination and coping orientations on social relationships within the household	no effect	the more concern about stigma, the more within-household support	the more concern about stigma, the more within-household support	no effect	no effect
Effect of devaluation-discrimination and coping orientations on social relationships with relatives and nonrelatives outside the household	no effect	the more concern about stigma, the less outside-the-household support	the more concern about stigma, the less outside-the-household support	no effect	no effect

[a] By "high" we mean that a majority tend to agree that stigma is a problem and that item and scale means are higher than their midpoints.

(1984). In their conception, the starting point for understanding interactions between a "marked" person (their term for a potentially stigmatizing social designation) and an "unmarked" person is each individual's expectations. Initial expectancies are influenced strongly by cultural conceptions as conveyed through the press, television, jokes, and the attitudes of important others. These expectations are brought to initial interactions and then influence them. Expectancies then are revised; new expectancies are brought to the next interaction, revised again, and so on.

We are interested in the influence of *patients'* initial, culturally derived expectancies of others' responses to them on their social support networks. We predict that patients' fear of devaluation and discrimination and their adoption of protective responses such as secrecy, withdrawal, and education are less relevant to interactions with household members than to interactions with nonhousehold members. Since patients are in direct, frequent contact with fellow household members, they are likely to have experienced repeatedly the process described by Jones et al. Their initial fears of devaluation and discrimination by "most people" become less relevant in this context. So do two approaches for coping with stigma: secrecy with household members is not possible and withdrawal leaves no place to go. This is not the case, however, for potential supporters outside the household. The Jones et al. process may not have occurred at all and is certainly less likely to have been repeated as frequently as for household members. Seeking supportive contact with such persons may mean engaging people who harbor the negative attitudes that patients fear. Furthermore, if patients do fear contact with people outside the household, they are more likely to rely on household members when supportive exchanges are required. With this reasoning, we predict that the expectation of devaluation-discrimination and reliance on the stigma coping approaches will increase the use of household supporters and decrease the use of nonhousehold supporters.

One further consideration is required with respect to the prediction concerning nonhousehold support. Nonrelative supporters can be chosen from a large pool of potential supporters, whereas relatives cannot. Patients can reconstitute their nonrelative support networks with people they have "tested" and found to be accepting or who are unlikely to reject them because they are current or former psychiatric patients themselves. Thus, it is possible for highly fearful patients to have a relatively robust network of nonrelatives. If patients withdraw, however, one would expect nonrelative support to be sparse because such people cope by withdrawing from interaction. Support networks consisting of relatives cannot be reconstituted in the same way as for nonrelatives because their numbers are predetermined and finite. Thus the greater the fear of rejection, the less likely that patients will have support from nonhousehold relatives.

Critics of labeling theory make different predictions from those based on our perspective. Because they claim that labeling and stigma are not a "severe problem" (Gove, 1982) and that former patients "enjoy nearly total acceptance in all but the most intimate relationships" (Crocetti et al., 1974), critics would expect beliefs that mental patients are rejected to be low to moderate (Step 1). In addition, patients should not feel the need to endorse secrecy, education, or withdrawal in the nearly stigma-free world that these critics envision (Step 3). Finally, there would be no reason to believe that official labeling should make beliefs about others' responses to mental patients personally relevant (Step 2) in such a way as to shape the nature of patients' social support networks (Step 4). This study was designed to ground the key elements of our theory in empirical facts. Since our predictions about these facts differ from those of critics, our study allows us to evaluate these two very different views about the importance of labeling and stigma.

METHOD

Sample

Samples of community residents ($N = 429$) and psychiatric patients ($N = 164$) from the Washington Heights section of New York City were administered two face-to-face interviews between 1980 and 1983 (Dohrenwend, Shrout, Link, & Skodol, 1985). We recruited the community respondents initially to participate in a methodological study of symptom scales and interviewed them approximately six months later for this research. In the original community sample, we enumerated households and contacted them to learn whether an eligible respondent between 19 and 59 years of age lived there. We also obtained information about ethnic background to permit us to sample roughly equal proportions of blacks, Hispanics, and non-Hispanic whites from this urban neighborhood in which the majority of residents is Hispanic. In 93 percent of the households, screening information was provided; and 68 percent contained one or more potential respondents. Of the 943 eligible individuals, 57 percent (541) were interviewed successfully.

The patient sample was selected from outpatient clinics and inpatient facilities in the same area of New York City. Since our goal was to select patients in two diagnostic categories—major depression and schizophrenia/schizophrenia-like psychotic disorders—all patients thought to belong to one of these diagnostic groups were referred to our project. In addition, we made a considerable effort to locate cases in their first episode of each of these types of disorder. While it was extremely difficult to locate first episode cases, we interviewed 164 patients in four groups: 50 first-episode major depression, 21 first-episode psychotic, 48 repeat major depression, and 44 repeat psychotic.

The Study Groups

To form the five groups, we required distinctions on psychiatric status and labeling exposure. We constructed the group of untreated community respondents with no evidence of psychopathology ($N = 171$) by subjecting all respondents to extensive screening. First, their scores on six symptom scales taken from the PERI interview needed to be low enough that they could be classified correctly as community respondents in a multiple-discriminant analysis (Shrout, Dohrenwend, & Levav, 1986). In addition, only individuals who had never undergone mental health treatment were eligible for this group. Finally, in the second interview subjects who scored high on a scale measuring psychological distress or demoralization were evaluated by a modified form of the Diagnostic Interview Schedule (DIS) (Robins, Helzer, Crougham, & Ratcliff, 1981), a standardized interview that yields psychiatric diagnoses according to *DSM-III* criteria. No individual who was found in this interview to have a diagnosable psychiatric disorder is included in the community respondents without psychopathology.

The untreated community case group can be formed in two different ways. One method uses multiple-discriminant analysis: A community case group is formed by community respondents who are "misclassified" in the analysis because they appear "just like" psychiatric patients in regard to the symptoms they express. The second way incorporates diagnostic procedures and uses the results from the modified DIS to generate *DSM-III* diagnoses. Further, because we wanted to identify untreated cases, we used information on treatment history to remove community cases who had had contact with a mental-health professional (psychiatrist, psychologist, or social worker) or who had been hospitalized in a mental hospital. We included in the untreated group individuals ($N = 142$) who were identified via the PERI discriminant function or via the modified DIS. Yet because this group can be defined in a variety of ways (i.e., discriminate function, DIS, both, or either) we check our results for each of these ways of defining this group.

The group of recently labeled first-treatment contact patients was generated from the community ($N = 11$) and from the patient sample ($N = 56$). Community respondents were defined as a first-contact patient if they reported a first-treatment contact with a psychiatrist, a psychologist, or a social worker during the year before the interview. To check if patient sample cases were experiencing their first-treatment contact, we examined both their self-reports and their clinic and hospital records.

The group of repeat-treatment contact patients ($N = 117$) also was generated from both the community ($N = 9$) and the patient ($N = 108$) samples. The small number of repeat-contact patients from the community consisted of individuals who reported their first contact to be more than a year ago and also reported current treatment. The group from the patient sample consisted of individuals who we determined had had a previous treatment contact.

All the past-treatment contact patients ($N = 96$) were drawn from the community sample. They reported past contact with a mental-health professional, but were not currently in treatment. Because this group of "former patients" was derived from the community sample, some were less like our patient samples and more like the "friends and supporters of psychotherapy" described by Kadushin (1969). Such persons seek treatment for personal growth or training within a context that values treatment seeking as a positive step in one's development. Thus such treatment does not constitute a potent labeling experience and could dilute stigma effects in this group.

Stigma Measures

Devaluation-discrimination. This measure consists of 12 six-point "strongly agree = 1" to "strongly disagree = 6" Likert items designed to assess the extent to which respondents believe that most people will devalue or discriminate against a person with a history of psychiatric treatment (see Table 3 below for wording of questions). All items (half are in the reverse direction) are scored so that a high score indicates a belief that mental patients will be devalued and discriminated against. The overall measure of devaluation-discrimination then is scored by adding the individual items and dividing by 12. This step allows us to locate the mean of the summative scale on the six-point agree-disagree scale. Because the midpoint of the scale is 3.5 and is located directly between the strongly agree–strongly disagree poles, a mean above 3.5 indicates that the average person tends to endorse an item or a pool of items (as with the summative scale).

Secrecy, withdrawal, and education. These three multiple-item measures were written to tap coping orientations that mental patients might use to deal with stigmatization. Thus they are appropriate only for individuals who have been officially labeled by treatment contact.

The items in these scales were answered with the same six-point Likert format used for the devaluation-discrimination measure. Items were recoded so that a high score indicated endorsement of a coping orientation (i.e., secrecy, withdrawal, or education). Summative scales were formed by adding the scores on individual items and dividing by the number of items in the scale so that each scale could vary from 1 to 6 with a midpoint of 3.5.

Measures of Social Network

We elicited measures of social network with Fischer's (1982) questions. We asked respondents to name individuals with whom they had or could have had supportive exchanges during the past year in nine areas of activity such as care of children, watching the house, discussing personal problems, borrowing money, and social-recreation activities. Note that for first-treatment contact patients this period comes before official labeling occurred, which is why we predict no labeling effects for these measures for this group. We focus on two types of measures generated from these data: extensiveness and availability of instrumental support (Dohrenwend, Shrout, Link, Martin, & Skodol, 1986). To construct the measures, our theory required we use information obtained from probes that asked whether each named person was a household member or a relative. This allowed us to develop network measures for household members, nonhousehold nonrelatives, and nonhousehold relatives.

Extensiveness. This variable represents the extent to which a network contains individuals who fulfill the supportive "tasks" identified in the nine questions. All respondents do not "need" all nine forms of supportive contact.

Therefore, we constructed the measure of extensiveness in the following way: the number of areas applicable to the respondent for which there was no coverage was subtracted from nine, the total. To that difference we added the weighted value (.5) of the number of areas for which backup support was available; these areas contained two or more supporters:

$$\text{Extensiveness} = (9 - \text{number of applicable areas not covered})$$
$$+ (.5 \times \text{number of areas with two or more}$$
$$\text{individuals named—backup support}).$$

Instrumental support. We focused on instances in which one person performed a task for another person or could be called on to lend money. The household member, nonhousehold relative, and nonhousehold, nonrelative measures are generated simply by adding the number of supporters specific to each of these categories.

RESULTS

With one exception, we organized results by presenting evidence concerning each step of our modified labeling theory in turn. Evidence for Step 2 is presented after Steps 1, 3, and 4 because Step 2 is the critical juncture at which the fate of labeled and unlabeled persons diverges (see Figure 1). Thus, we examine Step 1 first because it involves labeled and unlabeled respondents. Then we follow labeled persons through Steps 3 and 4 and finally return to test Step 2 by examining whether the fate of unlabeled persons is different.

Evidence Concerning Step 1: Beliefs about Devaluation and Discrimination in the Community and Patient Samples

Beliefs of unlabeled community respondents. Our labeling approach posits widespread endorsement of the belief that mental patients are devalued and discriminated against. Consistent with this, for 11 of the 12 items in Table 2 the mean is higher than the 3.5 midpoint of the six-point Likert scale both for untreated cases and for untreated well respondents. This trend across the 12 items is reflected in the summative scale of perceived devaluation-discrimination: the scale mean for both untreated cases and community well respondents is significantly higher than the 3.5 midpoint.

Clearly, any assessment of how negative an attitude is cannot be resolved by quantitative assessments of how much higher a mean is than a midpoint. The position of the mean in relation to the midpoint can be manipulated by item wording. Thus, it is important to examine the content of the items. If the questions focused on inconsequential forms of rejection or on mild slights, a mean higher than the midpoint would not be substantively significant, but we show in Table 2 that respondents tend to believe that a former patient will be excluded from close friendships, jobs, and intimate relationships.

To highlight this point, we translated the community sample's responses into percentages by grouping together all responses that fell into one of the

Table 2 Means (Standard Deviations) and One-Way Analysis of Variance Showing the Extent to Which Community Respondents, Former Patients, and Current Patients Believe That Mental Patients Will Be Devalued and Discriminated Against (six-point strongly agree = 1 to strongly disagree = 6; "R" indicates reverse scoring).

	First-Treatment Contact Patients (N = 61)[a]	Repeat-Treatment Contact Patients (N = 115)[a]	Formerly Treated Community Respondents (N = 95)[a]	Community Untreated Cases (N = 142)[a]	Community Respondents without Psychopathology (N = 169)[a]	P-value One-Way Analysis of Variance
1. Most people would willingly accept a former mental patient as a close friend.	4.11* (1.57)	3.94* (1.64)	4.43* (1.44)	4.23* (1.57)	4.31* (1.56)	n.s.
2. Most people believe that a person who has been in a mental hospital is just as intelligent as the average person.	3.93 (1.82)	3.66 (1.62)	4.03* (1.55)	4.05* (1.51)	3.95* (1.61)	n.s.
3. Most people believe that a former mental patient is just as trust worthy as the average citizen.	3.97* (1.56)	4.09* (1.44)	4.27* (1.58)	4.46* (1.42)	4.19* (1.67)	n.s.
4. Most people would accept a fully recovered former mental patient as a teacher of young children in a public school.	4.31* (1.39)	4.40* (1.38)	4.91* (1.63)	4.76* (1.26)	4.76* (1.50)	p < .05
5. Most people feel that entering a mental hospital is a sign of personal failure (R).	3.62 (1.65)	4.14* (1.45)	3.83 (1.80)	3.51 (1.68)	3.41 (1.72)	p < .01

6. Most people would not hire a former mental patient to take care of their children, even if he or she had been well for some time (R).	4.38* (1.65)	4.47* (1.52)	4.61* (1.55)	4.44* (1.57)	4.45* (1.69)	n.s.
7. Most people think less of a person who has been in a mental hospital (R).	4.13* (1.57)	4.48* (1.32)	4.20* (1.51)	4.07* (1.42)	4.02* (1.50)	n.s.
8. Most employers will hire a former mental patient if he or she is qualified for the job.	3.23 (1.52)	3.57 (1.61)	3.99* (1.48)	3.32 (1.47)	3.53 (1.50)	p <.05
9. Most employers will pass over the application of a former mental patient in favor or another applicant (R).	4.43* (1.37)	4.71* (1.30)	4.65* (1.50)	4.34* (1.49)	4.38* (1.69)	n.s.
10. Most people in my community would treat a former mental patient just as they would treat anyone.	3.53 (1.64)	3.65 (1.68)	3.86* (1.71)	3.74 (1.55)	3.57 (1.65)	n.s.
11. Most young women would be reluctant to date a man who has been hospitalized for a serious mental disorder (R).	4.64* (1.50)	4.41* (1.55)	4.44* (1.55)	4.48* (1.40)	4.51* (1.58)	n.s.

(continued)

Table 2 Continued

	First-Treatment Contact Patients (N = 61)[a]	Repeat-Treatment Contact Patients (N = 115)[a]	Formerly Treated Community Respondents (N = 95)[a]	Community Untreated Cases (N = 142)[a]	Community Respondents without Psychopathology (N = 169)[a]	P-value One-Way Analysis of Variance
12. Once they know a person was in a mental hospital, most people will take his or her opinions less seriously (R).	4.07* (1.54)	4.23* (1.45)	4.17* (1.42)	4.11* (1.37)	4.15* (1.53)	n.s.
13. Devaluation-discrimination (sum of items 1 through 12 divided by 12).	4.03* (.86)	4.14* (.89)	4.33* (.92)	4.13* (.73)	4.08* (.80)	n.s.

[a] The Ns given are for the number of valid cases for the summed devaluation-discrimination measure. Eleven respondents with fewer than 8 valid responses were assigned missing values. For respondents with one to four missing values, the valid responses were prorated. Reports for individual items include all valid responses (maximum N = 584, minimum N = 577).

* The mean is significantly higher than the midpoint at $p < .05$.

three "agree" categories versus all responses falling into one of the "disagree" categories. Notably, the results show that 75 percent of the community sample agreed that employers will discriminate against former mental patients; 80 percent and 66 percent subscribe to similar expectations with regard to dating relationships and close friendships respectively; 71 percent agreed that former patients will be seen as less trustworthy, 62 percent that they will be seen as less intelligent, and 70 percent that their opinions will be taken less seriously. Finally, results for the full 12-item scale show that only 19 percent of the untreated community respondents score below the 3.5 midpoint and a mere 2 percent below 2.5, a score which would indicate a strong refutation of the notion that mental patients face devaluation-discrimination. In contrast, 28 percent of the respondents score above 4.5, indicating a strong belief that patients can expect devaluation-discrimination. Therefore, it is clear that most people expect patients to be devalued and discriminated against at least in some ways, and that more than one-fourth of the respondents (those scoring above 4.5) believe that this reaction occurs consistently across many important aspects of a patient's life.

Beliefs of labeled respondents: first-contact, repeat-contact, and former patients. Our theory specified that patients and former patients will share the nonpatient public's views. We show in Table 2 that with only one exception, all means for these patient groups exceed the 3.5 midpoint, indicating that the average patient believes that mental patients may face severe devaluation and discrimination. The mean of the summative scale is significantly higher than the midpoint for all three patient groups.

We also show in Table 2 that differences in perceptions among the five groups are minimal and inconsistent. Contrary to the claims of some labeling critics, we find that current patients, former patients, and nonpatients agree that mental patients will be rejected by most people.

Evidence Concerning Step 3: Responses to Labeling in First- and Repeat-Contact Patients

According to our approach, one determinant of patients' outcomes is the protective maneuvering they use in response to labeling. Therefore, it is important to determine the extent to which coping orientations such as secrecy, withdrawal, and education are deemed advisable by patients. Moreover, their endorsement of such approaches is further evidence that they feel stigmatized by their patient status. Otherwise, why would they report that these approaches are necessary?

Recall that we could ask questions about stigma coping orientations only of our patient sample ($N = 164$). Therefore, the results in Table 3 are restricted to these respondents. Most items measuring secrecy, withdrawal, and education are endorsed strongly by patients; mean scores generally are above the 3.5 midpoint of the items. Only three exceptions occur. Two of the secrecy items (Items 2 and 5) and one of the withdrawal items (Item 3) have means below the midpoint, but even with these questions, over 40 percent

Table 3 Means and Standard Deviations of Items Measuring Secrecy, Education, and Withdrawal in the Patient Sample (Maximum N = 158)[a] (six-point strongly agree = 1 to strongly disagree = 6; "R" indicates reverse scoring.)

Item	Mean (standard deviation)		Percent Endorsing Strategy
Secrecy			
1. In order to get a job, a former mental patient will have to hide his or her history of hospitalization (R).	4.26*	(1.65)	70.5
2. There is no reason for a person to hide the fact that be or she was mental patient at one time.	3.25	(1.84)	40.1
3. If yon have been treated for a serious mental illness, the best thing to do is to keep it a secret (R).	3.85*	(1.79)	61.1
4. If I had a close relative who had been treated for a serious mental illness, I would advise him or her not to tell anyone about it (R).	3.70	(1.77)	58.6
5. I rarely feel the need to hide the fact that I have been in psychiatric treatment.	3.25	(1.68)	41.8
Education			
1. I've found that it's best to help the people close to me understand what psychiatric treatment is like (R).	5.07*	(1.28)	91.1
2. If I thought a friend was uncomfortable with me because I had been in psychiatric treatment, I would take it upon myself to educate him or her about my treatment (R).	4.55*	(1.50)	78.8
3. If I thought an employer felt uneasy hiring a person who had been in psychiatric treatment, I would try to make him or her understand that most ex-patients are good workers (R).	4.35*	(1.65)	78.2
4. After I entered psychiatric treatment, I often found myself educating others about what it means to be a psychiatric patient (R).	3.80*	(1.77)	62.0
5. I would participate in an organized effort to teach the public more about psychiatric treatment and the problems of people who seek the help of psychiatrists (R).	4.87*	(1.47)	85.4
Withdrawal			
1. It is easier for me to be friendly with people who have been psychiatric patients (R).	3.80*	(1.65)	61.3
2. If I thought that someone I knew held negative opinions about psychiatric patients, I would try to avoid him or her (R).	3.62	(1.69)	51.6
3. After being in psychiatric treatment, it's a good idea to keep what you are thinking to yourself (R).	3.14	(1.78)	42.3
4. If I was looking for a job and received an application which asked about a history of psychiatric treatment, I wouldn't fill it out (R).	3.87*	(1.84)	58.0
5. If I thought an employer was reluctant to hire a person with a history of psychiatric treatment, I wouldn't apply for the job (R).	3.85*	(1.84)	57.3
6. If I believed that a person I knew thought less of me because I had been in psychiatric treatment, I would try to avoid him or her (R).	4.15*	(1.69)	67.7
7. When I meet people for the first time, I make a special effort to keep the fact that I have been in psychiatric treatment to myself (R).	4.33*	(1.76)	71.3

[a]Questions in this table were asked only of respondents from the patient sample. Thus 19 individuals from the community sample who were classified originally as first- or repeat-contact patients are excluded. The minimum number of cases on any item was 156.
*The mean is significantly higher than the midpoint at $p < .05$.

reported that they employed or would employ the approach. Moreover, the means of summative scales measuring withdrawal and education are significantly higher than the midpoint, whereas the means of secrecy is above the midpoint but not significantly so. Finally, first- and repeat-contact patients do not differ significantly in their endorsement of the coping orientations (not shown); this finding suggests a widespread belief that such protective responses are required.

It is also important to note the wording of some of the items because these orientations to coping may show how negative labeling effects emerge. Items 2 and 5 of the withdrawal scale, for example, indicate that a patient would avoid a person or would decline to apply for a job if he or she believed that rejection might be the result. Because many patients believe that "employers" will discriminate against them and that "most people" will value them less (see Items 7 and 9 of Table 2), the strong endorsement of these "withdrawal" items suggests the plausibility of Step 4 of our model, which specifies that efforts designed to cope with stigma may have negative consequences for a patient's life chances.

Evidence Concerning Step 4: Repeat-Treatment Contact Patients

We now test the effects of stigma among repeat-treatment contact patients, using two measures of network-based social support for three types of supporters: relatives outside the household, nonrelatives outside the household, and household members. Before we report on these six measures, we note that overall (irrespective of the type of supporter), repeat-treatment contact patients have fewer instrumental supporters and less extensive task coverage, than do either well community respondents or untreated cases. The comparison of the repeat-treatment contact patients to the untreated case group supports the labeling perspective because the label seems to be the most salient factor distinguishing the two groups. Critics of labeling theory, however, are correct in countering that untreated cases are less severely impaired, on average, and that attempts to control such differences statistically are subject to regression artifacts that bias toward finding support for labeling (see Link, 1982).

Our analysis goes beyond such group comparisons by asking whether stigma variables affect specific types of social network ties within groups of patients who are relatively homogeneous in the nature and severity of their disorder. Most of the difficulty in interpreting labeling effects arises when one attempts to equate labeled and unlabeled groups statistically on psychiatric condition (Link, 1982).

Multivariate hypothesis tests. The most global test of our hypotheses asks whether the four stigma measures (devaluation-discrimination, secrecy, withdrawal, and education), when considered together, have an effect on the six social support network variables. To test this hypothesis we used multivariate multiple regression analysis, a procedure that tests the significance of the relationships between the two sets of variables using a multivariate F-test. We found a highly significant association between the four stigma measures and the six support network variables.

We do not yet know, however, which of the six outcome measures are affected by the stigma variables or whether the effects are in the direction predicted in Table 1 (i.e., more stigma concern, more household support—more stigma concern, less nonhousehold support).

We address these more refined questions by examining the six univariate (single dependent variable) multiple-regression equations that formed the basis of the omnibus multivariate test reported above. In presenting these equations, we faced an issue raised by the degree of overlap between the stigma variables. Although the four stigma variables predicted substantial proportions of variance as a group, they often failed to show significant unique effects when considered singly, with the other three held constant. To conclude from this that no effects exist constitutes what Gordon (1968) called the "partialling fallacy." When significant empirical overlap exists among variables, much of the predictive power can reside in the shared variance that is partialled from consideration. In our study, for example, secrecy was correlated with both devaluation-discrimination ($r = .575$) and withdrawal ($r = .405$), such that a full 43 percent of the variance in secrecy—more than half its reliable variance (alpha = .71)—was accounted for by these two variables. To avoid the partialling fallacy we chose to retain devaluation-discrimination and withdrawal and to drop the other two measures. Aside from its centrality in our theory, devaluation-discrimination is the one measure that was asked of all groups, and withdrawal has clear theoretical significance for the study of social connectedness. Moreover, even with the other stigma variables partialled, these two variables showed unique effects for at least one of the six outcome variables, whereas secrecy and education never did.

Effects of stigma measures on household-based support networks. According to our theory, we should not expect that the stigma dimensions will be associated with a *reduction* in the availability of household members for socially supportive contacts. In fact, we expect a greater reliance on these individuals in the presence of a strong fear that most people will be rejecting. As shown in Table 4 insofar as there are any significant associations between household support and stigma, more stigma concern results in greater reliance on household support. Specifically, if patients believe that they will be devalued and discriminated against, they are more likely to have important tasks covered by household members.

Effects of stigma measures on nonhousehold network members. In Table 5 we show significant relationships between social network ties outside the household and both perceived devaluation-discrimination and withdrawal when we control for relevant sociodemographic characteristics. The more one fears devaluation and discrimination, the less likely one is to have instrumental supporters and extensive task coverage among nonhousehold *relatives*. Withdrawal is related inversely to support from *nonrelatives*

Table 4 Multiple Regression Analyses Showing the Effect of Stigma Dimensions on the Number of Instrumental Supporters and the Extensiveness of Task Coverage among Household Members (repeat-treatment contact patients N = 103)

	Number of Instrumental Supporters		Extensiveness of Task Coverage	
	Regression coefficient	Standardized coefficient	Regression coefficient	Standardized coefficient
Control Variables				
Children under 14 at home (1 = yes, 0 = no)	.226	.056	−.732	−.111
Currently employed (1 = yes, 0 = no)	−.095	−.030	−1.510**	−.278
Diagnosis (1 = depression, 0 = schizophrenia)	.408	.134	.492	.093
Marital status (1 = married, 0 = other)	−.172	−.043	2.502**	.355
Age (years)	−.041**	−.334	−.070***	−.321
Education (years)	−.041	−.093	.076	.100
Black	−.678*	−.220	−.834	−.155
Hispanic	−.068	−.017	.003	.001
Stigma Variables				
Perceived devaluation-discrimination	.236	.143	.732**	.255
Withdrawal	.013	.008	−.223	−.080
Increment to variance explained due to stigma variables	1.9%		5.8%	
Variance explained by entire equation	18.2%		29.3%	

*$p < .05$.
**$p < .01$.
***$p < .001$.

outside the household are available to provide instrumental support. Thus, as predicted, nonhousehold network ties are related negatively to stigma dimensions.

Evidence Concerning Step 4: Former Patients from the Community Sample

Data on ex-patients in the community provide further assessment of Step 4 in our approach. Contrary to our expectations, former patients are similar to the group with little psychopathology in number of instrumental supporters and in the extensiveness of their task coverage. However, the former patient group may include people whom Kadushin (1969) calls "the friends and

Table 5 Multiple Regression Analyses Showing the Effect of Stigma Dimensions on the Number of Instrumental Social Supporters and the Extensiveness of Task Coverage of Relatives and Nonrelatives Living outside the Household (repeat-treatment contact patients $N = 103$)

	Number of Instrumental Supporters				Extensiveness of Task Coverage			
	Nonhousehold relatives		Nonhousehold nonrelatives		Nonhousehold relatives		Nonhousehold nonrelatives	
	Regression coefficient	Standardized coefficient	Regression coefficient	Standardized coefficient	Regression coefficient	Standardized coefficient	Regression coefficient	Standardized coefficient
Control Variables								
Children under 14 at home (1 = yes, 0 = no)	−.311	−.078	.579	.120	−1.774**	−.286	−.091	−.014
Currently employed (1 = yes, 0 = no)	.192	.062	.497	.134	−.473	−.099	.416	.081
Diagnosis (1 = depression, 0 = schizophrenia)	.232	.077	.467	.129	.809	.174	.517	.104
Marital status (1 = married, 0 = other)	1.023*	.256	−.941*	−.195	2.585***	.417	−1.775*	−.264
Age (years)	.001	.001	−.003	−.020	.038*	.191	−.027	−.134
Education (years)	.018	.042	.114*	.222	.003	.005	.106	.149
Black	.114	.037	−.652	−.178	.405	.086	−.351	−.069
Hispanic	.157	.041	−.324	−.070	−.139	−.023	−1.064	−.168
Stigma Variables								
Perceived devaluation-discrimination	−.549**	−.336	.134	.068	−.621*	−.246	.062	.023
Withdrawal	−.030	−.019	−.481**	−.253	.121	.044	−.295	−.112
Increment to variance explained due to stigma variables	10.7%		5.5%		5.3%		1.1%	
Variance explained by entire equation	17.1%		32.4%		26.5%		23.0%	

* $p < .05$; ** $p < .01$; *** $p < .001$.

supporters of psychotherapy" and who consequently have not been exposed to a potent labeling experience. When we examined those who reported having been hospitalized ($N = 19$)—a substantial labeling experience—we found that they had significantly fewer instrumental supporters and less extensive task coverage than other former patients. In fact, their support networks closely resemble those of repeat-treatment contact patients and differ significantly from the group with little evidence of psychopathology.

Evidence Concerning Step 2: The Importance of Official Labeling

According to Step 2, official labeling makes patients' beliefs about devaluation-discrimination personally relevant and activates coping strategies such as secrecy, withdrawal, and education. Below we present two tests of Step 2: one involves first-treatment contact patients; the other, nonpatient community respondents.

First-treatment contact patients. Recall that there was no reason to expect that the networks of first-treatment contact patients would be affected by the stigma measures we developed. Their exposure to labeling is new and thus cannot have affected the network questions that were asked about the period *before* they entered treatment. Because we found effects among repeat-contact patients, we wanted to determine whether there were, in fact, no significant effects among first treatment contact patients. Therefore, we performed the same multivariate tests of stigma factors on social network measures among the 48 first-treatment contact patients from the patient sample. We found no significant multivariate association between stigma and network support. Moreover, when we examined the individual regression coefficients of the stigma variables, we found no evidence to suggest effects similar to those for repeat-contact patients.

Nonpatient community respondents. A second test of Step 2, conceptually similar to the test with first-treatment contact patients, can be achieved by focusing on our measure of perceived devaluation-discrimination and by directing attention to the association between this variable and social network ties among two groups: untreated community cases and community well respondents. Recall that the perceived devaluation-discrimination measure can be answered by patients and nonpatients alike. For labeled persons these beliefs about others' opinions are potentially applicable to themselves, whereas for unlabeled persons they are an innocuous array of beliefs about what others think of mental patients.

We assessed the effect of perceived devaluation-discrimination on the six network variables. We found no significant overall multivariate association in untreated cases, community well respondents, or the two groups combined. Nor did we find a significant effect when we used any of the other ways of defining untreated cases: positive on PERI symptom scales alone, positive on DIS alone, or positive on both.

DISCUSSION

Our results are consistent with the following explanation of the effects of labels, based on modified labeling theory. In the course of being socialized, individuals develop negative conceptions of what it means to be a mental patient and thus form beliefs about how others will view and then treat someone in that status. Typically this array of beliefs is fully in place before an individual enters treatment. As a result, when patients enter treatment for the first time, they are likely to confront the effects of stigma immediately because often they have internalized a generally negative view about what it means to be a mental patient. Moreover, they tend to endorse coping orientations such as secrecy, withdrawal, and education. With time, their beliefs about the implications of the label they carry and their way of dealing with it shape the nature of their social connectedness. Those patients who are most concerned with stigma are likely to have insular support networks consisting of safe and trusted persons on whom they rely extensively. At the same time, such patients have considerably less support available from individuals outside their immediate household. Our results are generally inconsistent with positions taken by critics of labeling theory and are not easily "explained away" by those investigators' major alternative explanations. This is true both for our attitudinal data (Steps 1 and 3) and our social support network data (Step 4).

With respect to attitudinal data, some researchers argue that the attitudes of the public (Crocetti et al., 1974) and of patients (Weinstein, 1983) are too positive to make any form of labeling theory believable. These investigators studied many, but certainly not all, potentially relevant attitudes. Because their findings usually were not intended as tests of labeling theory, the attitudes measured often were not the key theoretical concepts required to form an adequate test. In contrast, we identified a set of theoretically relevant attitudes—beliefs about how most people will treat mental patients—that turned out to be consistently but not uniformly negative. Thus, although our results do not directly contradict the attitudinal findings marshaled by critics of labeling theory, they do lead us to question strenuously the conclusion that labeling processes are unimportant.

In general, the findings concerning social networks—behavioral outcomes—support a modified labeling approach over an antilabeling position. The only result that might support the critics' view is the finding that stigma variables have no detectable effect on the support networks of former patients. This finding could indicate that the effect of labeling dissipates with time, as Gove's (1982) ideas about the "transitory" nature of stigma would suggest. Still, even if this is true, this and other research (Link, 1987) suggests that the short-term consequences can be powerful and unfortunate—a possibility most critics deny. Moreover, this finding might indicate that some of these former patients were "friends and supporters of psychotherapy" who never experienced a potent label to begin with. Consistent with this latter view is the finding that former hospital patients, who clearly did encounter a potent labeling experience, showed evidence of enduring stigma effects. The other predictions of the modified labeling approach were supported: significant effects of stigma when labeling preceded the outcome variables (repeat contact patients), and no effects either when labeling followed the period covered by the outcome variables (first-treatment contact patients) or when no labeling occurred (community untreated cases, community well respondents).

Moreover, these results cannot be explained away by invoking the leading alternative explanation offered by critics of labeling. According to critics, any untoward effects experienced by mental patients are more likely to be caused by psychopathology than by labeling. This plausible alternative, however, cannot explain our findings concerning social support networks. Our modified labeling perspective specifies variables that should have effects *within* groups of patients with severe disorders (major depression and schizophrenia). Behavior is held relatively constant in this way, and yet the variables specified as important by a modified labeling perspective remain important. Moreover, we used six PERI symptom scales to control for variability on severity within these patient groups, and still the stigma variables remained significant predictors of social support networks. Finally, we showed that the stigma variables had consistent effects across the two diagnostic groups (schizophrenia and major depression). This result suggests that even when psychopathology varies, the stigma variables have relatively constant effects. These findings make it difficult to explain the effects of the stigma variables by asserting that they are caused by psychopathology.

Our study strongly challenges the notion that labeling and stigma are inconsequential in the lives of psychiatric patients.

Perhaps the most important work that can be motivated by this and related studies is a test of the still-unexplored fifth step of the modified labeling perspective. If labeling and stigma are connected to outcome variables, such as self-esteem, employment status (Link 1987), and support networks (this paper), it will become more and more plausible to conceive of these factors as playing a role in producing a chronic course for some people; environmentally oriented investigators point to these variables as major risk factors for the onset of episodes of mental disorder. Therefore, it is possible that labeling and stigma can leave patients and former patients vulnerable to the likelihood of experiencing another episode of disorder. A modified labeling position offers the possibility of deepening our understanding of chronic mental disorder as a process within an influential social context.

References

Albrecht, Gary, Vivian Walker, and Judith Levy. 1982. "Social Distance from the Stigmatized: A Test of Two Theories." *Social Science and Medicine* 16:1319–27.

Crocetti, Guido, Herzl Spiro, and Iradj Siassi. 1971. "Are the Ranks Closed?: Attitudinal Social Distance and Mental Illness." *American Journal of Psychiatry* 127:1121–27.

————. 1974. *Contemporary Attitudes Towards Mental Illness*. Pittsburgh: University of Pittsburgh Press.

Cullen, Francis and John Cullen. 1978. *Toward a Paradigm of Labeling Theory*. Monograph No. 58. Lincoln: University of Nebraska Press.

Cumming, John and Elaine Cumming. 1965. "On the Stigma of Mental Illness." *Community Mental Health Journal* 1:135–43.

Dohrenwend, Bruce P., and Barbara Dohrenwend. 1981. "Socioenvironmental Factors, Stress, and Psychopathology." *American Journal of Community Psychology* 9:123–64.

Dohrenwend, Bruce P., Patrick Shrout, Bruce Link, John Martin, and Andrew Skodol. 1986. "Overview and Initial Results from a Risk-Factor Study of Depression and Schizophrenia." Pp. 184–215 in *Mental Disorders in the Community*, edited by James E. Barrett and Robert M. Rose. New York: Guilford.

Dohrenwend, Bruce P., Patrick Shrout, Bruce Link, and Andrew Skodol. 1985. "Risk Factors for Major Depression and Schizophrenia" [MRDF]. New York State Psychiatric Institute.

Farina, Amerigo, Donald Gliha, Louis Boudreau, Jon Allen, and Mark Sherman. 1971. "Mental Illness and the Impact of Believing Others Know about It." *Journal of Abnormal Psychology* 77:1–5.

Fischer, Claude. 1982. *To Dwell among Friends: Personal Networks in Town and City.* Chicago: University of Chicago Press.

Goffman, Irving. 1963. *Stigma: Notes on the Management of Spoiled Identity*. Englewood Cliffs, NJ: Prentice Hall.

Gordon, Robert. 1968. "Issues in Multiple Regression." *American Journal of Sociology* 73:592–616.

Gove, Walter. 1970. "Societal Reaction as an Explanation of Mental Illness: An Evaluation." *American Sociological Review* 35:873–84.

————. 1980. "Labeling and Mental Illness: A Critique." Pp. 53–109 in *Labeling Deviant Behavior*, edited by Walter Gove. Beverly Hills: Sage.

————. 1982. "The Current Status of the Labeling Theory of Mental Illness." Pp. 273–300 in *Deviance and Mental Illness*, edited by Walter Gove. Beverly Hills: Sage.

Gove, Walter and Terry Fain. 1973. "The Stigma of Mental Hospitalization: An Attempt to Evaluate Its Consequences." *Archives of General Psychiatry* 29:494–500.

Huffine, Carol and John Clausen. 1979. "Madness and Work: Short- and Long-Term Effects of Mental Illness of Occupational Careers." *Social Forces* 57:1049–62.

Jones, Edward, Amerigo Farina, Albert Hastorf, Hazel Markus, Dale Miller, and Robert Scott. 1984. *Social Stigma: The Psychology of Marked Relationships*. New York: Freeman.

Kadushin, Charles. 1969. *Why People Go to Psychiatrists*. New York: Atherton.

Lehman, Stanley, Virginia Joy, Dolores Kreisman, and Samuel Simmens. 1976. "Responses to Viewing Symptomatic Behaviors and Labeling of Prior Mental Illness." *Journal of Community Psychology* 4:327–34.

Lemert, Edwin. 1967. *Human Deviance, Social Problems, and Social Control*. Englewood Cliffs, NJ: Prentice Hall.

Link, Bruce. 1982. "Mental Patient Status, Work and Income: An Examination of the Effects of a Psychiatric Label." *American Sociological Review* 47:202–15.

————. 1987. "Understanding Labeling Effects in the Area of the Mental Disorders: An Empirical Assessment of the Effects of Expectations of Rejection." *American Sociological Review* 52:96–112.

Link, Bruce and Francis Cullen. 1983. "Reconsidering the Social Rejection of Ex-Mental Patients: Levels of Attitudinal Response." *American Journal of Community Psychology* 11:261–73.

Link, Bruce, Francis Cullen, James Frank, and John Wozniak. 1987. "The Social Rejection of Ex-Mental Patients: Understanding Why Labels Matter." *American Journal of Sociology* 92:1461–500.

Mead, George Herbert. 1934. *Mind, Self and Society.* Chicago: University of Chicago Press.

Palamara, Frances, Francis Cullen, and Joanne Gersten. 1986. "The Effect of Police and Mental Health Intervention on Juvenile Deviance: Specifying Contingencies in the Impact of Formal Reaction." *Journal of Health and Social Behavior* 27:90–105.

Robins, Lee, John Helzer, Jack Crougham, and Kathryn Ratcliff. 1981. "National Institute of Mental Health Diagnostic Interview Schedule: Its History, Characteristics and Validity." *Archives of General Psychiatry* 38:381–89.

Scheff, Thomas. 1966. *Being Mentally Ill: A Sociology Theory.* Chicago: Aldine.

———. 1984. *Being Mentally Ill: A Sociological Theory.* 2nd ed. Chicago: Aldine.

Schneider, Joseph and Peter Conrad. 1980. "In the Closet with Illness: Epilepsy, Stigma Potential and Information Control." *Social Problems* 28:32–44.

Shrout, Patrick, Bruce Dohrenwend, and Itzhak Levav. 1986. "Screening Cases of Diverse Diagnostic Types in the General Population: Preliminary Results from Jerusalem." *Journal of Consulting and Clinical Psychology* 54:314–19.

Thoits, Peggy. 1985. "Self-Labeling Processes in Mental Illness: The Role of Emotional Deviance." *American Journal of Sociology* 91:221–49.

Tringo, John. 1970. "The Hierarchy of Preference toward Disability Groups." *Journal of Special Education* 4:295–306.

Turner R. Jay. 1981. "Social Support as a Contingency in Psychological Well-Being." *Journal of Health and Social Behavior* 22:357–67.

Weinstein, Raymond. 1979. "Patient Attitudes toward Mental Hospitalization: A Review of Quantitative Research." *Journal of Health and Social Behavior* 20:237–58.

———. 1983. "Labeling Theory and the Attitudes of Mental Patients: A Review." *Journal of Health and Social Behavior* 24:70–84.

DISCUSSION

1. How does modified labeling theory differ from Scheff's original theory? What predictions do they share? What predictions differ?

2. Link and colleagues were not able to test all of the steps in their model in this analysis. What is missing from their test? How strong is the evidence for their theory in the absence of that test?

Stigma

Pescosolido, Bernice A., Jack K. Martin, Bruce G. Link, Saeko Kikuzawa, Giovani Burgos, Ralph Swindle, and Jo Phelan

With the 1996 Mental Health Module Team:

Carol A. Boyer, Brian Powell, Michaeline Bresnahan, Sharon Schwartz, Jeremy Freese, Ann Stueve, Kenneth Heller, Steven A. Tuch, John Monahan, and Jason Schnittker

Americans' Views of Mental Illness and Health at Century's End: Continuity and Change[†]

This selection includes excerpts from a report of a study on public attitudes toward mental illness that was conducted in 1996. Prior to this study, the most recent information on public attitudes came from a survey conducted in the 1950s by Shirley Star, a researcher at the National Opinion Research Center. This more recent study adopted some of Star's methods in order to facilitate comparisons over time. It established that, although public knowledge regarding mental illness has improved since the 1950s, public attitudes have not, and thereby stimulated a resurgence of interest in mental illness stigma.

OVERVIEW

The goal of this study is to examine the public's perceptions of mental illness and substance abuse, and to determine how individuals with these mental health problems recognize and seek help. In particular, we seek to understand how these views may have changed over time and whether stigma

Pescosolido, Bernice A., Jack K. Martin, Bruce G. Link, Saeko Kikuzawa, Giovanni Burgos, and Ralph Swindle. 2000. "Americans' Views of Mental Illness and Health at Century's End: Continuity and Change." Public Report on the MacArthur Mental Health Module, 1996 General Social Survey. Bloomington, Indiana: Indiana Consortium for Mental Health Services Research.

is still a major problem. Furthermore, we ask what people believe are the causes of mental illness and substance abuse, what can be done for persons with these problems, and their comfort level with persons who are mentally ill. We see this work as speaking to the interests of mental health advocates, policymakers, and professionals.

A major challenge to mental health and substance abuse policy is the repeated demonstration in epidemiological studies that more than two-thirds of individuals experiencing diagnosable mental health problems do not seek professional care. It is thought that lack of knowledge about mental illness, the stigma of mental illness, and ignorance about effective treatments play an important role in lack of treatment-seeking. Compounding this problem is a mismatch of professional's preference for working with the "worried well" and the compelling unmet needs for community-based treatment for the deinstitutionalized severely mentally ill. The original *Americans View Their Mental Health* study by Gerald Gurin, Joseph Veroff, and Sheila Feld (1957) supported an emphasis on national education about mental illness that was incorporated in the original 1960s and 70s Community Mental Health legislation. In the 1980s and 1990s, consumer groups added their voices and family stories in a call for stepped-up community support treatment programs, the search for new medications and a better understanding of the biology of mental illness, and the destigmatization of mental illness. These have been positive moves aimed at destigmatizing severe mental illness and matching treatment resources to the needs of the severely mentally ill and their families.

Possibly countering these positive trends, however, have been rare but highly visible acts of violence by mentally ill persons such as the Son of Sam murders, the assassination of John Lennon, assassination attempts on Presidents Ford and Reagan, and on George Harrison, and the Unabomber's terrorist campaign. There has been the epidemic of crack-related murders in the 90s. Rural America has been struck by an unprecedented rash of church arsons. School shooting rampages by students are threatening to turn schools into fortified enclaves. Finally, popular films such as *Taxi Driver, Swingblade, Son of Sam,* and *Psycho* (twice) epitomize an entertainment media that capitalizes on the rare but sensational, with widespread but unknown impacts on the public's views of mental illness.

In the 20 years that have passed since the AVTMH (*Americans View Their Mental Health*) was replicated, much has changed in mental health care: a dismantling of national mental health legislation in the 1980s; the development of new medications and therapeutic approaches; and the advent of a primary care-mental health carve-out system of health care. We have little idea how the historical literature on stigma and labeling now applies in current public conceptions. Much too has changed in the methodology of assessment.

In 1950, Shirley Star collected the first major survey on mental illness at the National Opinion Research Center (NORC), at the University of Chicago. While the results were never formally published and the final report never written, both the methodological and substantive findings of this work have been highly influential. In the mid-1950s Gerald Gurin, Joseph Veroff, and Sheila Feld (1957) fielded *Americans View Their Mental Health*. This survey, entitled "Study of Modern Living," asked about several domains of life (work, marriage, physical and mental health), the problems that individuals faced, and how they responded. In 1976, the AVTMH was replicated. Our current understandings of these issues make some of their methodological approaches out-of-date (in part because of the advances they made and future directions they suggested).[*] We used two new strategies. Rather than ask a diffuse, general question (e.g., How likely are persons with depression to hurt themselves?), we presented our sample of Americans with a case or vignette describing a person who, according to the criteria in the *Diagnostic and Statistical Manual-IV*, met criteria for either schizophrenia, major depression, alcohol dependence, or drug dependence. These cases were largely the inspiration of the module team members from the Columbia University School of Public Health. Second, we found a core of items in each survey that would allow us to mark changes in the public's understanding, experiences of and responses to mental health problems and issues over a 40 year period. Public knowledge, attitudes, and beliefs shape personal and policy decisions that have tremendous bearing on the quality of life of people who suffer from mental illness. A comparison over time facilitates our understanding of the changing public understanding of and response to mental illness, both in personal ways and in the way that they think about and support public policy change. These ideas, background work (including meeting with original researchers), and comparable coding were developed by the module team members associated with the Indiana Consortium for Mental Health Services Research. The issues and questions on competence, dangerousness, and coercion were inspired by the work of the MacArthur Law and Mental Health Network.

AMERICANS' RECOGNITION OF MENTAL HEALTH PROBLEMS IN 1996: CONTINUITY AND CHANGE SINCE THE 1950s

As noted, the last 50 years have witnessed dramatic changes in the public's perceptions and understanding of mental illness. One anticipated result of these changes is a presumed broadening of the public's definition of just what constitutes a mental health problem. In other words, it has been suggested that in defining mental health problems, contemporary Americans will be more likely to include less severe problems such as mild anxiety and mood disorders in that definition than were their counterparts five decades

---

[*] We thank Tom Smith and Patrick Bova at NORC for their assistance and advice on retrieving the original Star survey forms, and Toni Antonnucci, Elizabeth Douvan and Joe Veroff for the same on the AVTMH studies.

earlier. In order to assess this possibility, the 1996 General Social Survey (GSS) included an open-ended question identical to that asked by Shirley Star in 1950: "Of course, everyone hears a good deal about physical illness and disease, but now, what about the ones we call mental or nervous illness…When you hear someone say that a person is mentally ill, what does that mean to you?" Responses to this item in 1950 and 1996 are summarized in Figure 1.

In 1950, when asked the meaning of mental illness, the largest proportion of respondents mentioned behaviors indicative of either psychoses (reported by 40.7 percent) or anxiety/depression (reported by 48.7 percent), with very low percentages mentioning social deviance (7.1 percent), mental retardation (6.5 percent), or other nonpsychotic disorders (7.1 percent). These reports, however, have changed dramatically in the 1996 data. While it remains in 1996 that the largest percentage of respondents continue to mention behaviors consistent with psychoses (34.9 percent) or anxiety/depression (34.3 percent), such reports are sharply reduced from the earlier 1950 levels.

By contrast, the percentage of respondents whose descriptions of mental illness included references to antisocial or deviant behavior and mental retardation more than doubled from 1950 to 1996. This pattern is even more pronounced in the case of descriptions of mental illness that reference non-psychotic disorders, where the percentage of respondents defining these conditions as mental illness nearly tripled to 20.1 percent (up from 7.1 percent in 1950). Thus, while large numbers of Americans continue to view mental illness in more-or-less conventional terms (i.e., as psychotic or anxious/depressed behavior), over the last five decades it would appear that public definitions of what constitutes a mental health problem have indeed broadened.

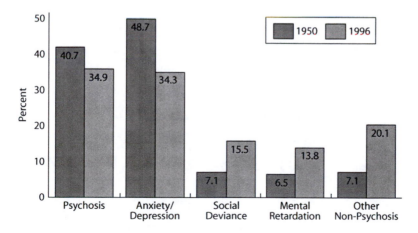

Figure 1 Classification of Americans' Responses to "What Is Mental Illness"
Adapted from: Phelan, J.C., B.G. Link, A. Stueve, and B.A. Pescosolido. 2000. "Public Conceptions of Mental Illness in 1950 and 1996: What is Mental Illness and is it to be Feared?" *Journal of Health and Social Behavior*, 41(2).

Another topic not adequately addressed in previous research, but a key issue for the 1996 GSS researchers, was the public's understanding of the meaning of the term "nervous breakdown" as compared to other concepts such as "mental illness". In order to examine this distinction, half of the 1996 respondents were asked to describe the characteristics of a mentally ill person, and the other half to describe a nervous breakdown. A comparison of responses to these two items is displayed in Figure 2.

Examination of the data in Figure 2 indicates that in the public mind a "nervous breakdown" corresponds most closely to neurotic and mood disorders. Commonly employed descriptors for a person who suffered a "nervous breakdown" included neurosis (mentioned by 65 percent), being unable to adjust to life (mentioned by 33.6 percent), neurasthenia (mentioned by 19.5 percent), loss of control (mentioned by 19.4 percent), and anxiety (mentioned

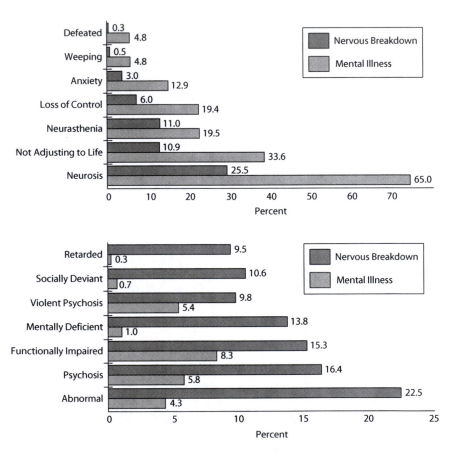

Figure 2. Percentage of Americans Mentioning Symptoms for Nervous Breakdown and Mental Illness

Adapted from: R. Swindle, K. Heller, B.A. Pescosolido, and S. Kikuzawa, 2000. "Responses to Nervous Breakdowns in America Over a 40-year Period: Mental Health Policy implications." *American Psychologist*, 55(7).

by 12.9 percent). A somewhat different picture emerges when examining how respondents described a person suffering from "mental illness." Here public perceptions are more likely to highlight more serious psychotic disorders and socially deviant behavior. For example, common descriptors included abnormal/disordered behavior (mentioned by 22.5 percent), psychosis (mentioned by 16.4 percent), functional impairment (mentioned by 15.3 percent), mental deficiencies (mentioned by 13.8 percent), social deviance (mentioned by 10.6 percent), violent psychosis (mentioned by 9.8 percent), and mental retardation (mentioned by 9.5 percent). It is also appropriate to note that three descriptors commonly used to characterize a "nervous breakdown" were also mentioned by a nontrivial percentage of the respondents who were asked to describe "mental illness." Specifically, when asked to describe "mental illness" 25 percent of respondents mentioned symptoms consistent with neurosis, 11 percent mentioned neurasthenia symptoms, and 10.9 percent mentioned adjustment problems.[1,2]

The 1996 data, then, provide some evidence for a broadening of the public's definition of what constitutes a mental illness. These data show, however, that the American public's definition of mental illness increasingly includes violence or other "frightening" characteristics. Table 1 provides data highlighting this trend. For example, in 1950 7.2 percent of Americans spontaneously described mental illness with terms referencing violent, dangerous, or frightening behavior.

Over the 50-year interval, however, the use of these terms had markedly increased. For example, in 1996 the proportion of respondents using terms indicative of violent or dangerous behavior to describe mental illness had increased significantly, nearly doubling to 12.1 percent (up from 7.2 percent in 1950). Similarly, the proportion of Americans describing mental illness in terms consistent with a diagnosis of violent psychosis also increased noticeably, up from 6.8 percent in 1950 to 12.4 percent in 1996. Thus, it would appear that while the American public has enlarged their definition of mental illness to include less severe problems such as mild anxiety and mood disorders, this broadening has also been accompanied by a somewhat contradictory increase in the public's perception that persons suffering from mental illness are likely to represent a threat for violent or dangerous behavior.[1]

In addition to examining past and present conceptions of mental illness, we agreed that it was important to determine whether or not Americans

Table 1 American's Perception of Violence as Part of Mental Illness

Responses to What Is Mental Illness	Star 1950 %	GSS 1996 %
Violent, Dangerous, Frightening	7.20	12.10
Describes Violent Psychosis	6.80	12.40

Adapted from: Phelan, J. C., B. G. Link, A. Stueve, and B. A. Pescosolido. 2000. "Public Conceptions of Mental Illness in 1950 and 1996: What Is Mental Illness and Is It to Be Feared?" *Journal of Health and Social Behavior,* 41(2): 188–207.

Table 2 Nature of Respondents' Contact with Persons with Mental Health Problems

Nature of Contact	% Yes	(N)
Knows Someone Who Was in a Hospital Because of a Mental Illness	50.2	(729)
Who was it?		(364)
Respondent	2.5	
Immediate Family	25.3	
Other Relative	27.2	
Close Friend	26.9	
Acquaintances	24.2	
Other	7.1	
Knows Other Seeing a Psychologist, Mental Health Professional Social Worker, or Counselor	57.9	(670)

based their perceptions, at least in part, on first-hand knowledge or personal interactions with persons suffering from mental health problems. To assess this question, the 1996 GSS asked respondents if they had ever known anyone hospitalized for a mental illness and their relationship to the hospitalized individual, and whether they had ever known anyone else (other than the hospitalized person) who was seeing a psychologist, mental health professional, social worker, or counselor. Responses to these items, summarized in Table 2, indicate that half (50.2 percent) of all Americans report having known someone who had been hospitalized due to a mental illness, with roughly a quarter of respondents indicating that the hospitalized person was a member of their immediate family, another relative, or a close friend. Moreover, an even larger percentage of respondents (57.9 percent) also reported knowing yet another person(s) who had received mental health services outside of a hospital setting. These data would suggest, then, that relatively large numbers of Americans today have at least some first-hand knowledge of persons suffering from mental health problems.

PUBLIC PERCEPTIONS OF THE CAUSES, LABELS, AND SEVERITY OF MENTAL ILLNESS AND SUBSTANCE ABUSE

What does the American public believe are the root causes of mental illness? Are Americans more likely to invoke biological, personal, or spiritual explanations when asked to account for the genesis of mental health problems? Does the public endorse different causal attributions for different types of mental health problems? Prior to the 1996 GSS, there had not been a large, national research effort to find answers to these obviously important questions.

In an attempt to shed much needed light on these and other important questions regarding public perceptions of mental illness, a team of investigators from Columbia University developed an experiment including vignettes and questions about vignettes, and brought to the drafting meetings for the 1996 Mental Health Module. From the vignettes they submitted, four were selected by the module members: schizophrenia, major depression, alcohol dependence, and troubled person. To these four a fifth was added to depict cocaine dependence. The questions about the vignettes were modified, improved and expanded by the module team. The history of and rationale for using vignettes to study public conceptions of mental illness is provided in Link et al. (1999). The mental health problems described in the vignettes were selected on the basis of severity, prevalence, and potential consequences of misidentification. After hearing one of the five vignette persons described, respondents were asked a series of interrelated questions that sought to assess whether or not the person described had a mental illness, how serious the person's problem is, the probable cause of the problem, etc.[3]

Turning first to how respondents defined the nature of the problem experienced by the person described in their vignette, Table 3 reports the percentage of respondents who indicated that the specific problem experienced was "very likely," or "somewhat likely" to be due to the normal "ups and downs" of life, a nervous breakdown, a mental illness, a physical illness, and the specific *DSM-IV* diagnostic disorder. According to these data, the vast majority of respondents correctly classified the specific disorder described in their vignette. For example, 97.8 percent of respondents hearing the depression vignette correctly indicated that the person was experiencing a major depression. Similar patterns were obtained for schizophrenia (84.8 percent

Table 3 Percentage of Americans Reporting on the Nature of the Problem in the Vignette

Respondent Report	Vignette Story				
	Alcohol Dependence %	Depression %	Schizophrenia %	Drug Dependence %	Troubled Person %
Ups and Downs of Life	62.0	79.6	40.0	40.8	96.2
Nervous Breakdowns	52.9	69.6	83.9	43.2	20.9
Mental Illness	48.6	69.1	88.2	43.5	21.5
Physical Illness	57.5	67.5	48.2	52.2	36.1
Alcohol Abuse	97.7	—	—	—	—
Depression	—	94.6	—	—	—
Schizophrenia	—	—	84.8	—	—
Drug Abuse	—	—	—	96.7	—

Adapted from: Link, B. G., J. C. Phelan, M. Bresnahan, A. Stueve, B. A. Pescosolido. 1999. "Public Conceptions of Mental Illness: Labels, Causes, Dangerousness, and Social Distance." *American Journal of Public Health* 89(9): 1328–33.

of respondents were correct), alcohol dependence (with 97.8 percent correct), and drug dependence (96.7 percent correct).[3]

The data in Table 3 point to several additional patterns of note. To begin, a clear majority of respondents (62 percent) feel that it is likely that persons experiencing alcohol dependence do so as part of the normal ups and downs of life, with an even higher percentage (79.6 percent) indicating that depression can be seen as the result of this same process. As might be expected, large majorities also believe that persons suffering from depression or schizophrenia are experiencing a nervous breakdown (69.6 percent and 83.9 percent, respectively), or a mental illness (69.1 percent and 88.1 percent, respectively). Finally, it is interesting to note that over half of respondents believe that alcohol dependent, drug dependent, and depressed persons are experiencing a type of physical illness.

While the data indicate that large numbers of Americans utilize multiple definitions for the types of problems they believe are being experienced by the vignette person, respondents are more-or-less uniform in their perceptions regarding the severity of these problems. Data relative to this issue are reported in Table 4. When asked to characterize the severity of the specific problem experienced by the person described in the vignette, for each of the four mental health problems a clear majority indicated the problem was "very serious." As might be expected, respondents were nearly unanimous in describing drug dependences as representing a very serious problem (97.9 percent), but it is interesting to note that over three-quarters of respondents indicated that schizophrenia (79.2 percent) and alcohol dependence (77.5 percent) are also very serious problems. Only in the case of the vignette describing a person experiencing major depression was the percentage of respondents answering "very serious" reduced somewhat, with 53.6 percent characterizing depression as a very serious problem. It should be pointed out, however, that in the case of depression an additional 40 percent of respondents viewed this condition as being at least "somewhat serious," with only 6.5 percent indicating that depression was "not very" or "not at all" serious. Indeed, when the "very serious" and "somewhat serious" responses are combined, for each of the four mental health problems

Table 4 Americans Report of the Severity of the Vignette

Vignette Story	Severity				
	Very Serious	Somewhat Serious	Not Very Serious	Not Serious at All	(N)
Alcohol Dependence	77.5	21.0	1.4	0.0	(276)
Depression	53.6	40.0	5.8	7.0	(295)
Schizophrenia	79.2	17.1	2.4	1.4	(293)
Drug Dependence	97.9	2.1	0.0	0.0	(289)
Troubled Person	4.5	28.5	44.9	22.1	(267)

well over 90 percent of respondents define these conditions as representing serious problems.

It would appear, then, that Americans are nearly uniform in their assessments of the severity of the problems experienced by persons with various forms of mental illness. There is far less uniformity, however, in how the public views the root causes of these problems. In Table 5 we turn our attention to this issue. In this table we ask, "Are contemporary attributions for the sources of mental health problems based primarily on genetic/medical, social structural, or individual-level causes?"

According to the data in Table 5, drug dependence is the only disorder for which the respondents' attribute an individual-level source—bad character (reported by 31.5 percent of respondents). For schizophrenia, on the other hand, chemical/biological attributions predominate, with nearly half of all respondents (46.9 percent) very likely to attribute the source of this disorder to a chemical imbalance. For depression and alcohol dependence, respondents tend to invoke social structural attributions (i.e., stress) as causal mechanisms. Indeed, a majority (54.5 percent) of respondents attribute depression and nearly 4 of 10 (36 percent) attribute alcohol dependency to problems related to dealing with daily stressors.[5]

The data displayed in Table 5 also indicate that with the exception of depression, there is no clear consensus regarding the source of drug dependence, alcohol dependence, or schizophrenia. For example, over one-fifth of respondents (20.8 percent) report chemical imbalance as a cause of drug

Table 5 Americans' Attributions Modal Category for Specific Mental Health Problems, Percentage Responding "Very Likely" to the Underlying Cause of the Problem (Panel 1), and Percentage Responding "Very Likely" That the Problem Is a Mental Illness (Panel 2).

Panel 1	Depression %	Schizophrenia %	Drug Dependence %	Alcohol Dependence %	Troubles %
Chemical	20.8	<u>46.9</u>	20.8	16.2	4.8
Genetic	13.3	20.7	5.7	12.3	5.2
Stress	<u>54.5</u>	33.8	25.5	<u>36.0</u>	<u>38.0</u>
Way Raised	11.5	8.2	10.7	11.1	13.2
Bad Character	11.2	14.1	<u>31.5</u>	20.2	9.0
God's Will	6.8	6.0	2.1	1.9	8.0
Panel 2					
"Very Likely" Mental illness	20.4	54.4	13.3	10.3	1.4

Source: Martin, J. K., B. A. Pescosolido, and S. A. Tuch. 2000. "Of Fear and Loathing: The Role of 'Disturbing Behavior', Labels, and Causal Attributions in Shaping Public Attitudes Toward Persons with Mental Illness." *Journal of Health and Social Behavior,* 41(2): 208–33. Also see Link, B. G., J. C. Phelan, M. Bresnahan, A. Stueve, and B. A. Pescosolido. 1999. "Public Conceptions of Mental Illness: Labels, Causes, Dangerousness, and Social Distance." *American Journal of Public Health* 89(9): 1328–33.

dependence, while another quarter (25.5 percent) mention stress. One-fifth of respondents (20.2 percent) see bad character as the underlying cause of alcohol dependence. Regarding the sources of schizophrenia, one-third of respondents (33.8 percent) point to stress, and an additional fifth (20.7 percent) identify genetic factors as the causal mechanism. Finally, it is interesting to note that only a small minority of respondents are likely to attribute the source of any of the four mental health problems as "God's will."[5]

PUBLIC VIEWS OF COMPETENCE AND DANGEROUSNESS OF PERSONS WITH MENTAL HEALTH PROBLEMS[4]

How do Americans assess the abilities of persons with mental health problems, and what threats do these individuals pose to society? In an attempt to provide answers to these questions, the 1996 GSS interview included two items tapping public perceptions of the competence of those suffering from mental health problems to manage treatment decisions and personal finances. An additional two items sought to assess the perceived level of threat for violence to self and others posed by persons with mental health problems. Responses to these items are summarized in Figures 3 and 4.

Figure 3 presents the percentage of respondents who indicated that the person described in their particular vignette was "very" or "somewhat able" to make treatment decisions and to manage finances. Examination of these data reveals several interesting patterns. To begin, as expected, nearly all respondents see the person described in the reference category (i.e., the

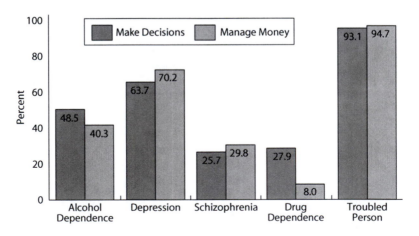

Figure 3 Percentage of Americans Reporting Vignette Person as Very or Somewhat Able to make Treatment Decisions or to Manage Money

Adapted from: Pescosolido, B.A., J. Monahan, B.G. Link, A. Stueve, and S. Kikuzawa. 1999. "The Public's View of the Competence, Dangerousness, and Need for Legal Coercion Among Persons with Mental Health Problems." *American Journal of Public Health* 89(9): 1339–1345.

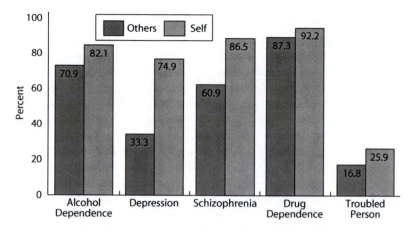

Figure 4 Percentage of Americans Reporting Vignette Person as Likely to do Something Violent to Others or Self

Adapted from: Pescosolido, B.A., J. Monahan, B.G. Link, A. Stueve, and S. Kikuzawa. 1999. "The Public's View of the Competence, Dangerousness, and Need for Legal Coercion Among Persons with Mental Health Problems." *American Journal of Public Health* 89(9): 1339–1345.

person with subthreshold "troubles"), to be competent to manage decisions regarding either treatment (93.1 percent), or finances (94.7 percent). Similarly, when asked to assess the competence of persons suffering from major depression, a majority of respondents indicate that a person with depression is either "very" or "somewhat able" to make decisions regarding treatment (63.7 percent) and money management (70.2 percent).

On the other hand, persons described as suffering from alcohol dependence, schizophrenia, and drug dependence are viewed as significantly less competent to manage decisions in either domain. In the case of alcohol dependence, for example, only a minority of respondents feel that the vignette person is at least "somewhat able" to make competent decisions regarding treatment (48.5 percent) or finances (40.3 percent). Moreover, this pattern is significantly more pronounced for persons described as suffering from schizophrenia or drug dependence. When the person described in the vignette presents symptoms consistent with a diagnosis of schizophrenia, only slightly more than a quarter of respondents (25.7 percent) believe that person to be competent to make decisions regarding treatment issues, and only 29.8 percent indicate that a person suffering from schizophrenia is competent to make financial decisions. Respondents' levels of skepticism, however, are highest when asked to rate the competence of those who are drug dependent. In this case, only 27.9 percent of respondents believe a drug dependent individual can make appropriate decisions regarding treatment, and less than 1 in 10 feel that a person with a drug habit is "somewhat" or "very able" to make competent decisions with regard to financial matters. Further, in a multivariate analysis of the correlates of perceptions of competence (data not shown)[4] assessments of the vignette person's competence did not vary as a function of the vignette person's individual attributes (i.e., age, education, ethnicity, or gender). In other words, regardless of the background characteristics of the person described as suffering from a specific mental health problem, it was the mental health problem alone that was predictive of the consistent public perception of reduced decision-making ability.[4]

Earlier we reported data to suggest that over the last 50 years the American public has become more likely to equate mental illness with a potential for violent or dangerous behavior. In Figure 4 we examine this finding in more detail by specifying a referent (i.e., violence toward self or others). According to the data displayed in Figure 4, Americans discriminate among the different mental health problems with respect to potential for dangerous behavior. Respondents perceive the highest potential for violent behavior among those who are either drug or alcohol dependent. For persons described as drug dependent, 92.2 percent of respondents report that person to be "very" or "somewhat likely to do violence to self, and 87.3 percent feel that a drug dependent person is likely to do violence to others. This pattern is somewhat reduced for those who are described as alcohol dependent, but it remains that over 8 of 10 respondents see the alcohol dependent individual as likely to do violence to self, and over 7 of 10 see this person as at least "somewhat likely" to do violence to others.[3,4]

When the vignette person is described as suffering from symptoms consistent with a diagnosis of schizophrenia, public perceptions of dangerousness to self are somewhat lower when compared to descriptions of individuals suffering from substance dependency. Nonetheless, over 6 of 10 respondents (60.9 percent) perceive a potential for violence toward others among individuals suffering from schizophrenia, and nearly 9 of 10 (86.5 percent) believe that individual is likely to commit violence toward him/herself. The proportion remains essentially unchanged for the depression scenario for the likelihood of violence toward self (74.9 percent believe the depressed individual is likely to do something violent toward him/herself), but changes dramatically when dangerousness toward others is considered. In this case, only a minority (33.3 percent) believes that the individual described as experiencing major depression would likely do violence toward others.[3,4]

The data reported in Figure 4, then, are clear. With regard to public perceptions of dangerousness, the vast majority of respondents believe that persons suffering from mental health problems represent a threat for violence toward themselves. Similarly, with the exception of persons suffering from depression, the public also believes that those experiencing mental health problems pose a threat for violence toward others.

PUBLIC WILLINGNESS TO INTERACT SOCIALLY WITH PERSONS WITH MENTAL HEALTH PROBLEMS[3,5]

In order to assess public attitudes toward interaction with the mentally ill, GSS respondents were asked a series of six "social distance" questions.

STIGMATOGRAPHY

The hospital had an address, 115 Mill Street. This was to provide some cover if one of us were well enough to apply for a job while still incarcerated. It gave about as much protection as 1600 Pennsylvania Avenue would have.

"Let's see, nineteen years old, living at 1600 Pennsylvania Avenue— Hey! That's the White House!"

This was the sort of look we got from prospective employers, except not pleased.

In Massachusetts, 115 Mill Street is a famous address. Applying for a job, leasing an apartment, getting a driver's license: all problematic. The driver's-license application even asked, Have you ever been hospitalized for mental illness? Oh, no, I just loved Belmont so much I decided to move to 115 Mill Street.

"You're living at One fifteen Mill Street?" asked a small, basement-colored person who ran a sewing-notions shop in Harvard Square, where I was trying to get a job.

"Uh-hunh"

"And how long have you been living there?"

"Oh, a while." I gestured at the past with one hand.

"And I guess you haven't been working for a while?" He leaned back, enjoying himself.

"No," I said. "I've been thinking things over."

I didn't get the job.

As I left the shop my glance met his, and he gave me a look of such terrible intimacy that I cringed. I know what you are, said his look.

What were we, that they could know us so quickly and so well?

We were probably better than we used to be, before we went into the hospital. At a minimum we were older and more self-aware. Many of us had spent our hospital years yelling and causing trouble and were ready to move on to something else. All of us had learned by default to treasure freedom and would do anything we could to get it and keep it.

The question was, What could we do?

Could we get up every morning and take showers and put on clothes and go to work? Could we think straight? Could we not say crazy things when they occurred to us?

Some of us could, some of us couldn't. In the world's terms, though, all of us were tainted.

There's always a touch of fascination in revulsion: Could that happen to me? The less likely the terrible thing is to happen, the less frightening it is to look at or imagine. A person who doesn't talk to herself or stare off into nothingness is therefore more alarming than a person who does. Someone who acts "normal" raises the uncomfortable question, What's the difference between that person and me? which leads to the question, What's keeping me out of the loony bin? This explains why a general taint is useful.

Some people are more frightened than others.

"You spent nearly two years in a loony bin! Why in the world were you in there? I can't believe it!" Translation: If you're crazy, then I'm crazy, and I'm not, so the whole thing must have been a mistake.

"You spent nearly two years in a loony bin? What was wrong with you?" Translation: I need to know the particulars of craziness so I can assure myself that I'm not crazy.

"You spent nearly two years in a loony bin? Hmmm. When was that, exactly?" Translation: Are you still contagious?

I stopped telling people. There was no advantage in telling people. The longer I didn't say anything about it, the farther away it got, until the me who had been in the hospital was a tiny blur and the me who didn't talk about it was big and strong and busy.

I began to feel revulsion too. Insane people: I had a good nose for them and I didn't want to have anything to do with them I still don't. I can't come up with reassuring answers to the terrible questions they raise.

Don't ask me those questions. Don't ask me what life means or how we know reality or why we have to suffer so much. Don't talk about how nothing feels real, how everything is coated with gelatin and shining like oil in the sun. I don't want to hear about the tiger in the corner or the Angel of Death or the phone calls from John the Baptist. He might give me a call too. But I'm not going to pick up the phone.

If I who was previously revolting am now this far from my crazy self, how much further are you who were never revolting, and how much deeper your revulsion?

Kaysen, Susanna. 1993. *Girl, Interrupted*. New York: Vintage Books. Pp. 123–125.

Specifically, respondents were asked how willing they would be to: "move next door" to the person described in their vignette; whether they would "spend an evening socializing" with that person; whether they would "make friends" with that person; whether they were willing to "work closely on the job" with that person; whether they were willing to have the vignette person "marry into their family"; and whether they were willing to have a "group home for people like the vignette person in their neighborhood." The percentage of respondents who indicated that they were "definitely" or "probably unwilling" to interact with a person suffering from mental health problems in these six settings is reported in Table 6.

Table 6 Percentage of Americans Reporting They Are "Definitely" or "Probably Unwilling" to Interact with Vignette Person

	Social Interaction						
Vignette Story	Move Next Door %	Spend an Evening Socializing with %	Make Friend with %	Work Close with on the Job %	Have a Group Home in Neighborhood %	Marry into Your Family %	Average % by Vignette Type
Alcohol Dependence	45.6	55.8	36.7	74.7	43.4	78.2	55.7
Depression	22.9	37.8	23.1	48.6	31.2	60.6	37.4
Schizophrenia	37.0	49.0	34.0	64.1	33.2	72.2	48.4
Drug Dependence	75.0	72.7	59.1	82.0	52.7	89.0	71.8
Troubled Person	9.5	14.9	10.0	21.0	27.7	41.9	20.8
Average % by Type of Interaction	38.0	55.8	32.6	58.1	37.6	68.4	46.8

Adapted From: Martin, J .K., B. A. Pescosolido, and S. A. Tuch. 2000. "Of Fear and Loathing: The Role of 'Disturbing Behavior,' Labels, and Causal Attributions in Shaping Public Attitudes toward Persons with Mental Illness." *Journal of Health and Social Behavior,* 41(2): 208–33.

Examination of the data in Table 6 provides little evidence to suggest that the public is willing to interact socially or occupationally with persons suffering from mental health problems. Overall, the highest level of social distance is desired from persons with substance dependency problems. Indeed, when averaged across the six interactional categories, nearly three-fourths (71.8 percent) prefer to avoid contact with people who are drug dependent, and a majority (55.7 percent) also prefer to avoid persons who are alcohol dependent. While attitudes toward persons with problems other than substance abuse are somewhat more tolerant, it remains that a significant percentage of the public indicates a desire to remain socially distant from persons who have either schizophrenia or major depression. For example, on average, nearly half of all respondents (48.4 percent) report an unwillingness to interact with the person described in the schizophrenia vignette, and nearly 40 percent (37.4 percent) indicate a similar unwillingness to interact with persons suffering from major depression.

Without regard to type of mental health problem, the average percentages by type of interaction summarized in the bottom row of Table 6 are also instructive with regard to those social environments in which the public is most willing and least willing to have contact with persons with mental health problems. According to these data, respondents are most willing to be friends with persons suffering from these problems. For example, fewer than a quarter of respondents (23.1 percent) are unwilling to have a depressed person as a friend. Indeed, across the four mental health problems, only somewhat more than a third of respondents (38.2 percent) are unwilling to be friends with a person having mental health difficulties.

While it is clear that the vast majority of Americans are willing to make friends with persons with mental health problems, it is equally clear that this tolerance does not extend to a willingness to accept these persons as either family members or coworkers. Across the four mental health problem categories, on average, 75 percent of respondents are unwilling to have someone suffering from drug or alcohol dependency, schizophrenia, or depression marry a family member, and a similarly high 67.4 percent are unwilling to have persons suffering from these problems as coworkers.[3, 5]

Looking within the body of Table 6, we see that Americans are most unwilling to have a person who is drug dependent marry into their family (89.0 percent). They are most willing to have the "troubled person" as their neighbor or friend. Only 9.5 percent and 10.0 percent, respectively, are unwilling to do so. Over a fifth of respondents reported an unwillingness to have the troubled person as a coworker (21.0 percent) or live in a nearby group home (27.7 percent), and nearly half do not want him/her to marry into their family (41.9 percent).[3,5]

With regard to the two traditional mental illness problems, depression and schizophrenia, the majority of respondents do not want to work alongside persons suffering from these problems, or have them marry into their family. Almost half are unwilling to have a person with depression as a close coworker (48.6%), and almost two-thirds (64.1 percent) report a similar unwillingness to work with persons with schizophrenia. Moreover, a large majority of respondents are unwilling to have persons with mental illness marry into their family (68.6 percent for depression, 72.2 percent for schizophrenia).

The preferences for social distance reported in Table 6, then, provide little evidence to suggest that the stigma of mental illness has been reduced in contemporary American society. Levels of social rejection of those with mental health problems have remained distressingly high.

SUMMARY

The complex picture of Americans' views of mental health and persons with mental health problems can be summarized along two dimensions: *differentiation* and *enduring stigmatization*. Encompassed within these themes are both positive patterns and causes for concern. In this section we comment on the overall sweep of the findings.

Differentiation. In the 1950s, Shirley Star's research demonstrated that Americans' views of mental illness were negative, one-dimensional, and typified by the exemplar of the person with paranoid schizophrenia. Our findings indicate that the current understanding of mental health problems has become more differentiated, and in some cases, more positive. With remarkable consistency, Americans now recognize and correctly identify schizophrenia, major depression, alcohol disorder, and drug abuse as types of mental health problems. Also on the positive side, the causes of mental health problems are increasingly viewed as a result of the combined effects of life stressors, genetic, and chemical imbalances, rather than upbringing or bad character. These various mental health disorders are also seen as very amenable to treatment, including both medication and psychotherapies.

Enduring stigmatization. Unfortunately, accompanying this differentiation, mental health problems and mental illnesses appear to be viewed along a continuum of severity that continues to carry very strong, stigmatizing attitudes. Americans' contemporary attitudes toward mental illnesses have apparently become more infused with concerns about violence associated with these illnesses. Our data show that mental health problems can roughly be ordered from least to most stigmatized as follows: personal troubles, nervous breakdowns, major depression, schizophrenia, alcohol disorder, and drug disorder. Alcohol and drug problems are seen as having the highest potential for violence, followed by schizophrenia and depression. Closely linked to these fears of violence is a social distancing—not wanting to associate with individuals with these problems; believing they cannot manage their own affairs; and believing that it is appropriate to coerce individuals into treatment. While there are more effective treatments for many of these conditions than ever before, the antipathy toward those with mental health problems remains distressing. These fears seem to fuel beliefs that it is appropriate to force individuals with substance abuse problems and schizophrenia into treatment, and to shun these individuals in work and in social life. Serious mental health problems continue to be stigmatizing and are coupled with fears of violence that appear to have increased significantly.

List of Scientific Publications, Papers, and Presentations

1. Phelan, J.C., B.G. Link, A. Stueve, and B.A. Pescosolido. 2000. "Public Conceptions of Mental Illness in 1950 and 1996: What is Mental Illness and Is It to be Feared?" *Journal of Health and Social Behavior* 41(2): 188–207.
2. Swindle, R., K. Heller, B.A. Pescosolido, and S. Kikuzawa. 2000. "Responses to 'Nervous Breakdowns' in America Over a 40-year Period: Mental Health Policy Implications." *American Psychologist*, 55(7).
3. Link, B.G., J.C. Phelan, M. Bresnahan, A. Stueve, and B.A. Pescosolido. 1999. "Public Conceptions of Mental Illness: Labels, Causes, Dangerousness, and Social Distance." *American Journal of Public Health* 89(9): 1328–1333.
4. Pescosolido, B.A., J. Monahan, B.G. Link, A. Stueve, and S. Kikuzawa. 1999. "The Public's View of the Competence, Dangerousness, and Need for Legal Coercion of Persons With Mental Health Problems. *American Journal of Public Health* 89(9): 1339–1345.
5. Martin, J.K., B.A. Pescosolido, and S.A. Tuch. 2000. "Of Fear and Loathing: The Role of 'Disturbing Behavior', Labels, and Causal Attributions in Shaping Public Attitudes Toward Persons With Mental Illness". *Journal of Health and Social Behavior* 41(2): 208–233.

TECHNICAL APPENDIX

A. The Vignettes

Vignette A: Alcohol Dependence. NAME is a RACE/ETHNICITY, MAN/ WOMAN, who has completed EDUCATION. During the last month NAME has started to drink more than his/her usual amount of alcohol. In fact, s/he has noticed that s/he needs to drink twice as much as s/he used to to get the same effect. Several times, s/he has tried to cut down, or stop drinking, but s/he can't. Each time s/he has tried to cut down, s/he became very agitated, sweaty, and s/he couldn't sleep, so s/he took another drink. His/her family has complained that s/he is often hungover, and has become unreliable, making plans one day, and canceling them the next.

Vignette B: Major Depressive Disorder. NAME is a RACE/ETHNICITY, MAN/ WOMAN, who has completed EDUCATION. For the last two weeks NAME has been feeling really down. S/he wakes up in the morning with a flat, heavy feeling that sticks with her/him all day long. S/he isn't enjoying things the way s/he normally would. In fact, nothing seems to give him/her pleasure. Even when good things happen, they don't seem to make NAME happy. S/ he pushes on through her/his days, but it is really hard. The smallest tasks are difficult to accomplish. S/he finds it hard to concentrate on anything. S/ he feels out of energy and out of steam. And even though NAME feels tired, when night comes s/he can't get to sleep. NAME feels pretty worthless, and very discouraged. NAME'S family has noticed that s/he hasn't been him/ herself for about the last month, and that s/he has pulled away from them. NAME just doesn't feel like talking.

Vignette C: Schizophrenia. NAME is a RACE/ETHNICITY, MAN/WOMAN, who has completed EDUCATION. Up until a year ago, life was pretty okay for NAME. But then, things started to change. S/he thought that people around him/her were making disapproving comments, and talking behind his/her back. NAME was convinced that people were spying on him/her and that they could hear what s/he was thinking. NAME lost his/her drive to participate in his/her usual work and family activities and retreated to his/ her home, eventually spending most of his/her day in his/her room. NAME became so preoccupied with what s/he was thinking that s/he skipped meals and stopped bathing regularly. At night, when everyone else was sleeping, s/ he was walking back and forth in his/her room. NAME was hearing voices even though no one else was around. These voices told him/her what to do and what to think. S/he has been living this way for six months.

Vignette D: Drug Dependence. NAME is a RACE/ETHNICITY, MAN/ WOMAN, who has completed EDUCATION. A year ago, NAME sniffed cocaine for the first time with friends at a party. During the last few months, s/he has been snorting it in binges that last several days at a time. S/he has lost weight and often experiences chills when binging. NAME has spent his/her savings to buy cocaine. When NAME'S friends try to talk about the changes they see, s/he becomes angry and storms out. Friends and family have also noticed missing possessions and suspect NAME has stolen them. S/he has tried to stop snorting cocaine, but can't. Each time s/he tries to stop, s/he feels tired, depressed, and is unable to sleep. S/he lost his/her job a month ago, after not showing up for work.

Vignette E: Troubled Person. NAME is a RACE/ETHNICITY, MAN/WOMAN, who has completed EDUCATION. Up until a year ago, life was pretty okay for NAME. While nothing much is going wrong in NAME'S life, s/he sometimes feels worried, a little sad, or has trouble sleeping at night. NAME feels that at times things bother him/her more than they bother other people and that when things go wrong, s/he sometimes gets nervous or annoyed. Otherwise, NAME is getting along pretty well. S/he enjoys being with other people and although NAME sometimes argues with his/her family, NAME has been getting along pretty well with his/her family.

DISCUSSION

1. The authors followed Star's strategy and used a vignette-based study design to elicit knowledge and attitudes about mental illness. Why might they have chosen that approach over direct questions about the acceptance or rejection of people with mental illness?

2. Based on the information from this study, how would you characterize public knowledge and attitudes toward mental illness? How accurate is public knowledge? How favorable or unfavorable are public attitudes? What public education campaigns are suggested by your answers?

3. In this study, the vignette persons with alcohol or cocaine dependence were rated as most dangerous. What might account for that high rating?

Help-Seeking and Utilization

Erving Goffman

The Moral Career of the Mental Patient

In this classic paper, Goffman introduces you to the value of considering the lives of people with mental illness in terms of their "career" as a mental patient. In particular, he highlights that the treatment process influences both a social dimension—such as the public stigma of mental illness and the negative societal treatment that often results—as well as deeper personal conceptualization of one's identity. Goffman's essay further highlights some of the critical junctures in self-related changes people with mental illness and clearly explores how these changes are deeply rooted in the nature of someone's involvement within the treatment system.

Traditionally the term *career* has been reserved for those who expect to enjoy the rises laid out within a respectable profession. The term is coming to be used, however, in a broadened sense to refer to any social strand of any person's course through life. The perspective of natural history is taken: unique outcomes are neglected in favor of such changes over time as are basic and common to the members of a social category, although occurring independently to each of them. Such a career is not a thing that can be brilliant or disappointing; it can no more be a success than a failure. In this light, I want to consider the mental patient.

One value of the concept of career is its two-sidedness. One side is linked to internal matters held dearly and closely, such as image of self and felt identity; the other side concerns official position, jural relations, and style of life, and is part of a publicly accessible institutional complex. The concept of career, then, allows one to move back and forth between the personal and the public, between the self and its significant society, without having to rely overly for data upon what the person says he thinks he imagines himself to be.

Goffman, Erving. 1959. "The Moral Career of the Mental Patient." *Psychiatry* 22:123–142.

This paper is an exercise in the institutional approach to the study of self. The main concern will be with the *moral* aspects of career—that is, the regular sequence of changes that career entails in the person's self and in his framework of imagery for judging himself and others.[1]

The category "mental patient" itself will be understood in one strictly sociological sense. In this perspective, the psychiatric view of a person becomes significant only in so far as this view itself alters his social fate—an alteration that seems to become fundamental in our society when, and only when, the person is put through the process of hospitalization.[2] I therefore exclude certain neighboring categories: the undiscovered candidates who would be judged "sick" by psychiatric standards but who never come to be viewed as such by themselves or others, although they may cause everyone a great deal of trouble;[3] the office patient whom a psychiatrist feels he can handle with drugs or shock on the outside; the mental client who engages in psychotherapeutic relationships. And I include anyone, however robust in temperament, who somehow gets caught up in the heavy machinery of mental hospital servicing. In this way the effects of being treated as a mental patient can be kept quite distinct from the effects upon a person's life of traits a clinician would view as psychopathological.[4] Persons who become mental hospital patients vary widely in the kind and degree of illness that a psychiatrist would impute to them, and in the attributes by which laymen

---

[1] Material on moral career can be found in early social anthropological work on ceremonies of status transition, and in classic social psychological descriptions of those spectacular changes in one's view of self that can accompany participation in social movements and sects. Recently new kinds of relevant data have been suggested by psychiatric interest in the problem of "identity" and sociological studies of work careers and "adult socialization."

[2] This point has recently been made by Elaine and John Cumming, *Closed Ranks* (Cambridge: Commonwealth Fund, Harvard University Press, 1957), pp. 101–2: *"Clinical experience supports the impression that many people define mental illness as 'that condition for which a person is treated in a mental hospital.' ... Mental illness, it seems, is a condition which afflicts people who must go to a mental institution, but until they go almost anything they do is normal."* Leila Deasy has pointed out to me the correspondence here with the situation in white-collar crime. Of those who are detected in this activity, only the ones who do not manage to avoid going to prison find themselves accorded the social role of the criminal.

[3] Case records in mental hospitals are just now coming to be exploited to show the incredible amount of trouble a person may cause for himself and others before anyone begins to think about him psychiatrically, let alone take psychiatric action against him. See John A. Clausen and Marian Radke Yarrow, "Paths to the Mental Hospital," *Journal of Social Issues*, XI (1955), pp. 25–32; August B. Hollingshead and Fredrick C. Redlich, *Social Class and Mental Illness* (New York: Wiley, 1958), pp. 173–74.

[4] An illustration of how this perspective may be taken to all forms of deviancy may be found in Edwin Lemert, *Social Pathology* (New York: McGraw-Hill, 1951), see especially pp. 74–76. A specific application to mental defectives may be found in Stewart E. Perry, "Some Theoretic Problems of Mental Deficiency and Their Action Implications," *Psychiatry*, XVII (1954), pp. 45–73, see especially pp. 67–68.

would describe them. But once started on the way, they are confronted by some importantly similar circumstances and respond to these in some importantly similar ways. Since these similarities do not come from mental illness, they would seem to occur in spite of it. It is thus a tribute to the power of social forces that the uniform status of mental patient cannot only assure an aggregate of persons a common fate and eventually, because of this, a common character, but that this social reworking can be done upon what is perhaps the most obstinate diversity of human materials that can be brought together by society. Here there lacks only the frequent forming of a protective group life by ex-patients to illustrate in full the classic cycle of response by which deviant subgroupings are psychodynamically formed in society.

This general sociological perspective is heavily reinforced by one key finding of sociologically oriented students in mental hospital research. As has been repeatedly shown in the study of nonliterate societies, the awesomeness, distastefulness, and barbarity of a foreign culture can decrease to the degree that the student becomes familiar with the point of view to life that is taken by his subjects. Similarly, the student of mental hospitals can discover that the craziness or "sick behavior" claimed for the mental patient is by and large a product of the claimant's social distance from the situation that the patient is in, and is not primarily a product of mental illness. Whatever the refinements of the various patients' psychiatric diagnoses, and whatever the special ways in which social life on the "inside" is unique, the researcher can find that he is participating in a community not significantly different from any other he has studied. Of course, while restricting himself to the off-ward grounds community of paroled patients, he may feel, as some patients do, that life in the locked wards is bizarre; and while on a locked admissions or convalescent ward, he may feel that chronic "back" wards are socially crazy places. But he need only move his sphere of sympathetic participation to the "worst" ward in the hospital, and this, too, can come into social focus as a place with a livable and continuously meaningful social world. This in no way denies that he will find a minority in any ward or patient group that continues to seem quite beyond the capacity to follow rules of social organization, or that the orderly fulfillment of normative expectations in patient society is partly made possible by strategic measures that have somehow come to be institutionalized in mental hospitals.

The career of the mental patient falls popularly and naturalistically into three main phases: the period prior to entering the hospital, which I shall call the prepatient phase; the period in the hospital, the inpatient phase; the period after discharge from the hospital, should this occur, namely, the ex-patient phase.[5] This paper will deal only with the first two phases.

---

[5] This simple picture is complicated by the somewhat special experience of roughly a third of ex-patients–namely, readmission to the hospital, this being the recidivist or "repatient" phase.

THE PREPATIENT PHASE

A relatively small group of prepatients come into the mental hospital willingly, because of their own idea of what will be good for them, or because of wholehearted agreement with the relevant members of their family. Presumably these recruits have found themselves acting in a way which is evidence to them that they are losing their minds or losing control of themselves. This view of oneself would seem to be one of the most pervasively threatening things that can happen to the self in our society, especially since it is likely to occur at a time when the person is in any case sufficiently troubled to exhibit the kind of symptom that he himself can see. As Sullivan described it,

> What we discover in the self-system of a person undergoing schizophrenic change or schizophrenic processes, is then, in its simplest form, an extremely fear-marked puzzlement, consisting of the use of rather generalized and anything but exquisitely refined referential processes in an attempt to cope with what is essentially a failure at being human—a failure at being anything that one could respect as worth being.[6]

Coupled with the person's disintegrative re-evaluation of himself will be the new, almost equally pervasive circumstance of attempting to conceal from others what he takes to be the new fundamental facts about himself, and attempting to discover whether others, too, have discovered them.[7] Here I want to stress that perception of losing one's mind is based on culturally derived and socially engrained stereotypes as to the significance of symptoms such as hearing voices, losing temporal and spatial orientation, and sensing that one is being followed, and that many of the most spectacular and convincing of these symptoms in some instances psychiatrically signify merely a temporary emotional upset in a stressful situation, however terrifying to the person at the time. Similarly, the anxiety consequent upon this perception of oneself, and the strategies devised to reduce this anxiety, are not a product of abnormal psychology, but would be exhibited by any person socialized into our culture who came to conceive of himself as someone losing his mind. Interestingly, subcultures in American society apparently differ in the amount of ready imagery and encouragement they supply for such self-views, leading to differential rates of self-referral; the capacity to take this disintegrative view of oneself without psychiatric

---

[6] Harry Stack Sullivan, *Clinical Studies in Psychiatry*, edited by Helen Swick Perry, Mary Ladd Gawel, and Martha Gibbon (New York: Norton, 1956), pp. 184–5.

[7] This moral experience can be contrasted with that of a person learning to become a marihuana addict, whose discovery that he can be "high" and still "op" effectively without being detected apparently leads to a new level of use. See Howard S. Becker, "Marihuana Use and Social Control," *Social Problems*, III (1955), pp. 35–44; see especially pp. 40–1.

prompting seems to be one of the questionable cultural privileges of the upper classes.[8]

For the person who has come to see himself—with whatever justification—as mentally unbalanced, entrance to the mental hospital can sometimes bring relief, perhaps in part because of the sudden transformation in the structure of his basic social situation; instead of being to himself a questionable person trying to maintain a role as a full one, he can become an officially questioned person known to himself to be not so questionable as that. In other cases, hospitalization can make matters worse for the willing patient, confirming by the objective situation what has theretofore been a matter of the private experience of self.

Once the willing prepatient enters the hospital, he may go through the same routine of experiences as do those who enter unwillingly. In any case, it is the latter that I mainly want to consider, since in America at present these are by far the more numerous kind.[9] Their approach to the institution takes one of three classic forms: they come because they have been implored by their family or threatened with the abrogation of family ties unless they go "willingly"; they come by force under police escort; they come under misapprehension purposely induced by others, this last restricted mainly to youthful prepatients.

The prepatient's career may be seen in terms of an extrusory model; he starts out with relationships and rights, and ends up, at the beginning of his hospital stay, with hardly any of either. The moral aspects of this career, then, typically begin with the experience of abandonment, disloyalty, and embitterment. This is the case even though to others it may be obvious that he was in need of treatment, and even though in the hospital he may soon come to agree.

The case histories of most mental patients document offenses against some arrangement for face-to-face living—a domestic establishment, a workplace, a semipublic organization such as a church or store, a public region such as a street or park. Often there is also a record of some *complainant*, some figure who takes that action against the offender which eventually leads to his hos-pitalization. This may not be the person who makes the first move, but it is the person who makes what turns out to be the first effective move. Here is the *social* beginning of the patient's career, regardless of where one might locate the psychological beginning of his mental illness.

The kinds of offenses which lead to hospitalization are felt to differ in nature from those which lead to other extrusory consequences—to imprisonment, divorce, loss of job, disownment, regional exile, non-institutional

---

[8] See Hollingshead and Redlich, *op. cit.,* p. 187, Table 6, where relative frequency is given of self-referral by social-class grouping.

[9] The distinction employed here between willing and unwilling patients cuts across the legal one of voluntary and committed, since some persons who are glad to come to the mental hospital may be legally committed, and of those who come only because of strong familial pressure, some may sign themselves in as voluntary patients.

psychiatric treatment, and so forth. But little seems known about these differentiating factors; and when one studies actual commitments, alternate outcomes frequently appear to have been possible. It seems true, moreover, that for every offense that leads to an effective complaint, there are many psychiatrically similar ones that never do. No action is taken; or action is taken which leads to other extrusory outcomes; or ineffective action is taken, leading to the mere pacifying or putting off of the person who complains. Thus, as Clausen and Yarrow have nicely shown, even offenders who are eventually hospitalized are likely to have had a long series of ineffective actions taken against them.[10]

Separating those offenses which could have been used as grounds for hospitalizing the offender from those that are so used, one finds a vast number of what students of occupation call career contingencies.[11] Some of these contingencies in the mental patient's career have been suggested, if not explored, such as socio-economic status, visibility of the offense, proximity to a mental hospital, amount of treatment facilities available, community regard for the type of treatment given in available hospitals, and so on.[12] For information about other contingencies one must rely on atrocity tales: a psychotic man is tolerated by his wife until she finds herself a boyfriend, or by his adult children until they move from a house to an apartment; an alcoholic is sent to a mental hospital because the jail is full, and a drug addict because he declines to avail himself of psychiatric treatment on the outside; a rebellious adolescent daughter can no longer be managed at home because she now threatens to have an open affair with an unsuitable companion; and so on. Correspondingly there is an equally important set of contingencies causing the person to by-pass this fate. And should the person enter the hospital, still another set of contingencies will help determine when he is to obtain a discharge—such as the desire of his family for his return, the availability of a "manageable" job, and so on. The society's official view is that inmates of mental hospitals are there primarily because they are suffering from mental illness. However, in the degree that the "mentally ill" outside hospitals numerically approach or surpass those inside hospitals, one could say that mental patients distinctively suffer not from mental illness, but from contingencies.

Career contingencies occur in conjunction with a second feature of the prepatient's career—the circuit of agents—and agencies—that participate

---

[10] Clausen and Yarrow, *op. cit.*

[11] An explicit application of this notion to the field of mental health may be found in Edwin Lemert, "Legal Commitment and Social Control," *Sociology and Social Research*, XXX (1946), pp. 370–78.

[12] For example, Jerome K. Meyers and Leslie Schaffer, "Social Stratification and Psychiatric Practice: A Study of an Outpatient Clinic," *American Sociological Review*, XIX (1954), pp. 307–10; Lemert, *op. cit.*, pp. 402–3; *Patients in Mental Institutions, 1941* (Washington, D.C.: Department of Commerce, Bureau of the Census, 1941), p. 2.

fatefully in his passage from civilian to patient status.[13] Here is an instance of that increasingly important class of social system whose elements are agents and agencies that are brought into systemic connection through having to take up and send on the same persons. Some of these agent roles will be cited now, with the understanding that in any concrete circuit a role may be filled more than once, and that the same person may fill more than one of them.

First is the *next-of-relation*—the person whom the prepatient sees as the most available of those upon whom he should be able to depend most in times of trouble, in this instance the last to doubt his sanity and the first to have done everything to save him from the fate which, it transpires, he has been approaching. The patient's next-of-relation is usually his next of kin; the special term is introduced because he need not be. Second is the *complainant*, the person who retrospectively appears to have started the person on his way to the hospital. Third are the *mediators*—the sequence of agents and agencies to which the prepatient is referred and through which he is relayed and processed on his way to the hospital. Here are included police, clergy, general medical practitioners, office psychiatrists, personnel in public clinics, lawyers, social service workers, schoolteachers, and so on. One of these agents will have the legal mandate to sanction commitment and will exercise it, and so those agents who precede him in the process will be involved in something whose outcome is not yet settled. When the mediators retire from the scene, the prepatient has become an inpatient, and the significant agent has become the hospital administrator.

While the complainant usually takes action in a lay capacity as a citizen, an employer, a neighbor, or a kinsman, mediators tend to be specialists and differ from those they serve in significant ways. They have experience in handling trouble, and some professional distance from what they handle. Except in the case of policemen, and perhaps some clergy, they tend to be more psychiatrically oriented than the lay public, and will see the need for treatment at times when the public does not.[14]

An interesting feature of these roles is the functional effects of their interdigitation. For example, the feelings of the patient will be influenced by whether or not the person who fills the role of complainant also has the role of next-of-relation—an embarrassing combination more prevalent, apparently, in the higher classes than in the lower.[15] Some of these emergent effects will be considered now.[16]

---

[13] For one circuit of agents and its bearing on career contingencies, see Oswald Hall, "The Stages of a Medical Career," *American Journal of Sociology*, LIII (1948), pp. 327–36.

[14] See Cumming and Cumming, *op. cit.*, p. 92.

[15] Hollingshead and Redlich, *op. cit.*, p. 187.

[16] For an analysis of some of these circuit implications for the inpatient, see Leila Deasy and Olive W. Quinn, "The Wife of the Mental Patient and the Hospital Psychiatrist," *Journal of Social Issues*, XI (1955), pp. 49–60. An interesting illustration of this kind of analysis may also be found in Alan G. Cowman, "Blindness and the Role of the

In the prepatient's progress from home to the hospital he may participate as a third person in what he may come to experience as a kind of alienative coalition. His next-of-relation presses him into coming to "talk things over" with a medical practitioner, an office psychiatrist, or some other counselor. Disinclination on his part may be met by threatening him with desertion, disownment, or other legal action, or by stressing the joint and exploratory nature of the interview. But typically the next-of-relation will have set the interview up, in the sense of selecting the professional, arranging for time, telling the professional something about the case, and so on. This move effectively tends to establish the next-of-relation as the responsible person to whom pertinent findings can be divulged, while effectively establishing the other as the patient. The prepatient often goes to the interview with the understanding that he is going as an equal of someone who is so bound together with him that a third person could not come between them in fundamental matters; this, after all, is one way in which close relationships are defined in our society. Upon arrival at the office the prepatient suddenly finds that he and his next-of-relation have not been accorded the same roles, and apparently that a prior understanding between the professional and the next-of-relation has been put in operation against him. In the extreme but common case, the professional first sees the prepatient alone, in the role of examiner and diagnostician, and then sees the next-of-relation alone, in the role of adviser, while carefully avoiding talking things over seriously with them both together.[17] And even in those non-consultative cases where public officials must forcibly extract a person from a family that wants to tolerate him, the next-of-relation is likely to be induced to "go along" with the official action, so that even here the prepatient may feel that an alienative coalition has been formed against him.

The moral experience of being third man in such a coalition is likely to embitter the prepatient, especially since his troubles have already probably led to some estrangement from his next-of-relation. After he enters the hospital, continued visits by his next-of-relation can give the patient the "insight" that his own best interests were being served. But the initial visits may temporarily strengthen his feeling of abandonment; he is likely to beg his visitor to get him out or at least to get him more privileges and to sympathize with the monstrousness of his plight—to which the visitor ordinarily can respond only by trying to maintain a hopeful note, by not "hearing" the requests, or by assuring the patient that the medical authorities know about these things and are doing what is medically best. The visitor then nonchalantly goes back into a world that the patient has learned is incredibly thick with freedom and privileges, causing the patient to feel that his next-of-relation is merely adding a pious gloss to a clear case of traitorous desertion.

Companion," *Social Problems*, IV (1956), pp. 68–75. A general statement may be found in Robert Merton, "The Role Set: Problems in Sociological Theory," *British Journal of Sociology*, VIII (1957), pp. 106–20.

[17] I have one case record of a man who claims he thought *he* was taking his wife to see the psychiatrist, not realizing until too late that his wife had made the arrangements.

The depth to which the patient may feel betrayed by his next-of-relation seems to be increased by the fact that another witnesses his betrayal—a factor that is apparently significant in many three-party situations. An offended person may well act forbearantly and accommodatively toward an offender when the two are alone, choosing peace ahead of justice. The presence of a witness, however, seems to add something to the implications of the offense. For then it is beyond the power of the offended and offender to forget about, erase, or suppress what has happened; the offense has become a public social fact.[18] When the witness is a mental health commission, as is sometimes the case, the witnessed betrayal can verge on a "degradation ceremony."[19] In such circumstances, the offended patient may feel that some kind of extensive reparative action is required before witnesses, if his honor and social weight are to be restored.

Two other aspects of sensed betrayal should be mentioned. First, those who suggest the possibility of another's entering a mental hospital are not likely to provide a realistic picture of how in fact it may strike him when he arrives. Often he is told that he will get required medical treatment and a rest, and may well be out in a few months or so. In some cases they may thus be concealing what they know, but I think, in general, they will be telling what they see as the truth. For here there is quite relevant difference between patients and mediating professionals; mediators, more so than the public at large, may conceive of mental hospitals as short-term medical establishments where required rest and attention can be voluntarily obtained, and not as places of coerced exile. When the prepatient finally arrives he is likely to learn quite quickly, quite differently. He then finds that the information given him about life in the hospital has had the effect of his having put up less resistance to entering than he now sees he would have put up had he known the facts. Whatever the intentions of those who participated in his transition from person to patient, he may sense they have in effect "conned" him into his present predicament.

I am suggesting that the prepatient starts out with at least a portion of the rights, liberties, and satisfactions of the civilian and ends up on a psychiatric ward stripped of almost everything. The question here is how this stripping is managed. This is the second aspect of betrayal I want to consider.

As the prepatient may see it, the circuit of significant figures can function as a kind of betrayal funnel. Passage from person to patient may be effected through a series of linked stages, each managed by a different agent. While each stage tends to bring a sharp decrease in adult free status, each agent may try to maintain the fiction that no further decrease will occur. He may even manage to turn the prepatient over to the next agent while sustaining this note. Further, through words, cues, and gestures, the prepatient is implicitly

[18] A paraphrase from Kurt Riezler, "Comment on the Social Psychology of Shame," *American Journal of Sociology,* XLVIII (1943), p. 458.

[19] See Harold Garfinkel, "Conditions of Successful Degradation Ceremonies," *American Journal of Sociology,* LXI (1956), pp. 420–4.

asked by the current agent to join with him in sustaining a running line of polite small talk that tactfully avoids the administrative facts of the situation, becoming, with each stage, progressively more at odds with these facts. The spouse would rather not have to cry to get the prepatient to visit a psychiatrist; psychiatrists would rather not have a scene when the prepatient learns that he and his spouse are being seen separately and in different ways; the police infrequently bring a prepatient to the hospital in a strait jacket, finding it much easier all around to give him a cigarette, some kindly words, and freedom to relax in the back seat of the patrol car; and finally, the admitting psychiatrist finds he can do his work better in the relative quiet and luxury of the "admission suite" where, as an incidental consequence, the notion can survive that a mental hospital is indeed a comforting place. If the prepatient heeds all of these implied requests and is reasonably decent about the whole thing, he can travel the whole circuit from home to hospital without forcing anyone to look directly at what is happening or to deal with the raw emotion that his situation might well cause him to express. His showing consideration for those who are moving him toward the hospital allows them to show consideration for him, with the joint result that these interactions can be sustained with some of the protective harmony characteristic of ordinary face-to-face dealings. But should the new patient cast his mind back over the sequence of steps leading to hospitalization, he may feel that everyone's current comfort was being busily sustained while his long-range welfare was being undermined. This realization may constitute a moral experience that further separates him for the time from the people on the outside.[20]

I would now like to look at the circuit of career agents from the point of view of the agents themselves. Mediators in the person's transition from civil to patient status—as well as his keepers, once he is in the hospital—have an interest in establishing a responsible next-of-relation as the patient's deputy or guardian; should there be no obvious candidate for the role, someone may be sought out and pressed into it. Thus while a person is gradually being transformed into a patient, a next-of-relation is gradually being transformed into a guardian. With a guardian on the scene, the whole transition process can be kept tidy. He is likely to be familiar with the pre-patient's civil involvements and business, and can tie up loose ends that might otherwise

---

[20] Concentration-camp practices provide a good example of the function of the betrayal funnel in inducing co-operation and reducing struggle and fuss, although here the mediators could not be said to be acting in the best interests of the inmates. Police picking up persons from their homes would sometimes joke good-naturedly and offer to wait while coffee was being served. Gas chambers were fitted out like delousing rooms, and victims taking off their clothes were told to note where they were leaving them. The sick, aged, weak, or insane who were selected for extermination were sometimes driven away in Red Cross ambulances to camps referred to by terms such as "observation hospital." See David Boder, *I Did Not Interview the Dead* (Urbana: University of Illinois Press, 1949), p. 81; and Elie A. Cohen, *Human Behavior in the Concentration Camp* (London: Jonathan Cape, 1954), pp. 32, 37, 107.

be left to entangle the hospital. Some of the prepatient's abrogated civil rights can be transferred to him, thus helping to sustain the legal fiction that while the prepatient does not actually have his rights he somehow actually has not lost them.

Inpatients commonly sense, at least for a time, that hospitalization is a massive unjust deprivation, and sometimes succeed in convincing a few persons on the outside that this is the case. It often turns out to be useful, then, for those identified with inflicting these deprivations, however justifiably, to be able to point to the cooperation and agreement of someone whose relationship to the patient places him above suspicion, firmly defining him as the person most likely to have the patient's personal interest at heart. If the guardian is satisfied with what is happening to the new inpatient, the world ought to be.[21]

Now it would seem that the greater the legitimate personal stake one party has in another, the better he can take the role of guardian to the other. But the structural arrangements in society that lead to the acknowledged merging of two persons' interests lead to additional consequences. For the person to whom the patient turns for help—for protection against such threats as involuntary commitment—is just the person to whom the mediators and hospital administrators logically turn for authorization. It is understandable, then, that some patients will come to sense, at least for a time, that the closeness of a relationship tells nothing of its trustworthiness.

There are still other functional effects emerging from this complement of roles. If and when the next-of-relation appeals to mediators for help in the trouble he is having with the prepatient, hospitalization may not, in fact, be in his mind. He may not even perceive the prepatient as mentally sick, or, if he does, he may not consistently hold to this view.[22] It is the circuit of mediators, with their greater psychiatric sophistication and their belief in the medical character of mental hospitals, that will often define the situation for the next-of-relation, assuring him that hospitalization is a possible solution and a good one, that it involves no betrayal, but is rather a medical action taken in the best interests of the prepatient. Here the next-of-relation may learn that doing his duty to the prepatient may cause the prepatient to distrust and even hate him for the time. But the fact that this course of action may have had to be pointed out and prescribed by professionals, and be defined by them as a moral duty, relieves the next-of-relation of some of the guilt he may

---

[21] Interviews collected by the Clausen group at NIMH suggest that when a wife comes to be a guardian, the responsibility may disrupt previous distance from in-laws, leading either to a new supportive coalition with them or to a marked withdrawal from them.

[22] For an analysis of these non-psychiatric kinds of perception, see Marian Radke Yarrow, Charlotte Green Schwartz, Harriet S. Murphy, and Leila Deasy, "The Psychological Meaning of Mental Illness in the Family," *Journal of Social Issues*, XI (1955), pp. 12–24; Charlotte Green Schwartz, "Perspectives on Deviance—Wives' Definitions of their Husbands Mental Illness," *Psychiatry*, XX (1957), pp. 275–91.

feel.[23] It is a poignant fact that an adult son or daughter may be pressed into the role of mediator, so that the hostility that might otherwise be directed against the spouse is passed on to the child.[24]

Once the prepatient is in the hospital, the same guilt-carrying function may become a significant part of the staff's job in regard to the next-of-relation.[25] These reasons for feeling that he himself has not betrayed the patient, even though the patient may then think so, can later provide the next-of-relation with a defensible line to take when visiting the patient in the hospital and a basis for hoping that the relationship can be re-established after its hospital moratorium. And of course this position, when sensed by the patient, can provide him with excuses for the next-of-relation, when and if he comes to look for them.[26]

Thus while the next-of-relation can perform important functions for the mediators and hospital administrators, they in turn can perform important functions for him. One finds, then, an emergent unintended exchange or reciprocation of functions, these functions themselves being often unintended.

The final point I want to consider about the prepatient's moral career is its peculiarly retroactive character. Until a person actually arrives at the hospital there usually seems no way of knowing for sure that he is destined to do so, given the determinative role of career contingencies. And until the point of hospitalization is reached, he or others may not conceive of him as a person who is becoming a mental patient. However, since he will be held against his will in the hospital, his next-of-relation and the hospital staff will be in great need of a rationale for the hardships they are sponsoring. The medical elements of the staff will also need evidence that they are still in the trade they were trained for. These problems are eased, no doubt unintentionally, by the case-history construction that is placed on the patient's past life, this having the effect of demonstrating that all along he had been becoming sick, that he finally became very sick, and that if he had not been hospitalized much worse things would have happened to him—all of which, of course, may be true. Incidentally, if the patient wants to make sense out of his stay

---

[23] This guilt-carrying function is found, of course, in other role complexes. Thus, when a middle-class couple engages in the process of legal separation or divorce, each of their lawyers usually takes the position that his job is to acquaint his client with all of the potential claims and rights, pressing his client into demanding these, in spite of any nicety of feelings about the rights and honorableness of the ex-partner. The client, in all good faith, can then say to self and to the ex-partner that the demands are being made only because the lawyer insists it is best to do so.

[24] Recorded in the Clausen data.

[25] This point is made by Cumming and Cumming, *op. cit.*, p. 129.

[26] There is an interesting contrast here with the moral career of the tuberculosis patient. I am told by Julius Roth that tuberculous patients are likely to come to the hospital willingly, agreeing with their next-of-relation about treatment. Later in their hospital career, when they learn how long they yet have to stay and how depriving and irrational some of the hospital rulings are, they may seek to leave, be advised against this by the staff and by relatives, and only then begin to feel betrayed.

in the hospital, and, as already suggested, keep alive the possibility of once again conceiving of his next-of-relation as a decent, well-meaning person, then he, too, will have reason to believe some of this psychiatric work-up of his past.

Here is a very ticklish point for the sociology of careers. An important aspect of every career is the view the person constructs when he looks backward over his progress; in a sense, however, the whole of the prepatient career derives from this reconstruction. The fact of having had a prepatient career, starting with an effective complaint, becomes an important part of the mental patient's orientation, but this part can begin to be played only after hospitalization proves that what he had been having, but no longer has, is a career as a prepatient.

How Stigma Interferes With Mental Health Care

Patrick Corrigan

I made an additional distinction about stigma that has been applied to more general work with all health conditions (Corrigan & Penn, 1999; Corrigan & Watson, 2002). I have distinguished *public stigma* (what a naive public does to the stigmatized group when they endorse the prejudice about that group) and *self-stigma* (what members of a stigmatized group may do to themselves if they internalize the public stigma). The ramification of this distinction for understanding the link between stigma and care seeking is important, although their impact is likely to interact with and augment each other.

PUBLIC STIGMA: HARM TO SOCIAL OPPORTUNITIES

Stigma harms people who are publicly labeled as mentally ill in several ways. Stereotype, prejudice, and discrimination can rob people labeled mentally ill of important life opportunities that are essential for achieving life goals. People with mental illness are frequently unable to obtain good jobs or find suitable housing because of the prejudice of key members in their communities: employers and landlords. Several studies have shown that public stereotypes and prejudice about mental illness have a deleterious impact on obtaining and keeping good jobs (Bordieri & Drehmer, 1986; Farina & Felner, 1973; Farina, Felner, & Bourdreau, 1973; Link, 1982, 1987; Olshansky, Grab, & Ekdhal, 1960; Wahl, 1999; Webber & Orcutt, 1984) and leasing safe housing (Aviram & Segal, 1973; Farina,

Thaw, Lovern, & Mangone, 1974; R. Hogan, 1985a, 1985b; Page, 1977, 1983, 1995; Segal, Baumohl, & Moyles, 1980; Wahl, 1999).

Stigma also influences the interface between mental illness and the criminal justice system. Criminalizing mental illness occurs when police, rather than the mental health system, respond to mental health crises, thereby contributing to the increasing prevalence of people with serious mental illness in jail (Watson, Ottati, Corrigan, & Heyrman, in press). Persons exhibiting symptoms and signs of serious mental illness are more likely than others to be arrested by the police (Teplin, 1984). Moreover, people with mental illness tend to spend more time incarcerated than those without mental illness (Steadman, McCarthy, & Morrissey, 1989). The growing intolerance of offenders in general has led to harsher laws and has hampered effective treatment planning for mentally ill offenders (Jemeka, Trupin, & Chiles, 1989; Lamb & Weinberger, 1998).

The negative impact of public stigma is also observed in the general health care system; people labeled mentally ill are less likely to benefit from the depth and breadth of available physical health care services than people without these illnesses. Druss and colleagues completed two studies on archival data that suggested people with mental illness receive fewer medical services than those not labeled in this manner (Desai, Rosenheck, Druss, & Perlin, 2002; Druss & Rosenheck, 1997). Moreover, studies by this group suggest that individuals with mental illness are less likely to receive the same range of insurance benefits as people without mental illness (Druss, Allen, & Bruce, 1998; Druss & Rosenheck, 1997). An additional study seems to implicate stigma more directly. Druss, Bradford, Rosenheck, Radford, and Krumholz (2000) examined the likelihood of a range of medical procedures after myocardial infarction in a sample of 113,653 individuals. Compared with the remainder of the sample, Druss et al. (2000) found that people identified with comorbid psychiatric disorder were significantly less likely to undergo percutaneous transluminal coronary angioplasty. Once again, mental illness is indicated as a barrier to receiving appropriate care.

Combined, this evidence suggests that public identification as "mentally ill" can yield significant harm. Research has suggested that people with concealable stigmas (people who are gay, of minority faith-based communities, or with mental illness) decide to avoid this harm by hiding their stigma and staying in the closet (Corrigan & Matthews, 2003). Alternatively, they may opt to avoid the stigma all together by denying their group status and by not seeking the institutions that mark them (i.e., mental health care). This kind of label avoidance is perhaps the most significant way in which stigma impedes care seeking.

SELF-STIGMA: HARM TO SELF-ESTEEM

People may also avoid the stigma of mental illness because of stigma's potential effects on one's sense of self. Living in a culture steeped in stigmatizing images, persons with mental illness may accept these notions and suffer diminished self-esteem, self-efficacy, and confidence in one's future (Corrigan, 1998; Holmes & River, 1998). Research shows that people with mental illness often internalize stigmatizing ideas that are widely endorsed within society and believe that they are less valued because of their psychiatric disorder (Link, 1987; Link & Phelan, 2001). Persons who agree with prejudice concur with the stereotype "That's right; I am weak and unable to care for myself!" Self-prejudice leads to negative emotional reactions; prominent among these is low self-esteem and low self-efficacy (Link, Struening, Neese-Todd, Asmussen, & Phelan, 2001; Markowitz, 1998). *Self-esteem* is typically operationalized as diminished views about personal worth (Corrigan, Faber, Rashid, & Leary, 1999; Rosenberg, 1965) and is often experienced as shame. Families frequently report an intense sense of shame secondarily as a result of a member's mental illness (Corrigan & Miller, 2004). *Self-efficacy* is defined as the expectation that one can successfully perform a behavior in a specific situation (Bandura, 1977, 1989). Low self-efficacy and demoralization has been shown to be associated with failing to pursue work or independent living opportunities at which people with mental illness might otherwise succeed (Link, 1982, 1987). Obviously, this kind of self-prejudice and self-discrimination significantly interferes with a person's life goals and quality of life.

Fundamental suppositions of social psychological research on prejudice suggest why self-stigma would dissuade people from being labeled and seeking treatment (Jost & Banaji, 1994). People in general are motivated to stigmatize others because of ego (Adorno, Frenkel-Bruns-wik, Levinson, & Sanford, 1950; Katz & Braly, 1935; Lippmann, 1922) or group enhancement (Tajfel, 1981). Instead of thinking "I am not competent," individuals buffer their self- or group's image against interpersonal failings by viewing others as incompetent; in this case, people with mental illness (among the many possible stigmatized groups) are deficient. Hence, people avoid being labeled mentally ill, thereby escaping the negative statements that lessen self-esteem and self-efficacy.

Research has shown a significant relationship between shame and avoiding treatment. The measures used in the study by Sirey, Bruce, Alexopoulos, Perlick, Raue, et al. (2001)—the Scale of Perceived Stigma (Link et al., 1989)—included a proxy of shame. Research participants who expressed a sense of shame from personal experiences with mental illness were less likely to be involved in treatment. Family shame was also a significant predictor of treatment avoidance. Results of the

Yale component of the ECA data (Leaf, Bruce, Tischler, & Holzer, 1987) showed that respondents with psychiatric diagnoses were more likely to avoid services if they believed family members would have a negative reaction to these services, that is, if they learned from their family that being identified as mentally ill disgraced themselves and/or their family. Conversely, positive attitudes of family members were associated with greater service use in a sample of more than 1,000 drawn from a representative community sample and a group from a mental health clinic (Greenley, Mechanic, & Cleary, 1987). Hence, the potential of self-stigma can yield label avoidance and decreased treatment participation. A point made earlier in this article is reiterated here. What is presented as self-stigma here is clearly influenced by public stigma. Hence, the two constructs, and their impact on care seeking, are best understood in interaction.

Patrick Corrigan. 1994. "How Stigma Interferes with Mental Health Care." *American Psychologist* 59(7):614–625.

THE INPATIENT PHASE

The last step in the prepatient's career can involve his realization—justified or not—that he has been deserted by society and turned out of relationships by those closest to him. Interestingly enough, the patient, especially a first admission, may manage to keep himself from coming to the end of this trail, even though in fact he is now in a locked mental hospital ward. On entering the hospital, he may very strongly feel the desire not to be known to anyone as a person who could possibly be reduced to these present circumstances, or as a person who conducted himself in the way he did prior to commitment. Consequently, he may avoid talking to anyone, may stay by himself when possible, and may even be "out of contact" or "manic" so as to avoid ratifying any interaction that presses a politely reciprocal role upon him and opens him up to what he has become in the eyes of others. When the next-of-relation makes an effort to visit, he may be rejected by mutism, or by the patient's refusal to enter the visiting room, these strategies sometimes suggesting that the patient still clings to a remnant of relatedness to those who made up his past, and is protecting this remnant from the final destructiveness of dealing with the new people that they have become.[27]

---

[27] The inmate's initial strategy of holding himself aloof from ratifying contact may partly account for the relative lack of group formation among inmates in public mental hospitals, a connection that has been suggested to me by William R. Smith. The desire to avoid personal bonds that would give licence to the asking of biographical questions could also be a factor. In mental hospitals, of course, as in prisoner camps,

Usually the patient comes to give up this taxing effort at anonymity, at not-hereness, and begins to present himself for conventional social interaction to the hospital community. Thereafter he withdraws only in special ways—by always using his nickname, by signing his contribution to the patient weekly with his initial only, or by using the innocuous "cover" address tactfully provided by some hospitals; or he withdraws only at special times, when, say, a flock of nursing students makes a passing tour of the ward, or when, paroled to the hospital grounds, he suddenly sees he is about to cross the path of a civilian he happens to know from home. Sometimes this making of oneself available is called "settling down" by the attendants. It marks a new stand openly taken and supported by the patient, and resembles the "coming-out" process that occurs in other groupings.[28]

Once the prepatient begins to settle down, the main outlines of his fate tend to follow those of a whole class of segregated establishments—jails, concentration camps, monasteries, work camps, and so on—in which the inmate spends the whole round of life on the grounds, and marches through his regimented day in the immediate company of a group of persons of his own institutional status.

Like the neophyte in many of these total institutions, the new inpatient finds himself cleanly stripped of many of his accustomed affirmations, satisfactions, and defenses, and is subjected to a rather full set of mortifying experiences: restriction of free movement, communal living, diffuse authority of a whole echelon of people, and so on. Here one begins to learn about the limited extent to which a conception of oneself can be sustained when the usual setting of supports for it are suddenly removed.

While undergoing these humbling moral experiences, the inpatient learns to orient himself in terms of the "ward system."[29] In public mental hospitals this usually consists of a series of graded living arrangements built around wards, administrative units called services, and parole statuses. The "worst"

the staff may consciously break up incipient group formation in order to avoid collective rebellious action and other ward disturbances.

[28] A comparable coming out occurs in the homosexual world, when a person finally comes frankly to present himself to a "gay" gathering not as a tourist but as someone who is "available." See Evelyn Hooker, "A Preliminary Analysis of Group Behavior of Homosexuals," *Journal of Psychology*, XLII (1956), pp. 217–25; see especially p. 221. A good fictionalized treatment may be found in James Baldwin's *Giovanni's Room* (New York: Dial, 1956), pp. 41–57. A familiar Instance of the coming-oat process is no doubt to be found among prepubertal children at the moment one of these actors sidles *back* into a room that had been left in an angered huff and injured *amour propre*. The phrase itself presumably derives from a *rite-de-passage* ceremony once arranged by upper-class mothers for their daughters. Interestingly enough, in large mental hospitals the patient sometimes symbolizes a complete coming out by his first active participation in the hospital-wide patient dance.

[29] A good description of the ward system may be found in Ivan Belknap, *Human Problems of a State Mental Hospital* (New York: McGraw-Hill, 1956), ch. ix, especially p. 164.

level often involves nothing but wooden benches to sit on, some quite indifferent food, and a small piece of room to sleep in. The "best" level may involve a room of one's own, ground and town privileges, contacts with staff that are relatively undamaging, and what is seen as good food and ample recreational facilities. For disobeying the pervasive house rules, the inmate will receive stringent punishments expressed in terms of loss of privileges; for obedience he will eventually be allowed to reacquire some of the minor satisfactions he took for granted on the outside.

The institutionalization of these radically different levels of living throws light on the implications for self of social settings. And this in turn affirms that the self arises not merely out of its possessor's interactions with significant others, but also out of the arrangements that are evolved in an organization for its members.

There are some settings that the person easily discounts as an expression or extension of him. When a tourist goes slumming, he may take pleasure in the situation not because it is a reflection of him but because it so assuredly is not. There are other settings, such as living rooms, which the person manages on his own and employs to influence in a favorable direction other persons' views of him. And there are still other settings, such as a workplace, which express the employee's occupational status, but over which he has no final control, this being exerted, however tactfully, by his employer. Mental hospitals provide an extreme instance of this latter possibility. And this is due not merely to their uniquely degraded living levels, but also to the unique way in which significance for self is made explicit to the patient, piercingly, persistently, and thoroughly. Once lodged on a given ward, the patient is firmly instructed that the restrictions and deprivations he encounters are not due to such blind forces as tradition or economy—and hence dissociable from self—but are intentional parts of his treatment, part of his need at the time, and therefore an expression of the state that his self has fallen to. Having every reason to initiate requests for better conditions, he is told that when the staff feel he is "able to manage" or will be "comfortable with" a higher ward level, then appropriate action will be taken. In short, assignment to a given ward is presented not as a reward or punishment, but as an expression of his general level of social functioning, his status as a person. Given the fact that the worst ward levels provide a round of life that inpatients with organic brain damage can easily manage, and that these quite limited human beings are present to prove it, one can appreciate some of the mirroring effects of the hospital.[30]

The ward system, then, is an extreme instance of how the physical facts of an establishment can be explicitly employed to frame the conception a per-

---

[30] Here is one way in which mental hospitals can be worse than concentration camps and prisons as places in which to "do" time; in the latter, self-insulation from the symbolic implications of the settings may be easier. In fact, self-insulation from hospital settings may be so difficult that patients have to employ devices for this which staff interpret as psychotic symptoms.

son takes of himself. In addition, the official psychiatric mandate of mental hospitals gives rise to even more direct, even more blatant, attacks upon the inmate's view of himself. The more "medical" and the more progressive a mental hospital is—the more it attempts to be therapeutic and not merely custodial—the more he may be confronted by high-ranking staff arguing that his past has been a failure, that the cause of this has been within himself, that his attitude to life is wrong, and that if he wants to be a person he will have to change his way of dealing with people and his conceptions of himself. Often the moral value of these verbal assaults will be brought home to him by requiring him to practice taking this psychiatric view of himself in arranged confessional periods, whether in private sessions or group psychotherapy.

Now a general point may be made about the moral career of inpatients which has bearing on many moral careers. Given the stage that any person has reached in a career, one typically finds that he constructs an image of his life course—past, present, and future—which selects, abstracts, and distorts in such a way as to provide him with a view of himself that he can usefully expound in current situations. Quite generally, the person's line concerning self-defensively brings him into appropriate alignment with the basic values of his society, and so may be called an apologia. If the person can manage to present a view of his current situation that shows the operation of favorable personal qualities in the past and a favorable destiny awaiting him, it may be called a success story. If the facts of a person's past and present are extremely dismal, then about the best he can do is to show that he is not responsible for what has become of him, and the term sad tale is appropriate. Interestingly enough, the more the person's past forces him out of apparent alignment with central moral values, the more often he seems compelled to tell his sad tale in any company in which he finds himself. Perhaps he partly responds to the need he feels in others of not having their sense of proper life courses affronted. In any case, it is among convicts, "winos," and prostitutes that one seems to obtain sad tales the most readily.[31] It is the vicissitudes of the mental patient's sad tale that I want to consider now.

---

[31] In regard to convicts, see Anthony Heckstall-Smith, *Eighteen Months* (London: Allan Wingate, 1954), pp. 52–3. For "winos" see the discussion in Howard G. Bain. "A Sociological Analysis of the Chicago Skid-Row Lifeway" (Unpublished M.A. thesis, Department of Sociology, University of Chicago, September 1950), especially "The Rationale of the Skid-Row Drinking Group," pp. 141–6. Bain's neglected thesis is a useful source of material on moral careers.

Apparently one of the occupational hazards of prostitution is that clients and other professional contacts sometimes persist in expressing sympathy by asking for a defensible dramatic explanation for the fall from grace. In having to bother to have a sad tale ready, perhaps the prostitute is more to be pitied than damned. Good examples of prostitute sad tales may be found in Henry Mayhew, *London Labour and the London Poor*, Vol. IV, *Those That Will Not Work* (London: Charles Griffin and Co., 1862), pp. 210–72. For a contemporary source, see *Women of the Streets*, edited by C. H. Rolph (London: Secker and Warburg, 1955), especially p. 6: "*Almost always, however,*

In the mental hospital, the setting and the house rules press home to the patient that he is, after all, a mental case who has suffered some kind of social collapse on the outside, having failed in some over-all way, and that here he is of little social weight, being hardly capable of acting like a full-fledged person at all. These humiliations are likely to be most keenly felt by middle-class patients, since their previous condition of life little immunizes them against such affronts, but all patients feel some downgrading. Just as any normal member of his outside subculture would do, the patient often responds to this situation by attempting to assert a sad tale proving that he is not "sick," that the "little trouble" he did get into was really somebody else's fault, that his past life course had some honor and rectitude, and that the hospital is therefore unjust in forcing the status of mental patient upon him. This self-respecting tendency is heavily institutionalized within the patient society where opening social contacts typically involve the participants' volunteering information about their current ward location and length of stay so far, but not the reasons for their stay—such interaction being conducted in the manner of small talk on the outside.[32] With greater familiarity, each patient usually volunteers relatively acceptable reasons for his hospitalization, at the same time accepting without open immediate question the lines offered by other patients. Such stories as the following are given and overtly accepted.

> I was going to night school to get a M.A. degree, and holding down a job in addition, and the load got too much for me.
> The others here are sick mentally but I'm suffering from a bad nervous system and that is what is giving me these phobias.
> I got here by mistake because of a diabetes diagnosis, and I'll leave in a couple of days. [The patient had been in seven weeks.]
> I failed as a child, and later with my wife I reached out for dependency.
> My trouble is that I can't work. That's what I'm in for. I had two jobs with a good home and all the money I wanted.[33]

The patient sometimes reinforces these stories by an optimistic definition of his occupational status. A man who managed to obtain an audition as a radio announcer styles himself a radio announcer; another who worked for

---

after a few comments on the police, the girl would begin to explain how it was that she was in the life, usually in terms of self-justification...." Lately, of course, the psychological expert has helped out the profession in the construction of wholly remarkable sad tales. See, for example, Harold Greenwald, *The Call Girl* (New York: Ballantine Books, 1958).

[32] A similar self-protecting rule has been observed in prisons. Thus, Alfred Hassler, *Diary of a Self-Made Convict* (Chicago: Regnery, 1954), p. 76, in describing a conversation with a fellow prisoner: *"He didn't say much about why he was sentenced, and I didn't ask him, that being the accepted behavior in prison."* A novelistic version for the mental hospital may be found in J. Kerkhoff, *How Thin the Veil: A Newspaperman's Story of His Own Mental Crack-up and Recovery* (New York: Greenberg, 1952), p. 27.

[33] From the writer's field notes of informal interaction with patients, transcribed as nearly verbatim as he was able.

some months as a copy boy and was then given a job as a reporter on a large trade journal, but fired after three weeks, defines himself as a reporter.

A whole social role in the patient community may be constructed on the basis of these reciprocally sustained fictions. For these face-to-face niceties tend to be qualified by behind-the-back gossip that comes only a degree closer to the "objective" facts. Here, of course, one can see a classic social function of informal networks of equals: they serve as one another's audience for self-supporting tales—tales that are somewhat more solid than pure fantasy and somewhat thinner than the facts.

But the patient's apologia is called forth in a unique setting, for few settings could be so destructive of self-stories except, of course, those stories already constructed along psychiatric lines. And this destructiveness rests on more than the official sheet of paper which attests that the patient is of unsound mind, a danger to himself and others—an attestation, incidentally, which seems to cut deeply into the patient's pride, and into the possibility of his having any.

Certainly the degrading conditions of the hospital setting belie many of the self-stories that are presented by patients, and the very fact of being in the mental hospital is evidence against these tales. And of course there is not always sufficient patient solidarity to prevent patient discrediting patient, just as there is not always a sufficient number of "professionalized" attendants to prevent attendant discrediting patient. As one patient informant repeatedly suggested to a fellow patient:

If you're so smart, how come you got your ass in here?

The mental-hospital setting, however, is more treacherous still. Staff have much to gain through discreditings of the patient's story—whatever the felt reason for such discreditings. If the custodial faction in the hospital is to succeed in managing his daily round without complaint or trouble from him, then it will prove useful to be able to point out to him that the claims about himself upon which he rationalizes his demands are false, that he is not what he is claiming to be, and that in fact he is a failure as a person. If the psychiatric faction is to impress upon him its views about his personal make-up, then they must be able to show in detail how their version of his past and their version of his character hold up much better than his own.[34] If both the custodial and psychiatric factions are to get him to co-operate in the various

---

[34] The process of examining a person psychiatrically and then altering or reducing his status in consequence is known in hospital and prison parlance as bugging, the assumption being that once you come to the attention of the testers you either will automatically be labeled crazy or the process of testing itself will make you crazy. Thus psychiatric staff are sometimes seen not as discovering whether you are sick, but as making you sick; and "Don't bug me, man" can mean, "Don't pester me to the point where I'll get upset." Sheldon Messinger has suggested to me that this meaning of bugging is related to the other colloquial meaning, of wiring a room with a secret microphone to collect information usable for discrediting the speaker.

psychiatric treatments, then it will prove useful to disabuse him of his view of their purposes, and cause him to appreciate that they know what they are doing, and are doing what is best for him. In brief, the difficulties caused by a patient are closely tied to his version of what has been happening to him, and if co-operation is to be secured, it helps if this version is discredited. The patient must "insightfully" come to take, or affect to take, the hospital's view of himself.

The staff also have ideal means—in addition to the mirroring effect of the setting–for denying the inmate's rationalizations. Current psychiatric doctrine defines mental disorder as something that can have its roots in the patient's earliest years, show its signs throughout the course of his life, and invade almost every sector of his current activity. No segment of his past or present need be defined, then, as beyond the jurisdiction and mandate of psychiatric assessment. Mental hospitals bureaucratically institutional-ize this extremely wide mandate by formally basing their treatment of the patient upon his diagnosis and hence upon the psychiatric view of his past.

The case record is an important expression of this mandate. This dos-sier is apparently not regularly used, however, to record occasions when the patient showed capacity to cope honorably and effectively with difficult life situations. Nor is the case record typically used to provide a rough average or sampling of his past conduct. One of its purposes is to show the ways in which the patient is "sick" and the reasons why it was right to commit him and is right currently to keep him committed; and this is done by extract-ing from his whole life course a list of those incidents that have or might have had "symptomatic" significance.[35] The misadventures of his parents or siblings that might suggest a "taint" may be cited. Early acts in which the patient appeared to have shown bad judgment or emotional disturbance will be recorded. Occasions when he acted in a way which the layman would consider immoral, sexually perverted, weak-willed, childish, ill-considered, impulsive, and crazy may be described. Misbehaviors which someone saw as the last straw, as cause for immediate action, are likely to be reported in detail. In addition, the record will describe his state on arrival at the hos-pital—and this is not likely to be a time of tranquillity and ease for him. The record may also report the false line taken by the patient in answering

---

[35] While many kinds of organization maintain records of their members, in almost all of these some socially significant attributes can only be included indirectly, being officially irrelevant. But since mental hospitals have a legitimate claim to deal with the "whole" person, they need officially recognize no limits to what they consider relevant, a sociologically interesting licence. It is an odd historical fact that persons concerned with promoting civil liberties in other areas of life tend to favor giving the psychiatrist complete discretionary power over the patient. Apparently it is felt that the more power possessed by medically qualified administrators and therapists, the better the interests of the patients will be served. Patients, to my knowledge, have not been polled on this matter.

embarrassing questions, showing him as someone who makes claims that are obviously contrary to the facts:

> Claims she lives with oldest daughter or with sisters only when sick and in need of care; otherwise with husband, he himself says not for twelve years.
> Contrary to the reports from the personnel, he says he no longer bangs on the floor or cries in the morning.
> ...conceals fact that she had her organs removed, claims she is still menstruating.
> At first she denied having had premarital sexual experience, but when asked about Jim she said she had forgotten about it 'cause it had been unpleasant.[36]

Where contrary facts are not known by the recorder, their presence is often left scrupulously an open question:

> The patient denied any heterosexual experiences nor could one trick her into admitting that she had ever been pregnant or into any kind of sexual indulgence, denying masturbation as well.
> Even with considerable pressure she was unwilling to engage in any projection of paranoid mechanisms.
> No psychotic content could be elicited at this time.[37]

And if in no more factual way, discrediting statements often appear in descriptions given of the patient's general social manner in the hospital:

> When interviewed, he was bland, apparently self-assured, and sprinkles high-sounding generalizations freely throughout his verbal productions.
> Armed with a rather neat appearance and natty little Hitlerian mustache this 45 year old man who has spent the last five or more years of his life in the hospital, is making a very successful hospital adjustment living within the role of a rather gay liver and jim-dandy type of fellow who is not only quite superior to his fellow patients in intellectual respects but who is also quite a man with women. His speech is sprayed with many multi-syllabled words which he generally uses in good context, but if he talks long enough on any subject it soon becomes apparent that he is so completely lost in this verbal diarrhea as to make what he says almost completely worthless.[38]

The events recorded in the case history are, then, just the sort that a layman would consider scandalous, defamatory, and discrediting. I think it is fair to say that all levels of mental-hospital staff fail, in general, to deal with this material with the moral neutrality claimed for medical statements and psychiatric diagnosis, but instead participate, by intonation and gesture if by no other means, in the lay reaction to these acts. This will occur in staff-patient encounters as well as in staff encounters at which no patient is present.

---

[36] Verbatim transcriptions of hospital case-record material.
[37] Verbatim transcriptions of hospital case-record material.
[38] Verbatim transcriptions of hospital case-record material.

In some mental hospitals, access to the case record is technically restricted to medical and higher nursing levels, but even here informal access or relayed information is often available to lower staff levels.[39] In addition, ward personnel are felt to have a right to know those aspects of the patient's past conduct which, embedded in the reputation he develops, purportedly make it possible to manage him with greater benefit to himself and less risk to others. Further, all staff levels typically have access to the nursing notes kept on the ward, which chart the daily course of each patient's disease, and hence his conduct, providing for the near present the sort of information the case record supplies for his past.

I think that most of the information gathered in case records is quite true, although it might seem also to be true that almost anyone's life course could yield up enough denigrating facts to provide grounds for the record's justification of commitment. In any case, I am not concerned here with questioning the desirability of maintaining case records, or the motives of staff in keeping them. The point is that, these facts about him being true, the patient is certainly not relieved from the normal cultural pressure to conceal them, and is perhaps all the more threatened by knowing that they are neatly available, and that he has no control over who gets to learn them.[40] A manly looking

---

[39] However, some mental hospitals do have a "hot file" of selected records which can be taken out only by special permission. These may be records of patients who work as administration-office messengers and might otherwise snatch glances at their own files; of inmates who had elite status in the environing community; and of inmates who may take legal action against the hospital and hence have a special reason to maneuver access to their records. Some hospitals even have a "hot-hot file," kept in the superintendent's office. In addition, the patient's professional title, especially if it is a medical one, is sometimes purposely omitted from his file card. All of these exceptions to the general rule for handling information show, of course, the institution's realization of some of the implications of keeping mental-hospital records. For a further example, see Harold Taxel, "Authority Structure in a Mental Hospital Ward" (Unpublished M.A. thesis, Department of Sociology, University of Chicago, 1953), pp. 11–12.

[40] This is the problem of "information control" that many groups suffer from in varying degrees. See Goffman, "Discrepant Roles," in *The Presentation of Self in Everyday Life* (New York: Anchor Books, 1959), ch. iv, pp. 141–166. A suggestion of this problem in relation to case records in prisons is given by James Peck in his story, "The Ship that Never Hit Port," in *Prison Etiquette,* edited by Holley Cantine and Dachine Rainer (Bearsville, N.Y.: Retort Press, 1950), p. 66:

"The hacks of course hold all the aces in dealing with any prisoner because they can always write him up for inevitable punishment. Every infraction of the rules is noted in the prisoner's jacket, a folder which records all the details of the man's life before and during imprisonment. There are general reports written by the work detail screw, the cell block screw, or some other screw who may have overheard a conversation. Tales pumped from stoolpigeons are also included.

"Any letter which interests the authorities goes into the jacket. The mail censor may make a photostatic copy of a prisoner's entire letter, or merely copy a passage. Or he may pass the letter on to the warden. Often an inmate called out by the warden or parole officer is confronted

youth who responds to military induction by running away from the bar-racks and hiding himself in a hotel-room clothes closet, to be found there, crying, by his mother; a woman who travels from Utah to Washington to warn the president of impending doom; a man who disrobes before three young girls; a boy who locks his sister out of the house, striking out two of her teeth when she tries to come back in through the window—each of these persons has done something he will have very obvious reason to conceal from others, and very good reason to tell lies about.

The formal and informal patterns of communication linking staff mem-bers tend to amplify the disclosive work done by the case record. A discred-itable act that the patient performs during one part of the day's routine in one part of the hospital community is likely to be reported back to those who supervise other areas of his life where he implicitly takes the stand that he is not the sort of person who could act that way.

Of significance here, as in some other social establishments, is the increasingly common practice of all-level staff conferences, where staff air their views of patients and develop collective agreement concerning the line that the patient is trying to take and the line that should be taken to him. A patient who develops a "personal" relation with an attendant, or man-ages to make an attendant anxious by eloquent and persistent accusations of malpractice, can be put back into his place by means of the staff meeting, where the attendant is given warning or assurance that the patient is "sick." Since the differential image of himself that a person usually meets from those of various levels around him comes here to be unified behind the scenes into a common approach, the patient may find himself faced with a kind of collusion against him—albeit one sincerely thought to be for his own ultimate welfare.

In addition, the formal transfer of the patient from one ward or service to another is likely to be accompanied by an informal description of his char-acteristics, this being felt to facilitate the work of the employee who is newly responsible for him.

Finally, at the most informal of levels, the lunchtime and coffee-break small talk of staff often turns upon the latest doings of the patient, the gossip level of any social establishment being here intensified by the assumption that everything about him is in some way the proper business of the hos-pital employee. Theoretically there seems to be no reason why such gossip should not build up the subject instead of tear him down, unless one claims that talk about those not present will always tend to be critical in order to maintain the integrity and prestige of the circle in which the talking occurs. And so, even when the impulse of the speakers seems kindly and generous, the implication of their talk is typically that the patient is not a complete

with something he wrote so long ago he had forgot all about it. It might be about his personal life or his political views—a fragment of thought that the prison authorities felt was danger-ous and filed for later use."

person. For example, a conscientious group therapist, sympathetic with patients, once admitted to his coffee companions:

> I've had about three group disrupters, one man in particular—a lawyer [*sotto voce*] James Wilson—very bright—who just made things miserable for me, but I would always tell him to get on the stage and do something. Well, I was getting desperate and then I bumped into his therapist, who said that right now behind the man's bluff and front he needed the group very much and that it probably meant more to him than anything else he was getting out of the hospital—he just needed the support. Well, that made me feel altogether different about him. He's out now.

In general, then, mental hospitals systematically provide for circulation about each patient the kind of information that the patient is likely to try to hide. And in various degrees of detail this information is used daily to puncture his claims. At the admission and diagnostic conferences, he will be asked questions to which he must give wrong answers in order to maintain his self-respect, and then the true answer may be shot back at him. An attendant whom he tells a version of his past and his reason for being in the hospital may smile disbelievingly, or say, "That's not the way I heard it," in line with the practical psychiatry of bringing the patient down to reality. When he accosts a physician or nurse on the ward and presents his claims for more privileges or for discharge, this may be countered by a question which he cannot answer truthfully without calling up a time in his past when he acted disgracefully. When he gives his view of his situation during group psychotherapy, the therapist, taking the role of interrogator, may attempt to disabuse him of his face-saving interpretations and encourage an interpretation suggesting that it is he himself who is to blame and who must change. When he claims to staff or fellow patients that he is well and has never been really sick, someone may give him graphic details of how, only one month ago, he was prancing around like a girl, or claiming that he was God, or declining to talk or eat, or putting gum in his hair.

Each time the staff deflates the patient's claims, his sense of what a person ought to be and the rules of peer-group social intercourse press him to reconstruct his stories; and each time he does this, the custodial and psychiatric interests of the staff may lead them to discredit these tales again.

Behind these verbally instigated ups and downs of the self is an institutional base that rocks just as precariously. Contrary to popular opinion, the "ward system" insures a great amount of internal social mobility in mental hospitals, especially during the inmate's first year. During that time he is likely to have altered his service once, his ward three or four times, and his parole status several times; and he is likely to have experienced moves in bad as well as good directions. Each of these moves involves a very drastic alteration in level of living and in available materials out of which to build a self-confirming round of activities, an alteration equivalent in scope, say, to a move up or down a class in the wider class system. Moreover, fellow inmates with whom he has partially identified himself will similarly be moving, but in different directions and at different rates, thus reflecting feelings of social change to the person even when he does not experience them directly.

As previously implied, the doctrines of psychiatry can reinforce the social fluctuations of the ward system. Thus there is a current psychiatric view that the ward system is a kind of social hothouse in which patients start as social infants and end up, within the year, on convalescent wards as resocialized adults. This view adds considerably to the weight and pride that staff can attach to their work, and necessitates a certain amount of blindness, especially at higher staff levels, to other ways of viewing the ward system, such as a method for disciplining unruly persons through punishment and reward. In any case, this resocialization perspective tends to overstress the extent to which those on the worst wards are incapable of socialized conduct and the extent to which those on the best wards are ready and willing to play the social game. Because the ward system is something more than a resocialization chamber, inmates find many reasons for "messing up" or getting into trouble, and many occasions, then, for demotion to less privileged ward positions. These demotions may be officially interpreted as psychiatric relapses or moral backsliding, thus protecting the resocialization view of the hospital; these interpretations, by implication, translate a mere infraction of rules and consequent demotion into a fundamental expression of the status of the culprit's self. Correspondingly, promotions, which may come about because of ward population pressure, the need for a "working patient," or for other psychiatrically irrelevant reasons, may be built up into something claimed to be profoundly expressive of the patient's whole self. The patient himself may be expected by staff to make a personal effort to "get well," in something less than a year, and hence may be constantly reminded to think in terms of the self's success and failure.[41]

In such contexts inmates can discover that deflations in moral status are not so bad as they had imagined. After all, infractions that lead to these demotions cannot be accompanied by legal sanctions or by reduction to the status of mental patient, since these conditions already prevail. Further, no past or current delict seems to be horrendous enough in itself to excommunicate a patient from the patient community, and hence failures at right living lose some of their stigmatizing meaning.[42] And finally, in accepting the hospital's version of his fall from grace, the patient can set himself up in the business of "straightening up," and make claims of sympathy, privileges, and indulgence from the staff in order to foster this.

Learning to live under conditions of imminent exposure and wide fluctuation in regard, with little control over the granting or withholding of this regard, is an important step in the socialization of the patient, a step that tells something important about what it is like to be an inmate in a mental hospital. Having one's past mistakes and present progress under constant moral

---

[41] For this and other suggestions, I am indebted to Charlotte Green Schwartz.
[42] See "The Underlife of a Public Institution," this book, fn. 167.

review seems to make for a special adaptation consisting of a less than moral attitude to ego ideals. One's shortcomings and successes become too central and fluctuating an issue in life to allow the usual commitment of concern for other persons' views of them. It is not very practicable to try to sustain solid claims about oneself. The inmate tends to learn that degradations and reconstructions of the self need not be given too much weight, at the same time learning that staff and inmates are ready to view an inflation or deflation of a self with some indifference. He learns that a defensible picture of self can be seen as something outside oneself that can be constructed, lost, and rebuilt, all with great speed and some equanimity. He learns about the viability of taking up a standpoint—and hence a self—that is outside the one which the hospital can give and take away from him.

The setting, then, seems to engender a kind of cosmopolitan sophistication, a kind of civic apathy. In this unserious yet oddly exaggerated moral context, building up a self or having it destroyed becomes something of a shameless game, and learning to view this process as a game seems to make for some demoralization, the game being such a fundamental one. In the hospital, then, the inmate can learn that the self is not a fortress, but rather a small open city; he can become weary of having to show pleasure when held by troops of his own, and weary of having to show displeasure when held by the enemy. Once he learns what it is like to be defined by society as not having a viable self, this threatening definition—the threat that helps attach people to the self society accords them—is weakened. The patient seems to gain a new plateau when he learns that he can survive while acting in a way that society sees as destructive of him.

A few illustrations of this moral loosening and moral fatigue might be given. In state mental hospitals currently a kind of "marriage moratorium" appears to be accepted by patients and more or less condoned by staff. Some informal peer-group pressure may be brought against a patient who "plays around" with more than one hospital partner at a time, but little negative sanction seems to be attached to taking up, in a temporarily steady way, with a member of the opposite sex, even though both partners are known to be married, to have children, and even to be regularly visited by these outsiders. In short, there is licence in mental hospitals to begin courting all over again, with the understanding, however, that nothing very permanent or serious can come of this. Like shipboard or vacation romances, these entanglements attest to the way in which the hospital is cut off from the outside community, becoming a world of its own, operated for the benefit of its own citizens. And certainly this moratorium is an expression of the alienation and hostility that patients feel for those on the outside to whom they were closely related. But, in addition, one has evidence of the loosening effects of living in a world within a world, under conditions which make it difficult to give full seriousness to either of them.

The second illustration concerns the ward system. On the worst ward level, discreditings seem to occur the most frequently, in part because of lack of facilities, in part through the mockery and sarcasm that seem to be the occupational norm of social control for the attendants and nurses who administer these places. At the same time, the paucity of equipment and rights means that not much self can be built up. The patient finds himself constantly toppled, therefore, but with very little distance to fall. A kind of jaunty gallows humor seems to develop in some of these wards, with considerable freedom to stand up to the staff and return insult for insult. While these patients can be punished, they cannot, for example, be easily slighted, for they are accorded as a matter of course few of the niceties that people must enjoy before they can suffer subtle abuse. Like prostitutes in connection with sex, inmates on these wards have very little reputation or rights to lose and can therefore take certain liberties. As the person moves up the ward system, he can manage more and more to avoid incidents that discredit his claim to be a human being, and acquire more and more of the varied ingredients of self-respect; yet when eventually he does get toppled—and he does—there is a much farther distance to fall. For instance, the privileged patient lives in a world wider than the ward, containing recreation workers who, on request, can dole out cake, cards, table-tennis balls, tickets to the movies, and writing materials. But in the absence of the social control of payment which is typically exerted by a recipient on the outside, the patient runs the risk that even a warmhearted functionary may, on occasion, tell him to wait until she has finished an informal chat, or teasingly ask why he wants what he has asked for, or respond with a dead pause and a cold look of appraisal.

Moving up and down the ward system means, then, not only a shift in self-constructive equipment, a shift in reflected status, but also a change in the calculus of risks. Appreciation of risks to his self-conception is part of everyone's moral experience, but an appreciation that a given risk level is itself merely a social arrangement is a rarer kind of experience, and one that seems to help to disenchant the person who undergoes it.

A third instance of moral loosening has to do with the conditions that are often associated with the release of the inpatient. Often he leaves under the supervision and jurisdiction of his next-of-relation or of a specially selected and specially watchful employer. If he misbehaves while under their auspices, they can quickly obtain his readmission. He therefore finds himself under the special power of persons who ordinarily would not have this kind of power over him, and about whom, moreover, he may have had prior cause to feel quite bitter. In order to get out of the hospital, however, he may conceal his displeasure in this arrangement, and, at least until safely off the hospital rolls, act out a willingness to accept this kind of custody. These discharge procedures, then, provide a built-in lesson in overtly taking a role without the usual covert commitments, and seem further to separate the person from the worlds that others take seriously.

The moral career of a person of a given social category involves a standard sequence of changes in his way of conceiving of selves, including, importantly, his own. These half-buried lines of development can be followed by studying his moral experiences—that is, happenings which mark a turning point in the way in which the person views the world—although the particularities of this view may be difficult to establish. And note can be taken of overt tacks or strategies—that is, stands that he effectively takes before specifiable others, whatever the hidden and variable nature of his inward attachment to these presentations. By taking note of moral experiences and overt personal stands, one can obtain a relatively objective tracing of relatively subjective matters.

Each moral career, and behind this, each self, occurs within the confines of an institutional system, whether a social establishment such as a mental hospital or a complex of personal and professional relationships. The self, then, can be seen as something that resides in the arrangements prevailing in a social system for its members. The self in this sense is not a property of the person to whom it is attributed, but dwells rather in the pattern of social control that is exerted in connection with the person by himself and those around him. This special kind of institutional arrangement does not so much support the self as constitute it.

In this paper, two of these institutional arrangements have been considered, by pointing to what happens to the person when these rulings are weakened. The first concerns the felt loyalty of his next-of-relation. The prepatient's self is described as a function of the way in which three roles are related, arising and declining in the kinds of affiliation that occur between the next-of-relation and the mediators. The second concerns the protection required by the person for the version of himself which he presents to others, and the way in which the withdrawal of this protection can form a systematic, if unintended, aspect of the working of an establishment. I want to stress that these are only two kinds of institutional rulings from which a self emerges for the participant; others, not considered in this paper, are equally important.

In the usual cycle of adult socialization one expects to find alienation and mortification followed by a new set of beliefs about the world and a new way of conceiving of selves. In the case of the mental hospital patient, this rebirth does sometimes occur, taking the form of a strong belief in the psychiatric perspective, or, briefly at least, a devotion to the social cause of better treatment for mental patients. The moral career of the mental patient has unique interest, however; it can illustrate the possibility that in casting off the raiments of the old self—or in having this cover torn away—the person need not seek a new robe and a new audience before which to cower. Instead he can learn, at least for a time, to practise before all groups the amoral arts of shamelessness.

References

Adorno, T. W., Frenkel-Brunswik, E., Levinson, D. J., & Sanford, R. N. (1950). *The authoritarian personality.* New York: Harper & Row.

Aviram, U., & Segal, S. P. (1973). Exclusion of the mentally ill: Reflection on an old problem in a new context. *Archives of General Psychiatry, 29,* 126–131.

Bandura, A. (1977). Self-efficacy: Toward a unifying theory of behavioral change. *Psychological Review, 84,* 191–215.

Bandura, A. (1989). Regulation of cognitive processes through perceived self-efficacy. *Developmental Psychology, 25,* 729–735.

Bordieri, J. E., & Drehmer, D. E. (1986). Hiring decisions for disabled workers: Looking at the cause. *Journal of Applied Social Psychology, 16,* 197–208.

Corrigan, P. W. (1998). The impact of stigma on severe mental illness. *Cognitive and Behavioral Practice, 5,* 201–222.

Corrigan, P. W., & Matthews, A. K. (2003). Stigma and disclosure: Implications for coming out of the closet. *Journal of Mental Health, 12,* 235–248.

Corrigan, P. W., Faber, D., Rashid, F., & Leary, M. (1999). The construct validity of empowerment among consumers of mental health services. *Schizophrenia Research, 38,* 77–84.

Corrigan, P. W., & Miller, F. E. (2004). *Shame, blame, and contamination: A review of the impact of mental illness stigma on family members.* Manuscript submitted for publication.

Corrigan, P. W., & Penn, D. L. (1999). Lessons from social psychology on discrediting psychiatric stigma. *American Psychologist, 54,* 765–776.

Corrigan, P. W., & Watson, A. C. (2002). The paradox of self-stigma and mental illness. *Clinical Psychology—Science and Practice, 9,* 35–53.

Desai, M. M., Rosenheck, R. A., Druss, B. G., & Perlin, J. B. (2002). Mental disorders and quality of care among postacute myocardial infarction outpatients. *Journal of Nervous and Mental Disease, 190,* 51–53.

Druss, B. G., Allen, H. M., & Bruce, M. L. (1998). Physical health, depressive symptoms, and managed care enrollment. *American Journal of Psychiatry, 155,* 878–882.

Druss, B. G., Bradford, D. W., Rosenheck, R. A., Radford, M. J., & Krumholz, H. M. (2000). Mental disorders and use of cardiovascular procedures after myocardial infarction. *JAMA: Journal of the American Medical Association, 283,* 506–511.

Druss, B. G., & Rosenheck, R. (1997). Mental disorders and access to medical care in the United States. *American Journal of Psychiatry, 155,* 1775–1777.

Farina, A., & Felner, R. D. (1973). Employment interviewer reactions to former mental patients. *Journal of Abnormal Psychology, 82,* 268–272.

Farina, A., Felner, R. D., & Bourdreau, L. A. (1973). Reaction of workers to male and female mental patient job applicants. *Journal of Consulting and Clinical Psychology, 41,* 363–372.

Farina, A., Thaw, J., Lovern, J. D., & Mangone, D. (1974). People's reactions to a former mental patient moving to their neighborhood. *Journal of Community Psychology, 2,* 108–112.

Greenley, J. R., Mechanic, D., & Cleary, P. (1987). Seeking help for psychological problems: A replication and extension. *Medical Care, 25,* 1113–1128.

Hogan, R. (1985a). Gaining community support for group homes. *Community Mental Health Journal, 22,* 117–126.

Hogan, R. (1985b). *Not in my town: Local government in opposition to group homes.* Unpublished manuscript.

Holmes, E. P., & River, L. P. (1998). Individual strategies for coping with the stigma of severe mental illness. *Cognitive and Behavioral Practice, 5,* 231–239.

Jemeka, R., Trupin, E., & Chiles, J. A. (1989). The mentally ill in prisons: A review. *Hospital and Community Psychiatry, 40,* 481–491.

Jost, J. T., & Banaji, M. R. (1994). The role of stereotyping in system-justification and the production of false consciousness. *British Journal of Social Psychology, 33,* 1–27.

Katz, D., & Braly, K. (1935). Racial prejudice and racial stereotypes. *Journal of Abnormal and Social Psychology, 30*, 175–193.

Lamb, H., & Weinberger, L. E. (1998). Persons with severe mental illness in jails and prisons: A review. *Psychiatric Services, 49*, 483–492.

Leaf, P. J., Bruce, M. L., Tischler, G. L., & Holzer, C. E. (1987). The relationship between demographic factors and attitudes toward mental health services. *Journal of Community Psychology, 15*, 275–284.

Link, B. G. (1982). Mental patient status, work and income: An examination of the effects of a psychiatric label. *American Sociological Review, 47*, 202–215.

Link, B. G. (1987). Understanding labeling effects in the area of mental disorders: An assessment of the effects of expectations of rejection. *American Sociological Review, 52*, 96–112.

Link, B. G., Cullen, F. T., Struening, E. L, Shrout, P. E., & Dohrenwend, B. P. (1989). A modified labeling theory approach to mental disorders: An empirical assessment. *American Sociological Review, 54*, 400–423.

Link, B. G., & Phelan, J. C. (2001). Conceptualizing stigma. *Annual Review of Sociology, 27*, 363–385.

Link, B. G., Struening, E. L., Neese-Todd, S., Asmussen, S., & Phelan, J. (2001). Stigma as a barrier to recovery: The consequences of stigma for the self-esteem of people with mental illness. *Psychiatric Services, 52*, 1621–1626.

Lippmann, W. (1922). *Public opinion.* New York: Macmillan.

Markowitz, F. E. (1998). The effects of stigma on the psychological well-being and life satisfaction of persons with mental illness. *Journal of Health and Social Behavior, 39*, 335–348.

Olshansky, S., Grab, S., & Ekdahl, M. (1960). Survey of employment experiences of patients discharged from three state mental hospitals during period 1951–1953. *Mental Hygiene New York, 44*, 510–522.

Page, S. (1977). Effects of the mental illness label in attempts to obtain accommodation. *Canadian Journal of Behavioural Science, 9*, 85–90.

Page, S. (1983). Psychiatric stigma: Two studies of behaviour when the chips are down. *Canadian Journal of Community Mental Health, 2*, 13–19.

Page, S. (1995). Effects of the mental illness label in 1993: Acceptance and rejection in the community. *Journal of Health and Social Policy, 7*, 61–68.

Rosenberg, M. (1965). *Society and the adolescent self image.* Princeton, NJ: Princeton University Press.

Segal, S. P., Baumohl, J., & Moyles, E. W. (1980). Neighborhood types and community reaction to the mentally ill: A paradox of intensity. *Journal of Health and Social Behavior, 21*, 345–359.

Sirey, J. A., Bruce, M. L., Alexopoulos, G. S., Perlick, D. A., Raue, P., Friedman, S. J., & Meyers, B. S. (2001). Perceived stigma as a predictor of treatment discontinuation in young and older outpatients with depression. *American Journal of Psychiatry, 158*, 479–481.

Steadman, H. J., McCarthy, D. W., & Morrissey, J. P. (1989). *The mentally ill in jail: Planning for essential services.* New York: Guilford Press.

Tajfel, H. (1981). *Human groups and social categories.* Cambridge, England: Cambridge University Press.

Teplin, L. A. (1984). Criminalizing mental disorder: The comparative arrest rate of the mentally ill. *American Psychologist, 39*, 794–803.

Wahl, O. F. (1999). Mental health consumers' experience of stigma. *Schizophrenia Bulletin, 25*, 467–478.

Watson, A., Ottati, V., Corrigan, P., & Heyrman, M. (in press). Mental illness stigma and police decision making. *Community Mental Health Journal*.

Webber, A., & Orcutt, J. D. (1984). Employers' reactions to racial and psychiatric stigmata: A field experiment. *Deviant Behavior, 5*, 327–336.

DISCUSSION

1. Goffman uses the concept of "career" to help identify the common social processes and contingencies that shape the self-concepts and social experiences of people who enter treatment for mental illness. What are the most important forces that influence the experiences of people with mental illness?

2. What are the major similarities and differences in the pre-patient and inpatient phases of the moral career of a mental patient? To what extent and in what ways, do individuals entering treatment influence the course of their careers?

3. In what ways is the process described by Goffman similar to and different from the labeling perspective discussed in the readings by Scheff, Gove, and Link, et al.?

Bernice A. Pescosolido, Carol A. Boyer, and Keri M. Lubell

The Social Dynamics of Responding to Mental Health Problems[†]

In more recent years, as the mental health system has become more organizationally complex, sociologists have become more interested in the multiple ways people identify mental health problems in themselves and/or others and enter into psychiatric treatment. In this selection, Pescosolido and colleagues provide an overview of several early theories of "help seeking" and "utilization behavior" in the case of mental illness. They highlight how different theories have identified many of the complex junctures that organize mental illness careers and conclude by offering a more general analytic framework, called the Network-Episode Model, to guide our thinking and study of the complex "pathways" into and out of the treatment system and the myriad of factors that influence an individual's mental illness career.

Pescosolido, Bernice A., Carol A. Boyer, and Keri M. Lubell. 1999. "The Social Dynamics of Responding to Mental Health Problems." Pp. 441–460 in *Handbook of Sociology of Mental Health*, edited by C. S. Aneshensel and J. C. Phelan. New York: Kluwer Academic-Plenum Publishers.

INTRODUCTION

Since social scientists first directed their attention to understanding how individuals recognize and respond to mental illness, they have struggled to capture both the underlying process or dynamic that drives the search for care and the social, cultural, medical, and organizational characteristics that shape the fate of persons dealing with mental health problems. At the present time, the dominant approaches to studying what many people call "help seeking" or "decision making," and others more generally call "illness behavior" or "service use" focus on well-developed but essentially correlation models of the factors associated with use, compliance and outcomes. The Health Belief Model (Strecher, Champion, & Rosenstock, 1997), the Theory of Reasoned Action and its close counterpart, the Theory of Planned Behavior (Maddux & DuCharme, 1977), and the Behavioral Model of Health Service Utilization (Aday & Awe, 1997; Andersen, 1995) share an approach of outlining a comprehensive set of factors that shape the use of both preventive and curative services. Although these models do not ignore the underlying *process* of service use, key assumptions focus primarily on the factors that facilitate or discourage entry into formal treatment (for a review, see Gochman, 1997; Pescosolido, 1991, 1992; Pescosolido & Boyer, 1999). Rarely are the dynamics of coping with health problems a part of the empirical study of illness behavior. With the dynamics *assumed*, empirical studies in this tradition collect information on the extent and volume of use, and on a wide range of factors thought to influence the behavior of those entering care and treatment.

Our approach here is less traditional as we trace the theoretical and empirical work describing the process of coping with mental illness and the patterns of using different systems of care. As the health care system is fundamentally transformed, understanding how individuals respond to mental illness, what pathways they travel, and what factors shape their trajectories requires a step backward to reevaluate what is known about service use and where further research is needed. We begin by describing two classic studies that initially invoked an "illness career" approach and by highlighting their fundamental lessons. Later, we explore the recognition of mental illness, different modes of entry into the formal system of care, the availability and use of diverse systems of care, and the patterns and pathways to care. We conclude by focusing on the Network– Episode Model that combines the strengths of previous process and contingency models of utilization. New empirical findings are drawn from past studies as well as ongoing studies of persons with serious mental illness, from samples in the general population that report mental health problems, and from others who offer their opinions on the nature and cause of mental health problems.

THE PROCESS OF RESPONDING TO MENTAL HEALTH PROBLEMS

Parsons's Illness Career and Clausen and Yarrow's Pathways to the Mental Hospital

A concern with process was fundamental in early studies of how individuals coped with illness and their use of formal medical services. The emphasis was fairly implicit in these theories and was targeted mostly at a macrosociological level. The major transition from agrarian to modern societies set the conditions for individuals to turn to relatively new forms of scientific medical care and away from older forms of folk or indigenous treatments. Influenced by industrialization, higher standards of living, and increased education, urban residents were more likely to use modern medical services. Their rural counterparts, without the benefit of changing circumstances and access to newer treatments, were likely to respond in traditional ways to medical problems within their own families or local communities. Larger social forces changed how individuals responded to illness and the availability of medical services. Though not entirely rational, individuals who became ill were assumed to want to take advantage of the specialized knowledge and technological changes associated with the rise of modern medical practice (see Pescosolido, 1992; Pescosolido & Kronenfeld, 1995). The assumptions of this analysis of the transition to using modern medicine were oversimplified, but the experience of illness and entering treatment was embedded in social life and framed as a causal, time-ordered process.

Talcott Parsons is credited with developing the first major social science schema for understanding people's behavior when they are ill. His concept of the "sick role," with accompanying rights (role release, nonresponsibility) and obligations (undesirability and help seeking), dominated social science approaches from the 1950s to the 1970s. What is less well understood about Parsons's (1951) work in *The Social System* is that embedded in it was an implicit model of an "illness career" that laid out stages and mechanisms for the transition between stages. Our visual understanding of this model is presented in Figure 1.

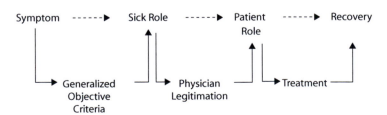

Figure 1 Diagrammatic representation of Parson's (1951) illness career model.

For Parsons, the illness career began with the onset of symptoms. In the first stage, which Suchman (1964) also called "the decision that something is wrong," the sick person evaluated "generalized objective criteria," weighing the severity of a problem, the prognosis, the frequency of its occurrence and normal "well-role" expectations. For Parsons, individuals would rationally and scientifically evaluate their circumstances, make a claim to those around them in the community, and proceed either to enter the sick role or return to normal roles. Upon entering the sick role, individuals would receive benefits and take on the obligations associated with the role. Because the obligation of seeking help from a competent professional (i.e., a physician) was an essential part of the sick role, individuals would proceed to make a claim to enter the patient role. At this stage, which Suchman called "the decision to seek professional advice," the "gatekeepers" are physicians who legitimate only "true" claims of illness, protecting society from "malingers" who might inappropriately seek the secondary gains of the patient role. Once in the patient role, the "decision to accept professional treatment," individuals with similar medical problems are treated equally. Once recovered, individuals reenter the world of the well, resume normal roles, and relinquish the rights and obligations of the roles associated with the illness career.

Across 20 years and hundreds of articles in the sociomedical sciences, researchers filled in the details of this model and showed where Parsons's theoretical, deductive, and logical scheme represented modern society's faith in the promise of modern medicine (e.g., see Segall, 1997; Siegler & Osmond, 1973). The sick role represented an "ideal type," not the social reality of sickness and the process of being treated. This voluminous research on the sick role yielded a large set of contingencies, or variables, for the now-dominant correlational models of health service use that shifted an emphasis from dynamic process to more static associations. Downplayed was Parsons's focus on the importance of the community as the adjudicator of the sick role. The patient role (being in treatment) was also often confused in practice with the sick role (a shift in status granted in the lay community). Both Parsons's approach and the multidimensional contingency theories that developed from it shared a view of service use as essentially "help seeking" focused more on acute, physical illness rather than on chronic and long-term health and behavioral problems.

At about the same time, John Clausen and his colleagues at the Laboratory of Socio-Environmental Studies, within the research branch of the National Institute of Mental Health, used an inductive approach to study how people came to use formal services. Focusing on men who were hospitalized and diagnosed with psychotic disorders, they described a social process that looked substantially different from the Parsons model. In their own words, they aimed "to delineate the process whereby families adapt to mental illness and to distinguish variables in personality, culture, or in the social situations which significantly affect this process" (4) (Clausen & Yarrow, 1955). Rather than a rational evaluation of psychiatric symptoms, Clausen and his colleagues described long scenarios of confusion, the use of coercion (from family and friends, as well as bosses and police), and accounts that varied from Parsons's ideal type. These researchers found that mental illness "seldom manifests itself in the guise of the popular stereotype of 'insanity'" (4), and individuals struggled to understand and attach meaning to the unfolding of a serious mental illness.

Figure 2 depicts our understanding of Clausen and Yarrow's description of the process preceding a first hospitalization at St. Elizabeth's in Washington, D.C. The stories of the men in their study, who were white and 20–60 years old, were told by their wives. For these women, the onset of the illness was rarely clearly demarcated. After marrying, the wives noticed things that they attributed to a variety of factors unrelated to mental illness. About six months into their marriage, one wife noticed that her husband, a 35-year-old cab driver, had irregular work habits and complained of constant headaches. Although she occasionally thought this behavior "wasn't right," she adjusted her expectations and attributed his behavior to his personality ("a nervous person"), his past experiences ("Worrying about the war so much...has gotten the best of him"), and the subcultural norms of his occupation ("Most cab drivers loaf"). For the next 2 years, she shifted her definitions of their marriage, her husband's behavior, and their circumstances. She thought that he was lazy at one point and later, that he was seeing another woman. She developed strategies to deal with instances of odd behavior. When her husband spoke of existing plots of world domination, she learned that confronting him simply increased his agitation and escalated the situation, so she adapted by "chang[ing] the subject." Despite these accommodations, this "accumulation of deviant behavior" strained the wife's level of tolerance, which nevertheless remained below her "threshold" as long as she was able to bring some understanding to these incidents.

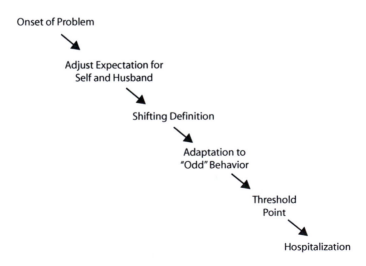

Figure 2 Diagrammatic representation of Clausen and Yarrow's (1955) process model of entry into formal care.

With a "trigger" event, she reached a threshold where she was confronted with defining his behavior as an illness. At this point, her husband had stopped bathing and changing clothes; he chased her around the house and growled like a lion. She later learned that he went to a local church, made a scene, and was taken to the hospital by the police. Even though she had forced him earlier to go to a physician, she was not involved in the decision-making process for entry into formal psychiatric care. Only with his involuntary admission to a psychiatric hospital did she frame his problem as a psychiatric one. Describing this story as the "process of help seeking" for a mental health problem is problematic.

From this classic study, four important aspects of dealing with mental health problems (and perhaps most illnesses, especially chronic ones) are apparent. First, mental health problems are poorly understood by most people. Typical "symptoms" of schizophrenia, and more so those associated with depression, are not easily or quickly recognized as illness. Families often normalize situations adapting to and accommodating behavior. Second, others beyond the family (e.g., police, bosses, teachers) are often the first to see the person's behavior as a mental health problem. Third, the image of entering treatment voluntarily is not entirely accurate. Fourth, the idea of an orderly progression through well-defined and logical stages is contradicted by the stories of people who faced, either for themselves or for their family members, mental health problems.

The following issues have been examined in research on illness behavior (Mechanic, 1968); the lay attribution of illness, the role of "others" in facing illness; the use of coercion in mental health treatment; and the refinement of stage models to reflect the complexity of the possible pathways to formal care. However, more studies have been conducted using correlation models than those focusing on process and on entering the formal medical care system in Western countries, not on community-based ethnographic, multimethod studies (Pescosolido & Kronenfeld, 1995). Nevertheless, anthropologists concerned with societies that had traditional, indigenous systems of treatment analyzed how different forms of care were used by individuals and dealt with by governments. Studies of illness behavior beyond the Western world and the sustained interest in understanding communities have also invigorated the continued focus on process and complexity.

ACKNOWLEDGING THE COMPLEXITIES: LEVELS OF ILLNESS BELIEFS

Several different literatures have evolved that attempt to understand the social "realities" faced by patients, families, and others who interact with the person with psychiatric symptoms or a diagnosed mental illness. Lay accounts of problem definition and the process of entering treatment are contained in a proliferating literature of first-person accounts, case studies, and surveys. The process by which a behavior, such as a delusion, is transformed and responded to as a symptom, the cognitive and emotional factors affecting its interpretation, and the process of referral and entry into treatment are of relevance to social scientists and clinicians alike. Ultimately, compliance could be enormously enhanced by learning more about how people make sense of psychiatric symptoms and their social selection into various pathways to prevention and treatment.

The recognition and definition of behavior as a symptom of mental illness is a complex, sometimes illogical, perplexing, and generally distressing and protracted process (Furnham, 1994; Horwitz, 1982). Only limited understanding or agreement exists about when behaviors are serious enough to require psychiatric treatment. Misconceptions about the illness and the person with a mental illness are common. One study of lay beliefs about persons with schizophrenia showed that they were regarded with apprehension, as potentially dangerous, amoral, egocentric, and as "dropouts" or vagrants (Furnham & Rees, 1988). The recognition of mental illness by professionals is delayed because self- and other appraisals are not always consistent with the medical model or clinical interpretations.

Complicating the lay recognition of symptoms of mental illness is stigma. The negative cultural stereotypes associated with the label of a mental illness and the fear of discrimination and rejection prompt defenses against acknowledging symptoms and behaviors as mental illness. In their efforts to manage difficult behaviors, families and mentally ill persons themselves deny, withdraw, conceal, or normalize symptoms of psychiatric illness (Clausen & Yarrow, 1955; Link, Mirotznik, & Cullen, 1991). Within some communities and families, a high tolerance for disturbing behaviors can delay early recognition of mental illness. In other cases, symptoms and behaviors may not be seen as treatable or worthy of medical intervention (Freidson, 1970).

A direct pathway to specialty mental health care does not logically follow from the onset of symptoms or even with relapse when prior symptoms reappear. It is not unusual for two or more years to elapse between the onset of symptoms and hospitalization (Clausen & Yarrow, 1955; Horwitz, 1977a). Close relatives are more likely to deny the initial symptoms, whereas more distant relatives and friends are more willing to interpret symptoms and behavior within a psychiatric framework (Horwitz, 1982). Selection into care is also strongly influenced by gender. Women are more likely than men to recognize their problem as an emotional one and to be labeled with a psychiatric problem by family and friends (Horwitz, 1977b). This gender difference in recognition separates men from women in the process of decision making and entering care. Based on attributions about symptoms, people will also engage in self-medication and seek advice from friends and relatives long before entering medical or psychiatric treatment. Even with referrals from primary care to specialty mental health care, the process of selection is defined as much by social as clinical indicators (Morgan, 1989).

ACKNOWLEDGING THE COMPLEXITIES: DIFFERENT MODES OF ENTRY

Theories about how individuals use services are based primarily on an underlying assumption that a proactive choice is made, that they "seek" care. The case from Clausen and Yarrow's study suggests that "help seeking" and "decision making" do not accurately describe the social process of entering the medical or mental health system. As suggested by Pescosolido, Gardner, and Lubell (1998), taking a broader view of how individuals enter treatment, especially mental health care, reveals two distinct literatures on health service use. The main literature is referred to as "utilization," "help seeking" or "health care decision making," where the focus is on the individual and implicitly on "choices" even in the face of restricted access. The second research tradition comes from those more concerned with the interface between the legal and mental health systems. Often referred to as "law and mental health," this area focuses more on the power of legal systems to force individuals into treatment and on pressure, however well intended, from others in the community to receive care.

Data from a number of studies support "the two faces" of mental health service use. Researchers who focus on legal "holds" and court-ordered treatments report that many individuals with mental health problems are "pushed" into care by friends, relatives, and coworkers. They enter the treatment system not on their own volition but by the actions of police, other institutional agents (e.g., teachers), or through mechanisms of emergency detention and involuntary commitment (Bennett et al., 1993; Miller, 1988; Perelberg, 1983).

Researchers distinguish between legal coercion (i.e., formal measures such as involuntary hospitalization used to compel service use and compliance) and extralegal coercion (i.e., pressures from family, clinicians, and friends to get and stay in treatment). The official distinction between "voluntary" and "involuntary" commitment is problematic. According to Lidz and Hoge (1993), many individuals hospitalized for mental health problems are persuaded to "sign themselves in" to increase their freedom in leaving the hospital. Furthermore, the recent series of reports from the MacArthur Coercion Study show that almost 40 percent of those who were admitted voluntarily believed that they would have been involuntarily committed had they not "agreed" to admission (Dennis & Monahan, 1996). Of all the patients studied in two mental hospitals, 46 percent of individuals report no pressures to enter care, 38 percent report efforts to "persuade," and 10 percent report the use of "force" (Dennis & Monahan, 1996).

Such coercion is not limited to those who are perceived by others to require intensive, inpatient care. In our ongoing longitudinal study (the Indianapolis Network Mental Health Study) of how "community" influences early illness careers of individuals with mental health problems and their families, individuals were asked to tell the "story" of how they first came to be treated in a public or private hospital or a Community Mental Health Center (CMHC).

Some of the individuals were later diagnosed with a major mental illness (e.g., schizophrenia, bipolar disorder), and others were diagnosed with "adjustment disorders." Similar to the MacArthur study, fewer than half of the stories (45.9 percent) match the notion of choice underlying dominant theories of health services use. Almost one-fourth of the respondents (22.9 percent) reported coercion. These stories were also examined for an additional kind of entry that has been called "muddling through." In about one-third (31.2 percent) of the cases, agency was virtually absent. Individuals neither resisted nor sought care and often struggled haphazardly to cope with a change in their mental health status, most likely perceived as resulting from a change in their social circumstances, such as divorce, job loss, or other life event. Often, it is unclear how they reached the mental health system at all.

Entry into care is shaped by both the type of mental health problems and the nature of the social contacts. For individuals with bipolar disorders, conflict with others is likely, and these individuals often describe a "supercharged" state. They are surprised and agitated when others around them want them to seek (and eventually pressure them into) medical care. The use of coercion appears also to be shaped by the availability of community ties. Larger social networks closely tied together have the social capacity to get individuals into the specialty sector even in the face of resistance (Pescosolido, Gardner, & Lubell, 1998).

Support for the use of legal coercion to get individuals with mental health problems into the formal system of care is substantial. According to results from the 1996 GSS, almost two-thirds of the public are willing to use legal means to force individuals with drug abuse problems to see a doctor, almost half report a willingness to do so with individuals described in the vignette as meeting criteria for schizophrenia, and over one-third agree for individuals with alcohol dependence. Interestingly, fewer individuals respond in a similar way to major depression, but still over one-fifth of Americans report a willingness to coerce those with major depression into medical treatment. A few (about 7 percent) were willing to use legal coercion for the person with "troubles" who did not meet criteria for any mental health problem (Pescosolido, Monahan, Link, Steuve & Kikuzawa, forthcoming).

ACKNOWLEDGING THE COMPLEXITIES: DIFFERENT SYSTEMS OF CARE

The differential response to mental health problems and to all illnesses is not a process that occurs in isolation. Many individuals with varying backgrounds and expertise can be involved in the process of identifying a mental health problem, providing advice or consultation, and taking part in the person's illness career. Kleinman (1980) has described three systems of care; the lay system, the folk system, and the formal medical care system. Table 1 offers a more detailed listing of the options, types of advisors, and examples of the different kinds of possibilities that exist in most, if not all, societies. The set of possibilities is the same whether the problem is physical or mental, in part because mental health problems are often first understood as physical problems. For others, the problem may be defined in terms of social relations, such as a problem with a significant other that may be handled with advice from a psychic rather than a psychiatrist. According to the stories in the Indianapolis Network Mental Health Study, few individuals saw the problem initially as a mental health problem. Rather, they attributed the problems to a wide variety of stressors in their lives such as bad marriages, difficult bosses, troubled children, and conflicts with their parents.

Reforms in health care and in medical practice are directed to decreasing mental health treatment costs by training general practitioners to recognize, diagnose, and treat problems rather than refer patients to expensive specialists, such as psychologists or psychiatrists. These changes also underscore the movement toward community-level innovations to fill in the gaps left by a reformed medical care system (Peterson, 1997). As Table 1 also indicates,

Table 1 The Range of Choices for Medical Care and Advice

Option	Advisor	Examples
Modern medical	M.D.'s, osteopaths (general practitioners, specialists), allied health professions	Physicians, psychiatrists, podiatrists, optometrists, nurses, midwives, opticians, psychologists, druggists, technicians, aides
Alternative medical practitioners	"Traditional" healers	Faith healers, spiritualists, shamans, curanderos, diviners, herbalists, acupuncturists, bone-setters, granny midwives
	"Modern" healers	Homeopaths, chiropractors, naturopaths, nutritional consultants, holistic practitioners
Nonmedical professionals	Social workers	
	Legal agents	Police, lawyers
	Clergymen	
	Supervisors	Bosses, teachers
Lay advisors	Family	Spouse, parents
	Neighbors	
	Friends	
	Co-workers, classmates	
Other	Self-care	Nonprescription medicines, self-examination procedures, folk remedies, health foods
None		

Source: Pescosolido (1992). Reprinted with permission.

individuals may try to deal with illness on their own, engaging in a variety of coping practices to alleviate symptoms (Pearlin & Aneshensel, 1986). They may resort to vitamins, over-the-counter medications, home remedies, prayer, exercise, or folk practices.

ACKNOWLEDGING THE COMPLEXITIES: THE RICH VARIETY OF PATHWAYS

As one of the first large-scale, population-based, representative sample surveys using a dynamic, community-based perspective of health care use, the Puerto Rican Study also provides new and important information not only on the nature and extent of the use of a wide variety of advisors and practices, but also on the ordering of these contacts. A wide variety of advisors were contacted initially. Almost two-thirds of those who talked to a relative did so first (65.4 percent in Wave 1 and 64.2 percent in Wave 2), but over one-third also went first to physicians (36.3 percent in Wave 1 and 39.1 percent in Wave 2). A similar percentage consulted a mental health provider (e.g., psychiatrist, social worker, mental health clinician) for their preliminary medical care contact (30.6 percent in Wave 1 and 35.3 percent in Wave 2). The only substantial difference between the two waves, was that 39 percent in Wave 1 and 26.7 percent in Wave 2 contacted a friend initially. Between one-fifth and one-fourth of those reporting mental health problems went initially to the clergy (243 percent and 20 percent, respectively).

These findings reflect two different ideas not usually taken into account in discussions of "help seeking." First, initial contact reflects the wide range of possible attributed causes and descriptions of the nature of mental health problems. Second, because not all people enter the treatment system voluntarily, the first person who "identifies" a mental health problem (e.g., the police, a crisis clinician) starts the illness career rather than being a logical end point in a "search" for care.

In acknowledging multiple pathways, Romanucci-Ross (1977) suggested two distinct "hierarchies of resort." For those she studied in Melanesia, an "acculturative" sequence started with physicians or nurses. If no relief occurred, individuals moved to Western religious healers, practitioners, and advisors. Finally, if the search continued, native religious practitioners and advisors were sought. In the "counteracculturative" sequence, individuals tried home remedies first, followed by visits to traditional, indigenous healers, finally going to a hospital if all else failed. Romanucci-Ross suggests that those acculturated to modern approaches to illness choose formal services first and will fall back on older cultural modes of responding when a "cure is not forthcoming" or "earlier choices are exhausted." Both Janzen's (1978) study of the "quest for therapy" in Zaire and Young's (1981) investigation of the "decision process" in a small Mexican village followed this tradition of describing and modeling the illness process. Young found four critical factors in structuring the process of dealing with an illness: (1) the seriousness of the illness; (2) knowledge about an appropriate home remedy; (3) faith in the effectiveness of folk treatment as opposed to medical treatment for that illness; and (4) the balance between the expense of alternatives and available resources.

Some mental health models (e.g., help-seeking decision-making model; Goldsmith, Jackson, & Hough, 1988) merge a concern with charting stages with the focus on correlates of use from models such as the Health Belief Model (Strecher et al., 1997) and the Sociobehavioral Model of Health Care (Andersen, 1995). Two problems still exist. First, although these models acknowledge that individuals might skip over stages or repeat them, a step-by-step ordering pervades the analyses of entering treatment and resembles Parsons's original scheme. The complexity of skipping stages is not modeled in the analytic design. Second, there is little guidance about how, when, and why different factors from the correlation models "kick in" to affect the process of coping with illness. Is social class more pronounced in interpreting the meaning of a "symptom" than in evaluating whether or not to seek formal care? In essence, attempts to blend dynamic and correlational models move in the right direction but are trapped in the theoretical "boxes" that faced Parsons and those who developed contingency models. These blended models still impose a single, logical order and decision-making framework on a process that is often disorderly and lacks rational stage-by-stage planning.

THE DYNAMIC, SOCIAL ORGANIZATION OF MENTAL HEALTH CONTACTS

This prior work suggests a need to study process without abandoning the search for how use is shaped by a variety of social, cultural, medical, and economic contingencies, and a need to consider multiple possibilities for the types of advisors and pathways to and from different systems of care. Prior quantitatively oriented attempts to incorporate process did not eliminate the "boxes" of contingencies that are so fundamental to these theories and to efforts to provide graphical displays of theories. In contrast, qualitatively oriented approaches failed to connect rich and textured descriptions of illness behavior to the larger, structural features that shape the process of responding to physical and mental health problems. Furthermore, theoretical, methodological, or statistical tools were also not available for venturing beyond descriptive, qualitative models or correlational, quantitative models.

The Network-Episode Model

The recently proposed Network-Episode Model (NEM) draws from the strengths of both dynamic and contingency models (Pescosolido, 1991, 1992; Pescosolido & Boyer, 1999; see Figure 3). The model moves away from "boxes" of contingencies and stages to "streams" of illness behavior

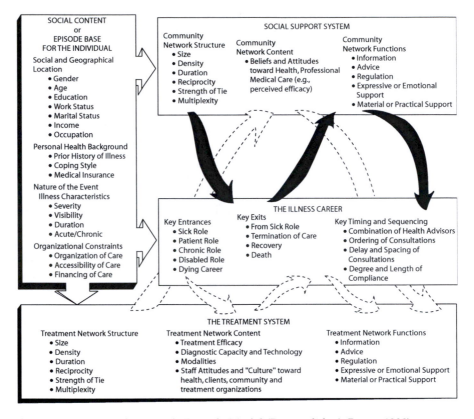

Figure 3 The revised Network-Episode Model (Pescosolido & Boyer, 1999).

incorporating changing community conditions and treatment system possibilities.

The NEM has three basic characteristics. First, rather than impose a rigid ordering of the process of coping with illness or the nature of the process, important research questions target understanding the illness career as patterns and pathways to and from the community and the treatment system; the degree to which individuals resort to different pathways; the continued use of services and outcomes; and when, how, and under what conditions individuals shift from invoking standard cultural routines and move into a rational choice-based calculus. Second, these patterns and pathways are not static, nor are they random. Both the social support system and the treatment system are ongoing streams that influence and are influenced by the illness career. Dealing with any health problem is a social process that is managed through contacts or social networks that individuals have in the community, the treatment system, and social service agencies, including self-help groups, churches, and jails. People face illness in the course of their day-to-day lives by interacting with other people who may recognize (or deny) a problem; send them to (or provide) treatment; and support, cajole or nag them about appointments, medications, or lifestyle. What this social support system looks like and what it offers is critical. The treatment sector represents the provision of clinical services that can be characterized as well by a set of networks of people who provide care, concern, pressure, and problems (Pescosolido, 1997). The NEM conceptualizes the medical system as a changing set of providers and organizations with which individuals may have contact when they are ill. Thinking about treatment in social network terms allows us to break down the treatment experience by charting the kinds (physicians, rehabilitation therapists, billing staff) and nature (supportive, antagonistic, cold or warm) of experiences that people have in treatment that affects whether they return, take their medications, or get better. Social networks in treatment create a climate of care that affects both patients and providers alike (Pescosolido, 1997). Third, the characteristics of the person and the illness (see the left-hand side of Figure 3) shape the illness career and its trajectory. All three streams are anchored in the social locations, histories, and problems of people and networks (for details, see Pescosolido 1991, 1992; Pescosolido & Boyer, 1999).

CHALLENGES TO THE SOCIOLOGICAL STUDY OF SERVICE USE: A MOVE TO UNDERSTANDING TREATMENT EFFECTIVENESS

Using the specialized mental health sector early and continuously until a problem is "solved" or "managed" should produce better outcomes for individuals and for the public health. To that end, models of service use that end at the door of the clinic do not tell us enough about what happens before individuals get there or what happens to them later. The chronicity of mental illness and of more and more physical problems requires a refocusing on illness careers that connect social interactions and communities that ultimately influence trajectories and outcomes. In this chapter, we have attempted to review the relevant literature and present new theories that provide direction for rethinking models of service use. As dramatic changes occur in the organization of the health care system, with new incentives and restricted choices, efforts to understand what happens to patients and their families in the process of entering treatment present a major challenge for mental health services research.

References

Aday, L. A., & Awe, W. C. (1997). Health service utilization models. In D. S. Gochman (Ed.), *Handbook of health behavior research: I. Personal and social determinants* (pp. 153–172). New York: Plenum Press.

Andersen, R. (1995). Revisiting the behavioral model and access to care: Does it matter? *Journal of Health and Social Behavior, 36,* 1–10.

Bennett, N. S., Lidz, C. W., Monahan, J., Mulvey, E., Hoge, S. K., Roth, L. H., & Gardner, W. (1993). Inclusion, motivation and good faith: The morality of coercion in mental hospital admission. *Behavioral Science and the Law, 11,* 295–306.

Clausen, J., & Yarrow, M. (1955). Introduction: Mental Illness and the family. *Journal of Social Issues, 11,* 25–32.

Dennis, D. L., & Monahan, J. (1996). *Coercion and aggressive community treatment.* New York: Plenum Press.

Freidson, E. (1970). *Profession of medicine.* New York: Dodd Mead.

Furnham, A. (1994). Explaining health and illness: Lay perceptions on current and future health, the causes of illness and the nature of recovery. *Social Science and Medicine, 39,* 715–725.

Furnham, A., & Rees, J. (1988). Lay theories of schizophrenia. *International Journal of Social Psychiatry, 34,* 212–220.

Gochman, D. S. (1997). Personal and social determinants of health behavior: An integration. In D. S. Gochman (Ed.), *Handbook of health behavior research: I. Personal and social determinants* (pp. 381–400). New York: Plenum Press.

Goldsmith, H. F., Jackson, D. J., & Hough, R.(1988). Process model of seeking mental health services: Proposed framework for organizing the literature on help-seeking. In H. F. Goldsmith, E. Lin, & R. A. Bell (Eds.), *Needs assessment: Its future* (pp. 49–64). DHHS Pub.No. (ADM) 88–1550. Washington. DC: U.S. Government Printing Office.

Horwitz, A. V. (1977a). Social networks and pathways into psychiatric treatment. *Social Forces, 56,* 86–106.

Horwitz, A. V. (1977b). The pathways into psychiatric treatment: Some differences between men and women. *Journal of Health and Social Behavior, 18,* 169–178.

Horwitz, A. V. (1982). *The social control of mental illness.* New York: Academic Press.

Janzen, J. M. (1978). *The quest for therapy in Lower Zaire.* Berkeley: University of California Press.

Kleinman, A. (1980). *Patients and healers in the context of culture.* Berkeley: University of California Press.

Lidz, C. W., & Hoge, S. K. (1993). Introduction to coercion in mental health care. *Behavioral Sciences and the Law, 11,* 237–238.

Link, B., Phelan, J., Bresnahan, M., Steuve, A., & Pescosolido, B. A. (forthcoming). Public conceptions of mental illness: Labels and causes. *American Journal of Public Health.*

Link, B. G., Mirotznik, J., & Cullen, F. T. (1991). The effectiveness of stigma coping orientations: Can negative consequences of mental illness labeling be avoided. *Journal of Health and Social Behavior, 32,* 302–320.

Maddux, J. E., & DuCharme, K. A. (1997). Behavioral intentions in theories of health behavior. In D. S. Gochman (Ed.), *Handbook of health behavior research: I. Personal and social determinants* (pp. 133–152). New York: Plenum Press.

Mechanic, D. (1968). *Medical sociology.* New York: Free Press.

Miller, R. D. (1988). Outpatient civil commitment of the mentally ill: An overview and update. *Behavioral Science and the Law, 6,* 99–118.

Morgan, D. (1989). Psychiatric cases: An ethnography of the referral process. *Psychological Medicine, 19,* 743–753.

Parsons, T. (1951). *The social system.* Glencoe, IL: Free Press.

Pearlin, L. I., & Aneshensel, C. S. (1986). Coping and social supports: Their functions and applications. In D. Mechanic & L. H. Aiken (Eds.), *Applications of social science* to clinical medicine and health policy (pp. 417–437). New Brunswick, NJ: Rutgers University Press.

Perelberg, R. J. (1983). Mental illness, family and networks in a London borough. *Social Science and Medicine, 17,* 481–491.

Pescosolido, B. A. (1991). Illness careers and network ties: A conceptual model of utilization and compliance. In G. Albrecht & J. Levy (Eds.), *Advances in medical sociology* (Vol. 2, pp. 164–181). Greenwich, CT: JAI Press.

Pescosolido, B. A. (1992). Beyond rational choice: The social dynamics of how people seek help. *American Journal of Sociology, 97,* 1096–1138.

Pescosolido, B. A. (1997). *Bringing people back in: Why social networks matter for treatment effectiveness research.* Unpublished paper. Bloomington: Indiana University Press.

Pescosolido, B. A., & Boyer, C. A. (1999). How do people come to use mental health services? Current knowledge and changing perspectives. In A. V. Horwitz & T. Scheid (Eds.), *Sociology of mental illness.* Cambridge, UK: Cambridge University Press.

Pescosolido, B. A., Gardner, C. B., & Lubell, K. M. (1998). How people get into mental health services: Stories of choice, coercion and "muddling through" from "first timers". *Social Science and Medicine, 46*(2), 275–286.

Pescosolido, B. A., & Kronenfeld, J. J. (1995). Health, illness and healing in an uncertain era: Challenges from and for medical sociology. *Journal of Health and Social Behavior, 36*(Extra Issue), 5–33.

Pescosolido, B. A., Monahan, J., Link, B. G., Steuve, A., & Kikuzawa, S. (forthcoming). The public's view of individuals with mental health problems: Competence, dangerousness and the need for coercion in health care. *Americian Journal of Public Health.*

Peterson, M. A. (1997). Community: meaning and opportunity and learning for the future. *Journal of Health Politics, Policy and Law, 22,* 933–936.

Romanucci-Ross, L. (1977). The hierarchy of resort in curative practices: The Admiralty Islands, Melanesia. In D. Landy (Ed.), *Culture, disease and healing* (pp. 481–486). New York: Macmillan.

Segall, A. (1997). Sick role concepts and health behavior. In D. S. Gochman (Ed.), *Handbook of Health behavior research: I. Personal and social determinants* (pp. 289–300). New York: Plenum Press.

Siegler, M., & Osmond, H. (1973). The 'sick role' revisited. *Hastings Center Report, 1,* 41–48.

Strecher, V. J., Champion, V. L., & Rosenstock, I. M. (1997). The health belief model and health behavior. In D. S. Gochman (Ed.), *Handbook of health behavior research: I. Personal and social determinants* (pp. 71–92). New York: Plenum Press.

Suchman, E. (1964). Sociomedical variations among ethnic groups. *American Journal of Sociology, 70,* 319–331.

Young, J. C. (1981). *Medical choices in a Mexican village.* New Brunswick, NJ: Rutgers University Press.

DISCUSSION

1. How, and in what ways, is the Network-Episode Model an improvement over earlier theoretical perspectives on help-seeking and utilization? What

are the key factors that the Network-Episode Model draws on from earlier theories and what unique insights does it add to our understanding?

2. The Network-Episode Model is a useful conceptual tool for thinking about the careers of people who face mental health challenges. What do you see as the major strengths and potential challenges associated with trying to apply this model as a guide for empirical research in the sociology of mental health and illness?

Karp, David A

Illness and Identity[†]

In his book, Speaking of Sadness, sociologist David Karp examines the experience of major depression, one of the most common and more severe mental disorders, using qualitative data gathered through in-depth interviews with people who have been or are currently in psychiatric care. A major emphasis in Karp's work is the profound effects that experiencing mental illness and its treatment can have on individuals' self-concepts. In this chapter, Karp offers an empirical description of the self-identity change processes that individuals with depression go through and highlights some of the factors that lead people to respond social psychologically to depression in different ways.

You know, I was a mental patient. That was my identity. . . . Depression is very private. Then all of a sudden it becomes public and I was a mental patient. . . . It's no longer just my own pain. I am a mental patient. I am a depressive. *I am a depressive* (said slowly and with intensity). This is my identity. I can't separate myself from that. When people know me they'll have to know about my psychiatric history, because that's who I am.

Female graduate student, aged 24

At the time we spoke, Karen, whose words open this chapter, had been doing well for more than two years, but described being badly frightened by a recent two-week period during which the all-too-familiar feelings of depression had begun to reappear. Aside from the terror she felt at the prospect of becoming sick, Karen realized that if depression returned, it would mean recasting her identity yet again. After two years with nothing but the "normal" ups and downs of life, she had started to feel that it might be possible to leave behind the mental patient identity she earlier thought she never could shed. By the time of our interview, only her family and a few old friends knew of her several hospitalizations. Her current roommates thought of her

Karp, David. 1996. "Illness and Identity." Pp. 50–77 in *Speaking of Sadness*. New York: Oxford University Press.

simply as Karen, one of about eight students in the large house they shared. She told me, "No one in my life right now knows...I'm so eager to talk to you about it [in this interview] because I can't talk about it with people." I said, "It must be hurtful not to be able to talk about so critical a part of your biography," and Karen responded, "Yes, but I don't want to test it with people.... [If I told them] they might not say anything, but their perception of me would change."

Karen was willing to be interviewed because I was one of those who knew about her history with depression. Years previously, while taking one of my undergraduate courses, she had confided that she was having a terrible time completing her course work. After much tentative discussion, the word depression finally entered the conversation. She seemed embarrassed by the admission until I opened my desk drawer and showed her a bottle of pills I was taking for depression. With this, we began to trade depression experiences and thereby formed the kind of bond felt by those who go through a common difficulty. As her undergraduate years passed, Karen came to my office periodically and during these visits we often spoke about depression. Our shared identity as depressed persons blurred the age and status distinctions that otherwise might have prevented our friendship. Karen's story is worth telling in brief because it so well reflects the more general process through which most of those interviewed eventually come to define themselves as depressed and then interpret the meaning of that identity.

Although we had shared thoughts often, my interview with Karen was the first time I heard her depression biography in a complete way. As the interview moved along, Karen also commented on the fact that it was the only time she herself had ever "recited the history." She occasionally had to pause, explaining "It is very hard [to recount these things]. It chokes me up. And when I recite the history [I realize] it's so fucked up." After another pause, she restated with emphasis, "What an awful history!" My interview with Karen was only the second for this project and I was, in fact, shocked by her account. Since the worst of my own depression did not happen until my early thirties, I was unprepared for descriptions of a childhood so pained that it included suicide attempts by early adolescence. Unfortunately, by the time all 50 interviews were completed, such stories no longer seemed unusual.

Like nearly everyone whom I talked with, Karen could pinpoint the beginning of her depression career. Although she described a "home filled with feelings of sadness" for as long as she could remember, it was, she said, "the beginning of the ninth grade that touched off...ten years of depression." She elaborated with the observation, "I was always sad or upset, but I was so busy and social [that the feelings were muted]. You know, things were not doing so well at home, but at school no one knew how much of a hell-hole I lived in." She described a home life that was fairly stable until her father became ill when she was a sixth grader. "When he came back from the hospital," she said, "he was very different, unstable [and] extremely violent." Till then Karen had been able to keep the misery of her home life apart from her school world, which served as a refuge. By the ninth grade, however, she "could no longer keep the two worlds separate" and in both places the same intrusive questions, feelings, and ruminations colonized her mind. Now she didn't feel safe anywhere in the world and had these relentless thoughts: "I'm miserable. [There is] such a feeling of emptiness. What the hell am I doing? What is my life all about? What is the point?" "And that," she said, "basically started it."

In the ninth grade Karen had no word for the "it" that had started. When I asked whether she recognized her pain as depression then, she replied, "Did I say this was depression [then]? Did I know [what it was]? It was pain, but I don't think I would have called it depression. I think I would have called it *my* pain." There was another factor that contributed to the anonymity of her misery and kept her pain from having a name—Karen was determined to keep her torment hidden. She said, "I lived with that for...a couple of years, from the ninth grade until the eleventh grade. [I lived] with that feeling....But it was all very private. I kept it quiet. It was something inside. I didn't really talk about it. I might have talked about it with some of my friends, but no one understood."

During this time, though, a subtle transformation was taking place in her thinking about "it." Previously, Karen felt that her pain came exclusively from her difficulties at home, but by the eleventh grade she was beginning to suspect that its locus might be elsewhere. She told me, "My family life might have been hell, but it was always, 'Oh [I feel this way] because my father is crazy. It's because of something outside of me.' But it was the first time I'm feeling awful about myself." By the eleventh grade Karen's new consciousness was that there was something really wrong with *her*. Now, her feelings about the pain took a critical turn when she began to say to herself, "I can't live like this. I will not survive. I will not be here. I can't live with the pain. If I have to live with the pain I will eventually kill myself." Despite such a shift in thinking Karen still succeeded in keeping things private until she experienced a very public crisis. It was, moreover, a "crash" that she understood as a major "turning point" in her identity. Here's what she said:

My whole family life just fell apart. There was no anchor. There was no anchor.... [Now] I was able to label it and say it was depression when I crashed in the eleventh grade and was hospitalized. You know, in ninth grade I told you about an experience where I was conscious of feeling pain, or whatever, but no one else knew about it....It is sort of like what my life is like now. I couldn't tell people about it. How can you tell people about it? What do you say?...But then it was like the two worlds just crashed in the eleventh grade. I did not want to be hospitalized because that meant for me [that] I could no longer deny that I was depressed. Everyone knew it. Everyone in my class...And I was a mental patient....And I'll tell you, that depression in the eleventh grade...it came to a head and I have never crashed so much. First of all, landing in a hospital, going into a hospital, in a way it was a relief because I didn't have to have that pretense. I really could crash. For three days I didn't even get out of that bed. I just remember being like in the fetal position. I wanted to die. It was like dying.

Then the interview turned to a lengthy discussion about psychiatric hospitals, doctors, and power—all of it negative. She expressed hostility toward doctors who wanted her to "open up" and toward institutional rules that seemed authoritarian and arbitrary. She said, "Psychiatrists and mental health workers have the power to decide when you are going to leave, if you're going to leave, if you can go out on a pass, if you're good, if you're not good." This first hospitalization (eventually there would be four) also started a long history with medications of all sorts. When I asked whether she was treated with medications she replied, "Yup, always medication. That's the big thing....Oh my God, I've had so many....I don't think they really affected me that much. By the time I left I was doing okay. Did I have these problems solved? No, [but] I had an added one. Now I felt crazy." I used Karen's observation about "feeling crazy" as a cue for asking if she had a disease. I said, "Did you now think of yourself as having an illness in the medical sense?" and her answer reflected the ambivalence and confusion I would later routinely hear when I asked this same question of others.

> I think of it less as an illness and more something that society defines. That's part of it, but then, it is physical. Doesn't that make it an illness? That's a question I ask myself a lot. Depression is a special case because everyone gets depressed....I think that I define it as not an illness. It's a condition. When I hear the term illness I think of sickness...[but] the term mental illness seems to me to be very negative, maybe because I connect it with hospitalization....I connect it with how people define people who have been hospitalized. I see so many people in psychiatric facilities...that are just like you and me. What makes them any different is just a diagnosis. Sometimes the diagnosis can keep people sicker. Sometimes the diagnosis can keep people there, you know. Yuh, I had a physical problem. Yuh, it affects my emotions. It's something that I can deal with. It's something that I can live with. I don't have to define it as a problem. But the thing about mental illness is that it lasts....Once a diagnosis always a diagnosis. And that's what I was saying [earlier] that it has only been within the last two years that I have been able to say, "I'm something beyond being mentally ill."

Before it ended, my interview with Karen covered other difficult emotional terrain, including a major suicide attempt, additional periods of hospitalization, stays in halfway houses, a traumatic college experience, failed relationships with therapists, job interviews that required lies about health history, and a personal spiritual transformation. As indicated at the outset, things had gotten better by the time of our interview and Karen believed she was pretty much past her problem with depression. She told me, "A couple of years ago, three years ago, four years ago, I would feel a need to tell people about it because I still felt depressed, because I still felt mentally ill. But now I no longer see myself in that way. I'm other things. I'm Karen the grad student. I'm Karen the one who loves to garden, the one who's interested in a lot of things. I'm not just Karen the mentally ill person." Still, such optimism about being past depression was sometimes distressingly eroded by periods of bad feelings and the ever-present edge of fear that "it" might return in its full-blown, most grotesque form.

THE SOCIAL CONSTRUCTION OF ILLNESS IDENTITIES

Karen's illness biography, even briefly documented, previews many of the issues that, as a sociologist, I find conceptually interesting and practically significant about illness in general and depression in particular. Especially insightful is her comment that depression is something of a "special case" because, as she put it, "everyone gets depressed." Indeed, the phrase "I'm so depressed," is so common in everyday discourse that one might presume depression to be a normal rather than a pathological condition. Sigmund Freud himself raised the question of "normal pain" with his often quoted observation that the purpose of psychotherapy was to "transform hysterical misery into everyday unhappiness." While no one can doubt that Karen suffered greatly, her experience, like my own and everyone else's in this study, raises the very difficult question, "Just when does the discomfort inevitably a part of living become acute enough to call it a disease?" As a sociologist inclined to see reality as a "social construction,"[1] I assume that the answer to the question is surely as much political and cultural as it is medical.

Attention to the connection between definitions of illness and power is more than an interesting theoretical issue since illness labels can have profound consequences for individuals. Even when there is no dispute about the presence of disease, as in the case of AIDS, the treatment of those afflicted is inseparable from fears, prejudices, and moral evaluations that have an exclusively social origin. The role of social expectations and human judgments is, of course, even greater when there is no demonstrable biological pathology for the human conditions and behaviors termed illness. This is what makes the case of mental illness so especially fuzzy and warrants deep concern about the exclusive legitimacy of psychiatry to decide who shall be labeled mentally ill and how they ought best be treated. Such reservations seen well-advised in light of what has been justified historically in the name of science and psychiatric medicine. Those deemed mentally ill have, at different moments in history, been subject to castration, involuntary incarceration, bloodletting, brutal "electric shock" treatments, mind-numbing drugs inducing permanent neurological damage, and a variety of brain surgeries.[2]

A CAREER VIEW OF THE DEPRESSION EXPERIENCE

As in many areas of social life, the notion of career seems an extremely useful, sensitizing concept. In his voluminous and influential writings on work, Everett Hughes showed the value of conceptualizing career as "the moving perspective in which the person sees his life as a whole and interprets the meanings of his various attitudes, actions, and the things which happen to him."[3] Hughes' definition directs attention to the subjective aspects of the career process and the ways in which people attach evaluative meanings to the typical sequence of movements constituting their career path. Here I shall be concerned with describing the career features associated with an especially ambiguous illness—depression.

Hughes' definition also suggests that each stage, juncture, or moment in a career requires a redefinition of self. The depression experience is a heuristically valuable instance for studying the intersection of careers and identities. The following data analysis illustrates that much of the depression career is caught up with assessing self, redefining self, reinterpreting past selves, and attempting to construct a future self that will "work" better. Although all careers require periodic reassessments of self, illness careers are especially characterized by critical "turning points" in identity. In his discussion of identity transformations, Anselm Strauss[4] comments on the intersection of career and identity turning points:

> In transformations of identities a person becomes something other than he or she once was. Such shifts necessitate new evaluations of self and others, of events, acts, and objects....Transformation of perception is irreversible; once having changed there is no going back. One can look back, but evaluate only from the new status....Certain critical incidences occur to force a person to recognize that "I am not the same as I was, as I used to be." These critical incidents constitute turning points in the onward movement of persons' careers.

The shape, predictability, and duration of different career paths vary considerably. For example, those following organizational careers may be provided with very clear formal and informal time clocks detailing where they "ought" to be in their careers at different ages.[5] Consequently, those pursuing such organizational careers can clearly feel that they are "on time," "off time," or even "running out of time." While the experiences of the respondents point to clear regularities in the sequencing of the depression experience, people differ considerably in the length of time they spend in any particular phase. For instance, some respondents describe years of discomfort before they even arrive at the definition of themselves as depressed; others move through the sequence described below in only a few years. To a large degree, of course, such variations depend on whether "acute" depression first occurs in childhood, as it did for Karen, or later, as in my life, and whether the depression is characterized by plainly defined episodes or greater chronicity. In my analysis, some attention is paid, as well, to the social and structural features of peoples' lives that influence their ability to recognize, to name, and to respond to their "problem."

While there is considerable variation in the timing of events, all the respondents in this study described a process remarkably similar to the one implicit in Karen's account. Every person I interviewed moved through these identity turning points in their view of themselves and their problem with depression:

1. A period of *inchoate feelings* during which they lacked the vocabulary to label their experience as depression.
2. A phase during which they conclude that *something is really wrong with me.*
3. A *crisis stage* that thrusts them into a world of therapeutic experts.
4. A stage of *coming to grips with an illness identity* during which they theorize about the cause(s) for their difficulty and evaluate the prospects for getting beyond depression.

Each of these career moments assumes and requires redefinitions of self.

Inchoate Feelings

The ages of respondents in this study range from the early twenties to the middle sixties. All these people described a period of time during which they had no vocabulary for naming their problem. Many traced feelings of emotional discomfort to ages as young as three or four, although they could not associate their feelings with something called "depression" until years later. It was typical for respondents to go for long periods of time feeling different, uncomfortable, marginal, ill-at-ease, scared, and in pain without attaching the notion of depression to their situations. A sampling of comments indicating an inchoate, obscure experience includes these:

> Well, I knew I was different from other children. I should say that from a very early age it felt like I had this darkness about me. Sort of shadow of myself. And I always had the sense that it wasn't going to go away so easily. And it was like my battle. And so, from a very early age I felt okay, "There's something going on here, [but] don't ask me for a word [for it]." It hurts me. I feel sad. My parents can't give me as much as I [would have] liked them to. And there was a feeling of helplessness in some ways. I knew that I was too young to understand what was going on. And I knew that when I got older I would understand things. There was always that sense that I would. [female travel agent, aged 41]

> If I think about it, I really can't pinpoint a moment [when I was aware that I was depressed]....It was just something I felt I was living with or had to live through, and maybe that goes back as far as graduate school. [male professor, aged 48]

Most of those reporting bad feelings from an early age could not conclude that something was "abnormal" because they had no baseline of normalcy for comparison. As might be expected, several respondents in this sample came from what they now describe as severely dysfunctional family circumstances, often characterized by alcoholism and both physical and emotional abuse. These individuals described feeling unsafe at home and often devised strategies to spend as much time as they could elsewhere. Some took refuge in the homes of friends. One man made a point of becoming friendly with the school custodians so that he could extend the school day in their company. Another woman went to the library every day after school where "the librarian got to know me...and started to look out for me." These children knew they were uncomfortable at home but still did not have wide enough experience to see their lives as unusual.

For most respondents the phase of inchoate feelings was the longest in the eventual unfolding of their illness consciousness. Particularly salient in terms of personal identity is the fact that initial definitions of their problem centered on the "structural conditions" of their lives instead of on the structure of their selves. The focus of interpretation was on the situation rather than on the self. Their emerging definition was that escape from the situation would make things right. Over and again individuals recounted fantasies of escape from their families and often from the community in which they grew up. However, initially at least, they felt trapped without a clear notion of how the situation might change.

> I remember from like five, starting to subtract five from eighteen, to see how many years I have left before I could get out [of the house]. So, I would say the overwhelming feeling was that I felt powerless. I felt a lot of things early. And I felt that I was stuck in this house and these people controlled me, and there wasn't anything I could do about it, and I was stuck there. So I just started my little chart at about four and a half or five, counting when I could get out. [female baker, aged 41]

> I felt sort of overwhelmed by the situation, and I was kind of sad that I was living the way I was living, and I didn't quite know how to get myself out of it...I guess a sense of feeling trapped. I think it was a recognition that this was not the way I wanted to live, but also the fact that I did not know how to get myself out of it. So it was feeling kind of trapped and kind of panicky. Now what do I do? [female nurse, aged 37]

Not everyone, of course, described his or her childhood as unhappy. However, even when ill feelings did not emerge until later in life, individuals initially chalked up their difficulty to their immediate life circumstances. A professor viewed his struggle to gain tenure as the source of his malaise. A 27-year-old man at first saw his bad feelings as resulting exclusively from an unstable occupational situation. Another woman thought that her feelings of depression would go away once she got over a failed relationship. A business deal gone sour was defined as precipitating depression in another case. And so on. In each of these instances, people held the view that as soon as the situation changed their discomfort would also disappear.

Therefore, a decisive juncture in the evolution of a "sickness" self-definition occurs when the circumstances individuals perceive as troubling their lives change, but mood problems persist. The persistence of problems in the absence of the putative cause requires a redefinition of what is wrong. A huge cognitive shift occurs when people come to see that the problem may be internal instead of situational; when they conclude that something is likely wrong with *them* in a manner that transcends their immediate situation.

Something Is Really Wrong with Me

In 1977, Robert Emerson and Sheldon Messinger published a paper entitled "The Micro-Politics of Trouble"[6] that analyzes the regular processes through which individuals come to see a personal difficulty as sufficiently troublesome a problem that something ought to be done about it. The materials offered in this chapter affirm the general process they describe. The process begins with a state of affairs initially "experienced as difficult, unpleasant, irritating, or unendurable."[7] At first, sufferers try an informal remedy, which sometimes works. If it doesn't, they seek another remedy. The decision that a consequential problem exists warranting a formal remedy typically follows a "recurring cycle of trouble, remedy, failure, more trouble, and a new remedy, until the trouble stops or the troubled person forsakes further efforts."[7] Here, then, is their description of the transformation from vague, inchoate feelings to a clearer sense that one is sufficiently troubled to seek a remedy.

> Problems originate with the recognition that something is wrong and must be remedied. Trouble, in these terms, involves both definitional and remedial components....On first apprehension troubles often involve little more than vague unease....An understanding of the problem's dimensions may only begin to emerge as the troubled person thinks about them, discusses the matter with others, and begins to implement remedial strategies.[7]

Despite the difficulties they have in naming their feelings as a problem, all of the respondents eventually conclude that something is *really wrong* with *them*. To be sure, many used identical phrases in describing their situations. The phrases "something was really wrong with me" and "I felt that I could no longer live like this" were repeated over and over. Respondents commented in nearly identical ways on the heightened feeling that "something is really wrong with me."

> When it really became apparent that I was just a mess was in January of 1989. I made the decision really quickly at the end of 1988 to go to school at [names a four year college] and live with my father and my stepmother and commute. And I packed up all my stuff in my car and went. I was miserable. I cried every day. Every single day I cried. I think I went to two classes [at the new school] and lasted there only a month. I was absolutely miserable. There was a lot of different factors that were involved with it [but] I just didn't feel right. There was something wrong with me, you know. [unemployed female, aged 23]

> Well, you know, you sort of get immobilized. You can't go to work. That's when it starts hitting you [that something is really wrong]. You're not sleeping or you're sleeping all the time. That kind of says something to you. [unemployed male waiter, aged 33]

> Probably my experience at that time was that there was something not right with me. As I look back on it, basically, you know, one of the struggles is like, is it *really me or is it them?* I mean, that's still a struggle, really *knowing in your gut*

that there is something wrong with me. . . . Definitely something is not right, you know. [female physical therapist, aged 42, my emphasis]

These quotes suggest a fundamental transformation in perception and identity at this point in the evolution of a depression consciousness. Respondents now located the source of their problem as somewhere within their bodies and minds, as deep within themselves. Such a belief implies a problematic identity far more basic and immutable than those associated with social statuses. If, for example, someone has a disliked occupational identity, the possibilities for occupational change exist. If the occupational identity becomes onerous enough, it is possible to quit a job. Similarly, without minimizing the difficulties of change, we can choose to become single if married, to change from one religion to another, and, these days, even to change our sex if the motivation is great enough. However, to see oneself as somehow internally flawed poses substantially greater problems for identity change or remediation because one's whole personhood is implicated. Getting rid of a sick self poses far greater problems than dropping certain social statuses. The important point here is that the rejection of situational theories for bad feelings is a critical identity turning point. Full acceptance that one has a damaged self requires acknowledgment that "I am not the same as I was, as I used to be."

Another important dimension of the career process that becomes apparent at this point is the issue of whether to keep the problem private or to make it public, especially to family and friends The private/public distinction was a dominant theme in respondents' talk throughout the history of their experience with depression. The question of being private or public is, of course, central to one's developing self-identification. As Peter Berger and Hansfried Kellner[8] point out in describing the "social construction of marriage" and Diane Vaughan[9] indicates in analyzing the process of "uncoupling" from a relationship, the moment a new status becomes public is a definitive one in solidifying a person's new identity. In the cases of both creating and disengaging from relationships, people are normally very careful not to make public announcements until they are certain they arc ready to adopt new statuses and identities. The significance attached to public announcements of even modest shifts in life style is indicated by the considerable thought people sometimes give to making public such relatively benign decisions as going on diets or quitting cigarettes.

Decisions about "going public" are, of course, greatly magnified when the information to be imparted is negative and, in the case of emotional problems, potentially stigmatizing. As Emerson and Messinger note, the search for a remedy necessarily involves sharing information with others. Still, at this early juncture of dealing with bad feelings, most respondents elected to keep silent about their pain. Both the stigma attached to mental illness and what respondents perceived to be the inherent incommunicability of their internal experience kept them quiet. In one case, however, silence was the only politically acceptable choice.

Whether or not they made their feelings public, this second phase of their illness career involved the recognition that they possessed a self that was working badly in *every* situation. Although everyone continued to identify the kinds of *social* situations that had caused their bad feelings in the past and precipitated them in the present, the qualitative change at this juncture was in the locus of attention from external to internal causes. At this point respondents were struggling to live their lives in the face of debilitating pain. This stage ended, however, when efforts to control things became impossible.

Crisis

Nearly everyone could pinpoint the precise time, situation, or set of events that moved them from the recognition that something was wrong to the realization that they were desperately sick. They could often remember in vivid detail the moment when things absolutely got out of hand.

> So I went to law school in the fall. I was at Columbia and in the best of times Columbia is a depressing place. I mean, it's a shithole. And you know, I was pretty messed up when I got there...I remember Columbia was a nightmare....So, I was getting to the point where I was paranoid about going to class and so someone talked to the dean and said, "Hey, you've got to do something about this guy, he's off the deep edge." [male administrator, aged 54]

> I'll never forget it as long as I live, when I got fired and I went and picked up my last paycheck. I was looking at it and I could just feel my pupils were dilating. I could feel the physiological difference in who I was. What is this? What is this? And I remember calling my parents. I remember telling them I had lost my job and I just started crying there. [unemployed male waiter, aged 33]

> My husband would drive, we'd drive together, and he would be ready to drop me off on his way into to work....I would sit in the car and try to nerve myself up to get out the door and force myself up the stairs (to work]....Like I would freeze, and be unable to move. And I'd say "Okay, I'm going to open the door now," and I'd look at my hand, and say "I'm going to make my hand move to the door handle and open it," and it wouldn't go. And so I'd actually have to pick it up with my other hand and put it on the door handle....And then I'd force myself up the stairs. And I couldn't do it everyday. So I'd just start to scream and rock back and forth. So things got very bad at that point. I began to want to try to hurt myself [female software quality control manager, aged 31]

At the crisis point, people fully enter a therapeutic world of hospitals, mental health experts, and medications. For many, entrance into this world is simultaneous with first receiving the "official" diagnosis of depression.[7] It is difficult to overstate the critical importance of official diagnoses and labeling. The point of diagnosis was a double-edged benchmark in the illness career. On the one hand, knowing that you "have" something that doctors regard as a specific illness imposes definitional boundaries onto an array of behaviors and feelings that previously had no name. Acquiring a clear conception of what one has and having a label to attach to confounding feelings and behaviors was especially significant to those who had gone for years without being able to name their situation. To be diagnosed also suggests the possibility that the condition can be treated and that one's suffering can be diminished. At the same time, being a "depressive" places one in the devalued category of those with mental illness. On the negative side, respondents made comments like these:

> I kept going to doctor after doctor, getting like all these new terms put on me....My family was dysfunctional and I was an alcoholic with an eating disorder and bulimia and depression and it was just all these labels. "Oh my God!" [unemployed female, aged 22]

> My father went to his allergy doctor who referred us to a guy who turned out to be a reasonable psychiatrist. I'll never forget. He said, "Your daughter is clinically depressed." I remember sitting in his office. He saw us on a Saturday like at six o'clock. He did us a favor. And I remember I just sat there. It was a sort of darkened office. It was the first time I ever cried in front of anybody. [female social worker, aged 38]

And on the liberating side:

> They gave me a blood test that measures the level of something in the blood, in the brain. And they pronounced me, they said "Mr. Smith [a pseudonym], you're depressed." And I said "Thank God," you know. I wasn't as batty as I thought. It was like the cat was out of the bag. You know? It was a breakthrough....[Before that] depression wasn't in my vocabulary....It was the beginning of being able to sort out a lifetime of feelings, events...my entire life. It was the chance for a new beginning. [male salesman, aged 30]

> It [getting a diagnosis] was a great relief. I said, "You mean there is something wrong with me. Its not some sort of weird complex mental thing." I was like tying myself up in knots trying to figure out what strange mechanism in my mind was producing unhappiness from this set of circumstances....It's like, "No, you're sick! (sigh) There was an enormous relief. [female software quality control manager, aged 31]

It is impossible to consider the kinds of profound identity changes occasioned by any mental illness without paying special attention to the experience of hospitalization. It is one thing to deal alone with the demons of depression, or to privately see a psychiatrist for the problem, but once a person "shuts down" altogether and seeks asylum or is involuntarily "committed," he or she adds an institutional piece to their biography that is indelible. Social scientists have properly given a great deal of attention to the identity consequences of hospitalization for mental illness.[10]

A few interviewees described the hospital as truly an asylum that provided relief and allowed them to "crash." Being hospitalized enabled them to give up the struggle of trying to appear and act normally. One person, in fact, described the hospital as a "wonderful place" where "I was taken care of, totally taken care of." Another was relieved "to go somewhere where I won't do anything to myself, where I can get in touch with this." Someone else explained, "I was glad to be there, definitely. It was a break from everything." Sometimes people were glad to be hospitalized since it provided dramatic and definitive evidence that something was really wrong with them when family and friends had been dismissing their complaints. More usual, though, were the responses like that of the person who said that "the experience of hospitalization was devastating to me" and the several who reported that being hospitalized made them feel like "damaged goods."

I found particularly chilling Sam's account. Sam was a person I first met at a depression support group. At age 58, he seemed anxious to recount what hospital treatment was like "before they even had antidepressants." I knew from our previous casual conversation and his distinctive accent that Sam had grown up in the South. During the interview I learned more about his religious upbringing. His father had been a minister and his mother, although a stern figure, "was dependable." Sam first became sick enough to be hospitalized when he was a high school senior. He remembers that after his two-month stay, "You went back with the stigma on you because people who went off their rocker went to [names a state hospital]. You know how kids are. They make jokes about crazy people.... The cops also knew about this and had me marked down as a crazy person from then on." However, it wasn't remembrance of his return home that startled me. I could barely listen to his description of the hospitalization itself. Although Sam did not blame anyone for his treatment, saying, "It's not that they were cruel or anything. They just didn't know," I could not imagine being a 17-year-old and living through an experience like Sam's.

Although Sam's story was the most disturbing I heard, many of the 29 people who spoke of their time in hospitals spontaneously acknowledged the extraordinary impact of the experience on the way they thought about themselves. Sometimes they were themselves shocked that they had landed in a hospital. Several mentioned that hospitalization caused them to confront for the first time just how sick they were.

> I remember being put onto the floor that was probably for the worst people of the sickness, because it was one of those floors where everything was really locked up. So I guess I was in pretty bad shape. [male administrator, aged 54]

> So I went to [names hospital] and I remember praying that I would get out. To me it seemed at the time as if the door would close—It was a secure facility—and I would never leave. I know I'm a basket case at this point.... The experience of having that severe depression, going to the hospital, and most of all being given shock treatments.... It made me feel...like damaged goods, impaired in some way that I was just not normal. It did make me feel impaired. [male professor, part-time, aged 48]

Among the identity-related comments about the hospitalization experience, one set of observations, although made by only a few individuals, caught my attention. Once in the hospital these persons surveyed their environment, both the oppressive physical character of the place and the sad shape of their fellow "inmates," many of whom seemed to them destined for an institutionalized life. However awful their condition, these respondents made a distinction between their trouble and patients who were overtly psychotic. Unlike those unfortunates, they had a choice to make, as they saw it. Either they would capitulate completely to their depression and possibly, therefore, to a life in the mental health system or they would do whatever necessary to leave the hospital as quickly as possible.

Giving up completely did have some appealing features. Full surrender meant relief from an exhausting battle and absolution from personal responsibility. One woman said, "I saw these people going back and forth [in and out of the hospital] for their whole lives [and] that I could be one [of them]. If I went in that direction, it somehow absolved me from responsibility. And I teetered on the edge for a long time. It involved a conscious decision... [about whether] I'm going to become a [permanent] part of the system because it's safe and where I belong." Another person described giving up as seductive because "you don't have to go out there and live by the rules of life. You never have to go out and risk things because you're in a safe environment." In effect, hospitalization posed for these individuals a consequential identity choice; a kind of "to be or not to be" moment in which they would see themselves as either hopelessly mentally ill or as salvageable. The starkness of the choice is caught in the following comment.

> I spent a month there....I saw people who really were insane. People who wanted to live their lives but had their lives constantly interrupted by having to come back here. And I saw what it was like to have my life taken away from me. Because for the first week or two they always keep you on a secure floor to make sure you're not nuts enough to hurt yourself. Which at that time I wasn't. But, the unsecure floor where I was supposed to be promoted almost immediately was full up. I spent about ten days to two weeks on a secure floor with my sharps taken away from me. And having to be let in and out of the unit to go to lunch and dinner. And I think it sort of sank in that...I was going to have to redefine my choices. And that's what it took. It took being up against what it would be like to be an insane person.... [It was] seeing what being mentally ill was like, and saying, "This is not for me." [female software quality control manager, aged 31]

Another critical feature of this career juncture was the recommendation that as "patients" they ought to begin taking antidepressant medications. one outstanding uniformity in the interviews was the initially strong negative reaction people had to taking drugs. One person was "leery of it" and others variously described the idea of going on medications as "revolting," "certainly not my first choice," and "embarrassing." Others elaborated on the recommendation that they begin drug therapy in ways similar to the nurse who said: "I didn't want to be told that I had something that was going to affect the rest of my life and that could only be solved by taking pills. And there was sort of a rebellion in that: 'No, I'm not like that. I don't need you and your pills.'" Underneath these common responses was the shared feeling that taking drugs was yet another distressing indication of the severity of a problem they could not control by themselves. The concurrent events of crisis, hospitalization, and beginning a drug regimen worked synergistically to concretize and dramatize respondents' status as patients with an illness that required ongoing treatment by therapeutic experts.

Coming to Grips with an Illness Identity

Whether people are hospitalized or not, involvement with psychiatric experts and medications is the transition point to a number of simultaneous processes, all with implications for the reformulation of identity. They are (1) reconstructing and reinterpreting one's past in terms of current experiences, (2) looking for causes for one's situation, (3) constructing new theories about the nature of depression, and (4) establishing modes of coping behavior. All of these activities require judgments about the appropriate metaphors for describing one's situation. Especially critical to ongoing identity construction is whether respondents approve of illness metaphors for describing their experience. A few individuals were willing clearly to define their condition as a mental illness:

> I know I have a mental illness. I'm beginning to feel that. [But] actually, there is a real relief in that. It's a sense of "Whew! Okay, I don't have to masquerade." I mean, sure I'll masquerade with work, because, listen, I've got to get the bread and butter on the table. But I don't have to masquerade in other ways. . . . It's sort of like mentally ill people in some ways . . . are my people. There is a fair amount of really chronically mentally ill people at [names hospital where she works]. They're all on heavy-duty meds and I figure like "I know what it's like for you." I mean, I can imagine what it's like. I know some of that pain. I'm sure I don't know all of it, because, you know, I'm not that bad off, but there is sort of a sense like they could understand me and I could understand them in something that's really, really painful. [female physical therapist, aged 42]

> I do think of it now very much . . . as an illness. I don't know what its base is, what its origin is. . . . Is it because I have a fucked-up family, or is there a screw up in my synapses? But I think, you know, I have an illness. . . . It's something that I see myself living with for the rest of my life. And it's something I see myself having to construct my life around, as opposed to being able to flush it down the drain, and say, "Okay, got rid of it." And because of that, I see it as an illness and not in any way related to my will or wants. [female mental health worker, aged 27]

Most, however, wanted simultaneously to embrace the definition of their problem as biochemical in nature while rejecting the notion that they suffer from a "mental" illness.

> I don't see it as an illness. To me, it seems like part of myself that evolved, part of my personality. And, I mean, it sounds crazy, but it is almost like a dual personality, the happy side of me and the sad side of me. And I mean, that's how I referred to it a lot when I was growing up. I mean biologically, I would have

to say, "Yeah, I have a permanent illness or whatever." But I don't like to look at that. I would prefer not to think of it that way. I mean, if there was another word, I wouldn't use illness. I guess, disorder. (pause) I'm comfortable with mental disorder. [female nanny, aged 22]

If you say illness, that means there's something wrong with you...especially a psychiatric label. That means I'm defective. If you told me I was diabetic I wouldn't think of it as bad. That would be acceptable and I would do whatever I have to live with that. But to tell me I had a mental illness, that made me feel defective. [female nurse, aged 37]

Adopting the view that one is victimized by a biochemically sick self constitutes a comfortable "account" for a history of difficulties and failures and absolves one of responsibility. On the negative side, however, acceptance of a victim role, while diminishing a sense of personal responsibility, is also enfeebling. To be a victim of biochemical forces beyond one's control gives force to others' definition of oneself as a helpless, passive object of injury. James Holstein and Gale Miller comment that "victimization...provides an interpretive framework and a discourse that relieves victims of responsibility for their fates, but at a cost. The cost involves the myriad ways that the victim image debilitates those to whom it is applied."[11] The interpretive dilemma for respondents was to navigate between rhetorics of biochemical determinism and a sense of personal efficacy.

There was a sense of relief when I started finding out that the medication was helpful, because then I could say it was a chemical problem and that I'm not looney tunes and that, you know, it's not a mental illness which sounds real bad to me....So, in a sense it was very comforting to be able to use the word chemical imbalance as opposed to mental illness. [male salesman, aged 30]

The illness thing I suppose I finesse to a certain degree....I mean, when a depression becomes profound enough to require hospitalization, I'd say I'm in the category of the ill or the emotionally ill, but I don't think of myself as an ill person generally. I think of myself as a pretty high functioning person who has some experiences like this along the way. [male professor, part-time, aged 48]

Respondents generally fall into two broad categories regarding their hopes that they can put depression behind them. First are those who view having depression as a life condition that they will never fully defeat and second are those who believe that either they are now past the depression forever or that they can attain such a status. As might be expected, the two categories are generally formed by those who have experienced depression as an ongoing chronic thing, on the one hand, in contrast to those who have had periods of depression punctuated by wellness. The role of medications is interesting in establishing for some the idea that depression is something they can leave behind. Among the words that reappeared in comments about drugs was "miracle." Although, as noted, most of those interviewed at first took medication reluctantly, several reported that often for the first time in their lives they felt okay after a drug "kicked in." Generally, subjects were split between those who felt that while there was always the possibility of a reoccurrence, they essentially could get past depression and those who have surrendered to its inevitability and chronicity in their lives. The following comments summarize the two positions:

> I've stopped thinking, "OK I'm going to get over this depression. I'm going to finally, like, do this primal scream thing, or whatever.... [At one point] I did buy into [the idea] of the pursuit of happiness and the pursuit of fulfillment. I hate that word. And the mental health equivalent to finding fulfillment is to fill up the gaps inside of you and everything grows green. And that's what [psychiatry] is really striving for... and that's the standard life should be lived on.... But then I finally realized that well, maybe I'm in a desert. Maybe your landscape is green, but, you know, I'm in the Sahara and I've stopped trying to get out.... I'd rather cure it if I had my choice, but I don't think that is going to happen. My choice is to integrate it into my life. So, no, I don't see it going away. I just see myself becoming, you know, better able to cope with it, more graceful about it. [female mental health worker, aged 27]

> I would say that this particular period of my life is a period where I don't have the fear or feeling [that depression will reoccur]. That's why, for me at least, I'm more inclined now to take the depression as an aberration and to take me in my more expansive, expressive state as the norm. For me, maybe I'm deluding myself, the way I feel now, and it's been three years since the hospitalization and I take no medications of any kind, [is] that I may be out of the woods, so to speak.... At the moment I don't have a fear of reoccurrence, but I do remember having it. [male professor, part-time, aged 48]

Unfortunately, the norm is for people to have repeated bouts with depression. In this regard, the process described here has a feedback-loop quality to it. Individuals move through a crisis with all its attendant identity-altering features, come to grips with the meaning of their experience by constructing theories about causation, and then sometimes reach the point where they feel they have gone beyond the depression experience. A new episode of depression, of course, casts doubt on all the previous interpretive work and requires people to once again move through a process of sense-making and identity construction. In this way, depression is like a virus that keeps mutating since each reliving of an experience, as the philosopher Edmund Husserl tells us, is a new experience. Chronically depressed people are constantly in the throes of an illness that is tragically familiar, but always new. As such, depression often involves a life centered on a nearly continuous process of construction, destruction, and reconstruction of identities in the face of repeated problems.

CONCLUSION

Chronic emotional illness poses especially difficult problems of sense-making because the source of the problem is unclear and its course uncertain.

The interview material presented illustrates that peoples' experience with clinical depression is an exercise in negotiating ambiguity and involves the evolution of an illness consciousness often extending over many years. The effort to describe how those living with depression interpret and respond to their problem over time complements the large volume of survey research studies on depression that neglect the processes through which illness realities are socially constructed.

Conceptually, the chapter's analysis focused on the intersection of the ideas of career and identity. Following the lead of sociologists who have demonstrated the value of the career concept for framing a range of human processes, this chapter was organized around four generic stages through which all respondents moved as they tried to comprehend their puzzling life condition. Everyone initially felt discomfort and emotional pain, which they could not name as depression. This was followed by the recognition that something was "really" wrong with them. In turn, people experienced a crisis that thrust them into a therapeutic world of mental health professionals. Finally, the crisis precipitated a stage of coming to grips with a mental illness diagnosis. Each stage corresponds to ongoing identity shifts as individuals come to view themselves as damaged and in need of repair by psychiatric experts. These identity transformations hinge, for example, on the way individuals reinterpret their pasts in the face of the depression diagnosis, deal with information control about their problem, experience hospitalization, understand the meaning of taking medication, and evaluate the validity of the illness metaphor.

References

1. Berger, P., and Luckman, T. 1967. *The Social Construction of Reality*. Garden City, NY: Doubleday.
2. Foucault, M. 1973. *Madness and Civilization: A History of Insanity in the Age of Reason*. Translated from the French by Richard Howard. New York: Vintage Books.
3. Hughes, E. 1958. *Men and Their Work*. New York: Free Press.
4. Strauss, A. 1992. "Turning Points in Identity." In *Social Interaction*, edited by C. Clark and H Robboy. New York: St. Martin's.
5. Karp, D., and W. Yoels. 1981. "Work, Careers, and Aging." *Quantitative Sociology* 4:145–166.
6. Emerson, R., and S. Messinger. 1977. "The Micro-politics of Trouble." *Social Problems* 25:121–133.
7. Brown, P. 1987. "Diagnostic Conflict and Contradiction in Psychiatry." *Journal of Health and Social Behavior* 28:37–50
8. Vaughan, D. 1986. *Uncoupling: Turning Points in Intimate Relationships*. New York: Oxford.
9. Berger, P., and Kellner, H. 1964. "Marriage and the Construction of Reality." *Diagnoses* 46:1–25.
10. Stanton, A., and M. Schwartz. 1954. *The Mental Hospital*. New York: Basic Books.
11. Holstein, J., and G. Miller. 1990. "Rethinking Victimization: An Interactional Approach to Victimology." *Symbolic Interaction* 13:103–122.

DISCUSSION

1. How does the self-identity of individuals experiencing depression change over the course of their illness career? What are the key experiences—internal and external—the influence these social psychological processes?

2. What is the difference between an "illness career" and an "illness identity"? Do all of Karp's respondents adopt an "illness identity" as a result of their experiences with depression?

3. How, and in what ways, might the theoretical stages described by Karp vary depending on the nature of psychiatric symptoms or diagnosis? That is, would the process he describes be the same or different for people who struggle with schizophrenia, bipolar disorder, or some other psychiatric diagnosis?

THE HISTORY AND SOCIAL ORGANIZATION OF MENTAL HEALTH POLICY AND TREATMENT

The social organization of psychiatric care and treatment has undergone significant changes over the years. Prior to the 18th and 19th centuries, social responses to mental illness in Europe and the United States varied from community to community and were deeply intertwined with prominent local cultural beliefs. In part because the behaviors and symptoms characteristic of what we now think of as mental illness could not be easily explained, communities often relied on the supernatural for explanations. In some societies, people who exhibited strange or bizarre behavior were believed to be possessed by spirits and were socially shunned, reviled, tortured, or even killed. In other communities, common psychiatric symptoms, such as visual or auditory hallucinations, were viewed as being indicative of special powers or a supernatural presence. Because of the reliance on these types of explanations, religious leaders and institutions often played a significant role in the care and treatment of people with mental illnesses. Unfortunately, families were often unable to care for their mentally ill relatives, and many people with mental illness were abandoned and left to fend for themselves. Others were warehoused in small community-based "institutions" such as local jails, almshouses, and poor houses.

In the 19th century, a more organized societal response emerged. Small groups of reformers began to question the societal treatment of the sick and infirm, including people with mental disorders. Many reformers argued that society had a responsibility to care for people with "mental deficiencies" and worked to establish dedicated private and public "asylums." These reformers had a major impact on mental health policy in the United States. By the end of 19th century, virtually every state and many territories in the United States and western European nations had established asylums or hospitals for the "treatment of the insane." With the ascendance of medical authority, a growing body of scientific knowledge regarding the brain and the causes of mental disorders, and changes in societal attitudes about the appropriate care and treatment of people with mental illness, mental health treatment, and policy has continued to change over the course of the 20th and early 21st centuries. In the 1950s, asylums and psychiatric hospitals received widespread criticism for being "inhumane" and providing ineffective "treatment" for people with mental illness. The result was deinstitutionalization—a widespread policy to close or downsize psychiatric hospitals and to rely on care provided in community-based settings that persists even today. The first three readings trace the major changes in mental health policy and treatment in the United States over the past 150 years.

As we have emphasized throughout this reader, the sociological and psychiatric perspectives on mental illness differ markedly. Most psychiatric research on mental health treatment focuses on evaluating the relative efficacy or effectiveness of discrete interventions, such as a specific psychiatric medication or behavioral intervention. Sociologists involved in mental health services research, in contrast, are generally more interested in the social forces that influence the development and expansion of particular treatment modalities or how the social organization of treatment influences the life experiences of people formally labeled as having a psychiatric illness. The second group of readings in this section provides you with an overview of the structure of contemporary mental health systems in the United States and highlights some important sociological dimensions of the organization or consequences of mental health care.

Sociohistorical Perspectives on Mental Health Treatment and Policy

David J. Rothman

The New World of the Asylum

In this chapter from his classic book, The Discovery of the Asylum, social historian David Rothman introduces you to the "New World of the Asylum." He traces many of the early reformers' philosophical beliefs and how they shaped the establishment and design of some of most famous asylums and hospitals in the United States. Rothman's description offers an important historical perspective on the social organization of 19th century psychiatric care.

The sturdy walls of the insane asylum became familiar landmarks in pre-Civil War America. They jutted out from flat rural landscapes or rose above the small houses of new suburbs, visible for some distance and unmistakably different from surrounding structures. Their growth was rapid and sudden. Before 1810, only a few eastern seaboard states had incorporated private institutions to care for the mentally ill, and Virginia alone had established a public asylum. All together they treated less than 500 patients, most of whom came from well-to-do families. Few departures from colonial practices occurred in the first 40 years after independence; the insane commonly languished in local jails and poorhouses or lived with family and friends. But in the course of the next few decades, in a dramatic transformation, state after state constructed asylums. Budding manufacturing centers like New York and Massachusetts erected institutions in the 1830s, and so did the agricultural states of Vermont and Ohio, Tennessee, and Georgia. By 1850, almost every northeastern and midwestern legislature supported an asylum; by 1860, 28 of the 44 states had public institutions for the insane.

Rothman, David J. 2002. "The New World of the Asylum." Pp. 130–154 in *Discovery of the Asylum: Social Order and Disorder in the New Republic*. Hawthorne, NY: Aldine de Gruyter.

Although not all of the mentally ill found a place within a hospital, and a good number among the aged and chronic poor remained in almshouses and jails, the institutionalization of the insane became the standard procedure of the society during these years. A cult of asylum swept the country.[1]

The movement was not born of desperation. Institutionalization was not a last resort of a frightened community. Quite the opposite. Psychiatrists and their lay supporters insisted that insanity was curable, more curable than most other ailments. Spokesmen explained that their understanding of the causes of insanity equipped them to combat it, and the asylum was a first resort, the most important and effective weapon in their arsenal.

The program's proponents confidently and aggressively asserted that properly organized institutions could cure almost every incidence of the disease. They spread their claims without restraint, allowing the sole qualification that the cases had to be recent. Practitioners competed openly with one another to formulate the most general and optimistic principle, to announce the most dramatic result. One of the first declarations came from the superintendent of the Massachusetts asylum at Worcester, Samuel Woodward. "In recent cases of insanity," he announced in 1834, "under judicious treatment, as large a proportion of recoveries will take place as from any other acute disease of equal severity." In his own institution, he calculated, 82.25 percent of the patients recovered. Still, Woodward's tone was judicious and moderate in comparison to later assertions. Dr. Luther Bell, from Boston's McLean Hospital, had no doubt that all recent cases could be remedied. "This is the general rule," he insisted in 1840; "the occasional instance to the contrary is the exception." Performance ostensibly kept pace with theoretical statements. John Galt reported from Virginia in 1842 that, excluding patients who died during treatment, he had achieved 100 percent recoveries. The following year, Dr. William Awl of the Ohio asylum simply announced without qualification 100 percent cures.[2]

These statistics were inaccurate and unreliable. Not only was there no attempt to devise criteria for measuring recovery other than release from an institution, but in some instances a single patient, several times admitted, discharged, and readmitted, entered the lists as five times cured. At Pennsylvania's Friends' asylum, for example, 87 persons contributed 274 recoveries. It was not until 1877 that the first major attack on these exaggerated claims appeared, and only at a time when the widespread faith in curability had already begun to evaporate.

Before the Civil War, these extraordinary pronouncements were widely accepted at face value, and no sceptical voices tried to puncture the balloon of inflated hopes. Psychiatrists, confident of having located the origins of the disease, were fully prepared to believe and to testify that the incredible number of cures was the just fruit of scientific investigation. Personal ambition as well as intellectual perspective made them eager to publicize these findings. The estimates were self-perpetuating; as soon as one colleague announced his grand results, others had little choice but to match or excel him. With supervisory committees of state legislatures and boards of trustees using the number of recoveries as a convenient index for deciding appointments and promotions, medical superintendents were under great competitive pressure to report very high rates. And professionals and laymen alike desperately wanted to credit calculations that would glorify American science and republican humanitarianism. A cure for insanity was the kind of discovery that would honor the new nation.[3]

The consistency of the claims quickly established their validity. With an almost complete absence of dissenting opinion, the belief in the curative powers of the asylum spread through many layers of American society. Given the hyperbolic declarations of the professionals, laymen had little need to exaggerate their own statements. The most energetic and famous figure in the movement, Dorothea Dix, took the message from Massachusetts to Mississippi. With passion and skill she reported in painful detail on the wretched condition of the insane in poorhouses and jails—"Weigh the iron chains and shackles, breathe the foul atmosphere, examine the furniture, a truss of straw, a rough plank"—and next recited the promise of the asylum. Her formula was simple and she repeated it everywhere: first assert the curability of insanity, link it directly to proper institutional care, and then quote prevailing medical opinion on rates of recoveries. Legislators learned that Dr. Bell believed that cure in an asylum was the general rule, incurability the exception, and that Drs. Ray, Chandler, Brigham, Kirkbride, Awl, Woodward, and Earle held similar views.[4] Legislative investigatory committees also returned with identical findings. Both Massachusetts and Connecticut representatives heard from colleagues that insanity yielded as readily as ordinary ailments to proper treatment. The most tax-conscious assemblyman found it difficult to stand up against this overwhelming chorus. One after another, the states approved the necessary funds for erecting asylums.[5]

The institution itself held the secret to the cure of insanity. Incarceration in a specially designed setting, not the medicines that might be administered or the surgery that might be performed there, would restore health. This strategy for treatment flowed logically and directly from the diagnosis of the causes of the disease. Medical superintendents located its roots in the exceptionally open and fluid quality of American society. The American environment had become so particularly treacherous that insanity struck its citizens with terrifying regularity.

One had only to take this dismal analysis one step further to find an antidote. Create a different kind of environment, which methodically corrected the deficiencies of the community, and a cure for insanity was at hand. This, in essence, was the foundation of the asylum solution and the program that came to be known as *moral treatment*. The institution would arrange and administer a disciplined routine that would curb uncontrolled impulses without cruelty or unnecessary punishment. It would recreate fixity and stability to compensate for the irregularities of the society. Thus, it would rehabilitate the casualties of the system.[6] The hospital walls would enclose a new world for the insane, designed in the reverse image of the one they had left. The asylum would also exemplify for the public the correct principles of organization. The new world of the insane would correct within its restricted domain the faults of the community and through the power of example spark a general reform movement.[7]

The broad program had an obvious similarity to the goals of the penitentiary, and both ventures resembled in spirit and outlook the communitarian movements of the period, such as Brook Farm and New Harmony. There was a utopian flavor to correctional institutions. Medical superintendents and penitentiary designers were almost as eager as Owenites to evolve and validate general principles of social organization from their particular experiments.

The central problem for these first psychiatrists was to translate the concept of a curative environment into reality. Rehabilitation demanded a special milieu, and they devoted almost all of their energy to its creation. The appropriate arrangement of the asylum, its physical dimensions, and daily routine, monopolized their thinking. The term for psychiatrist in this period, *medical superintendent*, was especially apt. Every detail of institutional design was a proper and vital subject for his consideration. His skills were to be those of the architect and the administrator, not the laboratory technician.

The writings of Thomas Kirkbride, head of the prestigious Pennsylvania Hospital for the Insane from 1840 until his death in 1883, testified to the significance of this perspective. He published one of the leading textbooks on insanity, *On the Construction, Organization, and General Arrangements of Hospitals for the Insane, with some Remarks on Insanity and Its Treatment;* and the title was ample evidence of the volume's intellectual focus and ordering of priorities.[8] Kirkbride gave the book over to the location of ducts and pipes in asylums, and to accounts of daily routines. He first discussed the proper size and location for the buildings, the right materials for constructing walls and making plaster, the best width for rooms and height for ceilings, the most suitable placement of water closets and dumbwaiters; then he analyzed how to group patients, to staff the hospital, to occupy the inmates during the day. This type of treatise, it is true, was very useful at a time when building and managing institutions was an infant skill. Still, the objective needs of the situation were only a part of the inspiration for a book like Kirkbride's. Far more important to him was the conviction that in settling these technical matters of construction and maintenance, he was confronting and solving the puzzle of curing insanity.

His attitude was not idiosyncratic. The Association of Medical Superintendents, organized in 1844, had a membership composed exclusively of heads of asylums. Institutional affiliation, not research or private practice, defined the profession; the association's committees were predominantly concerned with administrative and architectural questions. There was a committee on construction, on the proper number of patients for one institution, on the best role of chapels and chaplains in the asylum, on separate structures for colored persons, on the comparative advantages of hospital and home treatment. The association also published the *American Journal of Insanity,* a periodical devoted to a wide range of issues. But the primary focus of the group was on the structure of institutions. In 1851 it produced its first major policy statement, a definition of the proper asylum architecture. Resolution number eight, for example, declared: "Every ward should have in it a parlor, a corridor...an associated dormitory...a clothes room, a bath room, a water closet...a dumb waiter, and a speaking tube." In 1853 it issued a second declaration on administrative organization; Rule number seven captured its spirit: "The matron, under the direction of the superintendent, should have a general supervision of the domestic arrangements."[9] In fact, the association was never able to widen its concerns. In the 1870s, when new ideas begin to revolutionize the field, it remained unalterably fixed to its original program, becoming a stumbling block to experimentation and innovation.

There was a functional quality to this narrowness of perspective. Medical superintendents lacked any guidelines with which to design and administer the first mental hospitals. Never before had Americans attempted to confine large numbers of people for long periods of time, and the difficulties were all the greater since their goals extended far beyond simple restraint. Eighteenth-century practices had little relevance to 19th-century officials. The almshouse and the jail represented all that medical superintendents wished to avoid in an institution.

Contemporary European practices were not very much more helpful. American superintendents frequently crossed the ocean to examine Continental institutions, but their visits were usually unproductive. Pliny Earle, who first headed the Friends' asylum in Philadelphia and then Bloomingdale in New York, toured the Continent in 1838–39 and then again in 1845, and his reports illuminated the unique problems and special opportunities confronting Americans, who were at once more free to innovate and yet felt more keenly the lack of precedents. European asylums, Earle discovered, were frequently nothing other than a new name carved in an ancient doorway. Each structure had a long history of different uses—a 14th-century monastery became later a 16th-century fort, and still later an 18th-century almshouse, and finally a 19th-century mental hospital. Earle methodically noted how in Prussia the asylums at Siegburg and at Brieg and at Owinsk were all former monasteries; in Halle, the hospital occupied the quarters of the old prison. The Austrian town of Ybbs, he found, turned a building that had served successively as a barracks, a military hospital, and an almshouse into an asylum. So, too, the German town of Sonnestein converted a onetime castle into a place for the insane and the village of Winnental made over to them a nobleman's palace that had once been a monastery.[10] But Americans, in marked contrast, had to start from scratch. "There were no old halfruined monasteries," observed one Englishman, "to be converted into asylums for their insane poor....Americans had to build their own asylums." They had the opportunity to create something new, and the predicament of precisely how to go about it.[11]

Medical superintendents received little assistance from their countrymen. No groups of specialists—architects, engineers, bureaucrats—possessed requisite skills for constructing and administering a mental hospital. There were no large-scale organizations in the country whose designs and procedures could be easily emulated. One result of these circumstances was that every new asylum became the immediate focus of attention for other officials. Medical superintendents and legislative investigatory committees from neighboring states seemed to have arrived at the door of a new institution along with its first patients. No sooner did New York State appoint a board of commissioners to construct an insane asylum in 1839 than the committee visited the institutions in Massachusetts, Pennsylvania, and other nearby states; two years later the first trustees of the new Utica asylum made an exhaustive review of procedures in all leading mental hospitals. The tour of inspection was as necessary as it was popular.[12]

But an even more important result of these circumstances was that the concepts shared by medical superintendents exercised an exceptional degree of influence in the actual construction and administration of the first insane asylums. With few precedents to guide them, they experimented with their own ideas; with no inherited structures to limit them, they built institutions according to their particular designs. Hence, reformatory theory and practical needs fit well together, perhaps too well. It may be that part of the enthusiasm for environmental solutions reflected the lack of experience. Still, this concentrated attention to institutional organization established the guidelines for translating confinement into cure.

The first postulate of the asylum program was the prompt removal of the insane from the community. As soon as the first symptom of the disease appeared, the patient had to enter a mental hospital. Medical superintendents unanimously and without qualification asserted that treatment within the family was doomed to fail. They recognized the unusual nature of their doctrine and its apparent illogic. Since families had traditionally lodged the insane, it might seem a cruel and wanton abdication of responsibility to send a sick member to a public institution filled with other deranged persons. But they carefully explained this fundamental part of their program. Isaac Ray, chief of Rhode Island's asylum, conceded that "to sever a man's domestic ties, to take him out of the circle of friends and relatives most deeply interested in his welfare...and place him...in the hands of strangers, and in the company of persons as disordered as himself—at first sight, would seem...little likely to exert a restorative effect." Yet he and his colleagues insisted that isolation among strangers was a prerequisite for success. Although the strategy might increase the momentary pain of the disease, it promised an ultimate cure. "While at large," Ray declared, "the patient is every moment exposed to circumstances that maintain the morbid activity of his mind...[and] the dearer the friend, the greater the emotion....In the hospital, on the other hand, he is beyond the reach of all these causes of excitement."[13] How else, asked Edward Jarvis, could the insane escape "the cares and anxieties of business...the affairs of the town...the movements of religious, political and other associations....Hospitals are the proper places for the insane....The cure and care of the insane belong to proper public institutions."[14]

Second, the institution itself, like the patients, was to be separate from the community. According to medical superintendents' design, it was to be built at a distance from centers of population. Since it was dependent upon the city for personnel and supplies, it could not completely escape contact. But the institution was to have a country location with ample grounds, to sit on a low hillside with an unobstructed view of a surrounding landscape. The scene ought to be tranquil, natural, and rural, not tumultuous and urban. Moreover, the asylum was to enforce isolation by banning casual visitors and the patients' families. If friends and relatives "were allowed the privilege they seek," cautioned Ray, "the patient might as well be at large as in the hospital, for any good the latter may do him by way of seclusion." Correspondence was also to be strictly limited. Even the mails were not to intrude and disrupt the self-contained and insular life.[15]

But the most important element in the new program, the core of moral treatment, lay in the daily government of the mentally ill. Here was the institution's most difficult and critical task. It had to control the patient without irritating him, to impose order but in a humane fashion. It had to bring discipline to bear but not harshly, to introduce regularity into chaotic lives without exciting frenetic reactions. "Quiet, silence, regular routine," declared Ray, "would take the place of restlessness, noise and fitful activity." Superintendents had to walk a tightrope, making sure that they did not fall to the one side of brutality or the other of indulgence. "So long as the patient is allowed to follow the bent of his own will," insisted Ray, he exacerbated his illness; outside the asylum, the "only alternative was, either an unlimited indulgence of the patient in his caprices, or a degree of coercion and confinement which irritated his spirit and injured his health." The charge of the asylum was to bring discipline to the victims of a disorganized society. To this end it had to isolate itself and its members from chaotic conditions. Behind the asylum walls medical superintendents would create and administer a calm, steady, and rehabilitative routine. It would be, in a phrase that they and their lay supporters repeated endlessly, "a well-ordered institution."[16]

The asylum's designers often labored under severe financial limitations, when legislatures and private philanthropists were not generous with appropriations. Sometimes public officials interfered with their policies, setting down admission requirements that limited administrators' prerogatives. In Massachusetts, for example, the state hospital had to admit the most troublesome and least curable cases first; legislators were more impressed with the convenience than the effectiveness of the institution. And many superintendents were discontented with one facet or another of the asylum's architecture or procedures. Nevertheless, there was usually a close correspondence between founders' ideals and the asylum reality.

No principle was more easily or consistently enacted than the physical separation of the asylum from the community. Almost all the institutions constructed after 1820 were located at a short distance from an urban center. New York erected its state asylum one and one-half miles west of the town of Utica, and Massachusetts built its mental hospital outside Worcester, on a hill overlooking the surrounding farmland. In this same spirit, Connecticut's Hartford asylum went up one mile from the city, with a fine view of the countryside. In Philadelphia, the Pennsylvania Hospital, which had long kept a ward for treating the insane, decided in this period to construct a separate facility for them. The city now surrounded the old institution so that the conditions which made the move seem necessary also simplified the raising of money. The hospital sold off some adjoining lots, at a great profit, and used the proceeds to erect an asylum two miles west of Philadelphia on a 101-acre farm. Midwestern states followed eastern practices. Ohio's officials, for example, located the mental hospital on the outskirts of Columbus, choosing a site that offered a broad natural panorama.[17]

There was, to be sure, a close fit between medical superintendents' desires and the more practical concerns of legislators and trustees. Land outside the city was not only more rural but it was cheaper. So, too, under this arrangement, no established community felt threatened by the intrusion of an asylum, or complained that a lunatic hospital would disturb its peace, safety, and real estate values. To the contrary, budding towns and growing suburbs competed for the right to have the institution in their midst, confident that the resulting income would more than compensate for any nuisance. By common agreement, and to everyone's satisfaction, the mental hospital secured its quiet and separate location.

The isolation of patients was more difficult to achieve. Medical superintendents had to balance a policy which was to the immediate benefit of the individual inmate with considerations of the long-range interest of mental hospitals in the nation. The asylum was a new institution, and citizens had to be assured that cruel practices would be prohibited. To exclude all of the interested and curious public from its buildings would not only keep distrust alive but even stimulate it. Under these conditions, legislative appropriations and charitable gifts would be curtailed and families would be loath to commit sick members. Some kind of balance had to be struck between isolation and publicity. Superintendents dared not seal off the institution from society.

The most common solution was to allow, and even encourage, tours of the asylum by the ordinary public while making every effort to curtail contact between patient and family. This arrangement would exhibit the institution to the largest number of persons at the least personal cost to the patient. The private Pennsylvania asylum explained to would-be visitors that "the visits of strangers among the patients, are often much less objectionable than those of friends and relatives." Managers would be "glad to show every part of the establishment, and to explain the details of treatment," to anyone genuinely interested in hospitals for the insane. But at the same time they carefully instructed relatives that "the welfare of the patient often demands that they should be completely interdicted." The presence of a family member could provoke an excitement that would take weeks to overcome and delay the recovery.[18]

A public institution, like the Utica asylum, opened its doors still more widely to strangers. Aware that many in the state were concerned about the institution's accommodations and management, officials uncomplainingly guided some 2,700 visitors around the grounds in a typical year, and even took special groups from different sections of the state through the patients' sleeping quarters. Yet they too asked relatives to avoid coming to the institution. The family, they noted, should not "throw any obstacles in the way of recovery, by frequent visits, or requesting friends and relatives to visit."[19] Medical superintendents also discouraged the exchange of letters, fearing that news from home might intrude on the calm and regular routine of the asylum and upset the patients' stability. They did not exclude all reading material, newspapers, and periodicals from the asylum. But they were eager to preserve the insularity of their domain. "Long and tender letters," warned Ohio's Superintendent William Awl, "containing some ill-timed news, or the melancholy tidings of sickness and death...may destroy weeks and months of favorable progress."[20]

Superintendents' ability to enforce rigid rules was limited. If regulations were too stringent, the family might vacillate and keep the patient at home too long, or commit and then remove him too soon. The chronic and poverty-stricken insane were captive patients; but psychiatrists, convinced of their ability to cure the disease and eager to make the asylum a first resort, wished to treat the recently sick and those from comfortable households as well. Unwilling to frighten away potential patients, and yet determined to assert control, superintendents adopted two tactics. They discouraged but did not *forbid* relatives to visit and they insisted that a patient be committed for a minimum period—at least three or six months. This strategy was well conceived and in the best institutions, successful. Doctors calmed family fears and gained time to effect a cure, or at least to demonstrate progress. The detailed records of the Pennsylvania Hospital, for example, reveal the loss of only a handful of patients by removal annually.[21] Thus, once medical superintendents received a patient, they were usually able to separate him fairly systematically from the outside world.

To isolate the insane more rapidly and effectively from the sources of his illness, medical superintendents were also eager to leave commitment laws as simple and as uncomplicated as possible. Most superintendents preferred to allow relatives to bring the patient directly to the institution and arrange for commitment on the spot; only a few believed that prior judicial examination or jury decisions were necessary. The managers of the Utica asylum, for example, objected strenuously to legal formalities in its incorporation act that made the certification of insanity under oath by two "respectable physicians," a prerequisite for admission.[22]

Their attitudes were not difficult to understand. Confinement, they believed, was not a punishment but a cure, and hence there was as little cause to begin a legal proceeding before the insane entered an asylum as there was to require it for persons going to any other type of hospital. Furthermore, they found no need to rely upon legal processes when they themselves could easily differentiate between sanity and insanity and every cumbersome requirement might discourage someone from sending a patient to the asylum, a risk which medical superintendents wanted to minimize. Finally, judicial routines too often consumed valuable time, and the longer the delay in admissions, the less the likelihood of a cure; better for the insane to sit in the asylum than in the courtroom.[23] These objections were generally persuasive. Managers were comparatively free to confine the mentally ill at their own discretion.

The internal organization of the asylum also represented medical superintendents' attempts to realize the idea of moral treatment. They designed and implemented an orderly and disciplined routine, a fixed, almost rigid calendar, and put daily labor at the heart of it. A precise schedule and regular work became the two chief characteristics of the best private and public institutions, and in the view of their managers, the key to curing insanity. The structure of the mental hospital would counteract the debilitating influences of the community. As one New York doctor explained, "the hours for rising, dressing and washing...for meals, labor, occupation, amusement, walking, riding, etc., should be regulated by the most *perfect precision*....The utmost *neatness* must be observed in the dormitories; the meals must be *orderly* and comfortably served....The physician and assistants must make their visits at *certain* hours."[24] Steady labor would also train inmates to proper habits, bringing regularity to disordered lives. "Useful employment, in the open air," explained the Vermont asylum superintendent, "affords the best moral means for the restoration of many of our patients." Luther Bell, head of the McLean Hospital, fully concurred: "*systematic, regular*, employment in useful body labor...is one appliance of moral treatment, which has been proved immeasurably superior to all others."[25] Precision, certainty, regularity, order—these became the bywords of asylum management, the main weapons in the battle against insanity.

From this perspective, the Pennsylvania Hospital arranged the patients' day. They rose at 5:00, received their medicines at 6:00, and breakfast at 6:30; at 8:00 they went for a physical examination, and then to work or to some other form of exercise. At 12:30 they ate their main meal and then resumed work or other activities until 6:00, when everyone joined for tea. They passed the evening indoors, and all were in bed by 9:30. This careful division of the day into fixed segments of time to rationalize the inmate's life was the creation of the 19th century.[26]

The procedures adopted at Pennsylvania were followed almost exactly in other hospitals. At the Worcester asylum, patients rose at 5:30 in the summer, 5:45 in the winter; after breakfast, according to the managers, "everything is put in readiness for the visit of the superintendent...which commences at precisely *eight* o'clock at all seasons." At Utica, patients awoke to a morning bell at 5:00, ate at 6:30, and officials strictly instructed the attendants to be punctual. One typical rule; "Breakfast is always to be placed upon the table precisely one hour and a half after the ringing of the bells."[27] These regulations had some administrative advantages, enabling superintendents to oversee a more efficient operation. But they reflected even more the strength of a theory that ascribed a therapeutic value to a rigid schedule.

Of all the activities, asylums prized labor the most, going to exceptional lengths to keep patients busy with manual tasks. The Pennsylvania Hospital offered a choice of farming, simple workshop crafts, or household tasks; and superintendent Thomas Kirkbride boasted that many who previously "had unfortunately never been accustomed to labour, nor to habits of industry," were now regularly at work. He encouraged his private patients to do any task; it did not matter whether they planted a garden, husked corn, made baskets or mattresses, cooked, sewed, washed, ironed, attended the furnace or cleaned up the grounds. Outdoor chores were probably most healthy and pleasant, but the critical thing was to keep at the job. This regimen, Kirkbride and his colleagues believed, inculcated regular habits, precisely the trait necessary for patients' recovery, and thus "rarely failed to contribute to the rapidity and certainty of their cure."

The proof for this was apparent in case histories and so exemplary tales abounded. One man, in a typical story, had suffered violent fits at least once a month; he took up gardening, applied himself vigorously, and subsequently was free of recurring attacks. Indeed, medical superintendents sounded very much like penitentiary wardens when claiming that their institutions succeeded, where society had failed, in teaching the virtue of steady labor. Kirkbride was certain that careful administration and a planned "monotony of the parlors and the halls" (wardens talked about the dullness of cells), would lead patients to regard work as a welcome diversion, a privilege and not a punishment. At that moment, every student of deviancy agreed, the inmate was well along the road to rehabilitation.[28]

Public asylums were even more eager to set patients to work. Administrators' needs seemed to fit neatly with inmates' welfare. Just as it was to the superintendent's personal interest to oversee an economical and efficient operation, so too the patient would benefit from a disciplined and fixed routine. The Worcester asylum had the insane clearing the dining-room tables, washing dishes, cleaning corridors, doing laundry, as well as tilling the adjoining farm; and Superintendent Samuel Woodward unhesitantly defended the hospital's right to utilize and even profit from their efforts. After all, this schedule was the best mode of treatment, and it was striking testimony to the asylum's "system of discipline that the labor of this class of individuals can be made available for any valuable purpose." The institution was entitled to the reward for having brought the insane to this stage of improvement. The managers of the Utica asylum followed an identical course. They reported enthusiastically how patients helped remove the enormous quantities of rubble that had accumulated during the period of construction, how they cleaned and scrubbed the institution daily, and how they raised some of their own food. Their pride in keeping costs down and a belief in the medical value of these tasks gave a self-congratulatory tone to officials' remarks. The well-ordered asylum was a hard-working one.[29]

The institution achieved its good order and enforced labor discipline without frequently resorting to the coercion of physical punishment or chains, straitjackets, and other bizarre contrivances. Superintendents everywhere stressed the importance of avoiding harsh penalties and punitive discipline, and their public statements gave first priority to the importance of benign treatment. Of course, declarations of ideals did not always coincide with actual performance, and there were asylums whose professions had little relationship to the hard truth of their practices. Still, many institutions in their first years did live up to these principles. Private asylums in Philadelphia, New York, and Boston were able to avoid in almost all instances artificial restraints and unusual punishment, to well maintain the balance between laxity and cruelty. It demanded great diligence, skillful planning, and painstaking administration, but they achieved the goal.

Pennsylvania's first step was to classify the patient population, dividing the noisy and violent from the quiet and passive, and housing them accordingly. The most dangerous group, those who were most likely to need restraint, entered separate and specially designed buildings. Their rooms were constructed with windows high on the walls, beyond inmates' reach, and could be opened or closed only from an outside hallway. The furiously disordered could not annoy or threaten milder patients, or endanger their own lives. Superintendent Kirkbride chose his attendants well, employed a good number of them—roughly one for every six inmates—and indoctrinated them thoroughly. "We insist," he informed them, "on a mild and conciliatory manner under all circumstances and roughness or violence we never tolerate." A total patient population of about 200 allowed Kirkbride to reserve for his medical staff the decision to use restraints. Convinced that attendants, no matter how rigorously trained or closely supervised were invariably too eager to apply them—thinking it would save them time and aggravation—Kirkbride gave them no discretion. The physicians, he expected, would first exhaust all other remedies. In fact, the staff usually secluded the violent or suicidal inmate in a guarded room and only if his life seemed in danger did it prescribe some form of restraint. Thus, through wise construction, expenditure of funds, and administrative regulations, Kirkbride minimized physical punishments. In a typical year, 1842, he happily reported that with the exception of one woman confined to her bed for a few nights, and seven men kept in wristbands or mittens for a few days, "we have found no reason for applying even the milder kinds of apparatus in a single one of the 238 cases under care."[30]

New York's Bloomingdale Asylum achieved a similar success through identical means. Classification was thorough and intricate for the 150 patients; there were six categories for men, four for women, and two separate buildings to lodge the violent of each sex. The superintendent, Pliny Earle, methodically schooled his attendants, and employed them in adequate numbers, one for approximately every seven inmates. A state legislative committee, after inspecting the institution in 1840, unhesitantly concluded: "The patients appear to have been remarkably well taken care of. There were none fettered, even with straitjackets. A pair of stuffed gloves for one patient, and stuffed chairs, with partial restraint for the arms, were the only restraints on any of the whole number in the establishment."[31]

In Boston, the McLean Hospital also managed to enforce discipline without harsh contrivances. Officials gave exceptional attention to classification, convinced that its importance "can not be overrated." They insisted that proper categorization together with "the extensive architectural arrangements...has enabled us to dispense almost entirely with restraining measures or even rigid confinement." With a dozen groupings to differentiate among the patients, and with such special facilities as a heated and padded room to calm frenzied inmates, McLean did not have to use mechanical constraints with even one percent of its population. Superintendent Luther Bell screened and selected the attendants very judiciously, considering himself especially fortunate not to "feel the want...of a proper kind of assistants." There were in New England, he declared, "a class of young men and women of respectable families, adequate education, and refined moral feelings," who were prepared to devote a few years to asylum employment. Bell hired them in large numbers, on the average of one for every four or five of his 150 patients. He carefully established precise regulations and severely circumscribed their discretionary powers. "No restraint, even of the slightest kind," announced the asylum rules, "should ever be applied or removed except under the direction of an officer." There is every indication that McLean followed both the letter and the spirit of the law.[32]

Public asylums attempted to emulate this performance. Superintendents, regardless of where they served, shared a revulsion against severe discipline, and tried to administer their institutions by the same standards as private asylums. State hospitals were generally less successful in this effort, unable to duplicate the record of Pennsylvania, Bloomingdale, or McLean. Nevertheless, their trustees and managers measured themselves against the criterion of a strict but not cruel discipline, organized a routine, and made necessary revisions to conform better to it. There were lapses and failures, but in the first years of the asylums they were not gross ones. Most mental hospitals in the 1830s and 1840s abolished the whip and the chain and did away with confinement in cold, dank basements and rat-infested cellars—no mean achievement in itself. And often they accomplished more, treating patients with thoughtfulness and humanity.

From its inception, the Utica asylum pledged to avoid corporal punishment, chains, and long periods of solitary confinement to control patients, and during its first years, it kept much of the promise. Managers delighted in describing how quickly they removed the rags and chains that so often bound a new patient, how they bathed and dressed him, and gave him freedom of movement. Almost invariably, they claimed, the patient became quiet, orderly, and responsible. To insure consistent treatment, Utica's regulations also reserved all disciplinary powers to the superintendent, requiring him to keep an official log of every restraint prescribed. Utica's managers instructed attendants precisely and explicitly in their duties: "Under all circumstances," they insisted, "be tender and affectionate; speak in a mild, persuasive tone of voice....A patient is ever to be soothed and calmed when irritated....*Violent hands are never to be laid upon a patient, under any provocation.*"[33]

Nevertheless, the organization and structure of the institution prevented full compliance. Attendants were too few—only 1 for every 15 patients—to allow close supervision to obviate mechanical restraints. No separate buildings existed for noisy and violent inmates—just makeshift rooms—and patients were hardly classified. Not surprisingly, superintendents in the 1840s resorted to some odd forms of discipline, such as a warm bath immediately followed by a cold shower; and they themselves complained about overcrowding, tumult, and filth within the institution. These conditions did not go entirely uncorrected. A new manager in the 1850s introduced more intricate classification and abolished the shower-bath treatment. He, too, however, frequently utilized tight muffs and strapped beds to maintain order. If Utica was by no means a model institution, it did demonstrate a real dedication to the idea of mild punishment.[34]

The Worcester asylum had a similar record. Superintendent Samuel Woodward was intent on demonstrating that the influence of fear and brutal physical force were unnecessary in treating the insane. Despite his good intentions, the asylum did not enjoy consistent success. Performance in its opening years, the mid-1830s, was unsatisfactory. Woodward complained bitterly that the buildings were too few, that classification was impossible, and that attendants were difficult to train. To his extreme displeasure, convalescing patients mingled with violent ones, inmates damaged much of the asylum property, the atmosphere was disorderly, and the patients were clearly not under firm control. Soon, however, the institution entered a second stage, solving within the decade some of these problems. With greater experience and some new facilities, Woodward instilled a steady discipline, so that trustees, including such men as Horace Mann, could boast of "the kindness, the patience, the fidelity, the perseverance and the skill with which the officers and assistants have discharged their duty."[35]

But conditions again degenerated, and by the end of the 1840s trustees and managers were unhappy with internal procedures. Separation and classification became problems as the number of chronic inmates increased, and violent ones inflicted, in Woodward's opinion, "positive injury" on others, and themselves received inadequate care. But their dissatisfactions notwithstanding, they believed that their asylum represented a fundamental improvement over local poorhouses and jails for the insane. So certain were they of this judgment that they refused to discharge a violent or dangerous patient, even when he was unquestionably incurable, to such places. There he would be chained or handcuffed or locked in a dungeonlike cell. At Worcester, for all its faults, he would enjoy greater comfort and care.[36]

The ideals of other public institutions were no different. The directors of the Kentucky asylum insisted that restraints not be utilized, and the managers of the Indiana State Hospital for the Insane diligently instructed attendants to treat patients with "kindness and good will," to "speak to them in a mild, persuasive tone of voice.... Violent hands shall never be laid upon patients... and a blow shall never be returned." The superintendent at the Eastern Lunatic Asylum at Williamsburg, Virginia, pledged to establish a routine in which "kindness coupled with firmness, are the prominent char-acteristics." Practice often fell below these standards, but despite the lapses, the world of the antebellum asylum was a universe apart from local jails and almshouses. Medical superintendents' theories and responses brought a new standard of treatment to the insane.[37]

But the asylum system was highly regimented and repressive. Medical superintendents, carrying out the logic of a theory of deviancy, administered an ordered routine and hoped to eliminate in a tightly organized and rigid environment the instabilities and tensions causing insanity. Their program did resemble that of the penitentiary. Proponents of both institutions insisted on strictly isolating the inmates from society, on removing them as quickly as possible to the asylum, on curtailing relatives' visits and even their correspondence. They both gave maximum attention to matters of design, and both institutions organized their daily routines in exact and punctual fashion, bringing an unprecedented precision and regularity to inmate care.

Superintendents' language, it is true, retained many 18th-century usages. Their favorite metaphor was a family one, and they borrowed freely from family vocabulary to describe asylum procedures. The superintendent at the Utica hospital explained his classification system by noting that "our household" was divided into "ten distinct families." When the Worcester asylum was enjoying its most successful years, Samuel Woodward delight-edly announced that his 230 patients "form a quiet and happy family, enjoying social intercourse, engaging in interesting and profitable employ-ments, in reading, writing and amusements." At Bloomingdale, Pliny Earle reported that "the internal arrangements of the Asylum are nearly the same as those of a well-regulated family."[38] Patients, unlike convicts, wore ordi-nary clothing, and medical superintendents even instructed relatives to send along good items to bolster inmates' self-respect. There were no spe-cial haircuts, no head-shaving, no identification badges, no number-wear-ing in the mental hospital; patients walked from place to place, they did not march about or group in formations. By the same token, psychiatrists were very careful not to use penitentiary terminology. Pennsylvania's Thomas Kirkbride, for example, instructed attendants to avoid certain expressions: "No insane hospital should ever be spoken of as having a cell or a keeper within its walls." A household terminology, he assumed, would help to quiet the patients.[39]

Medical superintendents, however, had very special qualities in mind when they spoke about the family. The routine that they would create in the asylum would bear no resemblance to a casual, indulgent, and negli-gent household that failed to discipline its members or to inculcate a respect for order and authority. Convinced that the primary fault of the contempo-rary family lay in its lax discipline and burdensome demands—so that chil-dren grew up without limits to their behavior or their ambitions—medical superintendents were determined to strike a new balance between liberty and authority, in a social sense. They did not wish to abandon the benevo-lent side of family organization, but they hoped to graft onto it a firm and regulatory regimen. They took their inspiration from the colonial period, believing that they were restoring traditional virtues. But to a surprising degree, the result was more in tune with their own era. Regularity, order, and punctuality brought the asylum routine closer to the factory than the village.

If passersby might easily have mistaken an 18th-century institution for an ordinary dwelling, there was no confusing a 19th-century asylum with a private residence. "The slightest reflection will render it obvious," declared the officials planning the Worcester hospital, "that an edifice designed for the residence of the insane must be materially different, both in form and in interior arrangement, from ordinary habitations."[40] To protect, confine, separate, and treat the insane demanded special architectural forms. Managers looked hard for their answers, and since the search was unprecedented, solutions at times differed. But despite some variety, a common pattern emerged. Typically, a central structure of several stories stood in the middle of the asylum grounds, and from it radiated long and straight wings. The main edifice, and usually the most ornate one, was an administration building, fronted with a columned portico and topped with a cupola of height and distinction. Here the superintendent lived, and here the similarity between a fine home and the asylum was most complete. The wings, however, where the inmates resided, had bare and unrelieved façades. Along their length the windows of the patients' rooms divided the space into regular and exact sequences, giving a uniform and repetitious appearance floor after floor. The design of the Hartford Retreat, one of the better institutions of the period, seemed to one later observer exceptionally "plain and factory-like."[41]

There were alternative designs available to medical superintendents. They might have constructed a series of small houses or cottages, each sleeping 5 to 10 patients. Classification would have been simplified, construction costs not significantly higher, and married couples could have supervised each lodging, giving a familylike quality to the units. But in fact, they welcomed the regimented quality of the wing design because it fit so neatly with their ideas on order and regularity. Its precise divisions, its uniformity and repetitiousness, symbolized superintendents' determination to bring steady discipline into the lives of the insane and to inspire private families to emulation. Since superintendents did not wish to recreate a prisonlike atmosphere, and wanted no one to confuse an asylum with a place of punishment, they carefully disguised window bars behind sashes and in a few of the more prosperous private institutions, carpeted the long hallways. They retained, however, regularity of appearance. This represented, in visual form, their faith in the ability of a fixed order to cure the insane.

Medical superintendents' confidence in the therapeutic effects of a rigid schedule also introduced a punctuality into the asylum routine. The institution brought a bell-ringing precision into inmates' lives. Officials' careful classification and supervision of inmates also gave the asylum a fixed and orderly quality. There would be no informal family government or easy mixing of its members here. The mental hospital grouped its patients, assigned them to different buildings, all men to one side of the wings, all women to the other, the noisy and bothersome to the outside, the calm and quiet to the inside. Each class of patients had its own particular obligations and privileges, and a hierarchy of officials watched their behavior, ready to move them from one category to another. Superintendents were determined not to impose a harsh system, but they saw nothing severe or unwarranted in regularity and regimentation. "Nothing is so important," wrote one psychiatrist, "as discipline and subordination, rules and order, in the government of an insane hospital." These virtues would enable patients to escape their disease.[42]

Thus the insane asylum, like other corrective institutions in the Jacksonian period, represented both an attempt to compensate for public disorder in a particular setting and to demonstrate the correct rules of social organization. Medical superintendents designed their institutions with 18th-century virtues in mind. They would teach discipline, a sense of limits, and a satisfaction with one's position, and in this way enable patients to withstand the tension and the fluidity of Jacksonian society. The psychiatrists, like contemporary penologists, conceived of proper individual behavior and social relationships only in terms of a personal respect for authority and tradition and an acceptance of one's station in the ranks of society. In this sense they were trying to recreate in the asylum their own vision of the colonial community. The results, however, were very different. Regimentation, punctuality, and precision became the asylum's basic traits, and these qualities were far more in keeping with an urban, industrial order than a local, agrarian one. The mental hospital was a rebuke to the casual organization of the household and a self-conscious alternative to the informality of earlier structures like the almshouse. It was, in essence, an institution—at its best uniform, rigid, and regular. This was the new world offered the insane. They were among the first of their countrymen to experience it.

Endnotes

1. For asylums' dates of origin, see John M. Grimes, *Institutional Care of Mental Patients in the United States* (Chicago, 1934), 123–125. Brief histories of the nineteenth-century asylums can be found in Henry M. Hurd, *The Institutional Care of the Insane in the United States and Canada* (Baltimore, 1916, 4 vols.). A useful survey also is Albert Deutsch, *The Mentally Ill in America: A History of Their Care and Treatment* (New York, 1937).
2. A convenient summary of the optimistic statements is in Pliny Earle, *The Curability of Insanity* (Philadelphia, 1887). The quotations are from pp. 23, 27–29; see too, pp. 38–39, 209, table VI. Earle helped to puncture the myth, but he too had once been guilty of perpetuating it: *Visit to Thirteen Asylums,* 130–131. Almost every memorial of Dorothea Dix repeated these declarations.

3. Pliny Earle, *Curability of Insanity,* was the most important statement; see especially pp. 9, 41–42. Some officials did admit to their techniques: Pennsylvania Hospital, *Fifth Annual Report* (Philadelphia, 1846), 25. For the defensiveness of most superintendents, see Worcester Lunatic Hospital, *First Annual Report* (Boston, 1833), 3, 22–23.

4. Dorothea Dix, *Memorial to the Legislature of Pennsylvania,* 3; quotation is condensed from the original. For other examples of her appeal, see *Memorial Soliciting an Appropriation for the State Hospital for the Insane at Lexington [Kentucky]* (Frankfort, K.Y., 1846), 10–11; *Memorial Praying a Grant of Land,* 25–27; *Memorial Soliciting a State Hospital for the Insane Submitted to the Legislature of New Jersey* (Trenton, N.J., 1845), 36–37.

5. *Report of Commissioners to Superintend the Erection of a Lunatic Hospital at Worcester* (Boston, 1832), 19–20; *Report of the Committee on the Insane Poor in Connecticut* (New Haven, C.T., 1838), 3–4. See too Philadelphia Citizens Committee on an Asylum for the Insane Poor, *An Appeal to the People of Pennsylvania* (Philadelphia, 1838), 9; Pliny Earle, *Insanity and Insane Asylums* (Louisville, 1841), 34–39; "Investigation of the Blooming-dale Asylum," *N.Y. Assembly Docs.,* 1831, I, no. 263, pp. 30–31.

6. For an introduction to the literature on moral treatment, see Norman Dain, *Concepts of Insanity,* chs. 1, 5; see, also, J. Sanbourne Bockoven, "Moral Treatment in American Psychiatry," *Journal of Nervous and Mental Disease,* 124 (1936), 183–194, 299–309.

7. *Report of the Insane Poor in Connecticut,* 4–5.

8. (Philadelphia, 1880, 2nd ed.). The volume first appeared in 1847. The entire first part was given over to physical details, the second to administrative details. In this same spirit, see Pennsylvania Hospital, *Second Annual Report* (Philadelphia, 1843), 31–32; Ohio Lunatic Asylum, *Thirteenth Annual Report* (Columbus, O.H., 1852), 60–61.

9. *History of the Association of Medical Superintendents of American Institutions for the Insane,* John Curwen, compiler (n.p., 1875), 4–7, 24–26, 28–30.

10. Pliny Earle, *Institutions for the Insane in Prussia, Austria, and Germany* (Utica, N.Y., 1853), *passim,* and pp. 107–122, 150–151. Earle traveled in 1849. His trip was not an uncommon one; the regularity with which he and his colleagues went to Europe for investigatory purposes ought to warn intellectual historians about taking the notions of a corrupt old world too literally.

11. Sir James Clark, *A Memoir of John Conolly* (London, 1869), 149. Just as Europeans were more cautious about linking civilization with insanity, so they were wary about a cult of institutionalization; see John Conolly, *An Inquiry Concerning the Indications of Insanity* (London, 1830; reprinted, London, 1964).

12. "Report of the Commissioners to Build a Lunatic Asylum," *N.Y. Senate Docs.,* 1839, I, no. 2, pp. 1–2; N.Y. Lunatic Asylum, "Annual Report," *N.Y. Senate Docs.,* 1842, I, no. 20, pp. 1–2, Appendix A, 47 ff. (Hereafter, "Description of Asylums in the U.S."). This survey of hospital practices is an invaluable compendium of information about the pre-Civil War asylums.

13. Isaac Ray, *Mental Hygiene,* 316; Butler Hospital, *Annual Report for 1856* (Providence, R.I., 1857), 19.

14. Edward Jarvis, *Address at Northampton,* 21–23, 25; Pennsylvania Hospital, *Second Annual Report,* 22–23; Philadelphia Citizens Committee, *An Appeal to the People,* 10–11; Ohio Lunatic Asylum, *Thirteenth Annual Report,* 17, 21; B.P.D.S., *Thirteenth Annual Report* (Boston, 1838), 200; and *Fifteenth Annual Report* (Boston, 1840), 420–421.

15. Thomas Kirkbride, *On the Construction of Hospitals for the Insane*, 36–38; *History of the Association of Medical Superintendents*, 24; Isaac Ray, *Mental Hygiene*, 24; Butler Hospital, *Annual Report for 1856*, 24.

16. Butler Hospital, *Annual Report for 1850* (Providence, R.I., 1851), 23; *Annual Report for 1856*, 19; and *Annual Report for 1855*, 13–14, 18. See also Edward Jarvis, *Visit to Thirteen Asylums*, 136, and his *Address at Northampton*, 26; Philadelphia Citizens Committee, *An Appeal to the People*, 10–11; Connecticut Retreat, *Thirty-Ninth Annual Report*, 27.

17. On location of asylums, see N.Y. Lunatic Asylum, "Description of Asylums in the United States," 47–49, 55–56. For the Philadelphia story, Pennsylvania Hospital, *First Annual Report* (Philadelphia, 1842), 17, and *Second Annual Report*, 6; cf. New Hampshire Asylum for the Insane, *Annual Report for 1843* (Concord, N.H., 1843), 20.

18. Pennsylvania Hospital, *Second Annual Report*, 27–28. See also Connecticut Retreat, *Twenty-Eighth Annual Report* (Hartford, 1852), 30, and *Thirty-First Annual Report* (Hartford, 1855), 21.

19. N.Y. Lunatic Asylum, "Annual Report," 1842, 29–30, 32, and "Annual Report," *N.Y. Assembly Docs.*, 1843, III, no. 50, pp. 52–53, 55.

20. Ohio Lunatic Asylum, *Second Annual Report* (Columbus, O.H., 1840), 40–42.

21. N.Y. Lunatic Asylum, "Description of Asylums in the U.S.," 66, 132; New Hampshire Asylum, *Annual Report for 1843*, 19; N.Y. Lunatic Asylum, "Annual Report," *N.Y. Senate Docs.*, 1847, I, no. 30, pp. 18–19. See also Connecticut Retreat, *Twenty-Eighth Annual Report*, 29. On Pennsylvania Hospital and premature removals, see *Fourth Annual Report* (Philadelphia, 1845), 8–9.

22. Edward Jarvis, *The Law of Insanity and Hospitals for the Insane in Massachusetts* (pamphlet reprinted from the *Law Reporter*, Boston, 1859), 16–17. The best survey of commitment practices is N.Y. Lunatic Asylum, "Description of Asylums in the U.S.," 63, 81–82, 93, 123, 149. The New York incident is recounted in the N.Y. Lunatic Asylum, "Annual Report," 1843, 56–59.

23. Francis Bowen, "The Jurisprudence of Insanity," *North American Review*, 60 (1845), 1–37. Most legal discussions of insanity centered on the issue of criminal responsibility, not on procedures for protecting the insane.

24. N.Y. Lunatic Asylum, "Descriptions of Asylums in the U.S.," 185, letter of Dr. James Macdonald, in response to the trustees' request for a plan of organization (italics added).

25. *Ibid.*, 63, 220–221 (italics added).

26. Pennsylvania Hospital, *First Annual Report*, 23–24.

27. Worcester Lunatic Hospital, *Seventh Annual Report*, 86–87; there too, bell-ringing accompanied every shift, N.Y. Lunatic Asylum, "Annual Report," 1842, 30–31. An excellent study of the origins and routine of the Worcester institution is Gerald N. Grob, *The State and the Mentally Ill: A History of the Worcester State Hospital in Massachusetts, 1830–1920* (Chapel Hill, N.C., 1966). See chs. 2–3 for its daily functioning.

28. Pennsylvania Hospital, *First Annual Report*, 27–29. See also its *Seventh Annual Report* (Philadelphia, 1848), 32–33.

29. Worcester Lunatic Hospital, *Seventh Annual Report*, 86–87; quotation is on p. 94; N.Y. Lunatic Asylum, "Annual Report," 1843, 46–49.

30. Pennsylvania Hospital, *First Annual Report*, 13–14, 22, 26; *Second Annual Report*, 41–44; *Fourth Annual Report*, 33–34.

31. "Comptroller's Investigation of Several Institutions of New York State," *N.Y. Assembly Docs.*, 1840, IV, no. 214, p. 90; Governors of the N.Y. Hospital, "Annual

Report," *N.Y. Assembly Docs.*, 1842, V, 8–9. See too William L. Russell, *The New York Hospital: A History of the Psychiatric Service, 1771–1936* (New York, 1945), chs. 13–16.

32. N.Y. Lunatic Asylum, "Description of Asylums in the U.S.," 87–90.

33. N.Y. Lunatic Asylum, "Annual Report," 1842, 5–6, 21–23, 27; "Annual Report," 1843, 51–52.

34. *Ibid.*, "Annual Report," 1843, 51–52, 63; "Annual Report," *N.Y. Senate Docs.*, 1851, I, no. 42, pp. 43–45.

35. Worcester Lunatic Hospital, *Third Annual Report* (Boston, 1836), 9, 29–30; *Fourth Annual Report* (Boston, 1837), 21; *Fifth Annual Report*, 10–11; *Sixth Annual Report*, 81. The Horace Mann quotation is from the *Ninth Annual Report* (Boston, 1842), 8.

36. *Ibid., Thirteenth Annual Report* (Boston, 1846), 6–7; *Fourteenth Annual Report* (Boston, 1847), 6–8. For discharge policies, see *Fifth Annual Report*, 6–7. For details, see Gerald N. Grob, *The State and the Mentally Ill*, chs. 3–4.

37. Kentucky Asylum, *Annual Report for 1845* (Frankfort, K.Y., 1846), 27 ff.; Indiana State Central Hospital for the Insane, *First Annual Report* (Indianapolis, I.N., 1849), 43; N.Y. Lunatic Asylum, "Description of Asylums in the U.S.," 126.

38. N.Y. Lunatic Asylum, "Annual Report," 1851, 44; Worcester Lunatic Hospital, *Ninth Annual Report*, 69; Governors of the New York Hospital, "Annual Report," 1842, 7.

39. N.Y. Lunatic Asylum, "Annual Report," 1843, 55–56; Indiana State Central Hospital for the Insane, *First Annual Report*, 36–37; Pennsylvania Hospital, *First Annual Report*, 12. For Kirkbride's instructions, see Pennsylvania Hospital, *Fourth Annual Report*, 35.

40. See the 1832 *Report of Commissioners to Superintend the Erection of a Lunatic Hospital at Worcester*, 1–2.

41. For designs see N.Y. Lunatic Asylum, "Description of Asylums in the U.S.," 72 (McLean), 122–123, 128–129 (Virginia), 165 (Pennsylvania), 169–170 (Bloomingdale). For Utica, see N.Y. Lunatic Asylum, "Annual Report," 1843, 39–41; for Connecticut Retreat, *Forty-Fifth and Forty-Sixth Annual Reports* (Hartford, 1869–1870), 21. The first annual reports of an asylum invariably contained a picture or a verbal description of the structure. See too Thomas Kirkbride, *On the Construction of Hospitals for the Insane, passim*.

42. N.Y. Lunatic Asylum, "Description of Asylums in the U.S.," 126. In a letter to the New York trustees, Philip Barbiza, chief of the Virginia institution, displayed all the ambivalence one might expect on this issue. For example: "The law of kindness should be the order of the house; nevertheless, discipline and restraint are absolutely necessary."

DISCUSSION

1. According to Rothman, what is "moral treatment"? Why did 19th century reformers believe that this type of treatment would provide better care, and, potentially, cure mental health problems? In what ways, was the concept of "moral treatment" grounded in broader historical trends occurring within U.S. society occurring during this same time period?

2. What was the typical structure of an asylum in the mid-19th century? To what extent and in what ways are these 19th century reformers' beliefs about the nature and treatment of mental illness reflected in the physical design and operational organization of these facilities?

Joseph P. Morrissey, Ph.D., and Howard H. Goldman, M.D., Ph.D.

Cycles of Reform in the Care of the Chronically Mentally Ill

In this selection, Morrissey and Goldman provide a broad historical overview of four major periods of reform in the care and treatment of people with mental illnesses, beginning with the 19th century asylum movement. They assert that each major reform initiative was deeply grounded in changing views of mental illness. In this regard, their analysis provides some insight into the changing nature of the public's and professionals' views of mental illness and what is and is not an appropriate social response. In addition, their study also highlights that mental health policy has become an increasingly important political issue and concern for public policy makers.

The history of public intervention on behalf of the mentally ill in America reveals a cyclical pattern of institutional reforms (1). The hallmark of each reform was a new environmental approach to treatment and an innovative type of facility or locus of care. The first cycle of reform, in the early 19th century, introduced moral treatment and the asylum (2–5); the second cycle, in the early 20th century, was associated with the mental hygiene movement and the psychopathic hospital (6–10); and the third cycle, in the mid-20th century, was spawned by the community mental health movement and the community mental health center (11–14). Although each reform was the result of a unique set of sociohistorical circumstances, a number of striking parallels can be discerned in their goals, their evolution, and their outcomes.

Each reform began with the promise that early treatment in the new setting would prevent the personal and societal problems associated with long-term mental disability. However, they were launched with little or no appreciation of the practical limits to which their core beliefs could be pushed. Consequently each reform movement and its special facility flourished for a few decades and then faltered in the face of changing and unanticipated circumstances.

At first championed as a generic solution for the treatment of the mentally ill, each intervention ultimately proved viable only with acute or milder—not chronic—forms of mental disorder. In each cycle, early optimism soon faded into despair over the increasing numbers of chronic patients who were considered incurable and who began to accumulate in acute treatment settings. The public's reluctance to allocate sufficient resources for an

Morrissey, Joseph P., and Howard H. Goldman. 1984."Cycles of Reform in the Care of the Chronically Mentally Ill." *Hospital and Community Psychiatry* 35:785–793.

ever-expanding population in need of mental health care, coupled with disappointment over the inability to meet exaggerated expectations, led to a period of pessimism, retrenchment, and neglect—especially of the chronically ill.

The residue of each reform set the stage for the next generation of innovators, with little cumulative impact on the problems to which the reforms were addressed. By shifting attention from one locus of care to another, from community to institution and back again, and from isolated to centralized to decentralized services, each reform movement expanded and diversified the American mental health system into today's pluralistic patchwork of public and private, acute and chronic, voluntary and involuntary service settings. Yet each reform failed to prevent chronicity or to alter the care of the severely mentally ill in any fundamental way.

While the lessons of history are often elusive and difficult to extrapolate to current circumstances, an understanding of the successes and failures of past efforts to deal with these issues can provide a perspective on the choices and challenges that must be confronted in the decades ahead. In this paper, we will review the history of earlier cycles of reform as a basis for evaluating emergent fiscal policies and their implications for the care of the chronically mentally ill in the United States.

Historical Reform Movements in Mental Health Treatment in the United States

Reform Movement	Era	Setting	Focus of Reform
Moral Treatment	1800–1850	Asylum	Humane, restorative treatment
Mental Hygiene	1890–1920	Mental hospital and clinic	Prevention, scientific orientation
Community Mental Health	1955–1970	Community mental health center	Deinstitutionalization, social integration
Community Support	1975–present	Community support	Mental illness as a social welfare problem (e.g., housing, employment)

Source: Table 2-10 in Chapter 2: Fundamentals of Mental Health and Mental Illness. U.S. Department of Health and Human Services. *Mental Health: A Report of the Surgeon General—Executive Summary.* Rockville, MD: U.S. Department of Health and Human Services, Substance Abuse and Mental Health Services Administration, Center for Mental Health Services, National Institutes of Health, National Institute of Mental Health, 1999.

MORAL TREATMENT AND THE ASYLUM

The first major effort to improve the care of the mentally ill in America occurred in the early 19th century as part of a broad-based social reform movement aimed at bettering the condition of the less fortunate members of society (2,4,5). The belief that man could be perfected by manipulating his social and physical environment, the reformist zeal of Evangelical Protestantism, and a spirit of noblesse oblige were prominent features of this humanitarian movement. In this ideological climate, the work of Philippe Pinel in France and William Tuke in England provided both the rationale and the organizational model for public intervention on behalf of the insane in this country. The "moral treatment" that they championed contributed to the growing acceptance of a medical-psychological rather than a theological model of mental illness and led to the establishment of asylums for its treatment. Influential laymen such as Horace Mann in Massachusetts were in the front ranks of this reform movement (2).

Moral treatment was essentially environmental in nature, encompassing a set of beliefs and practices akin to today's concepts of milieu therapy (15). The core belief was that new cases of insanity could be cured by segregating the "distracted" into small, pastoral asylums where they could receive humane care and instruction. The regimen called for the creation of a warm, familial atmosphere with medical treatment, occupational therapy, religious exercises, amusements and games, kind treatment by a staff headed by a resident superintendent, and in large measure a repudiation of all threats of physical violence.

Adopted first by private facilities such as the Friends Asylum in Pennsylvania (about 1817) and the Hartford Retreat in Connecticut (about 1824), moral treatment was soon advocated for use in state-supported asylums with the indigent insane, who languished unattended in local almshouses and jails. Superintendents of the early asylums often claimed success rates of 90 percent or more with patients who had been ill less than a year, and their optimism fueled the humanitarian zeal of a new generation of social reformers. Dorothea Lynde Dix, who was attracted to the cause of the insane poor in the 1840s, became the principal spokesperson and lobbyist for the construction and expansion of public asylums throughout the United States (16). Ironically, even as this new wave of asylum-building got under way, the social reality that supported the idea of a "moral asylum" was rapidly fading (4).

The therapeutic ideals of these hospitals remained viable only to the extent that their patients and staff shared common religious, ethnic, and cultural values; that their caseloads were held to a relatively small size so that intimate staff-patient relationships could be developed and sustained; that their admissions consisted of recent as opposed to long-term or chronic cases; that their sense of purpose was championed by charismatic superintendents and influential laymen; and that their governmental sponsors were willing to appropriate adequate funds for their operation. Beginning in the mid-19th century, each of these supports was undermined by social, economic, and intellectual forces beyond the control of hospital superintendents. Slowly but inexorably, public mental hospitals were transformed from small, therapeutic asylums into large, custodial institutions.

During the late 1840s and early 1850s, with the advent of industrialization and the influx of impoverished immigrant groups, pauperism or public dependency for the first time became a major social problem in America (2,5). As population growth accelerated, so to did the demands for institutional care. State legislatures responded to these pressures by expanding asylum capacity or erecting large facilities. Admissions began to be disproportionately drawn from the ranks of immigrant groups; many immigrant patients constituted the oldest and most advanced cases on mental illness and had the least chance of recovery. Superintendents were faced with a legal, administrative, and financial structure that limited their control over admissions and discharge policies and maximum institutional size (8 pp. 193–195).

Consequently the state-supported asylums began to be filled with ever-increasing numbers of chronic cases that overcrowded existing facilities and undermined therapeutic practices. Under these circumstances, cure rates dropped off precipitously, and increasingly, in both the public and the professional views, insanity became associated with pauperism and incurability (17).

These incipient social and intellectual currents did not converge into an explicit public policy for dealing with problems of mental illness in a rapidly industrializing and urbanizing society until the 1870s. The intervening years were a period of reassessment and exploration for alternatives to large public asylums. The most imaginative proposal was the idea of building small cottages to replace large centralized institutions. Originally suggested in the 1850s by John Galt, superintendent of the Virginia State Asylum at Williamsburg, the proposal was resurrected after the Civil War by Merrick Bemis, superintendent of the Worcester Asylum in Massachusetts, who was deeply influenced by the renowned colony for the insane in the Belgian town of Gheel (2,15,18).

Bemis advocated the decentralization of state asylums so that they could sustain their role in caring for all social classes and ethnic groups while providing humane custody for the chronically ill in family-like residences under the supervision of attendant staff. In 1869 he persuaded the Worcester trustees to adopt a Gheel-like cottage plan as the architectural design for a new facility, which would replace the antiquated and overcrowded building of the original asylum. Bemis' plan was opposed by fellow superintendents who saw the new type of institution as a threat to the central role of the psychiatrist as stipulated by the basic precepts of moral treatment, and by conservative members of the legislature who were persuaded it would be more costly to operate, and approval of the plan was rescinded. Shortly thereafter a large congregate care facility was erected, and the original buildings were converted into a separate asylum for the chronically insane.

While variants of the cottage plan caught hold in some other states (most notably at the Illinois State Asylum in Kankakee and the county asylums in Wisconsin and Pennsylvania), its rejection in Massachusetts set a national precedent of building new congregate care facilities as the need arose (8). Ultimately the Massachusetts experience also influenced the growth of a centralized administrative structure in each state to govern the increasing number of facilities.

Other trends dating from the 1850s were also solidified. As the state asylums became filled with lower-class patients, well-to-do families resorted to private facilities for the care of their mentally ill members. Private resources were increasingly used to build facilities for paying patients; public resources were allocated for the establishment of separate asylums for the indigent mentally ill. Private-sector facilities tended to specialize in providing treatment to wealthier, quiet, primarily voluntary patients, while the state asylums were left to provide long-term custodial care to poor; disturbed, involuntary patients. As the care system evolved over the next century, a two-class system emerged and became firmly entrenched (1).

By the 1870s, therefore, the functions of state asylums had been clearly delineated. Their central purpose was defined by state legislatures in terms of custodial care and community protection; treatment was of secondary importance. Emphasis was placed on the custody of the largest number of patients at the lowest possible cost. The small, pastoral retreat that offered hope and humane care had been transformed into a general purpose solution to the welfare burdens of a society undergoing rapid industrialization and stratification along social class and ethnic lines.

This institutional transformation was reinforced by the growing pessimism and therapeutic nihilism that began to envelop psychiatric theory and practice. With the deaths or retirement of the early moral therapists, the new generation of psychiatrists passively accepted the social role of these facilities while actively attending to their own professionalization (5,8). In time, both hospital staff and local communities came to believe that the majority of patients committed to state asylums, were destined to reside there for life. With overcrowding and staff shortages, a uniform routine was imposed on all patients, which ultimately led to an insidious process of "institutionalization" or total dependency on the asylum (19,20).

MENTAL HYGIENE AND THE PSYCHOPATHIC HOSPITAL

Despite the seemingly irreversible course that state policies and programs had followed, the voices calling for institutional reform had not been completely silenced. As early as the 1870s, American psychiatrists had come under attack from their British counterparts for the deteriorating conditions in state asylums, the overreliance on physical restraint to maintain order, and the general stagnation of the profession. These criticisms were met by denial and counter charges from asylum medical superintendents.

Gradually, however, these essentially intraprofessional disputes were trans-formed into a progressive social reform movement with a broad base outside of psychiatry. Neurologists, social workers, and lay reformers began to pub-licize some of the shortcomings that characterized American psychiatry in an effort to break the stranglehold of medical superintendents over the care of the insane (6–10).

Therapeutic pessimism soon gave way to the optimism of a new scientific psychiatry associated with turn-of-the-century figures such as Adolf Meyer. The work of Meyer and his students, reinforced by the development of psy-choanalysis, restored hope that the mentally ill could be effectively treated. The public was outraged by exposés of conditions in mental hospitals, but the 1908 publication of *A Mind That Found Itself,* Clifford Beers' account of his experiences as a mental patient, added a note of optimism to the prevailing criticism (21).

In 1909 Beers sought the support of Meyer and William James (the noted Harvard philosopher-psychologist) to help him found the National Committee for Mental Hygiene. This reform organization revived the notion of the treatability of mental disorder, especially by early intervention with acute cases (6). Mental hygienists advocated creating a "psychopathic hos-pital," an acute treatment or reception facility affiliated with university training and research institutes. Building upon the earlier concept of moral treatment and several later innovations in psychiatric care, the first psycho-pathic hospitals opened in Albany, Ann Arbor, Baltimore, and Boston (7,8).

The reform spread, and spawned other new mental health agencies such as psychiatric dispensaries and child guidance clinics. However, these new facilities were unable to eliminate chronic illness. They provided high-quality care for a few, but were unable to fundamentally reform American mental health care. As the movement matured, its original goal of improv-ing mental hospital care fell by the wayside. In its place, reformers began to champion the relevance of psychiatry in the care of the feebleminded, eugen-ics, control of alcoholism, management of abnormal children, treatment of criminals, prevention of prostitution and dependency, and the problems of industrial productivity (7,8,10).

As part of the received wisdom in the mental health field, it has been fashionable to think of the decades between 1890 and 1950 as the Dark Ages in the state care of the mentally ill. Recent historical scholarship, however, has begun to penetrate the myth that institutional care in this period was uniformly stagnant, repressive, and monolithic (8). While psychiatrists pushed the boundaries of their specialty outward into the community and attempted to broaden its functions and roles under the aegis of the mental hygiene movement, profound changes were also occurring within the state asylum system.

In 1890 New York's State Care Act established the precedent for states to assume full financial responsibility for the care and treatment of the men-tally ill. This legislation was designed to remedy the quality-of-care deficien-cies associated with asylums operated by municipalities and counties and to absolve these governmental units of the maintenance costs of asylum operation. It represented the culmination of efforts to rationalize public provisions for the mentally ill under a centralized regulatory structure; it also legitimized psychiatry's exclusive claims for care and management of this population (8). Consistent with this development, the official designation for these institutions was soon changed from state asylums to state mental hospitals.

Local officials, however, began to recognize the advantages in redefining insanity to include aged and senile individuals. By transferring such patients from local almshouses to the state hospitals, fiscal burdens associated with their care were shifted from local to state auspices. The result was a dramatic transformation in the patient case mix of state mental hospitals.

Prior to 1900, chronic or incurable patients and the aged senile were sent to county and local almshouses; state asylums had concentrated largely on acute cases institutionalized for less than 12 months (8). After the states monopolized provisions for the mentally ill, state mental hospitals gradually assumed responsibility for senile patients as well as for individuals suffering from a variety of diseases and conditions that required custodial care on a lifelong basis rather than treatment by specific psychiatric therapies. Concomitantly the almshouse declined in significance as a public institution.

As Grob (8, p. 181) points out, "What occurred, in effect, was not a deinstitutionalization movement, but rather a transfer of patients between different types of institutions. The shift, moreover, was less a function of medical or humanitarian concerns than a consequence of financial considerations." Between 1903 and 1950, the number of patients in state mental hospitals increased by 240 percent (from 150,000 to 512,500), a rate of growth nearly twice as large as the increase in the U.S. population as a whole.

While the small number of psychopathic hospitals had little direct impact on the changing volume and composition of state mental hospital caseloads, other outgrowths of the mental hygiene movement such as psychiatric social work, clinical psychology, and pastoral counseling were gradually melded to the staff complement of these institutions. To a large extent, however, the state hospitals were caught up in a vast holding operation. In the absence of specific treatments, mental disorders remained chronic illnesses, and state mental hospitals remained predominantly chronic care facilities providing long-term custody of the poor and disabled.

During these years, the state mental hospitals were portrayed as a throwback to an unenlightened and immature stage of psychiatric practice. The exhilaration of forging a marriage between the new scientific psychiatry and social activism deflected the attention of many psychiatrists from the custodial and managerial origins of their profession. As the preoccupations of organized psychiatry shifted from state hospitals to private office and outpatient treatment, recognition of a core reality was lost. That is, despite their very real shortcoming and failures, state mental hospitals did provide *minimum* levels of care (not otherwise available) for individuals unable to survive by themselves (8). It would take another generation, a new cycle of institutional reform, and the near-cataclysmic emptying of state mental hospitals for this fundamental truth to be fully appreciated by mental health policymakers.

COMMUNITY MENTAL HEALTH AND THE CMHC

World War II simultaneously marked the nadir in the decline of the mental hygiene movement and the turning point initiating the third cycle of reform. The finding that so many young Americans were mentally unfit for military duty, coupled with front-line successes of brief interventions in the treatment of "war neurosis" (22) stimulated renewed interest in prevention and new optimism for the treatment of mental illness (23).

The community mental health movement was born out of this enthusiasm for brief treatment techniques, which avoided the removal of patients to faraway hospitals. The psychiatrists returning to state mental hospitals from military service experimented with brief hospitalization and new psychosocial treatment techniques and by the mid-1950s they made extensive use of the new psychotropic medications (24). In the late 1940s and early 1950s, pioneer mental health professionals, like Erich Lindemann, adapted next techniques in brief therapy and psychiatric consultation for use in outpatient clinics, creating mental health centers in the community (25). At the same time, innovative state mental hospitals opened aftercare clinics to serve increasing numbers of discharged mental patients (26), and general hospitals opened acute psychiatric inpatient units (27). Again reformers offered the promise that early intervention in a community setting could prevent chronicity and long-term disability, rendering the state mental hospital obsolete.

This also was a period of significant federal government activity. In 1946 the National Mental Health Act created the National Institute of Mental Health to stimulate research and training efforts. The Mental Health Study Act of 1955 established the Joint Commission on Mental Illness and Health to analyze and evaluate the needs and resources of the mentally ill in the United States and make recommendations for a national mental health program. The final report of the Joint Commission in 1961, *Action for Mental Health*, promoted the concept of community mental health care (11). This concept became the "bold new approach" adopted by President Kennedy in the Community Mental Health Centers Act of 1963, which created the elaborate system of community mental health centers (CMHCs) in the mid-1960s.

The passage of the CMHC legislation marked the culmination of a political struggle to involve the federal government in the direct provision of mental health services (13,14). Throughout the 1950s proponents of the community mental health philosophy had waged a concerted battle against state mental health authorities for the right to define the shape of the postwar mental health services system. This struggle was sustained by two essentially antagonistic ideologies, one rooted in institutional psychiatry and the other in community mental health (28).

The first called for the regeneration of state mental hospitals as the hub of a mental health services network, while the second called instead for the early demise of these hospitals and their replacement by a new community-based and community-controlled mental health service delivery system. Both groups, however, were in agreement that their proposals required massive funding from the federal government. When federal policymakers came down on the side of the CMHC concept, state mental health authorities were pushed to the periphery of the planning process.

The near-term accomplishments of the community mental health movement seemingly rival the success claims advanced for the early asylums. Between 1955 and 1980, for example, the resident population of state mental hospitals was reduced by more than 75 percent, or by approximately 420,000 occupied beds, and since the mid-1960s more than 700 CMHCs, serving catchment areas representing 50 percent of the U.S. population, have been created (28). Upon closer scrutiny, however, it is clear that shifts in the locus of care did not solve the problem of chronic mental illness. Indeed, many observers have argued that the centers exacerbated the plight of the chronic patient (29–32).

In many communities, the CMHCs extended services to new populations of previously untreated individuals; largely ignoring the populations traditionally served by state mental hospitals (33). At the same time, the promise of the centers, especially for reducing the census of state mental hospitals and saving resources, helped to promote a policy of deinstitutionalization (34).

Deinstitutionalization policy took shape in response to civil-libertarian litigation over the state hospital commitment process, the Medicaid-Medicare amendments to the Social Security Act of 1965, and the fiscal crises that enveloped the states in the early 1970s (28). Similar to the state care acts of the late 19th and early 20th centuries, the Medicaid-Medicare amendments allowed for buck-passing from one governmental budget to another—in this case, from the states to the federal level. Within a short period of time, these fiscal and legal incentives led to the discharge of hundreds of thousands of mental patients from the state mental hospitals. CMHCs were almost totally unprepared (or unwilling, or both) to shoulder the responsibility of this chronic population. As with the psychopathic hospitals of an earlier era, CMHC leadership considered the centers' mission and promise to be preventing chronicity, not dealing with the failures of previous approaches to mental health care.

The problem for CMHCs was compounded by two additional factors. First, the concept of federal "seed money," with federal contributions decreasing annually, often meant that centers had to abandon poorer patients with a pattern of high service utilization (such as chronic patients) in favor of insured patients who might respond to brief interventions (35). Second, CMHC funding was through a federal-to-local-community grant mechanism that avoided state involvement. This attempt to circumvent state mental health agencies in order to avoid control of CMHCs by "institution-minded bureaucrats" also meant that the depopulation of state mental hospitals would proceed without coordination with the new centers (29,30).

By the mid-1970s the policy of deinstitutionalization was being severely criticized. Despite the optimism stimulated by the movement to deinstitutionalization mental health services, it was apparent that community care of the chronically mentally ill had brought with it new patterns of exclusion, neglect, and abuse. The many tragedies of deinstitutionalization were reported in vivid detail in mass-media descriptions of former hospital patients sleeping outdoors on heating grates and in doorways, living in squalid single-room occupancies, wandering the streets, and trying desperately to get back into institutions in which they could feel secure and safe (36,37).

Patients in effect asked, "Where is my home?" (38), and others decried the move "out of their beds and into the streets" (39) and from "back wards to back alleys" (40). Some observers felt that conditions in the communities were as bad as those in the institutions that proponents of deinstitutionalization were trying to replace. Others thought that current policies were creating the same pre-asylum conditions that led to the reformist efforts of Horace Mann and Dorothea Dìx in the first half of the 19th century.

Once again, rather than deinstitutionalization, a process of "transinstitutionalization" occurred. Supported largely by federal SSI and SSDI payments, thousands of former patients now live in nursing homes, board-and-care homes, adult homes, and other institutional settings in the community (41–44). These mostly private, profit-making facilities serve the custodial, asylum, and treatment functions that were once performed almost exclusively by state mental hospitals. The growth of what has been characterized as "social control entrepreneurialism" (45) has thereby perpetuated the segregation of the chronically mentally ill in a new ecological arrangement in the community. Numerous reports also indicate that many other patients are now incarcerated in local jails and correctional facilities (46–48).

In the late 1970s the community mental health movement entered a transitional phase. The change was occasioned by the political backlash to several years of rapid census decreases and a fuller realization that the abrupt closure of state hospitals was premature. In November 1977 the General Accounting Office issued the final report of a year-long study of state mental hospital deinstitutionalization (49). While the report contained little new information on the consequences of the rapid phase-down of state mental hospitals, it offered a devastating critique of the federal support for this policy and called for immediate efforts to deal with the needs of the thousands of chronic patients who were released to local communities without adequate provision for their care. The following year the President's Commission on Mental Health presented a similar assessment and called for a national mental health policy focused, in part, on the chronically mentally ill (50).

THE COMMUNITY SUPPORT PROGRAM

In response to this new wave of criticism, the National Institute of Mental Health launched its community support program (CSP) designed "to improve services for one particularly vulnerable population—adult psychiatric patients whose disabilities are severe and persistent but for whom long-term skilled or semi-skilled nursing care is inappropriate" (51, p. 319). A total of $3.5 million was allocated to contracts with 19 states for three-year pilot demonstration programs involving crisis care services, psychosocial rehabilitation services, supportive living and working arrangements, medical and mental health care, and case management for the chronically mentally ill (52).

The CSP effort was described as "a much needed social reform" that championed the concept of a "community support system" (CSS) as a solution to the problem of the chronically mentally ill in the community (51). To some observers the CSS movement has been a mid-course correction in the community mental health reform, an administrative "fix" for the problems of deinstitutionalization (53).

However, in other respects this movement may be viewed as the fourth cycle of institutional reform in that it proposed a fundamental change in attitude and approach to the chronically mentally ill. Unlike the earlier reform movements, it offers direct care and rehabilitation for the chronically mentally ill rather than focusing on preventing chronicity by the early treatment of acute cases. Further, its goals are predicated on the development of a *system* of support services among existing community agencies rather than the construction of a new type of facility.

In addition to stimulating and sponsoring the development of community support systems, the community support movement fostered the development of the National Plan for the Chronically Mentally Ill (54) and the passage of the Mental Health Systems Act of 1980. The former is a comprehensive blueprint for improving services for the chronically mentally ill, a plan developed but not endorsed by the Carter administration. The latter, the first major mental health legislation since the Community Mental Health Centers Act in the mid-1960s, enabled states and local agencies to establish community support systems and other community-based mental health services with federal funding. Thus in 1980 it appeared that the community support movement had succeeded in ushering in a major reform in mental health services for chronically mentally ill persons.

FISCAL THREATS TO THE CSS REFORM MOVEMENT

As with earlier reforms, however, economic realities and fiscal policies have begun to jeopardize this promising start. In 1981 the Omnibus Budget Reconciliation Act (P.L. 97–35) repealed the major provisions of the Mental

Health Systems Act. The authorization for using federal funds specifically to establish community-based services for the chronically mentally ill was eliminated. Instead all federal funds for alcohol, drug abuse, and mental health programs were consolidated into a block grant, funded at a level below previous appropriations (52). Shortly thereafter, Medicaid funds were capped, limiting the availability of federal funds for mental health services for the poor (55).

Advocates of community support systems and community-based care for the chronically mentally ill are concerned by these changes. They fear that they will lead to an erosion of the mental health reforms of the past 30 years and promote a return to the use of institutional services. Data from NIMH indicate that "new chronic patients" have continued to accumulate in state and county mental hospitals throughout the country (56), and statistics from New York (57) and several other states show a reversal in the downward trend of the overall resident census in public mental hospitals. These trend reversals preceded the fiscal limits of the early 1980s, but a recent analysis suggests that current budgetary restrictions are likely to increase institutionalization (58).

Early in 1981 the Social Security Administration advanced the implementation date for its three-year review of millions of cases of SSI and SSDI recipients and claimants, a review designed to save billions of dollars by applying a stricter interpretation of eligibility standards. The mentally disabled were disproportionately included among the SSI and SSDI recipients whose cases were reviewed, and thousands had their benefits terminated. These procedures threaten the community-based approach to care of the chronically mentally disabled, many of whom depend on SSI and SSDI to live independent of an institution.

In 1983 the Medicare Prospective Payment System was inaugurated. The enabling legislation authorized payment for hospitalization prospectively on the basis of preestablished rates for specific "diagnosis-related groups" (DRGs) rather than retrospectively on the basis of actual costs. Although designed to save Medicare resources in the Hospital Insurance Trust Fund by reducing the length and cost of hospitalization, the prospective payment system could also increase pressure on public general hospitals and long-term care facilities to provide for patients who might be discharged prematurely by other institutions on fiscal rather than clinical grounds.

Such clinically irresponsible behavior would lead to a shifting of costs rather than a savings of resources and would counter the trend away from unnecessary use of institutional services. Because of a lack of experience in and general uncertainty about applying DRG-based systems to mental disorders, psychiatric hospitals and psychiatric units in general hospitals were excluded from the prospective payment system until the applicability of DRGs to inpatient psychiatric care and treatment could be evaluated.

SUSTAINING THE FOURTH CYCLE OF REFORM

A critical response and considerable remedial action followed these fiscal threats to the community-based approach to the care of the chronically mentally ill. In fact, some of the new legislation and administrative policies created opportunities as well as problems, and the fourth cycle of reform may persist in spite of serious threats to its viability.

After the repeal of the Mental Health Systems Act, the NIMH community support program continued to receive an annual appropriation of approximately $6 million in fiscal years 1982 and 1983. Furthermore, the block grants contained provisions for funding community-based mental health services. However, resources are limited, and the CSP received no appropriation for fiscal 1984. In spite of that development, the community support and rehabilitation branch of NIMH continues to provide national leadership and technical assistance at the federal level, and almost every state has developed some type of community support program.

The Omnibus Budget Reconciliation Act, which repealed most of the Mental Health Systems Act, contained provisions for waivers permitting the use of Medicaid funds for home- and community-based care such as case management services, respite care, and partial hospitalization services. Many states have applied for these waivers. Provisions in the law stipulate that average costs may not exceed the costs of nursing home care, thus encouraging the use of community-based alternatives to institutional care.

The controversy surrounding the SSI and SSDI review process has led to a number of administrative adjustments. In June 1983, for example, Department of Health and Human Services Secretary Heckler announced immediate changes, including exempting from review two-thirds of all mental impairment cases and liberalizing the review process. In addition, the Social Security Administration has convened several work groups to propose changes in the mental impairment standards for disability determination and in the disability assessment process.

The exclusion of psychiatric units and hospitals from the Medicare prospective payment system provides an opportunity to study the applicability of prospective payment and DRGs to psychiatric hospitalization. Congress mandated a Department of Health and Human Services report to guide further legislation about the applicability to psychiatric care. As part of that report, the Health Care Financing Administration and NIMH plan to study the appropriateness of current classification systems for mental disorders for use in a prospective payment system. Various other professional and provider organizations are discussing independent studies as well. Of particular importance in the context of the fourth cycle of reform is the impact of a DRG-based system or any other prospective payment system on long-term care and services for chronic mental patients.

IMPLICATIONS

Even a cursory familiarity with the cycles of institutional reform in public mental health care leads one to affirm H. L. Mencken's acerbic aphorism: "For every problem there is one solution which is simple, neat, and wrong!" Hindsight suggests that the failures of institutional reform in America have often turned on unidimensional or particularistic "solutions" to the complex, multidimensional problems of mental health care. Foresight now demands that, as we tinker with the financing and delivery of mental health services in the 1980s, we remain skeptical of policies that ignore the long-term care needs of the chronically mentally ill. The experience of the last 150 years clearly indicates that fiscal and programmatic interventions based on considering mental illness exclusively an acute care problem are likely to produce undesirable consequences for the chronically mentally ill.

We have found the paradigm of cycles of reform useful for analyses of the enduring role of state mental hospitals (1), the functions of community support programs in the care of the chronically mentally ill (52), and the potential consequences of current fiscal policy. If the elusive goal of creating and sustaining a truly humane system of care for the dependent mentally ill is to be realized in this generation, then policymakers must avoid the trap of quick and partial fixes. Cycles of reform and retrenchment in public mental health care can be broken only by creative financing mechanisms focused on both the acute and the chronic care needs of the mentally ill.

References

1. Morrissey JP, Goldman HH, Klerman LV: The Enduring Asylum: Cycles of Institutional Reform at Worcester State Hospital. New York, Grune & Stratton, 1980
2. Grob GN: The State and the Mentally Ill: A History of Worcester State Hospital in Massachusetts, 1830–1920. Chapel Hill, University of North Carolina Press, 1966
3. Caplan RB, Caplan G: Psychiatry and the Community in Nineteenth-Century America. New York, Basic Books, 1969
4. Rothman DJ: The Discovery of the Asylum. Boston, Little, Brown, 1971
5. Grob GN: Mental Institutions in America: Social Policy to 1875. New York, Free Press, 1973
6. Deutsch A: The history of mental hygiene, in One Hundred Years of American Psychiatry. Edited by Hall JK, Zilboorg G, Bunker HA. New York, Columbia University Press, 1944
7. Rothman DJ: Conscience and Convenience: The Asylum and Its Alternatives in Progressive America. Boston, Little, Brown, 1980
8. Grob GN: Mental Illness and American Society, 1875–1940. Princeton, NJ, Princeton University Press, 1983
9. Quen JM: Asylum psychiatry, neurology, social work, and mental hygiene: an exploratory study in interprofessional history. Journal of the History of the Behavioral Sciences 13:3–11, 1977
10. Sicherman B: The Quest for Mental Health in America, 1880–1917. New York, Arno Press, 1980

11. Joint Commission on Mental Illness and Health: Action for Mental Health. New York, Basic Books, 1961
12. Levinson A, Brown B: Some implications of the community mental health center concept, in Social Psychiatry. Edited by Hoch P, Zubin J. New York, Grune & Stratton, 1967
13. Musto D: Whatever happened to community mental health? Public Interest 39:53–79, 1975
14. Foley HA, Sharfstein SS: Madness and Government: Who Cares for the Mentally Ill? Washington, DC, American Psychiatric Press, 1983
15. Dain N: The chronic mental patient in 19th-century America. Psychiatric Annals 10:323–327, 1980
16. Dix D: On Behalf of the Insane Poor: Selected Reports. Reprinted, New York, Arno Press, 1971
17. Deutsch A: The Mentally Ill in America: A History of Their Care and Treatment From Colonial Times. New York, Columbia University Press, 1937
18. Srole L: Gheel, Belgium: the natural therapeutic community, 1475–1975, in New Trends of Psychiatry in the Community. Edited by Serban G, Astrachan B. Cambridge, Mass, Ballinger, 1977
19. Goffman E: Asylums. New York, Doubleday, 1961
20. Gruenberg E: The social breakdown syndrome and its prevention, in American Handbook of Psychiatry, 2nd ed., vol 2. Edited by Arieti S. New York, Basic Books, 1974
21. Dain N: Clifford W Beers: Advocate for the Insane. Pittsburgh, University of Pittsburgh Press, 1980
22. Spiegel J, Grinker R: Men Under Stress. Philadelphia, Blakiston, 1945
23. Mechanic D: Mental Health and Social Policy. Englewood Cliffs, NJ, Prentice-Hall, 1969
24. Talbott JA: Twentieth-century developments in American psychiatry. Psychiatric Quarterly 54:207–219, 1982
25. Mora G: The history of psychiatry, in Comprehensive Textbook of Psychiatry, 1st ed. Edited by Freedman AM, Kaplan HI. Baltimore, Williams & Wilkins, 1967
26. Decentralization of Psychiatric Services and Continuity of Care. New York, Milbank Memorial Fund, 1962
27. Linn L: Frontiers in General Hospital Psychiatry. New York, International Universities Press, 1961
28. Morrissey J: Deinstitutionalizing the mentally ill: process, outcomes, and new directions, in Deviance and Mental Illness. Edited by Gove W. Beverly Hills, CA, Sage, 1982
29. Bassuk E, Gerson J: Deinstitutionalization and mental health services. Scientific American 238:46–53, 1978
30. Chu F, Trotter S: The Madness Establishment. New York, Grossman, 1974
31. Rose S: Deciphering deinstitutionalization: complexities in policy and program analysis. Milbank Memorial Fund Quarterly 57:429–460, 1979
32. Gruenberg E, Archer J: Abandonment of responsibility for the seriously mentally ill. Milbank Memorial Fund Quarterly 57:485–506, 1979
33. Windle C, Scully D: Community mental health centers and the decreasing use of state mental hospitals. Community Mental Health Journal 12:239–243, 1976
34. Bachrach LL: Deinstitutionalization: An Analytical Review and Sociologic Perspective. Rockville, MD, National Institute of Mental Health, 1976

35. Weiner RS, Woy JR, Sharfstein SS, et al: Community mental health center and the "seed money" concept: effect of terminating federal funds. Community Mental Health Journal 15:129–138, 1979
36. Koenig P: The problem that can't be tranquilized: 40,000 mental patient dumped in city neighborhoods. New York Times Magazine, May 21, 1978, pp 14–17
37. Drake D: The forsaken: how American has abandoned troubled thousands the name of social progress. Philadelphia Inquirer, July 18–24, 1982
38. National Institute of Mental Health: Where Is My Home? Proceedings of a Conference on the Closing of State Mental Hospitals, Scottsdale, AZ, 1974. Stanford Research Institute, 1974
39. Santiestevan H: Deinstitutionalization: Out of Their Beds and Into the Streets. Washington, DC, American Federation of State, County, and Municipal Employees, 1975
40. Trotter S, Kuttner B: The Mentally ill: from backwards to back alleys. Washington Post, February 24, 1974
41. Schmidt L, Reinhardt A, Kane R, et al: The mentally ill in nursing homes: new back wards in the community. Archives of General Psychiatry 34:687–691, 1977
42. Segal S, Aviram U: The Mentally Ill in Community-Based Sheltered Care. New York, Wiley, 1978
43. Lamb HR: The new asylums in the community. Archives of General Psychiatry 36:129–134, 1979
44. Shadish W, Bootzin R: Nursing homes and chronic mental patients. Schizophrenia Bulletin 7:488–498, 1981
45. Warren C: New forms of social control: the myth of deinstitutionalization. American Behavioral Scientist 6:724–740, 1981
46. Abrahamson M: The criminalization of mentally disordered behavior: a possible side effect of a new mental health law. Hospital and Community Psychiatry 23:101–105, 1972
47. Stelovich S: From the hospital to the prison: a step forward in deinstitutionalization? Hospital and Community Psychiatry 30:618–620, 1979
48. Whitmer G: From hospitals to jails; the fate of California's deinstitutionalized mentally ill. American Journal of Orthopsychiatry 50:65–75, 1980
49. General Accounting Office: Returning the Mentally Disabled to the Community: Government Needs to Do More. Washington, DC, General Accounting Office, 1977
50. President's Commission on Mental Health: Final Report. Washington, DC, US Government Printing Office, 1978
51. Turner J, TenHoor W: The NIMH community support program: pilot approach to a needed social reform. Schizophrenia Bulletin 4:319–348, 1978
52. Tessler RC, Goldman HH: The Chronically Mentally Ill: Assessing Community Support Programs. Cambridge, Mass, Ballinger, 1982
53. Lamb HR: What did we really expect from deinstitutionalization? Hospital and Community Psychiatry 32:105–109, 1981
54. National Plan for the Chronically Mentally Ill: Final Draft Report to the Secretary of Health and Human Services. Washington, DC, Department of Health and Human Services, 1980
55. Sharfstein SS: Medicaid cutbacks and block grants: crisis or opportunity for community mental health? American Journal of Psychiatry 139:466–470, 1982

56. Taube CA, Thompson JW, Rosenstein MJ, et al: The "chronic" mental hospital patient. Hospital and Community Psychiatry 34:611–615, 1983
57. Weinstein A: The pace of the resident patient decrease is slowing down. Statistical report. Albany, New York State Office of Mental Health, 1980
58. Sharfstein SS, Frank RG, Kessler LG: State Medicaid limitations for mental health services. Hospital and Community Psychiatry 35:213–215, 1984

DISCUSSION

1. What are the four major "cycles of reform?" What beliefs and historical circumstances were the principle drivers of reform during each period? To what extent do these changes reflect historical changes occurring in other areas of U.S. society?

2. What have been the biggest changes in the organization of care and treatment of people with mental illness? To what extent have these changes been driven by public attitudes versus scientific knowledge about psychiatric disorders?

Fred E. Markowitz

Psychiatric Hospital Capacity, Homelessness, and Crime and Arrest Rates[†]

Many critics of deinstitutionalization and the increased emphasis on the community-based treatment maintain that these policies have had a detrimental effect on the lives of people with mental illness and society. Indeed, numerous government studies and newspaper reports published in the last three decades of the 20th century found the increasing numbers of people with mental illness who were homeless and/or incarcerated. Often, these writers concluded that deinstitutionalization was a failure and that the community-based care reform movement resulted simply in the systematic "abandonment of the mentally ill." In this paper, sociologist Fred Markowitz takes an empirical look at the relationship between the availability of hospital care, homelessness, and crime and arrest rates and finds that the situation is more complicated than many critics have acknowledged.

Sociologists and criminologists have sought to explain the rise and expansion of formal institutions of social control, including the criminal justice, mental health, and welfare systems. Studies have focused largely on the role

Markowitz , Fred E. 2006. "Psychiatric Hospital Capacity, Homelessness, and Crime Arrest Rates." *Criminology* 44:45–72.

of socioeconomic conditions such as the contraction of labor markets and the size of minority populations as threats to the social order (Grob, 1994; Inverarity & Grattet, 1989; Jackson, 1989; Liska, 1992; Liska & Chamlin, 1984; Liska et al., 1999; Piven & Cloward, 1971; Scull, 1977; Sutton, 1991). However, comparatively less attention has been given to the consequences, or outcomes associated with the capacity of social control institutions. Classic work by Penrose (1939) demonstrated an inverse relationship between the prison and psychiatric hospital populations in European countries. Palermo and colleagues (1991) showed a similar relationship for the United States as a whole. The impact of psychiatric hospital capacity on crime and arrest rates across United States cities, however, has not been directly examined.

In recent decades, the inpatient capacity of public psychiatric hospitals has dropped dramatically. This has stimulated much individual-level research documenting the increasing numbers of persons with mental illness in jails and prisons, many of whom are homeless. Moreover, there has been increased attention to the risk of homelessness, violence, criminal behavior, and arrest among persons with severe mental illness. Building on this research, in an effort to understand the impact of psychiatric hospital capacity in terms of macro-level social control processes, I first discuss changes in the U.S. mental health care system over the last several decades and their impact on the criminal justice system. I then examine the relationships between psychiatric hospital capacity, homelessness, and crime and arrest rates for a sample of cities in the United States.

Psychiatric Deinstitutionalization

Until the 1960s, substantial numbers of persons with mental illness could be treated in large, publicly funded hospitals. Based on National Institute of Mental Health (NIMH) estimates, in 1960, about 563,000 beds were available in U.S. state and county psychiatric hospitals (314 beds per 100,000 persons), with about 535,400 resident patients. By 1990, the number of beds declined to about 98,800 (40 per 100,000) and the number of residents to 92,059 (NIMH, 1990). Several factors contributed to this drop. First, medications were developed that controlled the symptoms of the most debilitating mental disorders (for example, schizophrenia). Second, an ideological shift, advocating a more liberal position on confinement led to states adopting stricter legal standards for involuntary commitment (dangerousness to self or others). Third, fiscal policy changed, including the shifting of costs for mental health care from states to the federal government (for example, Medicare, Medicaid, Social Security Disability Income), followed by budget cuts and substantial underfunding of public mental health services (Gronfein, 1985; Issac & Armat, 1990; Kiesler & Sibulkin, 1987; Mechanic & Rochefort, 1990; Redick et al., 1992; Weinstein, 1990). These trends and associated policies are generally referred to as the deinstitutionalization of the mentally ill.

The sharp decline in public psychiatric hospital capacity has been offset to some extent by inpatient units in private psychiatric and general hospitals.

An important component to the changing nature of psychiatric hospitalization is the increasing role of general hospitals. Emergency rooms and psychiatric units in general hospitals provide acute treatment for those with mental illness and can bill Medicaid for doing so (Mechanic, McAlpine, & Olfson, 1998). Although these hospitals may contribute to cities' social control capacity, they still do not provide the long-term treatment found in public psychiatric hospitals. Therefore, as many have argued, the capacity for maintaining and treating America's mentally ill, especially the most severely impaired and economically disadvantaged patients, has substantially diminished (Ehrenkranz, 2001; Lamb & Bachrach, 2001; Torrey, 1995).

Many patients were discharged from state hospitals into the community. Others, as a result of stricter standards for involuntary commitment, were not even admitted—an "opening of the back doors" and "closing of the front doors." Moreover, in the early 1960s the average length of stay was about 6 months, but by the early 1990s it had declined to about 15 days. Overall, the rate of admissions increased slightly (NIMH, 1990). Thus, patients are often stabilized (given medication) and released back into the community, many times without adequate follow-up treatment and support (Wegner, 1990). Not surprisingly, substantial numbers of these patients end up being readmitted. This has been referred to as the "revolving door" phenomenon (Kiesler & Sibulkin, 1987).

Historically, psychiatric hospitals have functioned as a source of control of persons who are unable to care for themselves and whose behavior may be threatening to the social order (Grob, 1994; Horwitz, 1982). An important consequence of reduced hospital capacity is that a large portion of persons with severe mental illness now live in urban areas with less supervision and support. Although many do well, others lack "insight" into their disorders, go untreated, or have difficulty complying with medication regimens, and are unable to support themselves (Mechanic, 1999). This presents considerable difficulties for families and others who are often unable or unwilling to deal with persons whose behavior may at times be unmanageable or threatening (Avison, 1999).

Deinstitutionalization is hypothesized by many to have resulted in an increased number of persons at risk of homelessness and publicly troublesome behavior, increasing the burden on the criminal justice system (Finn & Sulllivan, 1988; Goldsmith, 1983; Grob, 1994; Dowdall, 1999; Issac & Armat, 1990; Johnson, 1990; Lewis et al., 1991; Mechanic & Rochefort, 1990; Morrisey, 1982; Task Force on Homelessness and Severe Mental Illness, 1992; Warner, 1989). Consequently, much individual-level research has focused on the increased proportion of mentally ill persons incarcerated, the likelihood of violent and criminal behavior among the mentally ill, the "criminalization" of mental illness, and the prevalence of mental illness among homeless persons. Despite the relevance of this research for macro-level social control processes, there has been no research directly examining the relationships of hospital capacity, homelessness, and crime at the city-level.

LIMITED HOSPITAL CAPACITY AND THE JUSTICE SYSTEM

In the aftermath of deinstitutionalization, several studies have investigated the extent to which prisons and jails have supplanted public psychiatric hospitals as institutions of social control of the mentally ill. These studies examined the frequency of arrest, jail, and imprisonment among people admitted into psychiatric hospitals before and during deinstitutionalization (Adler, 1986; Arvanites, 1988; Belcher, 1988; Cocozza, Melick, & Steadman, 1978; Goldsmith, 1983). A study in New York found that the percentage of patients with prior arrests increased from 15 percent in the 1946 to 1948 period to 32 percent in 1969 and to 40 percent by 1975 (Melick, Steadman, & Coccozza, 1979). A study of five states reported a 17-percent increase in the percentage of patients with prior arrests between 1968 and 1978 (Arvanites, 1988). Studies of imprisonment were less conclusive, however. For example, in a study of six states, Steadman and colleagues (1984) reported an overall increase (from 8 percent to 11 percent) in the percentage of prison inmates with prior mental hospitalization between 1968 and 1978. Although the increase occurred in only three states, it was enough to outweigh the decrease for the other three, yielding a net increase. Some researchers thus concluded that the mentally ill are being overarrested, but not overimprisoned, and instead are being warehoused in city and county jails (Adler, 1986; Lamb & Grant, 1982; Palermo et al., 1991, Pogrebin & Regoli, 1985; Teplin, 1990). However, a recent nationally representative survey of state and federal prisoners, jail inmates, and probationers indicates that persons who reported currently or ever having a "mental or emotional condition" are overrepresented in all those groups for both violent and property offenses, but not for drug offenses (Ditton, 1999). That study estimates that up to 16 percent of persons in prisons and jails may have a mental illness, many of whom have committed serious offenses. There are now more persons with mental illness in jails and prisons than in psychiatric hospitals (Torrey, 1995).

Because of a lack of appropriately trained staff and screening procedures, many persons are retained in jails and prisons without adequate treatment. These inmates are less likely than others to be released on bail, more likely to experience abuse from guards and other inmates, and are at an increased risk of suicide (Torrey, 1995). Thus, corrections facilities serve, in part, as alternatives to psychiatric hospitals. Although many jails and prisons provide mental health services, and several communities have programs to divert mentally ill offenders from jail to community treatment, the availability of these services and programs are limited relative to the need for them (Goldstrom et al., 1998; Morris, Steadman, & Veysey, 1997; Steadman, Morris, & Dennis, 1995).

The "Criminalization" of Mental Illness

How disproportionate numbers of the mentally ill end up in criminal justice settings can be understood in several interrelated ways. One is that it results from the "behavior" of the criminal justice system. That is, in the face of limited treatment options, disturbing behavior that might have been dealt with medically is now more likely to be treated as criminal behavior. For example, even though police may recognize some disruptive behavior as resulting from mental illness, they often have little choice but to use "mercy bookings" as a way to get persons into mental health treatment. Police are now one of the main sources of referral of persons into mental health treatment (Engel & Silver, 2001; Lamb et al., 2002). Also, police who see troublesome situations through the lens of their role as "law enforcers," are motivated to maintain their authority in conflict situations, often invoking the power of arrest to do so. These processes have led some to argue that mental illness has been "criminalized," with mentally ill suspects more likely to be arrested than suspects who are not mentally ill (Lamb & Weinberger, 1998; Lamb et al., 2002; Steury, 1991; Teplin, 1990).

The evidence in support of the criminalization hypothesis comes primarily from systematic observation of police-citizen encounters in major cities. One study showed that mentally ill suspects are about 20 percent more likely to be arrested than their counterparts (Teplin, 1984). However, a more recent study of police-citizen encounters in 20-four police departments in three metropolitan areas contradicts those findings (Engel & Silver, 2001). The study also showed that other factors, not considered in previous research, such as whether suspects are under the influence of drugs, are noncompliant, fight with officers or others, as well as the seriousness of their offense predict the likelihood of arrest. An important implication of their research is that if mentally ill persons are overrepresented in criminal justice settings, it is not solely attributable to discriminatory treatment on the part of police, but in part, due to a greater likelihood of arrest-generating behavior.

Much research has examined a second way that mentally ill persons are more likely than others to end up in criminal justice settings—that is, the direct relationship between mental disorder and the likelihood of violent and criminal behavior (Hiday, 1995; Hodgins, 1993; Link, Andrews, & Cullen, 1992; Link et al., 1999; Monahan, 1992; Steadman & Felson, 1984). Several strategies have been used. One approach samples jails or prisons and administers diagnostic inventories to determine the prevalence of mental illness among inmates. Estimates from these studies vary, but have shown that up to 20 percent of those incarcerated meet diagnostic criteria for a serious mental disorder, with about 5 percent having psychotic disorders (Roth, 1980; Steadman et al., 1987; Teplin, 1990, 1994), a rate higher than that of the general population. Another approach, using samples of those with a mental illness, finds a higher incidence of self-reported violence and arrest compared to the general population (Link et al., 1992; Steadman & Felson, 1984). One of the more rigorous approaches uses representative samples from the general population to estimate the prevalence of mental disorder and asks respondents about their involvement in violence and crime. These studies show that those who suffer from severe mental disorders are at an increased risk of violence and arrest (Link et al., 1992, 1999; Swanson et al., 1990). In many cases, those experiencing certain psychotic symptoms may misperceive the actions of others (including police officers) as threatening and respond aggressively (Link et al., 1999). These studies show, significantly, that the association between mental disorder and violence or arrest holds after controlling for comparable risk factors, such as sex, age, race, and socioeconomic status.

THE ROLE OF HOMELESSNESS

The effect of hospital capacity on crime and arrest rates at the city-level manifests itself in another set of ways. Psychiatric hospitals provide a place to stay (at least temporarily) for mentally ill persons. Given limited affordable housing options for the mentally ill, cities with less psychiatric inpatient capacity may have higher rates of homelessness (Bachrach, 1992; Jencks 1994; Mechanic & Rochefort, 1990). Studies estimate that approximately one-third of homeless persons meet diagnostic criteria for a major mental illness (Jencks, 1994; Lamb, 1992a; Shlay & Rossi, 1992). Including substance-related disorders, the figure is closer to 75 percent.

Homelessness is considered to be an important pathway to incarceration among the mentally ill (Lamb & Weinberger, 2001). Surveys of jail and prison inmates find that mentally ill offenders are more likely than other inmates to have been homeless at the time of arrest and in the year before arrest (DeLisi, 2000; Ditton, 1999; McCarthy & Hagan, 1991). Because of a lack of community treatment programs and limited staffing (critical for monitoring medication compliance), personal resources, and social supports, many mentally ill homeless persons are at increased risk of police encounters and arrest for not only "public order" types of offenses, such as vagrancy, intoxication, or disorderly conduct, but also for more serious types of crimes, such as assault (Dennis & Steadman, 1991; Hiday et al., 2001; Estroff et al., 1994; Hiday, 1995; McGuire & Rosenbeck, 2004; Mechanic & Rochefort, 1990; Steadman, McCarty, & Morrisey, 1989; Teplin, 1994; Teplin & Pruett, 1992).

Although the presence of homeless persons and public order offenses may be primarily a nuisance, they are a significant source of neighborhood disorder, generating fear and reducing social cohesion among neighborhood residents, thus facilitating more serious crime, such as robbery (see Markowitz et al., 2001; Skogan, 1990). In addition, high levels of urban disorder, including the visibility of homeless mentally ill persons, has led many cities (for example, New York) to take aggressive policing approaches that may contribute to the overrepresentation of mentally ill persons in jails and prisons.

The vulnerability of the homeless mentally ill also increases their risk of being the victims of crime (Dennis & Steadman, 1991). They are easier targets for offenders. Insights from routine activities theory suggest that homeless persons have reduced levels of "capable guardianship" necessary to protect themselves from crimes (Felson, 2002; Hagan & McCarthy, 1998). Moreover, the likelihood of victimization among homeless mentally ill persons is increased because of the risks of victimization associated with alcohol use more generally (Felson & Burchfield, 2004). For all of these reasons, cities with higher inpatient psychiatric capacity—with fewer homeless mentally ill persons on the streets—can be predicted to have lower crime and arrest rates.

The consequences of limited long-term care facilities are compounded by the fact that many mentally ill and homeless persons reside, temporarily, in group homes, shelters, or single-room occupancy hotels in more "socially disorganized" urban areas, where there are more economically disadvantaged persons, greater racial diversity, and more fragmented families. Social disorganization theory predicts that such structural characteristics lead to weakened social cohesion, thereby lessening the ability of communities to exert informal control over the behavior of their residents, resulting in increased crime (Bursik & Grasmick, 1993; Sampson & Groves, 1989; Sampson, Raudenbusch, & Earls, 1997). For persons with mental illness, living in such neighborhoods increases the risk of criminal offending beyond individual characteristics (Silver, 2000a, 2000b; Silver, Mulvey, & Monahan, 1999).

RESEARCH QUESTIONS

A key yet underexamined implication of the above research is that the capacity of mental health care systems to manage the behavior of persons with severe mental and addictive disorders—who are at increased risk of criminal offending—may be related to crime and arrest rates across macro-social units. I depart from the focus on individual variation in criminal or violent behavior as a result of mental illness. Instead, this analysis is concerned with the question of social control, conceptualizing hospital capacity and crime rates as social facts, asking whether cities with greater hospital capacity have lower crime and arrest rates. I examine both crime and arrest rates because arrest rates reflect political pressures and police activity in addition to levels of crime (O'Brien, 1996). Arrest rates may be sensitive to policing policies designed to reduce urban disorder, including the visibly homeless and mentally ill. I also examine the mediating role of homelessness in the relationship between psychiatric hospital capacity and crime and arrest rates. I predict that cities with greater hospital capacity will have lower levels of homelessness. Homelessness, in turn, is expected to be related to increased levels of crime and arrest.

METHODS

Sample

Questions regarding the macro-level relationships between psychiatric hospital capacity, homelessness, and crime/arrest rates raise important issues regarding the appropriate level of analysis. Most public psychiatric hospitals are state-controlled, thus the policy decisions determining the funding, staffing, and capacity of these institutions takes place at the state level.

However, crime and control of crime are generally considered local phenomenon. I therefore employ a strategy that apportions psychiatric hospital capacity to the city level using geographic information regarding catchment-area coverage.

The study is based on a sample of 81 U.S. cities with populations more than 50,000 where city-level estimates of homelessness from a variety of sources are available, which yield a sufficient number of cities for analysis. These cities represent a sample of mid-size to large urban areas where the processes of interest largely take place, and for which complete demographic, psychiatric hospital, and homelessness data are available. The sample is well-distributed geographically, with about 23 percent of cities located in the East, 25 percent in the Midwest, 21 percent in the West, and 31 percent in the South. The data examined are from 1989 to 1990. Thus, the period represented is one where the decline in hospital capacity was leveling off from the sharp declines from the 1960s to the 1980s, when crime rates were still comparatively high, before the crime drop of the mid-1990s. Further, in the early 1990s, the public mental health care system was just crossing a threshold where the majority of expenditures previously directed toward state hospital inpatient care were now directed toward community-based services (Lutterman & Hogan, 2000).

Measures

Psychiatric Hospital Capacity. The city-level measure of psychiatric hospital capacity comes from the annual *Guide to the Healthcare Field* (American Hospital Association, 1990). These data include the number of beds, admissions, patient census, personnel, average length of stay, source of funding, and expenditures for all hospitals in the United States and include community mental health centers with inpatient units. The level of error is likely low because the data are obtained from reports using a standardized instrument, with clearly identifiable variables that are closely monitored by hospital administrations. Capacity data were recorded for both private and public (state and county) psychiatric hospitals, aggregated to the city level, and expressed in terms of population proportions (number of beds per 100,000 residents). Most public psychiatric hospitals serve catchment areas—sets of counties including the ones in which they are located. Catchment area information was obtained from either the hospitals or the states' mental health departments. A similar procedure was used for cities served by hospitals outside the city.

Because local general hospitals are currently an important component of emergency and inpatient treatment, especially in light of Medicaid reimbursement, I also consider the effects of city population-proportionate number of psychiatric beds in general hospitals (per 100,000) that are reported at the state level and compiled by the Center for Mental Health Services and NIMH.

Crime and Arrest Rates. Crime and arrest rates come from the FBI Uniform Crime Reports (UCR). I focus on the Part I index offenses that include violent (homicide, assault, rape, and robbery) and property (burglary, theft, and motor vehicle theft) crimes. There are, of course, well-known limitations associated with UCR data, especially the underestimation of the "true" amount of crime (O'Brien, 1996).

Homelessness. Because there are well-known difficulties associated with measures of homelessness (Shlay & Rossi, 1992), I use three city-level measures from two sources. I use the U.S. Census Bureau's 1990 enumeration of persons visible in street locations and residing in shelters (per 100,000 persons). I also use Burt's 1989 homeless rate (number of shelter beds per 10,000), based on survey data from city administrators of the U.S. Department of Housing and Urban Development Comprehensive Homeless Assistance Plan (Burt, 1992). In the analysis, I combine the three correlated measures into a weighted factor score derived from principal components analysis.

Structural Variables. Throughout the analysis, I control for the following demographic structural variables associated with crime, the prevalence of mental illness, and homelessness: percent nonwhite, economic disadvantage (a factor score derived from principal components analysis of percent unemployed and percent of families in poverty), divorce rate, percentage age 15 to 34, and city population (Brenner, 1973; Catalano & Dooley, 1977, 1983; Elliot & Krivo, 1991; Fenwick & Tausig, 1994; Land, McCall, & Cohen, 1990; Sampson, 1987; Shlay & Rossi, 1992; Steffensmeier & Harer, 1999). All of these measures come from published U.S. Census Bureau figures.

RESULTS

National and Urban Levels of Psychiatric Hospital Capacity and Crime Rates

First, I compare the national level of psychiatric hospital capacity and crime rates to the urban sample. This is important because first, in terms of generalizability, I want to know how closely data from the urban sample reflects national estimates, and, second, I am concerned that the procedure for apportioning state and county hospital capacity to cities does not bias the data and model estimates. Table 1 shows the hospital capacity and crime rates (per 100,000) for both the nation and the urban sample. The level of city hospital capacity is very close to the national rate. As might be expected, crime rates are higher for the urban sample.

Bivariate Correlations between Hospital Capacity and Crime and Arrest Rates

Next, I examine the bivariate correlations between psychiatric hospital capacity and crime and arrest rates for both public and private hospitals, for violent, property, and both types of crime combined. In Table 2, correlations are shown for public hospitals. Consistent with the hypothesized relationships,

Table 1 Public Psychiatric Hospital Capacity and Crime Rates, 1990

Hospital Capacity		Index Crimes	
National Estimates	City Sample	National Estimates	City Sample
40	38	5820	9700

Note: Hospital capacity is the number of beds per 100,000. Index crimes include murder, robbery, assault, rape, burglary, larceny/theft, and auto theft (total per 100,000).

Table 2 Correlations between Psychiatric Hospital Capacity and Crime and Arrest Rates

	Violent		Property		Total	
	Crime	Arrest	Crime	Arrest	Crime	Arrest
Public Psychiatric	−.143*	−.145*	−.115	−.092	−.145*	−.142*
Private Psychiatric	−.049	.057	.249**	.338*	.184*	.267**
General Hospitals	−.073	−.042	−.139*	.005	−.082	.063

*$p < .05$ **$p < .01$ *$p < .10$

Note: Violent crimes include murder, robbery, assault, and rape (rates per 100,000). Property crimes include burglary, larceny/theft, and auto theft. Hospital capacity is measured as number of beds per 100,000.

the correlations of public hospital capacity with both crime and arrest rates are negative. For violent crimes, the correlation between hospital capacity and crime rate is very similar to the correlations involving arrest rates. For property crime however, the correlation between hospital capacity and crime rates are lower than the correlations involving arrest rates. As a result, the correlation between hospital capacity and total crime rate is slightly lower than correlation involving total arrest rates. In the regression analysis, I present results for violent and property crimes combined, but do so for crime and arrest rates separately.

Turning to the bivariate correlations between private psychiatric hospital capacity and crime and arrest rates (shown in Table 2), a pattern of relationships emerges that is generally opposite from that of public psychiatric hospitals. The correlations are mostly positive, indicating that private hospitals, more likely to serve those with private insurance, less severe disorders, and for shorter inpatient stays (Mechanic, 1999), may not provide the same crime-reducing function as public hospitals. Although seemingly anomalous, the positive correlation between private hospital capacity and crime and arrest rates is consistent with research indicating that where cities have more private hospitals and beds, police may be more likely to

arrest mentally ill offenders. This is due to the well-documented organizational reluctance among private hospitals to admit patients who are
uninsured, are covered by Medicaid, or have more severe mental illnesses
(Schlesinger & Gray, 1999). The correlations between psychiatric beds in
general hospitals and crime (see Table 2), show that, with the exception of a
small negative correlation with property crimes, there is very little bivariate relationship of crime and arrest rates with general hospital psychiatric
beds. The mostly private general hospitals with psychiatric bed allocation
may operate in a manner similar to private psychiatric hospitals, in terms
of providing only short-term care, thus having a limited crime-reducing
effect. Therefore, in the regression analysis, I focus mainly on public psychiatric hospitals, but comment on the sensitivity of the effects of public
psychiatric beds when private and general hospital beds are included in
the equations.

Hospital Capacity, Homelessness, and Crime and Arrest Regression Models

Table 3 presents the results of a series of OLS regression models for the relationships between public hospital capacity, homelessness, and crime and
arrest rates. Equation 1 shows the effects of hospital capacity and structural
variables on homelessness, followed by equations 2 through 5 estimating the
effects of hospital capacity and homelessness on crime and arrest rates. First,
the results from equation 1 show that hospital capacity has a statistically
significant negative effect on homelessness (beta = −.15). The effects of several structural variables are in the expected direction. Percentage nonwhite
and economic disadvantage are associated with increased homelessness. As
might be anticipated, homelessness is also more prevalent in larger cities.
Hospital capacity and the structural variables account for about 12 percent of
the variation in homelessness.

The hospital capacity effect on the crime rate (equation 2) is generally
similar to the bivariate correlation. The effect is negative and statistically
significant, with a standardized coefficient (beta) of −.13. The effects of the
structural variables are in the expected direction. Percentage nonwhite, economic disadvantage, percentage age 15 to 34, and divorce are associated with
increased crime rates.

When homelessness is introduced into the model (equation 3) the results
indicate that it has a statistically significant effect on crime rates (beta = .34).
Consequently, the hospital capacity effect is reduced by about 40 percent and
is no longer significant. Together, hospital capacity and structural variables
account for about 31 percent of the variation in crime rate. When the models
are estimated separately for violent and property crime rates, the results (not
shown) indicate a slightly stronger effect of homelessness on violent crime
compared to property crime. However, using a covariance structure model
with maximum likelihood estimation with violent and property crime rates
specified as endogenous, controlling for the other variables, I constrained

Table 3 Regression Models Relationships 1990

	Homelessness		Crime Rate				Arrest Rate			
	(1)		(2)		(3)		(4)		(5)	
Variables	b	Beta	b	Beta	b	Beta	b	Beta	b	Beta
Hospital capacity	−.01*	−.15	−6.90*	−.13	−4.17	−.08	−2.37*	−.17	−2.01'	−.14
Nonwhite	.02**	.31	47.84**	.27	28.40*	.16	5.30*	.13	8.47*	.24
Economic disadvantage	.17**	.17	730.89***	.23	674.23*	.29	36.97	.05	34.74	.05
Divorce	.04	.05	240.72*	.16	266.38'	.17	15.18	.15	18.22	.15
Age 15 to 34	.01	.02	83.77*	.12	89.54'	.13	37.58*	.15	36.34*	.12
Population (1,000s)	.01'	.15	.01	.04	.01	.01	.04	.05	.01	.04
Homelessness	—	—	—	—	134.95**	.34	—	—	62.50*	.12
R^2(n)		.12(80)		.20(79)		.31(79)		.10(75)		.12(75)

$p < .10$ $^*p < .05$ $^{**}p < .01$ $^{***}p < .001$.
Note: b = unstandardized regression coefficients; Beta = standardized regression coefficients.

the unstandardized effects of homelessness to be equal across the two equations and tested for model fit using the nested chi-sure test (Bollen, 1989). The results indicate no significant difference in the effect of homelessness across the two equations (chi-square, 1 d.f. = 2.72, p = .10).

Equations 4 and 5 in Table 3 present the results of regression models for the effects of hospital capacity and the control variables on arrest rates. In equation 4, excluding homelessness, the hospital capacity effect is similar to the bivariate correlation (beta = −.17). The coefficients for the other structural variables are in the expected direction. Comparing the effect of hospital capacity on crime and arrest rates (equations 2 and 4), the effect on crime rates is slightly greater (chi -square, 1 d.f. = 9.70, p = .003).

When homelessness is added to the arrest rate model (equation 5), the effect of hospital capacity is reduced (by about 15 percent), yet is still close to conventional levels of statistical significance. Together, hospital capacity and structural variables account for about 12 percent of the variation in arrest rate. When arrest rates are examined separately by types of crimes (not shown), homelessness is found to have a statistically significant and substantial effect on arrests for violent crime (beta = .19), but only a small and nonsignificant effect on arrests for property crime (beta = .08). Again using a covariance structure model with equality constraints on the unstandardized homelessness effect across equations, the difference this time is found to be statistically significant (chi-square, 1 d.f. = 9.82, p = .002). This might be expected given that property crimes are far less likely to be reported, let alone result in arrest.

To determine whether these results are affected by controlling for private and general psychiatric hospital capacity, I re-estimated the series of equations including these variables. When the private psychiatric hospital capacity is added, it is found to have no statistically significant effects on any of the dependent variables. The effects of public hospital capacity do increase slightly, but remain substantively unchanged. Moreover, to test for the possibility that the effects of public hospital capacity may be conditioned by private and general hospital capacity, product terms were formed between public capacity and each of these variables and added to the equations. Using nested F-tests, none of these effects were found to be significant.

DISCUSSION

In this study, I first tested the hypothesis that public psychiatric hospital capacity is inversely related to crime and arrest rates at the city level. The results are consistent with that hypothesis and with surveys of jail and prison inmates that find mentally ill offenders are overrepresented among those incarcerated, especially for violent crimes, which have a greater likelihood of resulting in arrest compared to property or drug offenses (Ditton, 1999). The findings are also consistent with arguments that when social control agents must deal with individuals whose behavior may be disturbing or troublesome, in the absence of hospitalization in public psychiatric institutions as an option, arrests may be more frequent, accounting for much of the "transinstitutionalization" that occurs (Adler, 1986; Belcher, 1988; Finn & Sullivan, 1988).

The public hospital capacity effect may be sensitive to outpatient services, which can affect patients' ability to successfully integrate into communities. If it is, I cannot be confident that the effect has been isolated. Unfortunately, standard measures of other mental health-related social service provision are not available in the same way that hospital data is.

Examining the relationships between psychiatric hospital capacity, homelessness, and crime and arrests, the results indicate a moderate link between public hospital capacity and homelessness at the city level that is not conditioned by private psychiatric beds, general hospital psychiatric beds or community-based expenditures. Although data on the proportion of mental illness among persons who are arrested and are homeless is not available for a city (or state) level analysis, the findings indicate that increased hospital capacity is associated with overall lower levels of homelessness, and increased homelessness is in turn associated with higher levels of crime and arrests for violent crime. The results indicated that part of the public hospital capacity effect on crime and arrest rates operates through its effect on homelessness.

I also estimated the equations including a variable capturing the ratio of private to public and general psychiatric hospital beds. The results indicated that, net of other factors in the equations, the predomination of private beds in cities is associated with statistically significant increases in crime (beta = .173) and arrest rates (beta = .359). This is consistent with the possibility that in cities where private hospital beds constitute a larger share of inpatient capacity, police have less access to facilities to readily take problematic persons and may be more likely to resort to arrest. However, police in such locales might be more inclined toward arrest generally.

The study complements our knowledge of the mental disorder and violence-crime association from individual-level research with a macro-level assessment of the relationship between the capacity for control of persons with psychiatric illness and crime and arrest rates. This relationship has several important implications for public policy related to community safety and the treatment of the mentally ill. Although some have raised the issue of a moratorium on deinstitutionalization (Lamb, 1992b), the results inform policy decisions regarding the impact of further reductions of psychiatric hospital capacity. The study suggests that modest increases in crime may be expected for given reductions in inpatient hospital capacity. This is especially important now that many states have implemented managed mental health care plans involving strict limitations on inpatient service expenditures (Mechanic, 1999). The exact effect of reduced hospital capacity on crime rates in any given city is difficult to predict, however, because this effect may depend on the availability and quality of a variety of fragmented community-based treatment and housing services that expenditure data alone may not fully capture.

Local jails often serve as conduits through which many mentally ill offenders pass before being transferred to psychiatric hospitals (Liska et al., 1999). Further reductions in psychiatric hospital capacity therefore increase the burden on law enforcement and corrections agencies. In fact, most jails in major metropolitan areas now provide some sort of mental health services. It is estimated that, nationally, corrections departments assume about one-third of the costs of mental health services provided in jails (Goldstrom et al., 1998). There have been increased efforts to provide services within correctional settings as well as support for community treatment alternatives, such as intensive case management, jail diversion programs, and mental health courts for mentally ill persons at risk of offending (Steadman, Joseph, & Bonita, 1999; Dvoskin, 1994; Morris et al., 1997; Steadman et al., 1995; Watson et al. 2001). In general, the evidence regarding the effectiveness of these often uncoordinated programs is somewhat limited (for a comprehensive review, see Fisher, 2003). In light of the findings of the present study, these types of programs may be insufficient to take the place of public institutions focusing specifically on the inpatient care needs of persons with serious mental illness and substance abuse disorders.

In sum, public psychiatric hospital capacity is an important source of control of those whose behavior or public presence may at times threaten the social order. Although controversial issues in mental health care such as easing standards for involuntary treatment, court-ordered medication compliance, and expanding custodial care continue to be debated (Lamb, 1992b; Mechanic, 1999; Miller, 1993; Torrey, 1997), the study suggests that reductions in public hospital capacity must be weighed against public safety concerns, tolerance, and the willingness to provide high-quality alternative community mental health and housing services.

References

Adler, Freda. 1986. Jails as a repository for former mental patients. *International Journal of Offender Therapy and Comparative Criminology* 30:225–236.

American Hospital Association. 1990. *Guide to the Healthcare Field*. Chicago: American Hospital Association.

Arvanites, Thomas M. 1988. The impact of state mental hospital deinstitutionalization on commitment for incompetency to stand trial. *Criminology* 26:225–320.

Avison, William R. 1999. The impact of mental illness on the family. In Carol S. Aneshensel and Jo C. Phelan (eds.), *Handbook of the Sociology of Mental Health*. New York: Kluwer Academic/Plenum.

Bachrach, Leona L. 1992. What we know about homelessness among mentally ill persons: An analytical review and commentary. *Hospital and Community Psychiatry* 43:453–464.

Belcher, John R. 1988. Are jails replacing the mental health system for the homeless mentally ill? *Community Mental Health Journal* 24:185–194.

Bollen, Kenneth A. 1989. *Structural Equations with Latent Variables*. New York: John Wiley & Sons.

Brenner, M. Harvey. 1973. *Mental Illness and the Economy*. Cambridge, MA: Harvard University Press.

Bursik, Robert J., Jr., and Harold G. Grasmick. 1993. *Neighborhoods and Crime*. New York: Lexington Books.

Burt, Martha R. 1992. *Over the Edge: The Growth of Homelessness in the 1980s*. New York: Russell Sage Foundation.

Catalano, Ralph, and C. David Dooley. 1977. Economic predictors of depressed mood and stressful life events in a metropolitan community. *Journal of Health and Social Behavior* 18:292–307.

Catalano, Ralph, and C. David Dooley. 1983. Health effects of economic instability: A test of the economic stress hypothesis. *Journal of Health and Social Behavior* 24:46–60.

Cocozza, Joseph, Mary E. Melick, and Henry J. Steadman. 1978. Trends in violent crime among ex-mental patients. *Criminology* 16:317–334.

DeLisi, Matt. 2000. Who is more dangerous? Comparing the criminality of adult homeless and domiciled jail inmates: A research note. *International Journal of Offender Therapy and Comparative Criminology* 44:59–69.

Dennis, Deborah L., and Henry J. Steadman. 1991. *The Criminal Justice System and Severely Mentally Ill Persons: An Overview*. Washington, DC: U.S. Department of Health and Human Services.

Ditton, Paula M. 1999. *Mental Health and Treatment of Inmates and Probationers*. NCJ 174463. Washington, DC: U.S. Department of Justice, Bureau of Justice Statistics.

Dowdall, George W. 1999. Mental hospitals and deinstitutionalization. In Carol S. Aneshensel and Jo C. Phelan (eds.), *Handbook of the Sociology of Mental Health*. New York: Kluwer Academic/Plenum.

Dvoskin, Joel A. 1994. Using intensive case management to reduce violence by mentally ill persons in the community. *Hospital and Community Psychiatry* 45:679–684.

Ehrenkranz, Shirley M. 2001. Emerging issues with mentally ill offenders: Causes and social consequences. *Administration and Policy in Mental Health* 28:165–180.

Elliot, Marta, and Lauren J. Krivo. 1991. Structural determinants of homelessness in the United States. *Social Problems* 38:113–131.

Engel, Robin Shepard, and Eric Silver. 2001. Policing mentally disordered suspects: A reexamination of the criminalization hypothesis. *Criminology* 39:225–252.

Estroff, Sue, Catherine Zimmer, William Lachotte, and Julia Benoit. 1994. The influence of social networks and social support on violence by persons with serious mental illness. *Hospital and Community Psychiatry* 45:669–679.

Felson, Marcus. 2002. *Crime and Everyday Life,* 3rd ed. Thousand Oaks, CA: Sage Publications.

Felson, Richard B., and Keri B. Burchfield. 2004. Alcohol and the risk of physical and sexual assault victimization. *Criminology* 42:837–860.

Fenwick, Rudy, and Mark Tausig. 1994. The macroeconomic context of job stress. *Journal of Health and Social Behavior* 356:266–282.

Finn, Peter E., and Monique Sullivan. 1988. *Police Response to Special Populations: Handling the Mentally Ill, Public Inebriate, and the Homeless.* Washington, DC: National Institute of Justice.

Fisher, William H. 2003. *Community-Based Interventions for Criminal Offenders with Severe Mental Illness.* New York: Elsevier.

Fisher, William H., Ira K. Packer, Lorna J. Simon, and David Smith. 2000. Community mental health services and the prevalence of severe mental illness in local jails: Are they related? *Administration and Policy in Mental Health* 27:371–382.

Goldsmith, Marsha F. 1983. From mental hospitals to jails: The pendulum swings. *Journal of the American Medical Association* 250:3017–3018.

Goldstrom, Ingrid, Marilyn J. Henderson, Alisa Male, and Ronald W. Manderscheid. 1998. Jail mental health services: A national survey. In Ronald W. Manderscheid and Marilyn J. Henderson (eds.), *Mental Health, United States, 1998.* Rockville, MD: Department of Health and Human Services, Substance Abuse and Mental Health Services Administration, Center For Mental Health Services.

Grob, Gerald N. 1994. *The Mad Among Us: A History of the Care of America's Mentally Ill.* New York: Free Press.

Gronfein, William. 1985. Psychotropic drugs and the origins of deinstitutionalization. *Social Problems* 32:437–455.

Hagan, John, and Bill McCarthy. 1998. *Mean Streets: Youth Crime and Homelessness.* New York: Cambridge University Press.

Hiday, Virginia A. 1995. The social context of mental illness and violence. *Journal of Health and Social Behavior* 36:122–137.

Hiday, Virginia A., Jeffrey W. Swanson, Marvin S. Swartz, Randy Borum, and H. Ryan Wagner. 2001. Victimization: A link between mental illness and violence? *International Journal of Law and Psychiatry* 24:559–572.

Hodgins, Sheilagh. 1993. *Mental Disorder and Crime.* London: Sage Publications.

Horwitz, Allan V. 1982. *The Social Control of Mental Illness.* New York: Academic Press.

Inverarity, James, and Ryken Grattet. 1989. Institutional responses to unemployment: A comparison of U.S. trends, 1948–1985. *Contemporary Crises* 13:351–370.

Issac, Rael Jean, and Virginia C. Armat. 1990. *Madness in the Streets: How Psychiatry and Law Abandoned the Mentally Ill.* New York: Free Press.

Jackson, Pamela 1. 1989. *Minority Group Threat, Crime, and Policing.* New York: Praeger.

Jencks, Christopher. 1994. *The Homeless.* Cambridge, MA: Harvard University Press.

Johnson, Ann B. 1990. *Out of Bedlam: The Truth About Deinstitutionalization.* New York: Basic Books.

Kiesler, Charles A., and Amy E. Sibulkin. 1987. *Mental Hospitalization: Myths and Facts about a National Crisis.* Newbury Park, CA: Sage Publications.

Lamb, H. Richard. 1992a. Deinstituionalization in the nineties. In Richard Lamb, Leona Bachrach, and Frederic Kass (eds.), *Treating the Homeless Mentally Ill.* Washington, DC: American Psychiatric Association.

Lamb, H. Richard. 1992b. Is it time for a moratorium on deinstitutionalization? *Hospital and Community Psychiatry* 43:669.

Lamb, H. Richard, and Leona L. Bachrach. 2001. Some perspectives on deinstitutionalization. *Psychiatric Services* 52:1039–1045.

Lamb, H. Richard, and R. Grant. 1982. The mentally ill in an urban jail. *Archives of General Psychiatry* 39:17–22.

Lamb, H. Richard, and Linda E. Weinberger. 1998. Persons with severe mental illness in jails and prisons: A review. *Psychiatric Services* 49:483–492.

Lamb, H. Richard, and Linda E. Weinberger. 2001. *Deinstitutionalization: Problems and Promise.* San Francisco: Jossey-Bass.

Lamb, H. Richard, Linda E. Weinberger, and Walter J. DeCuir, Jr. 2002. The police and mental health. *Psychiatric Services* 53:1266–1271.

Land, Kenneth C., Patricia L. McCall, and Lawrence E. Cohen. 1990. Structural covariates of homicide rates: Are there any invariances across time and social space? *American Journal of Sociology* 95:922–963.

Lewis, Dan A., Stephanie Riger, Helen Rosenberg, Hendrik Wagenaar, Arthur J. Lurigio, and Susan Reed. 1991. *Worlds of the Mentally Ill: How Deinstitutionalization Works in the City.* Carbondale: Southern Illinois University Press.

Link, Bruce G., Howard Andrews, and Francis T. Cullen. 1992. The violent and illegal behavior of mental patients reconsidered. *American Sociological Review* 57:275–292.

Link, Bruce G., John Monahan, Ann Steuve, and Francis T. Cullen. 1999. Real in their consequences: A sociological approach to understanding the association between psychotic symptoms and violence. *American Sociological Review* 64:316–332.

Liska, Allen E. 1992. *Social Threat and Social Control.* Albany: State University of New York Press.

Liska, Allen E., and Mitchell B. Chamlin. 1984. Social structures and crime control among macrosocial units. *American Journal of Sociology* 90:383–395.

Liska, Allen E., Fred E. Markowitz, Rachel Bridges-Whaley, and Paul E. Bellair. 1999. Modeling the relationships between the criminal justice and mental health systems. *American Journal of Sociology* 104:1744–1775.

Lutterman, Ted, and Michael Hogan. 2000. State mental health agency controlled expenditures and revenues for mental health services, FY 1981 to FY 1997. In Ronald Manderscheid and Marilyn Henderson (eds.), *Mental Health, United States, 2000.* Rockville, MD: Department of Health and Human Services, Substance Abuse and Mental Health Services Administration, Center for Mental Health Services.

Markowitz, Fred E., Paul E. Bellair, Allen E. Liska, and Jianhong Liu. 2001. Extending social disorganization theory: Modeling the relationships between cohesion, disorder, and fear. *Criminology* 39:293–320.

McCarthy, Bill, and John Hagan. 1991. Homelessness: A criminogenic situation. *British Journal of Criminology* 31:393–410.

McGuire, James F., and Robert A. Rosenbeck. 2004. Criminal history as a prognostic indicator in the treatment of homeless people with severe mental illness. *Psychiatric Services* 55:42–48.

Mechanic, David. 1999. *Mental Health and Social Policy: The Emergence of Managed Care.* Boston, MA: Allyn and Bacon.

Mechanic, David, Donna McAlpine, and Mark Olfson. 1998. Changing patterns of psychiatric inpatient care in the United States, 1988–1994. *Archives of General Psychiatry* 55:785–791.

Mechanic, David, and D.A. Rochefort. 1990. Deinstitutionalization: An appraisal of reform. *Annual Review of Sociology* 16:301–327.

Melick, Mary E., Henry J. Steadman, and Joseph C. Cocozza. 1979. The medicalization of criminal behavior among mental patients. *Journal of Health and Social Behavior* 20:228–237.

Miller, R. D. 1993. The criminalisation of the mentally ill: Does dangerousness take precedence over need for treatment? *Criminal Behavior and Mental Health* 3:241–250.

Monahan, John. 1992. Mental disorder and violent behavior: Perceptions and evidence. *American Psychologist* 47:511–521.

Morris, Suzanne M., Henry J. Steadman, and Bonita M. Veysey. 1997. Mental health services in United States jails. *Criminal Justice and Behavior* 24:3–19.

Morrisey, Joseph P. 1982. Deinstitutionalizing the mentally ill: Processes, outcomes, and new directions. In Walter R. Gove (ed.), *Deviance and Mental Illness*. Beverly Hills, CA: Sage Publications.

National Institute of Mental Health. 1990. *Mental Health, United States*. Washington, DC: U.S. Government Printing Office.

O'Brien, Robert M. 1996. Police productivity and crime rates: 1973–1992. *Criminology* 34:183–208.

Palermo, George B., M.B. Smith, and Frank J. Liska. 1991. Jails versus mental hospitals: A social dilemma. *International Journal of Offender Therapy and Comparative Criminology* 35:97–106.

Penrose, Lionel. 1939. Mental disease and crime: Outline of a comparative study of European statistics. *British Journal of Medical Psychology* 18:1–15.

Piven, Francis F., and Richard Cloward. 1971. *Regulating the Poor: The Function of Public Welfare*. New York: Vintage.

Pogrebin, Mark R., and Robert M. Regoli. 1985. Mentally disordered persons in jail. *Journal of Community Psychology* 13:409–412.

Redick, Richard W., Michael J. Witkin, Joanne Atay, and Ronald W. Manderscheid. 1992. Specialty mental health system characteristics. In Ronald Manderscheid and Mary Anne Sonnenschein (eds.), *Mental Health, United States, 1992*. Rockville, MD: U.S. Department of Health and Human Services, Substance Abuse and Mental Health Services Administration, Center For Mental Health Services.

Roth, L. H. 1980. Correctional psychiatry. In W. Curran, A. McGarry, and C. Petty (eds.), *Modern Legal Medicine, Psychiatry, and Forensic Science*. Philadelphia: Davis.

Sampson, Robert J. 1987. Urban black violence: The effect of male joblessness and family disruption. *American Journal of Sociology* 93:348–382.

Sampson, Robert J., and W. Byron Groves. 1989. Community structure and crime: Testing social disorganization theory. *American Journal of Sociology* 94:774–802.

Sampson, Robert J., Stephen W. Raudenbush, and Felton Earls. 1997. Neighborhoods and violent crime: A multilevel study of collective efficacy. *Science* 277:918–924.

Schlesinger, Mark, and Bradford Gray. 1999. Institutional change and its consequences for the delivery of mental health services. In Allan V. Horwitz and Teresa Scheid (eds.), *A Handbook for the Study of Mental Health: Social Context, Theories, and Systems*. Cambridge: Cambridge University Press.

Scull, Andrew. 1977. Madness and segregative control in the rise of the insane asylum. *Social Problems* 24:337–351.

Shlay, Anne B., and Peter H. Rossi. 1992. Social science research and contemporary studies of homelessness. *Annual Review of Sociology* 18:129–160.

Silver, Eric. 2000a. Extending social disorganization theory: A multilevel approach to the study of violence among persons with mental illnesses. *Criminology* 38:301–332.

Silver, Eric. 2000b. Race, neighborhood disadvantage, and violence among persons with mental disorders: The importance of contextual measurement. *Law and Human Behavior* 24:449–456.

Silver, Eric, Edward B. Mulvey, and John Monahan. 1999. Assessing violence risk among discharged patients: Towards an ecological approach. *Law and Human Behavior* 23:235–253.

Skogan, Wesley G. 1990. *Disorder and Decline: Crime and the Spiral Decay of American Neighborhoods*. New York: Free Press.

Steadman, Henry J., and Richard B. Felson. 1984. Self-reports of violence: Ex-mental patients, ex-offenders, and the general population. *Criminology* 22:321–342.

Steadman, Henry J., Joseph J. Cocozza, and Bonita M. Veysey. 1999. Comparing outcomes for diverted and nondiverted jail detainees with mental illnesses. *Law and Human Behavior* 23:615–627.

Steadman, Henry J., Dennis, W. McCarty, and Joseph P. Morrisey. 1989. *The Mentally Ill in Jail*. New York: Guilford.

Steadman, Henry J., Suzanne M. Morris, and Deborah L. Dennis. 1995. The diversion of mentally ill persons from jails to community-based services: A profile of programs. *American Journal of Public Health* 85:1630–1635.

Steadman, Henry J., S. Fabiasak, Joel Dvoskin, and Edward J. Holohean. 1987. A survey of mental disability among state prison inmates. *Hospital and Community Psychiatry* 38:1086–1090.

Steadman, Henry J., John Monohan, Barbara Duffee, Eliot Hartstone, and Pamela C. Robbins. 1984. The impact of state mental hospital deinstitutionalization on U.S. prison populations, 1968–1978. *Journal of Criminal Law and Criminology* 75:474–490.

Steffensmeier, Darrell, and Miles D. Harer. 1999. Making sense of recent U.S. crime trends, 1980 to 1996/1998: Age composition effects and other explanations. *Journal of Research in Crime and Delinquency* 36:235–274.

Steury, Ellen H. 1991. Specifying "criminalization" of the mentally disordered misdemeanant. *Journal of Criminal Law and Criminology* 82:334–359.

Sutton, John R. 1991. The political economy of madness: The expansion of the asylum in progressive America. *American Sociological Review* 56:665–678.

Swanson, Jeffrey W., Charles E. Holzer III, Vijay K. Ganju, and Robert T. Jono. 1990. Violence and psychiatric disorder in the community: Evidence from the epidemiological catchment area surveys. *Hospital and Community Psychiatry* 41:761–770.

Task Force on Homelessness and Severe Mental Illness. 1992. *Outcasts on Main Street: Report of the Federal Task Force on Homelessness and Severe Mental Illness*. Rockville, MD: U.S. Department of Health and Human Services.

Teplin, Linda A. 1984. Criminalizing mental disorder: The comparative arrest rate of the mentally ill. *American Psychologist* 39:794–803.

Teplin, Linda A. 1990. The prevalence of severe mental disorder among male urban jail detainees: Comparison with the Epidemiological Catchment Area Program. *American Journal of Public Health* 80:663–669.

Teplin, Linda A. 1994. Psychiatric and substance abuse disorders among male urban jail detainees. *American Journal of Public Health* 84:290–293.

Teplin, Linda A., and N. S. Pruett. 1992. Police as street-corner psychiatrist. *International Journal of Law and Psychiatry* 15:157–170.

Torrey, E. Fuller. 1995. Jails and prisons—America's new mental hospitals. *American Journal of Public Health* 85:1611–1613.

Torrey, E. Fuller. 1997. *Out of the Shadows: Confronting America's Mental Illness Crisis.* New York: John Wiley & Sons.

Warner, Richard. 1989. Deinstitutionalization: How did we get where we are? *Journal of Social Issues* 45:17–30.

Watson, Amy, Patricia Hanrahan, Daniel Luchins, and Arthur Lurigio. 2001. Mental health courts and the complex issue of mentally ill offenders. *Psychiatric Services* 52:477–481.

Wegner, Eldon L. 1990. Deinstitutionalization and community-based care for the chronically mentally ill. In James Greenley (ed.), *Research in Community and Mental Health,* vol. 6. Greenwich, CT: JAI Press.

Weinstein, Raymond M. 1990. Mental hospitals and the institutionalization of patients. In James Greenley (ed.), *Research in Community and Mental Health,* vol. 6. Greenwich, CT: JAI Press.

DISCUSSION

1. According to Markowitz, what are the prevailing theoretical views on why there may be a relationship between psychiatric hospital capacity and rates of homelessness, crime, and arrest?

2. What do Markowitz's findings suggest about structural weaknesses in our contemporary system of care and treatment for people with mental illness? Should we increase psychiatric hospital capacity? Given his findings, what would be the likely effects, if any, if we tried to expand the number of psychiatric hospital beds where you live?

Sociological Perspectives on Contemporary Mental Health Care and Treatment

Alisa Lincoln

Psychiatric Emergency Room Decision Making, Social Control and the 'Undeserving Sick'[†]

As discussed in more detail in the previous section, we can learn a great deal about the sociological dimensions of mental illness by studying the careers of people with mental illness and how they "enter" the mental health system. In this study, sociologist Alisa Lincoln examines decision making in the psychiatric emergency room and the motives, contingencies, and potential consequences of involuntary hospitalization. Like other sociological research on involuntary commitment, Lincoln finds that social factors play an important role in how treatment providers respond to psychiatric emergencies. Her research, however, also highlights how changes in the organization of the mental health system have made these decisions even more challenging.

INTRODUCTION

There is a strong history of sociological work related to the involuntary commitment of people with mental illness to treatment. However, dramatic changes in the organization and financing of the U.S. health care system, and the social context of mental illness and the mental healthcare system, make it necessary to re-examine the role of social factors in involuntary commitment decisions. This paper describes how these changes, specifically those in the mental health care system, have impacted on the ways that social factors influence involuntary hospitalisation decisions. In addition, I examine

Lincoln, Alisa. 2006. "Psychiatric emergency room decision-making, social control and the 'undeserving sick'." *Sociology of Health and Illness* 28:54–75.

the utility of previously-used theoretical frameworks for understanding the ways in which social factors influence involuntary commitment.

As one of the few forms of coercive state intervention in the health care system, the involuntary commitment process remains a particularly important area of focus. While the specifics of involuntary hospitalization laws vary from state to state, they are most often based on two standards: (1) the presence of a mental illness for which hospitalization is an appropriate treatment, and (2) potential danger to oneself (deriving from the *parens patriae* power) or to others (deriving from the police power). Based on the "rule of law," these standards alone should determine who receives coercive state intervention in the form of civil commitment.

Previous sociological work has examined the role of social factors in involuntary commitment from a social control framework. The application of social control theory to the involuntary commitment process suggests that people who have less power or fewer resources are more likely to receive coercive responses to their actions (Horwitz, 1982). Thus, for example, blacks have been reported to have disproportionately high rates of involuntary hospitalization (Rosenfield, 1984; Lindsey & Paul, 1989). However, the radical changes in the social context within which involuntary hospitalization decisions are made have altered the relationships between social factors and the mechanisms of social control.

This study examined two important questions related to involuntary hospitalization decisions. First, do the medical and legal criteria for involuntary hospitalization predict psychiatric emergency room decision making, as expected? Second, do social factors influence psychiatric emergency room decision making? And, if so, does the traditional use of social control theory still provide a helpful framework within which to examine these questions, or do new models better elucidate these relationships under the current sociohistoric conditions?

BACKGROUND

The medical and legal criteria for involuntary commitment include diagnoses and symptoms, as well as history and level of dangerousness. These factors have consistently been found to predict psychiatric emergency room (PER) decision making (Gerson & Bassuk, 1980; Marson et al., 1988; Rabinowitz et al., 1995), and provide evidence for the appropriate use of medical and legal characteristics in PER decision making. At the same time there is also ample evidence that social factors such as a person's race (Rosenfield, 1984; Lindsey & Paul, 1989; Strakowski et al., 1995), gender (Rosenfield, 1982), pathway to the emergency room (Rosenfield, 1984; Way et al., 1993) and level of family involvement (Marson, 1988; Gerson & Bassuk, 1980; Friedman et al., 1981) can influence PER decision making in several ways. First, social factors may operate solely as confounding or intervening variables in the relationship between medical or legal characteristics and involuntary commitment. This would be the case, for example, if men were more likely to be involuntarily committed than women because they had higher rates of psychiatric disorder or were more violent than women. If so, the relationship between social factors and decisions would simply be a byproduct of the application of the medical and legal criteria for involuntary commitment.

Social factors may also be used by doctors to make decisions deemed appropriate from a purely medical perspective. For example, these factors may identify patients who the doctors perceive to have a high "need for services" even if they do not meet the legal criteria for involuntary hospitalisation. Under these circumstances, there can be an incongruity between the law and the manifest function (Merton, 1968) of psychiatry: a clash between the medical mandate and legal institutions, in which physicians may find themselves in a position where they must circumvent the law in order to do their job. For instance, physicians may be more likely to hospitalize homeless patients who are sick but do not meet the dangerousness criteria because they know that people may be unable to recuperate in the streets. While this would be decision making influenced by a social factor it would also serve an intended function of psychiatry by treating a person who has a severe mental illness.

Social factors, however, may also create unintended consequences of PER decision making, influencing PER decision making in ways that derive neither from perceived medical need nor the legal criteria. Social factors may influence PER decision making by serving a latent function of psychiatry— that of social control. Under such circumstances, patients' social characteristics would operate to expose those at the bottom of the social structure to disproportionately harsh treatment that can not be justified by legal or medical criteria (Horwitz, 1982).

While social control is known to influence many aspects of medicine, the explicit coercive nature of involuntary commitment has led to the codification into law of the decision-making criteria, in order to minimize the influence of other factors on the involuntary hospitalization. In the past, however, blacks (Rosenfield, 1984; Lindsey & Paul, 1989), men (Rosenfield, 1982), and people arriving at the PER with a police officer (Rosenfield, 1984; Way et al., 1993) were more likely to be involuntarily hospitalized than whites, women, and people arriving with family members or alone. These findings are consistent with expectations from a social control framework, in which marginalized and powerless groups are more likely than powerful groups to receive undesired treatment, in this case coercive forms of treatment. To the extent that psychiatry serves a latent function of social control, those at the bottom of the social hierarchy would more frequently receive undesired and coercive forms of treatment. The greater likelihood of hospitalization for those accompanied to the emergency room by a police officer can be similarly understood from a social control perspective. As Way and colleagues state, "Police cases may be judged by emergency room staff as more dangerous, not by objective standards, but by simply due to the presence of a police officer" (1993, 395). It has been hypothesized that the more coercive treatment response experienced by blacks may also be due to disproportionate involvement with, and therefore label from, the police.

The role of the patient's sex is less clear. In most areas men are more likely to gain access to a desired resource than women (e.g., employment, education). However, in this setting men may be seen as the more difficult patients, given gender-linked perceptions about potential for violence (Coontz, Lidz, & Mulvey, 1994). In addition to the role of gender suggested by social control theory, women may be more likely to be seen as in need of care, or to be more vulnerable to victimization on the streets. Social control theory also offers several explanations for the influence of family members on involuntary commitment. Formal social control agents, in this case psychiatrists, will often act in accordance with the families' wishes. Formal social control is however also more likely when families are either unwilling or unable to respond. Evidence for this would be seen in higher rates of involuntary commitment among patients with no family involvement.

Changes in the Social Context of Involuntary Commitment

Major changes in the organization and financing of health care in the United States have radically altered the social context in which involuntary commitment decisions take place. Managed care has created new treatment decision incentives for physicians. Whereas in the past the central issue seems to have been coercion into treatment for those who don't want it, the central problem now seems to be the difficulty of getting into treatment if you want it. Indeed, in recent legal cases involving HMOs people with mental illness are fighting for access to treatment, not for the right to refuse treatment as in the earlier landmark cases (Hughes, 1996, 1333).

In addition to these health care system changes, the vast mental health care reforms of the second half of the 20th century have been well documented (Applebaum, 1994; Bachrach, 1980). Throughout the early nineties deinstitutionalization and advances in the development of psychotropic medication continued, while landmark cases broadened patients' rights and provided greater protection of individual liberties. An active consumer movement and advocacy groups have also greatly influenced mental health care in many ways. These include lobbying for policy changes, the mainstreaming of self-help groups in mental health care, and the continued work to empower mental health consumers and their families in psychiatric decision making. In addition, these organizations have played an important role in the changing societal attitudes and beliefs about mental illness. In fact, simultaneously with these structural changes to the organization and financing of mental health care, there have been changes in societal attitudes and beliefs about mental illness (Link et al., 1999). These changes in societal norms are also likely to influence PER decision making.

These changes have been of such a sweeping nature that in some settings the involuntary hospitalization process is seen as providing better due process protection of patient's rights than voluntary hospitalization (Hughes, 1996). This may influence medical staff to favor involuntary commitment as a means of admission, further restricting access to inpatient psychiatric treatment. Patients who are very sick but present no threat of harm to themselves or others may not be involuntarily hospitalized or admitted to an inpatient unit any other way. As Malone states "The ED, rather than being the catchall safety net for public health, mental health and social services that it has heretofore been in actual practice, shifts towards a much narrower role that involves only triage and care of illness and injuries that have clear cut medical boundaries and are relatively urgent" (Malone, 1998, 818).

These changes related to mental health and the mental health care system have simultaneously created an increase in the demand for care at psychiatric emergency rooms while restricting the availability of emergency departments and inpatient care. "The admission rate to public mental hospitals is at its lowest point in 100 years. On the other hand, visits to psychiatric emergency services increased by more than 150 per cent during the 1970s and early 1980s" (Fitzgerald, 1996, 233). The question then becomes: How do medical, legal, and social factors influence involuntary hospitalization decisions under these new social conditions?

A New Model?

Psychiatric hospitalisation has become a scarce resource in many public-sector mental health care systems. When an outcome is desired, and even more so when it is desired and restricted, social factors will predict who is able to access treatment. Physicians draw on these social factors in determining whether someone is deserving of, or appropriate for, treatment. With limited beds available, pressure is exerted on physicians to use their available resources effectively. Ironically, this means that people with less severe or less complicated illness may be more likely to get a bed. Poorer patients whose problems are more complex and time consuming may disproportionately be denied care (Malone, 1998). In addition, it is easier for people with greater social resources to negotiate the process of accessing treatment.

In this access model people at the bottom of the social structure may disproportionately be denied "needed services" to a greater extent than those of higher social status, particularly when they do not meet the legal criteria for involuntary hospitalization. This might create a group of patients who, based on social factors, physicians view as inappropriate for or undeserving of treatment: *the undeserving sick.*

Evidence supporting an access model would be found if the more advantaged patients were more likely to be hospitalized, including involuntarily, than less socially advantaged patients. For example, if white patients, patients who arrive with other people at the PER and people who have a family member advocating hospitalization are more likely to be hospitalized than less advantaged patients. This would suggest that the tremendous change in the social context of involuntary hospitalization has altered the specific mechanisms of the relationship between social status and involuntary hospitalization, but that the fundamental relationship of the influence of social factors on involuntary commitment remains. Thus, the same people who, in earlier studies, were found to receive the undesirable coercive outcome of involuntary hospitalization disproportionately will still be more likely to receive the undesirable outcome. However, the nature of the undesirable treatment outcome may have changed. The least socially advantaged group would no longer be disproportionately involuntarily hospitalized but instead might be disproportionately denied needed care.

This study therefore examined whether the previously-used operationalization of social control theory remained appropriate in understanding the influence of social factors on PER decision making, or whether a formulation focused on the "undeserving sick" and access to care, provided a better explanation.

HYPOTHESES

The hypothesis that psychiatric emergency room decisions are based only on the medico-legal criteria is supported when: (a) the medical and legal criteria predict psychiatric emergency room disposition and (b) the social and demographic factors are either not related to disposition, or any effects of the social and demographic variables on hospitalization disappear when medical and legal criteria are controlled for.

The hypothesis that psychiatric emergency room decisions are influenced by factors other than those in the medical and legal criteria is supported when: (a) there are relationships between sociodemographic factors and disposition and (b) they do not disappear when medico-legal criteria are controlled.

The traditional or *coercive* exclusion model of *social control* is supported when people who are more marginalized and have less power and prestige are disproportionately involuntarily hospitalized, and this is not explained by relationships between these groups and medical and legal criteria. An *access model* is supported when hospitalization is defined as a desired good and when people who are less marginalized and have more power or prestige are hospitalized more frequently than others and this is not explained by relationships between these groups and medical and legal criteria.

METHODS

The study was conducted in one of the busiest urban, public, teaching hospitals in the country. The PER receives 6,000 visits per year and serves as the admission service for 350 inpatient beds. These beds were at 100 percent plus capacity throughout the entire course of this study. The size of the facility, the high level of involvement with the criminal justice system and the racial and ethnic diversity of the patient population made this program an excellent setting in which to examine the study's hypotheses.

Cases were identified from the PER logbook from January, March, and June of 1995. There were a total of 1,546 visits during these months. Police-involved cases were over-sampled to guarantee adequate data on these cases, with every police-involved case and every fifth nonpolice-involved case included in the sample. Medical records were available on 67 percent of nonpolice involved cases and 66 percent of police-involved cases, thus differential loss to follow-up related to police involvement did not bias the results. This created a sample of 379 visits of which 13 were repeat visits and are excluded from these analyses. Finally, the police-involved cases included both emotionally disturbed persons (EDPs) for whom no criminal charges were pending and pre-arraignment cases. The pre-arraignment cases ($n = 79$) have been excluded from the analyses presented here since their ultimate disposition rested in the criminal justice system.

In order to assess changes in the social context of involuntary commitment, several sources of qualitative data were examined. First, all descriptions of the reason for the visit, dangerousness, violence, or rationale for the disposition were extracted from the medical records. In addition, using a snowball sampling design, key informants were identified and interviewed using a semi-structured interview. The director, assistant director, and two additional medical staff were interviewed. Topics included perceptions of how PER decisions were made, the role of social factors, and their thoughts about involuntary commitment as a treatment modality. Informal participant observation techniques were used over a one-year period of time. These observations were not however collected in a systematic way; notes were taken on informal conversations with staff and observed interactions, which were related to PER decision making. These data were intended as exploratory work in this area, and served as important evidence in the appropriateness of testing these study hypotheses. These data were not systematically analysed using qualitative analytic methods. Quotes from these data are used here for illustrative purposes.

For each sampled visit, the patient's sociodemographic characteristics and medical and legal characteristics were collected from the medical records. The medical and legal criteria were operationalized as variables for diagnosis, symptoms, and level of dangerousness.

The symptom coding was accomplished with very limited data because, although the Mental Status Exam was given to every patient, recording of these data was erratic. Four symptom groups were created: speech irregularities, suicidal/homicidal ideation, thought content disorders, and thought process disorders.

The final medical and legal decision-making variable used in these analyses was created from data collected on the precipitating events from the patient's chart. A person was coded as "dangerous" if they had attacked someone or something with or without a weapon or made a suicide attempt. A person was coded as "potentially dangerous" if they were described as being potentially dangerous to themselves or others. The third level included people with noted suicidal ideation. Finally, people described as having only bizarre behavior, without any indications of dangerousness, and who thus did not fall into any of the above categories, are described as "bizarre behaviour only." Multiple informant reports of the precipitating events were used whenever available to try to address potential bias in the recording of the precipitating events in the chart.

Data on patient race/ethnicity, sex, age, insurance status, and education level were obtained from the PER visit sheet. Homelessness was determined from physician notes in the PER visit sheet and variables were created for where the person lived (apartment/house, shelter, SRO (single room occupancy), street, etc.) and with whom (parents, spouse/partner, alone, other family member). This served as a cross-check of the person's actual living situation.

Data on people who arrived at the PER with the person seeking care were collected from the medical record, and confirmed with police reports. Several indicators of social support were created: (1) whether or not the patient was able to provide any name of a person for the medical staff to contact, (2) whether or not any family member was involved in this specific visit either directly by bringing them to the PER, or indirectly by calling the police or a social worker, and (3) living arrangements (alone or with others).

Variables were also created for the source of information present in the medical record. The mean age of the study subjects was 38 years. Table 1 contains other descriptive data for the important independent variables used in the study.

Possible dispositions for cases at the PER include emergency hold, involuntary commitment, voluntary admissions, transfer to other hospitals, transfer to state hospital or long-term care, and treated and released or discharged. Forty-six percent of the sample was hospitalized: 10 percent voluntarily, 36 percent involuntarily. Nine percent of the sample was ultimately transferred to long-term care, most frequently the state hospital. For the purposes of these analyses, voluntary hospitalization, involuntary hospitalization, and treated and released, are the outcomes used.

ANALYSES

The stratified sampling used in this study necessitated the use of SUDAAN in the final analyses. SUDAAN uses Taylor Series methods to calculate appropriate standard errors when such complex sampling designs are used. Throughout the paper all frequencies are unweighted (N) and all proportions have been computed using the weighted data. Univariate analyses and logistic regression models were used to test each hypothesis. The outcome

Table 1 Frequency Table for the Medico-Legal and Sociodemographic Variables
(*N* = 287)

	Weighted Proportion (%)	Unweighted *N*
Psychotic diagnosis	53.6	156
Affective diagnosis	34	94
Substance abuse disorder	55.2	155
Personality disorder	4.4	12
Anxiety disorder	5.3	12
Speech irregularity	21.9	73
Suicidal/Homicidal ideation	30.4	83
Thought content irregularity	45.5	134
Thought process irregularity	39.8	126
Attacks on people or objects	5.2	31
Threats of attacks on people or objects	17.1	60
Potentially threatening behavior to others or self	24.1	83
Suicidal ideation	29.4	68
Suicide attempt	5.9	22
Bizarre behavior	42.4	122
Seeking social services	7.6	17
Seeking medication	29.8	60
Sex		
Male	76.9	209
Female	23.1	78
Race		
White	32.1	96
Black	42.5	115
Hispanic	20.4	54
Other race/ethnicity	5.1	22
Living arrangement		
Apartment/house	37.2	115
SRO	3.3	10
Shelter	17.2	40
Street	26.8	76
Other	15	45
No family involvement	61.7	117
Living alone	64.7	174
Unemployed	77.4	217
Source to the PER		
Alone	65.1	122
Family	7.2	14
Police	17.6	131
Other	10	20

variable used when examining the appropriateness of traditional social control theory is involuntary hospitalization, because this operationalization of social control theory has focused on the importance of a coercive social response. The outcome variable used when testing the access hypothesis is any type of hospitalization, since hospitalization is the desired outcome and involuntary hospitalization is merely a mechanism used to obtain hospitalization. Finally a baseline model consisting of the medical and legal variables found to be a significant predictor of hospitalization and involuntary hospitalization was created. These groups of variables were then used as the control variables in testing the social and demographic hypotheses.

RESULTS

Evidence of a Change in the Role of Social Factors in the PER

The first step in testing the study hypotheses was to examine the data for evidence of a change in the social context of involuntary commitment at the PER. Qualitative data were examined for evidence of change in three areas: that hospitalizing a patient was a difficult process; that hospitalization, even if this necessitated involuntary hospitalization, was a desired outcome for people seeking care; and that physicians' attitudes toward involuntary commitment reflected changes in the social context of involuntary commitment.

If involuntary commitment decisions reflect a traditional coercive operationalization of social control, then hospitalizing marginalized or disenfranchised people should not be difficult. However, staff meetings were dominated by discussions of how to get people into the hospital and physicians were frustrated by their inability to provide needed services. "Generally, we no longer worry about who we falsely imprison, we worry more about people getting in or getting kicked out once they get in" (Dr. M). Physicians referred to surmounting the obstacles to admission as "case building." Building a case involved gathering information from as many sources as possible to show that a person had met the commitment criteria. Many medical records noted "suffering from major mental illness but not commitable at this time." Reimbursement mechanisms had a profound influence on people's ability to access care. "The patient walked in requesting guidance. Has been in detox for six weeks, feeling depressed and wants someone to talk to. But he has been very disappointed and dejected since they [other facilities he had been to today] only take MasterCard/Visa and major insurance and he only has Medicaid." At this public facility no one was denied care based on their insurance status however; the pressures on the physicians to try to find reimbursement for care was often discussed in team meetings.

Evidence that hospitalization, even involuntary commitment, was a desired outcome of people seeking care was found. When asked about the PER decision-making process Dr. R stated, "Let's say a black man, Mr. Smith, comes here. Dr. Jones, a white doctor sympathetic to the underclass, recommends involuntary admission..." Here the "sympathetic" thing to do is recommend involuntary admission. Dr. R stated that he did not think race played a role in the decision-making process at the PER although he chose to provide racial descriptors in the example.

Notes in the medical record often reflected peoples' desire for admission. Several patients were noted to have said, "Better hospitalisation than jail." Others saw the PER as a refuge where they could rest and regain their strength for the streets. One man wanted to be held "overnight to rest, but no longer!" People even threatened the medical staff to let them into the hospital: "the patient is currently intoxicated and threatening to get into the hospital." Patients seeking hospitalization, in this setting where voluntary hospitalizations were rare and difficult to obtain, often pushed for involuntary hospitalization as it remained the only means to admission. One man presented to the PER seeking admission early in the morning, and was told he did not meet the "threshold" for admission. He returned to the PER later that day, accompanied by two police officers, having thrown a brick through the window of a business in a neighbouring affluent shopping district, and stating, "Now can you keep me?" Notes in the medical record indicated that the physician attributed this behavior to the patient's efforts to be committed.

Finally, there was evidence that physicians' attitudes toward involuntary commitment reflected the current social context. The director described part of his job as "fighting the cynicism" of his staff that patients are trying to manipulate their way into the hospital for nonpsychiatric reasons. These included getting off the street, a meal, shoes, sleep, or avoidance of jail. The PER maintained a closet with shoes and clothes in order to return people to the streets with these items.

These exploratory qualitative data provided evidence of a change in the social context of involuntary commitment at the PER. It is therefore appropriate to test the study's hypotheses using these data.

The Medical and Legal Model

The most severe diagnoses and the most dangerous precipitating events did predict hospitalisation outcomes. The baseline models comprising the significant medical and legal predictors are presented in Table 2. Separate best-fit models were created for the two outcome variables, voluntary hospitalization and involuntary hospitalization. These models contained identical factors, except speech irregularities and suicidal/homicidal ideation, which were not significant predictors of involuntary hospitalization. These odds ratios should be interpreted as follows: people with a diagnosis of a psychotic disorder without substance abuse were more than 10 times as likely to be hospitalized as people who had neither a psychotic disorder nor substance abuse. Similarly, those deemed dangerous were between four and nine times more likely to be hospitalized than people not exhibiting the same types of dangerous behaviors. For example, people who arrived at the PER having

Table 2 The Best-Fit of the Medico-Legal Criteria: Logistic Regression Analysis of the Diagnostic, Symptom and Level of Dangerousness on Hospitalization and Involuntary Hospitalization ($N = 287$)

Variables	Hospitalized/Not Hospitalzed		Involuntarily Hospitalized/Not Involuntarily Hospitalized	
	OR	(95% C.I.)	OR	(95% C.I.)
Psychotic disorder without substance abuse ($N = 77$)	10.70**	(3.91,29.28)	11.00**	(4.18,28.93)
Psychotic disorder with comorbid substance abuse ($N = 78$)	8.23**	(3.33,20.39)	9.85**	(3.84,25.23)
Affective disorder ($N = 94$)	5.28**	(2.13,13.12)	5.18**	(2.25,12.03)
Speech irregularities ($N = 83$)	2.24+	(.86,5.80)	XXXX	XXXX
Suicidal/homicidal ideation (as symptom) ($N = 73$)	3.53**	(1.45,8.60)	XXXX	XXXX
Danger 1—attacks, threats and suicide attempt ($N = 97$)	3.99**	(1.32,12.00)	3.73**	(1.31,10.62)
Danger 2—potential danger to self or others ($N = 33$)	7.40**	(1.99,27.50)	8.73**	(2.53,30.17)
Danger 3—suicidal ideation as precipitating event ($N = 61$)	.54	(.16,1.88)	.20*	(.04,.93)
Danger 4—bizarre behavior only ($N = 64$)	2.16	(.67,6.98)	1.55	(.49,4.85)

+$p < .10$
*$p < .05$
**$p < .01$

just assaulted someone, threatened someone, or made a suicide attempt were 3.73 times more likely to be involuntarily hospitalized than people who did not exhibit these behaviors (see Table 2). The medical and legal criteria did predict hospitalization outcomes as expected, providing support for the first part of this hypothesis. Diagnosis, dangerousness, and their combined effects predicted both hospitalization and involuntary hospitalization.

Testing the Social Factors Hypotheses

Initial analyses were conducted to determine the univariate relationships between the social and demographic variables and the hospitalization outcomes. Being unemployed and having no permanent home did not significantly relate to the hospitalization outcomes; these variables were therefore not included in the final models. Race, source, living with a relative, and sex were each tested as predictors of the hospitalization outcomes, adjusting for the baseline models, and each was a significant predictor. The relationships between the social and demographic variables and the hospitalization outcome are substantial and remained significant after controlling for the

Table 3 Logistic Regression Analysis of Race, Living Arrangement, Source and Gender Controlling for the "Best-fit Models" and Age on Involuntary Hospitalization ($N = 287$)

Variables	Involuntarily Hospitalized/Not Involuntarily Hospitalized			
	Model 1		Model 2	
	Odds ratio	95% C.I.	Odds ratio	95% C.I.
Race—White ($N = 95$)	contrast		contrast	
Black ($N = 115$)	.82	(.37,1.81)	.36*	(.13,.95)
Hispanic ($N = 54$)	3.73**	(1.46,9.52)	1.72	(.59,5.06)
Asian/Other ($N = 22$)	2.84	(.56,14.44)	1.10	(.25,4.82)
Source—Self ($N = 122$)	contrast		contrast	
Other/Formal ($N = 20$)	20.81**	(.46,7.75)	29.38**	(.95,33.12)
Police ($N = 131$)	4.30**	(2.14,8.63)	3.57**	(1.50,8.54)
Family ($N = 14$)	1.90	(4.85,89.25)	5.60*	(4.85,179.7)
Living with parent or sibling ($N = 48$)	1.92	(.70,15.25)	1.04	(.36,3.0)
Gender (male $N = 209$)	.41**	(.19,.85)	.32**	(.12,.84)
Psychotic disorder without substance abuse ($N = 77$)			7.66**	(2.49,23.58)
Psychotic disorder with comorbid substance abuse ($N = 78$)			17.15**	(4.90,59.94)
Affective disorder ($N = 94$)			5.60**	(2.08,15.03)
Danger 1—attacks, threats and suicide attempt ($N = 97$)			2.70+	(.72,10.02)
Danger 2—potential danger to self or others ($N = 33$)			5.16+	(.96,27.88)
Danger 3— suicidal ideation as precipitating event ($N = 61$)			.09**	(.02,.43)
Danger 4—bizarre behavior only ($N = 64$)			1.42	(.32,6.35)

+ $p < .10$
* $p < .05$
** $p < .01$

baseline models (Tables 3 and 4). Based on these results, it is clear that factors other than the medical and legal factors predict hospitalization. What do the results tell us about the relative merit of social control as opposed to access explanations for deviations from the medical and legal model of PER decision making?

Race. Under the traditional assumptions of social control the most historically disadvantaged racial or ethnic group should have the highest rate of involuntary commitment. In the American literature this has been seen for black patients. Here the inverse is true—the likelihood of involuntarily

Table 4 Logistic Regression Analysis of Race, Living Arrangement, Source and Gender Controlling for the "Best-fit Models" and Age on Hospitalization ($N = 287$)

| | Hospitalized/Not Hospitalized | | | |
| | Model 3 | | Model 4 | |
Variables	Odds ratio	95% C.I.	Odds ratio	95% C.I.
Race: Black ($N = 115$)	contrast		contrast	
White ($N = 95$)	.78	(.37,1.62)	.88	(.34,2.32)
Hispanic ($N = 54$)	3.18**	(1.36,7.42)	2.41*	(1.03,5.68)
Asian/Other ($N = 22$)	3.43+	(.81,14.64)	2.56	(.66,9.90)
Source—Self ($N = 122$)	contrast		contrast	
Other/Formal ($N = 20$)	16.11**	(3.25,79.22)	14.89**	(2.50,87.53)
Police ($N = 131$)	3.05*	(1.60,5.78)	3.01*	(1.22,7.42)
Family ($N = 14$)	1.31	(.33,5.16)	2.50	(.44,14.14)
Living with parent or sibling ($N = 48$)	2.05	(.87,4.82)	1.67	(.61,4.62)
Gender (Male $N = 209$)	.70	(.34,1.44)	.50+	(.22,1.14)
Psychotic disorder without substance abuse ($N = 77$)			7.23**	(2.63,19.87)
Psychotic disorder with comorbid substance abuse ($N = 78$)			9.05**	(3.23,25.41)
Affective disorder ($N = 94$)			4.71**	(1.81,12.21)
Speech Irregularities ($N = 83$)			2.75*	(.95,7.91)
Suicidal/homicidal ideation ($N = 73$)			4.83**	(1.96,11.91)
Danger 1—attacks, threats and suicide attempt ($N = 97$)			2.66+	(.73,9.66)
Danger 2—potential danger to self or others ($N = 33$)			3.95+	(.84,18.71)
Danger 3—suicidal ideation as precipitating event ($N = 61$)			.54	(.54,7.99)
Danger 4—bizarre behavior only ($N = 64$)			2.08+	(.13,2.13)

$+ p < .10$
$* p < .05$
$** p < .01$

hospitalization for blacks is one-third that of whites after adjusting for the effects of medical and legal criteria (see Table 3.)

In order to test the access hypothesis, the dummy variables for race were recoded with blacks serving as the contrast group since, under these assumptions, blacks should have the lowest hospitalisation rates. No significant differences were found between blacks and whites, but Hispanics had almost three times the odds of being hospitalized as blacks. While not predicted within this theoretical framework, this would be in keeping with an access hypothesis if Hispanics were somehow more advantaged, or perceived as more advantaged or appropriate for treatment than blacks or whites. The increased odds ratios for those of other racial/ethnic background (mostly Asian) may be explained by different patterns of help-seeking behavior among these groups (Snowden & Chung, 1990), particularly the delaying of help-seeking until symptoms can no longer be tolerated within the community (see Table 4).

Source to the psychiatric emergency room. Patients arrived at the psychiatric emergency room with police, family members, alone, or were brought by another formal source (an outreach team or hospital transfer). Preliminary analysis determined that people who arrived alone had the lowest unadjusted involuntary hospitalization and hospitalization rate. The dummy variable was therefore coded with "self" as the contrast group.

People who were brought to the PER by a formal source (transfers or outreach teams) were the most likely to be hospitalized. This is consistent with both the social control and the access hypotheses (Tables 3 and 4).

Several of the relationships that support a social control model were found in the analysis of source. Police involvement increased the likelihood of involuntary hospitalization compared with arriving alone. This may be because those who arrived with police were previously labeled as dangerous or deviant, as suggested in earlier work (Lindsey & Paul, 1989). Police referrals may also reflect an aspect of dangerousness not specifically captured in these variables, or police involvement may have other alternative meanings.

People who arrived with family members had six times the odds of involuntary hospitalization compared with those who arrived alone. There are two possible interpretations of this finding that are in keeping with a social control model: (1) families are viewed as providing previous labels of mental illness or dangerousness, and (2) this effect reflects the influence of informal agents of social control (family members) on formal agents. There are also two possibilities in keeping with the access hypothesis: (1) families serve as advocates helping the patient negotiate for admission, and (2) the existence of family support provides the hospital with the likelihood of easier discharge planning.

Living arrangement. Living arrangement, coded as living with parent, sibling, spouse/partner, friend, other arrangement, or alone, was found to be a univariate predictor of involuntary hospitalization. Because of the small numbers in some of these cells, those living with family of origin (parent/sibling) were compared with those who were not. Living with a member of the family of origin significantly increased the likelihood of involuntary hospitalization in a reduced model with only the baseline variables. However, this relationship lost significance in the full model (see Tables 3 and 4). This finding did not support the social control hypothesis and, in combination with the important role family plays as a source to the psychiatric emergency room, suggests that the role of family needs to be examined for evidence of alternatives to the social control hypothesis. This provides possible support for the access hypothesis.

Sex. Men were significantly less likely than women to be involuntarily hospitalized (Table 3). It has been suggested (Horwitz, 1990) that higher rates of involuntary hospitalization among men might be consistent with a social control hypothesis; this finding therefore does not support the social control hypothesis. It may, however, support the access hypothesis, particularly if men are thought to be more difficult to treat or manage behaviorally, or if women are perceived as more in need of protection or deserving of care than men (Table 3).

The social factors in combination. As a final test of the hypotheses the social and demographic variables were examined in combination to determine whether their effects on involuntary hospitalization were independent of each other. For instance, was the race effect merely a reflection of the importance of police as a source to the psychiatric emergency room as found in earlier work (Lindsey & Paul, 1989; Rosenfield 1984)? This analysis (Table 3) shows that not only do the social and demographic variables predict involuntary hospitalization but that they do so independently. Only living arrangement is no longer a significant predictor of involuntary hospitalisation in this analytic framework.

The social and demographic variables were also examined in combination for their ability to predict both hospitalization outcomes above and beyond the medical and legal criteria (Tables 3 and 4). While some of the odds ratios decreased, Hispanics remained almost two-and-a-half times as likely as blacks to be hospitalized. Neither the impact of family as source to the PER or the relationship between living arrangement and hospitalization are any longer significant. Finally, male gender continued to decrease the likelihood of hospitalization in the elaborated model.

CONCLUSION

As expected, medical and legal factors were the strongest predictors of both voluntary and involuntary hospitalization in this study of the PER. People presenting with severe diagnoses and dangerous behaviour were more likely to be hospitalized than other people. Yet, while we know that social factors influence all medical decisions, the decision to involuntarily hospitalize a patient brings such powerful consequences that the decision-making criteria have been codified into law in order to minimize inappropriate influences on the decision. Nevertheless, social factors continue to play a role in who is involuntarily hospitalized and who is not. This study tested whether the ways in which these social factors influenced involuntary hospitalization have changed with the organizational and financing changes of the mental health system as well as the changes in mental health law.

This examination of two possible hypotheses to explain hospitalization decisions has highlighted many important social influences on psychiatric emergency room decision making. The first hypothesis, that medical and legal criteria are the only influences on psychiatric emergency room decision making, was not supported, as several social factors influenced hospitalization decisions. The alternative hypothesis, that there are social influences on hospitalization decisions, was supported. A person's race/ethnicity, living arrangement, family involvement, source to the PER, and gender all influenced whether or not they would be hospitalized.

There are important relationships between race/ethnicity and family variables, which influence hospitalization patterns that must be examined further. Many of the PER staff reported that they believed Hispanics were hospitalized more frequently because of their family structure and support. Further analyses showed that Hispanics were more likely than those from other racial/ethnic backgrounds to have family involvement, but none of the family involvement measures in this study explained the increased hospitalization rate among Hispanics. More work is needed to determine whether these rates are replicable in other studies and to explore possible explanations for these findings, such as the role of language and medical staff perceptions of Hispanic patients and their families.

The limitations of these data and methodologies, particularly the use of medical record review, the limitations of sample size on interpreting the confidence intervals of several important variables, and the lack of important insurance data, highlight the need for further investigation concerning the ways that social factors continue to influence involuntary hospitalization. In particular, future work should examine the role of insurance status as this is a potentially powerful predictor, which I was unable to examine in this study. Future studies should include more rigorous qualitative methods of data collection and analysis in order to expand our understanding of the social context of PER decision making.

Finally, this study, as well as most studies of PER decision making, took place in a busy, public, urban teaching hospital. These conclusions are therefore not generalizable to less urban or rural settings. While it is likely that social factors continue to influence PER decision making in all PER settings, it is important that future studies examine the ways in which social factors influence PER decision making in diverse PER settings. We can, however, be confident about this documented change, since the earlier studies suffered from these same, as well as additional, limitations. This re-examination of the social process of involuntary hospitalization showed that new mechanisms now explain the influence of social factors on PER decision making. The question in this setting has become, How is the limited resource of hospitalization, which has become predominantly involuntary, distributed among people who desire or need it?

Social control theory has provided helpful insights for understanding the ways that social factors, such as race and gender, have influenced PER decision making. However, social theories are developed and used in a sociohistorical context. As Donald Light writes, "Central at all times is the issue of control, and sociological theories about its nature have explicitly or implicitly framed our understanding of the health care system from one period to another. Ironically, sociologists present these theories in universal terms, when in fact each of them reflects the tenor of its time" (Light, 1989, 457). Social control theory provided a reasonable explanation for the role of social factors in PER decision making in the past. Consistent findings of an inverse relationship between social power and involuntary hospitalization rates (a coercive treatment response), that is the increased probability of involuntary hospitalization for blacks, those arriving with a police officer, those with few social connections and males, are all consistent with a traditional social control explanation.

Does social control continue to serve as a guiding theory in understanding these new relationships between social factors and PER decision making? While denying needed psychiatric treatment may be unjust it is difficult to categorize the treatment and release of patients seeking hospitalization as coercive. Traditionally, social control has focused on the importance of negative sanctions; however, a broader examination of social control theory (Horwitz, 1990) suggests that the traditional coercive treatment options served as social control because they excluded people from society. In this expanded model, involuntary hospitalization no longer serves as an easily accessible or cost-efficient form of exclusion from society. When people are denied needed psychiatric care, they may no longer be able to fulfill their societal roles and may ultimately be excluded and disconnected from social networks. If social control theory is based on exclusion and not strictly coercion, then the access hypothesis may reflect new forms of social control.

The previous focus on coercive social control occurred at a time when involuntary hospitalization was an easily accessible and seemingly endless resource. But now, psychiatric hospitalization is the best possible alternative, for many people when social services are scarce and the streets are dangerous. This gives involuntary hospitalization a very different meaning to those seeking care. At the same time, fiscal pressures, limited numbers of inpatient beds, and overwhelming demand are forcing PER, to limit the number of people they serve and the types of problems they address. "The narrowing role of the ED, in the absence of addressing the almshouse role it has traditionally filled for the dependent poor, amounts to de facto rationing on the basis of social worth" (Jecker in Malone 1998).

Despite all of the changes in the mental health care system and the law, the importance of social factors remains. What has not changed is that those people who are disempowered or marginalized are still likely to remain so. By preserving the best resources for the most powerful people psychiatric emergency room decisions continue to reflect the larger unintended consequences of psychiatry. Previous policies led to disproportionate rates of involuntary hospitalization among marginalized and powerless groups; these same groups are now disproportionately denied access to psychiatric inpatient treatment. While clearly not all of the patients required psychiatric hospitalization, very few were not suffering from mental illness. The rest may have been exaggerating their mental health needs for "ulterior motives," but they had legitimate psychiatric and social needs. What will happen to those patients who are not sick enough to meet the involuntary hospitalization criteria, who are unfortunate enough to be one of the "undeserving sick"?

References

Applebaum, P.S. (1994) *Almost a Revolution: Mental Health Law and the Limits of Change.* New York: Oxford University Press.

Bachrach, L.L. (1980) Is the least restrictive environment always the best? Sociological and semantic implications, *Hospital and Community Psychiatry,* 31, 2, 97–102.

Coontz, P.D., Lidz, C.W., and Mulvey, E.P. (1994) Gender and the assessment of dangerousness in the psychiatric emergency room, *International Journal of Law and Psychiatry,* 17, 4, 369–76.

Fitzgerald, M. (1996) Structuring psychiatric emergency services for smaller communities in response to managed care, *Psychiatric Services,* 47, 233–34.

Friedman, S., Feinsilver, D., Davis, G., Margolis, R., and David, O. (1981) Decision to admit in an inner city psychiatric emergency room: beyond dangerousness—the psychosocial factors, *Psychiatric Quarterly,* 53, 259–74.

Gerson, S. and Bassuk, E. (1980) Psychiatric emergencies: an overview, *American Journal of Psychiatry,* 137, 1–11.

Horwitz, A. (1982) *The Social Control of Mental Illness.* New York: Academic Press.

Horwitz, A. (1990) *The Logic of Social Control.* New York: Plenum Press.

Hughes, D.M. (1996) Implications of recent court rulings for crisis psychiatric emergency services, *Psychiatric Services,* 47, 12, 1332–3.

Kelsey, J. (1986) *Methods in Observational Epidemiology.* Oxford: Oxford University Press.

Light, D. (1989) Social control and the American health care system. In Freeman, H. and Levine, S. (eds) *Handbook of Medical Sociology,* 4th Edition. Englewood Cliffs, NJ: Prentice Hall.

Lindsey, K. and Paul, G. (1989) Involuntary commitments to public mental institutions: issues involving the overrepresentation of blacks and assessment of relevant functioning, *Psychological Bulletin,* 106, 171–83.

Link, B., Phelan, J., Bresnahan, M. *et al.* (1999) Public conceptions of mental illness: labels, causes, dangerousness and social distance, *American Journal of Public Health,* 89, 1293–460.

Malone, R. (1998) Whither the almshouse? Overutilization and the role of the emergency department, *Journal of Health Politics, Policy and Law,* 23, 795–832.

Marson, D.C., McGovern, M.P. and Pomp, H.C. (1988) Psychiatric decision making in the emergency room: a research overview, *American Journal of Psychiatry,* 145, 918–25.

Merton, R. (1968) *Social Theory and Social Structure.* New York: The Free Press.

Rabinowitz, J., Massad, A., and Fennig, S. (1995) Factors influencing disposition decisions for patients seen in a psychiatric emergency service, *Psychiatric Services,* 46, 7, 712–18.

Rosenfield, S. (1982) Sex roles and societal reactions to mental illness: the labeling of 'deviant' deviance, *Journal of Health and Social Behavior*, 23, 18–24.

Rosenfield, S. (1984) Race differences in involuntary hospitalization: psychiatric v. labeling perspectives, *Journal of Health and Social Behavior*, 25, 14–23.

Segal, S.P. (1996) Quality of care and use of less restrictive alternatives in the psychiatric emergency service, *Psychiatric Services*, 47, 6, 623–7.

Snowden, L. and Chung, F. (1990) Use of inpatient services by members of ethnic minority groups, *American Psychologist*, 45, 347–55.

Strakowski, S.M., Lonczak, H.S., Sax, K.W., West, S.A., Crist, A., Menta, R., and Thiehaus, O.J. (1995) The effects of race on diagnosis and disposition from a psychiatric emergency service, *Journal of Clinical Psychiatry*, 56, 3, 101–7.

Way, B., Evans, M., and Banks, S. (1993) Factors predicting referral to inpatient or outpatient treatment from psychiatric emergency services, *Hospital and Community Psychiatry*, 43, 7, 703–8.

DISCUSSION

1. What are the medical and legal criteria used to evaluate whether or not to commit someone? What do you see as the strengths and weaknesses of these criteria for balancing the individual rights of people with serious mental illness and the need to protect society from potentially disruptive or dangerous behavior?

2. What are the major social factors that influence the likelihood that someone will be involuntarily hospitalized or committed during a psychiatric emergency? In what ways do these social factors reflect broader social structures within American society? How do these factors help to define the special group that Lincoln defines as "the undeserving sick"?

3. According to Lincoln, when is involuntary hospitalization and commitment "the best possible option" for responding to the urgent, critical needs of people with serious mental illness? What are the implications of her research for people interested in improving the care and treatment of people with serious mental illness?

Sarah Rosenfield

Labeling Mental Illness: The Effects of Received Services and Perceived Stigma on Life Satisfaction

In this award-winning paper, Sarah Rosenfield raises interesting questions about the potential positive impact of psychiatric treatment. Traditionally, sociologists interested in mental illness have focused on the negative psychological and social outcomes of being labeled or treated for mental illness. Rosenfield's research suggests that it is more complicated and that psychiatric care can help to improve the quality of life of people with mental illness.

A conflict between proponents of the labeling perspective on mental illness and their critics has continued for several decades. Labeling theorists examine mental illness as a form of deviance: The label rather than the behavior per se shapes the fate of mentally ill persons, by creating chronic mental illness or by compromising the life chances of those so labeled (Link, 1982, 1987; Link et al., 1987; Link et al., 1989; Palamara, Cullen, & Gersten, 1986; Scheff, 1966, 1974). In contrast, from what is often called the psychiatric perspective, critics of labeling theory view mental illness as a form of individual pathology. The fate of people with mental illness depends primarily on the severity of their illness and their treatment rather than on extra-illness factors, such as labels (Huffine & Clausen, 1979; Kirk 1974; Lehman, Possidente, & Hawker 1986; Schwartz, Myers, & Astrachan, 1974).

A pivotal difference between these perspectives involves the importance of stigma. From a labeling perspective, the stigma attached to the illness is a central problem. A psychiatric label sets into action cultural stereotypes and negative images about mental illness that are applied to the person by others and by the person to himself or herself (Link, 1987; Link et al., 1987; Link et al., 1989; Thoits, 1985). These images devalue those with mental illness and result in discrimination—persons who have mental illnesses are evaluated as "not quite human" (Goffman, 1963:5). Originally, labeling theory held that the expectations attached to the label perpetuate the mental illness (Scheff, 1966, 1974). The theory was modified later to claim that the devaluation and discrimination created by the label interfere with a broad range of life areas, including access to social and economic resources and general feelings of well-being (Link et al., 1987; Link, 1982, 1987; Link et al., 1989).

Critics of labeling theory, however, question the claims of both the original and the modified labeling approaches. Perceptions of stigma among mental patients are seen as subjective and untrustworthy or, at the extreme,

---

Rosenfield, Sarah. 1997. "Labeling Mental Illness: The Effects of Received Services and Perceived Stigma on Life Satisfaction." *American Sociological Review* 62:660–672.

as distortions resulting from the pathology (Crocetti, Spiro, & Siassi, 1974). Other people are seen to be reluctant to label and stigmatize those with mental illness (Gove & Fain, 1973; Huffine & Clausen, 1979). Thus, stigma is deemed by labeling theory critics to be relatively inconsequential for the mentally ill (Gove, 1970, 1975, 1980, 1982; Killian & Bloomburg, 1975). In contrast, critics emphasize that being labeled mentally ill allows people to receive needed treatment. High-quality treatment provides persons suffering from psychiatric disorders with a range of services to improve symptoms, expand functioning, and enhance well-being (Gove & Fain, 1973; Linn, 1968).

In sum, the contrasting views of stigma offered by labeling theory and its critics imply opposite effects of psychiatric labels: Labeling theorists predict destructive outcomes, while psychiatric theorists claim beneficial results. Past research has found evidence for both positive and negative effects of labeling. However, this evidence comes from independent bodies of research that reflects the often adversarial relationship between the proponents of labeling and those with more traditional psychiatric concerns. Because no empirical study has examined the joint effects of services and stigma, the relative importance of each for the mentally ill is unknown (Link & Cullen, 1992).

I directly compare the effects of the receipt of services versus perceptions of stigma on the subjective quality of life for people with chronic mental illness. Quality of life is increasingly emphasized as an outcome of particular significance for persons with chronic illnesses—illnesses that medicine has a limited ability to cure (Lehman, 1983). Subjective quality of life or life satisfaction is a critical component of well-being, and well-being is damaged by stigma according to the modified labeling approach, but is improved by services according to the psychiatric view (Bradburn & Caplovitz, 1965; Gurin, Veroff, & Feld, 1960; Veroff, Kulka, & Douvan, 1981). Thus, along with symptomatology and objective quality of life or functioning, subjective quality of life is a crucial outcome for both the labeling and psychiatric perspectives.

Consistent with Link and Cullen (1992), I argue that labeling has both positive and negative effects on subjective quality of life. The label itself implies stigma; the positive effects are indirect, through the receipt of services. I contend that both stigma and services are consequential because they shape central aspects of self-concept, which is connected to life satisfaction. I test this perspective in a model treatment program for persons with chronic mental illness.

THEORETICAL FRAMEWORK

A sense of mastery and self-esteem are fundamental goals that protect and enhance the self and contribute to a general feeling of well-being (Pearlin et al., 1981). Low levels of perceived mastery and self-esteem compromise subjective quality of life by producing a sense of hopelessness and a tendency to give up in difficult times. These dimensions of self-concept prevent individuals from trying for and getting what they want, thus diminishing the chances for life satisfaction. Ample research documents the relationships between perceptions of mastery and self-esteem and feelings of psychological well-being and subjective quality of life (Pearlin et al., 1981; Rosenfield, 1992).

Modified labeling theory holds that the stigma of mental illness is problematic because it damages mental patients' sense of self-esteem and self-efficacy (Link, 1987). The degree to which the stigma of mental illness is incorporated into patients' self-concept increases with the likelihood that the illness is long term, which most chronic mental illnesses are. To the extent that stigma becomes a master status (Becker, 1963) or part of one's self-schema, it affects patients' basic evaluations of themselves. They reorganize their views of themselves and their self-knowledge in terms of what they are not and cannot do rather than what they are and what they can do (Jones et al., 1984). Thus, people with chronic mental illness often experience a profound sense of loss of the characteristics they valued in themselves and of cherished life goals and assumptions. The damage to these assumptions and ideals is seen as the basis of demoralization (Frank, 1973; Link, 1987; Sullivan, 1941), and by extension, such damage affects subjective quality of life.

Evidence links stigma specifically to self-esteem. Patients and their families indicate that strong perceptions of stigma are associated with low self-esteem (Link, 1987; Wahl & Harman, 1989). When patients know others are aware that they are in psychiatric treatment, they perform more poorly, feel less appreciated, and are more anxious in their interactions compared to patients whose labels are concealed (Farina et al., 1971).

In contrast to the effects of stigma, the receipt of certain services positively affects patients' self-conceptions. Feelings of low self-efficacy are a particular problem among people with chronic mental illness, who often feel ruled by forces beyond their control (Lamb, 1982; Mendel & Allen, 1978; Mosher & Menn, 1978). Some researchers propose that the major goal of therapeutic intervention is to enhance patients' sense of mastery (Lamb, 1982). Some evidence suggests that the receipt of services increases perceptions of control. Specifically, services that give patients greater power in terms of status or economic resources (Weber, 1946) improve patients' levels of self-efficacy (Rosenfield, 1992).

In sum, I argue that stigma and received services have independent and antithetical effects on quality of life through their opposing influences on self-concept. Evidence for this approach comes from separate lines of research on the consequences of stigma and the effects of mental health services.

Tests of modified labeling theory demonstrate the stigmatizing consequences of psychiatric labels for a number of outcomes. Comparisons of individuals who are similar in psychopathology but vary in exposure to treatment show that labeling has a negative impact on income and work status. Individuals who have been in treatment earn lower incomes and are less likely to be employed than those with similar symptoms who have not been in treatment (Link, 1982) A later study examined the effect of perceived stigma directly. Patients from several treatment groups (first-contact and repeat-contact or chronic patients) and untreated individuals were matched on psychopathology. Stronger perceptions of stigma, defined in terms of devaluation and discrimination, were associated with greater income loss and higher unemployment only for the treated groups (Link, 1987). The degree of stigma perceived by labeled persons and their adaptations to the stigma shaped patients' social relations and inhibited the support available from individuals outside their households (Link et al., 1989). Most important, perceived stigma was associated with greater demoralization among treated groups compared to non-labeled individuals (Link, 1987).

Evaluations of services show that certain programs influence a range of outcomes, including the mental status and quality of life of persons with chronic mental illness. These model programs include "Training in Community Living" in Madison, Wisconsin, and the Fountain House program in New York City. Compared to standard care, patients in these programs have fewer rehospitalizations, are more economically self-sufficient, and have more social relationships. In terms of subjective indicators, they are more satisfied with their work lives, their living situations, their relationships, and with their lives in general (Beard, 1978; Beard, Malamud, & Rossman, 1978; New South Wales Department of Health, 1983; Stein & Test, 1976, 1978, 1980; Stein, Test, & Marx, 1975). These programs combine traditional psychiatric treatment with psychosocial and vocational rehabilitation, supervision, and guidance; they also provide basic needs like housing, financial support, and medical care. The programs tend to share an approach to treatment that some term "empowerment," an approach that stresses personal rather than professional relationships and minimizes status differences between patients and staff. Staff encourage patients' strengths and take a partnership approach to treating mental illness. Empowerment is seen as an attempt to combat stigmatizing attitudes about mental patients, at least within the programs.

Recent work indicates that certain of these services improve patients' quality of life. For example, economic services, including vocational rehabilitation and financial support, and services providing greater status through empowerment increase life satisfaction. Furthermore, these services affect patients' subjective quality of life by increasing their perceptions of personal control (Rosenfield, 1992).

Thus, past research has found both positive and negative consequences of labeling. In simultaneously investigating the impact of stigma relative to services, I build on these findings. I predict that perceived stigma and received services shape the subjective quality of life through their effects on dimensions of self-concept. This hypothesis is examined in a model treatment program for people with chronic mental illness.

METHODS

Research Strategy

Ideally, to evaluate the relative effects of stigma and received services, the full range of treatment and stigma experiences would be studied, including detailed measures of services provided and a uniform measure of stigma in diverse settings. However, the practical problems of such an investigation are formidable. Model treatment programs offer an opportunity to assess whether received services and stigma have simultaneous effects in opposite directions. Based on their clients' low rehospitalization rates and high quality of life, several model programs offer high quality treatment in a context specifically designed to combat stigma (Beard, 1978; Rosenfield, 1992; Stein & Test, 1978). Labeling theorists, who generally downplay or ignore the positive effect of treatment, would expect such positive effects to emerge only when

Community Spotlight

Fountain House Clubhouse
New York City

The year was 1948 and a group of courageous New Yorkers with mental illness, some having been locked away in hospitals or other institutions for more than three decades, was about to change their own lives and the lives of countless others around the world.

Galvanized by their creed, "We Are Not Alone," these visionaries embraced a then-revolutionary idea—that by openly joining together and working side-by-side rather than retreating in isolation, they would encourage one another to make effective new lives outside of the hospital. From their efforts, Fountain House—the world's first Clubhouse

True to their vision, the founders created a membership organization run for and by persons with mental illness. They searched for a meeting place with no bars on the windows and, more importantly, no limitations on the dreams of the members. Over time, they found a home with a small fountain in the back that served as a constant symbol of hope and renewal, and from it came the Clubhouse's name.

More than 50 years later, the original vision is alive and a true community has grown up, consisting of more than 16,000 members who have both found a place to belong and discovered that they are not alone. Helping link that community to the broader metropolitan area is a network of corporate employers offering real jobs at competitive wages; schools and colleges providing pathways to the completion of educations; physicians and psychiatrists offering a full array of community-based care; and a dedicated staff and Board working tirelessly to pursue common goals.

This community is open and available 365 days a year and provides a comprehensive range of services designed to foster self-worth and facilitate reintegration into the mainstream of life. As Kenneth Dudek, Executive Director, says, "What Fountain House has always been about is hope."

Through the years, Fountain House has grown into a complex of modern, attractive buildings on W. 47th Street, as well as four other residences throughout New York City and a 480-acre farm in New Jersey. Like all Clubhouses, Fountain House is run by members and staff working side-by-side every day.

Members carry out many of the functions of the Clubhouse, from routine clerical duties to a unique research program through which mental health consumers and professional academics (including some former members) collaborate on important grant-funded research on essential Clubhouse programs. Says Mr. Dudek, "We've always believed strongly in the people behind the illness, and in the relationships between the staff and our members. That is our founding principle."

Fountain House currently serves roughly 1,300 members, ranging from 16 to 80 years of age. One of its newest programs is the Young Adult Initiative, which includes intensive college outreach. This program identifies and works with young people at an early stage of their illness, in order to provide resources that will enable them to stay in school and keep their lives together.

Like all Clubhouses, Fountain House places an intense emphasis on employment programming, in the belief, according to Mr. Dudek, that "Work is what gives people their identity." Strong programs exist for Transitional, Supported, and Independent Employment, based on partnerships with such high-profile corporations as American Express Publishing, Dow Jones, and *Newsweek*.

Two recurring special events center on the partnerships Fountain House has developed to provide employment opportunities for persons with serious and persistent mental illness. The "Employers' Evening," which is more than 20-years-old, is a celebration for employers from around New York City who employ Clubhouse members through Fountain House employment programs. Attendance runs into the hundreds, as both front-line company supervisors and senior corporate officials mix with Fountain House members. Says Mr. Dudek, "This event is a way for the corporate world to get to know us better up close and become even more a part of our community."

For the past four years, Fountain House has also hosted a special "Corporate Awards Dinner", both to honor major employment partners and to raise funds for the organization. Honorees have included such companies as HBO and Dow Jones, and attendees include corporate giants such as D'Arcy, Masius, Benton, and Bowles, one of the country's largest ad agencies and a committed employment partner for more than 20 years. The most recent dinner honored Vincent Mai, husband of Board President Anne Mai and developer of jobs for many Fountain House members through the years.

One of Fountain House's most recent initiatives is a public art gallery located in a storefront on 9th Avenue. Members, many of whom have dreams of becoming working artists and photographers, create all items displayed. Works are both shown and sold. A primary idea underlying the gallery's development is that given the proper display, members' evident talent can do much to help combat the public stigma of mental illness.

A unique feature of Fountain House is High Point Farm, the 480-acre New Jersey property. Members rotate through this working farm, given to Fountain House by a farmer whose son had mental illness. High Point encompasses both a tree farm and a home for alpaca, llamas, and other animals. The farm provides members not only with an opportunity to do meaningful work, but also with a healing rural environment where they can swim, hike, and go boating.

Fountain House is also home to the Advocacy Resource Center, in which people learn to successfully advocate for themselves, for others, and for improvements in the mental health system. One of the center's recent successes was its major role in securing passage of the MTA Half Fare Fairness Act, which required the Metropolitan Transit Authority to end a discriminatory practice by expanding its Reduced Fare Program to S.S.I. recipients with serious mental illness.

Frances Olivero, a member of Fountain House and Co-Chair of the Advocacy Resource Center, and Fred Levine, Counsel to Fountain House's Executive Director, spearheaded the Clubhouse's effort. They traveled to Albany together to meet with legislators, held rallies, and distributed literature to increase support throughout New York's mental health community.

After the bill was passed, a celebration was held at Fountain House with the legislative sponsors, Senator Frank Padavan (R- Queens) and Assemblyman James Brennan (D- Brooklyn). Sadly, Mr. Olivero passed away just days before Governor George Pataki actually signed the bill making the Half Fare Fairness program effective.

Speaking about his partnership with Mr. Olivero, Fred Levine—who was himself diagnosed with bipolar illness in 1975—notes, "Every day I worked with Frances was a gift. He was insightful, energetic, passionate about human rights, and he had a unique ability to bring people together and make them listen. He was the heart and soul of the Fairness Campaign."

Clearly, Mr. Levine believes that important things can happen when persons with mental illness are empowered.

Perhaps the best testament to Fountain House occurred immediately after the September 11 tragedy. Located in the heart of New York City, Fountain House had a unique opportunity for service as the result of that day's horrific events.

Says Mr. Dudek, "We stayed open all night. It seemed as though everyone connected with Fountain House over the past 15 years and who was in Manhattan that day came flooding through our doors. They obviously thought of us as their safe haven."

It is evident that the vision and hope of Fountain House's original members—"We Are Not Alone"—is still a guiding principle at Fountain House today.

Visit Fountain House online at www.fountainhouse.org.

Source: Center for Reintegration. "Community Spotlight: Fountain House, New York City." North Bergen, New Jersey. Retrieved: July 27, 2008 <http://www.reintegration.com/reint/community/fountain.asp>

contrasting the extremes of treatment, that is, comparing individuals receiving very high quality treatment to those receiving very low quality treatment. Similarly, the critics of labeling theory, who downplay the importance of stigma, would expect to find any effects of stigma only when comparing those individuals who are highly stigmatized to those experiencing very low stigma. Thus, if services have positive effects and stigma has negative effects in a sample of participants in a model program, labeling theorists would have to acknowledge positive effects of treatment even when gross variations in treatment quality are not present, and the critics of labeling would have to acknowledge that stigma has effects even when large variations in stigma are not present. Consequently, support for the predicted outcomes should be convincing to labeling theorists and their critics.

Labeling need not be defined dichotomously (i.e., by comparing people who are officially labeled and thus have contact with both services and stigma to those who are not labeled and have contact with neither services nor stigma). Rather, labeling can be conceptualized as a continuum that exposes people to the possibility of stigma and the possibility of services: Patients can experience varying degrees of services and stigma. Indeed, there is substantial variation in perceptions of stigma and in the receipt of services among persons who are labeled (Link, 1987; Rosenfield, 1992). The services received as well as perceived stigma vary substantially even within one program. My strategy examines the effects of such variations in experiences and perceptions among individuals who are officially labeled.

Research Site

This research was conducted at The Club/Habilitation Services program, which was funded in 1973 as a model program for people with chronic mental illness. It is a unit of the University of Medicine and Dentistry of New Jersey-Community Mental Health Center in Piscataway, New Jersey. This program offers ongoing, intensive rehabilitative care for mentally ill adults within the psychosocial clubhouse model, based on the Fountain House prototype (Beard, 1978; Lenoil, 1982). The program serves all patients with chronic mental illness in the Community Mental Health Center's catchment area. In an evaluation, this program's rehospitalization rate (20 percent over a year period) was comparable to that of effective model programs (Rosenfield, 1992).

In a day-program format, The Club offers vocational rehabilitation; supervision and guidance; services providing basic needs; and training in psychosocial skills including daily living skills and social skills. The program also arranges for psychiatric treatment and provides social contacts and a structure of activities. The Clubhouse model holds an empowerment approach to treatment termed "mutual empowerment." This approach emphasizes the development of independence, decision-making skills, and individual responsibility as well as personal, supportive relationships between staff and patients. All program activities are performed by members and staff working together, and members participate in most aspects of decision making within the program.

The data were collected from face-to-face interviews with patients conducted by psychiatric social workers and psychiatric nurses who were independent of the program and unaware of the research hypotheses. Interviews averaged one and one-half hours. The population included all patients active in The Club program for at least one entire month over a one-year period (1988–1989). The total number of respondents in the sample was 157, or 93 percent of the eligible patients.

Measures

Subjective quality of life is assessed using Lehman's measure of life quality developed for people with chronic mental illness (Lehman, 1983; Lehman et al., 1986; Lehman, Ward, & Linn, 1982). Two items ask patients to rate their levels of satisfaction with life as a whole. Patients are also asked about their satisfaction with specific areas of their lives, including their living arrangements, family relations, social relations, leisure activities, financial situations, employment status, safety, and health. The scales combining these items—as well as measures described below—are discussed more fully elsewhere (Rosenfield, 1992; Rosenfield & Neese-Todd, 1993). The reliability of each scale, using alpha coefficients, is .85 or above. I present results for overall satisfaction with life, noting consistencies or discrepancies with results for the specific life areas.

To measure *received services*, patients were asked whether they received specific services in the last month, including psychiatric services, services for daily living skills, social skills, vocational rehabilitation, structured activities, social contacts, and basic needs. For example, vocational rehabilitation services include learning work responsibilities, expectations, and skills. Services for developing a structure of activities involve help from staff with planning time on week nights, weekends, and holidays. For most of the scales measuring program services, the reliabilities are .60 or above. Exceptions are services for daily living skills (.57), for planning time (.56), and for social skills (.49). For these areas, I analyze separate items.

Mutual empowerment is measured using a scale of 21 items focusing on patients' decision-making power and supportive interactions. For example, patients were asked how much influence they felt they had in the program, how much their opinions and ideas counted, how much they felt cared about, and how much the staff accepted them the way they are (alpha = .82).

Stigma is measured using Link's (1987, 1989) scale of devaluation-discrimination (alpha = .88). This scale consists of 12 items asking respondents' opinions about the extent to which *most people* would accept a former mental patient as a friend, teacher, worker, or caretaker of their children. It also covers whether former patients are seen as less trustworthy or less intelligent than others. This scale focuses on perceptions of stigma rather than stigmatizing experiences, thus allowing assessments across labeled and unlabeled groups. According to modified labeling theory, this assessment of stigma should have effects because labeled individuals—and only labeled individuals—apply perceived stigma to themselves, as evidenced by the damage to a range of life areas found among labeled persons but not among unlabeled persons (Link, 1987). Furthermore, asking about stigma in this general way avoids the pain of recounting personal experiences that could deter candid reporting.

Self-esteem is measured by Rosenberg's (1984) scale, which surveys feelings of worthlessness, uselessness, and failure (alpha = .82).

Mastery is measured using the scale developed by Pearlin et al. (1981), which covers feelings of helplessness, control over forces affecting oneself, and the ability to change or to solve problems (alpha = .73).

In the analyses, I control for race, years of education, age, and sex. I included one item to control for the influence of recent events by asking whether anything happened in the last year that upset the respondent a lot or made him or her very unhappy. I adjust for clinical characteristics using scales based on staff-reported functioning levels in areas corresponding to the services offered (e.g., daily living skills, social skills, etc. [alphas ≥ .80]), and staff-reported symptomatology (covering hallucinations, delusions, paranoia, depression, social isolation, lack of motivation, and fear of success [alphas ≥ .90]).

Hypotheses are tested using regression analysis. In examining the importance of stigma for quality of life, background and clinical characteristics are entered into the equation first; stigma is entered in the second step. Received services are investigated in a similar manner: Control variables are entered in the first step, and services are entered second. I note that the correlations between these independent variables and the control variables are relatively low (r < .25). For the comparative test, measures of stigma and received services are entered simultaneously in the second step. To examine self-concept as an explanatory mechanism, measures of self-esteem and mastery are entered in the final stage of the analysis.

RESULTS

The Relationship of Perceived Stigma and Received Services to Quality of Life

How much stigma do patients perceive? A majority of patients (65 percent) feel that former mental patients are not accepted by most people as friends, that they are not seen as being as intelligent or trustworthy as other people (57 percent and 53 percent, respectively), and that their job applications would be passed over by employers (77 percent). Overall, slightly more than one-half of the respondents believe that mental patients are stigmatized. Thus, nearly one-half of respondents disagree that stigma exists, which leaves adequate variation for analyses of the effects of stigma.

Table 1 shows the relationship of perceptions of stigma and received services to quality of life, controlling for demographic and clinical characteristics. Perceived stigma is significantly and negatively associated with patients' evaluations of life as a whole: The greater the perception of devaluation and discrimination among mental patients, the lower their satisfaction with life in general. These results also hold in analyses of the specific quality-of-life areas (not shown).

Table 1 also shows the services that are significantly and positively related to overall quality of life. Services that increase economic resources—vocational rehabilitation and financial services (which approaches statistical significance at $p < .06$)—enhance overall life satisfaction. Services that raise patients' status—empowerment ideology and groups for mentally ill chemical abusers (which are based on an empowerment approach)—also improve subjective quality of life. Finally, time spent in activities and staff help with structuring free time positively affect satisfaction with life as a whole.

The central issue here, however, concerns the importance of stigma relative to services for people with mental illness. In evaluating the effects of labeling, I hypothesized that the relationships between perceived stigma and quality of life will hold even when the effects of received services are considered, and vice-versa. To test this, I examine stigma in relation to services found to be effective for overall life satisfaction. For the most part, perceptions of stigma and received services are not related to each other.

Table 2 presents coefficients for regressions that include specific services that are effective for increasing life satisfaction and perceptions of stigma, controlling for background and clinical characteristics. Table 2 also shows

Table 1 Coefficients from Regressions of Overall Subjective Quality of Life on Perceived Stigma or Received Services: Mental Health Patients, 1988–89

Independent Variable	Coefficient		R²
	Unstandardized	Standardized	
Stigma	−.6979*	−.23	.199
	(.2649)		
Received Services			
Vocational rehabilitation	.2008*	.21	.182
	(.0838)		
Financial support	.8033ª	.23	.198
	(.4293)		
Empowerment	.7094*	.19	.178
	(.3198)		
Mental illness/ chemical abuse groups	.1947*	.20	.191
	(.0916)		
Time in leisure activities	.2349*	.29	.238
	(.0846)		
Structure for leisure time	.6909*	.22	.199
	(.2797)		

Note: Numbers in parentheses are standard errors. Number of cases range from 141 to 144 owing to missing data. All regressions control for clinical characteristics and demographic characteristics. A separate regression is run for each independent variable.

ªCoefficient for financial support approaches statistical significance ($p < .06$, two-tailed test).

*$p < .05$ (two-tailed tests)

the results of a regression of stigma and services combined on quality of life. This combined measure counts the total number of services associated with quality of life that patients received. Individuals receive one point each for receiving vocational services, using financial services, obtaining services for structuring leisure time, attending MICA group meetings, reporting high levels of empowerment, and spending time in leisure activities within the program. The measure thus ranges from 0 to 6 and has adequate reliability (alpha = .72).

Examining received services first, Table 2 demonstrates that each of the services is significantly related to life satisfaction when stigma is controlled. That is, vocational rehabilitation, financial support, empowerment, MICA groups, and structure for leisure time contribute to overall quality of life even when the effect of stigma is controlled. The combined services measure is highly and significantly related to quality of life, holding perceived stigma constant. Thus, examining services separately or in combination, the positive impact of services received on overall quality of life is not reduced by perceptions of stigma.

Table 2 also demonstrates that the impact of stigma on life satisfaction remains significant when services are included in the regression. Controlling

Table 2 Coefficients for Regressions of Overall Subjective Quality of Life on Perceived Stigma *and* Specific Received Services: Mental Health Patients, 1988–89

Independent Variable	Coefficient		R^2
	Unstandardized	Standardized	
Vocational rehabilitation	.2298*	.24	
	(.0815)		
Stigma	−.7372*	−.24	.245
	(.2612)		
Financial support	.8160*	.23	
	(.4200)		
Stigma	−.6815*	−.22	.246
	(.2721)		
Empowerment	.7138*	.19	
	(.3223)		
Stigma	−.6225*	−.21	.228
	(.2623)		
Mental illness/chemical abuse groups	.2176*	.23	
	(.0894)		
Stigma	−.7220*	−.24	.244
	(.2627)		
Time in leisure activities	.2202*	.27	
	(.0832)		
Stigma	−.6394*	−.22	.287
	(.2695)		
Structure for leisure time	.6865*	.22	
	(.2778)		
Stigma	−.5992*	−.20	.239
	(.2693)		
All services combined	2.5201*	.44	
	(.7186)		
Stigma	−.6803*	−.23	.398
	(.2717)		

Note: All regressions control for clinical characteristics and demographic characteristics. Numbers in parentheses are standard errors.

* $p < .05$

for vocational or financial services, empowerment, or for services structuring leisure time, stigma retains its significant negative association with global quality of life. Stigma is also significantly related to life quality controlling for these services combined.

Thus, analyses comparing the effects of services and stigma show that both perceived stigma and received services are strongly related to overall quality of life, but in opposite directions. The results are similar for most of the specific areas of life quality (not shown). These analyses support the prediction of an independent impact of stigma and received services on subjective quality of life.

Perceived Stigma, Received Services, and Self-Concept

The last prediction to be tested is that perceived stigma as well as received services are important for patients' quality of life because both affect self-conceptions. Table 3 presents coefficients from regressions that include measures of mastery and self-esteem as explanatory factors.

Controlling for the two dimensions of self-concept reduces the relationship between stigma and quality of life shown in Table 1 to nonsignificance. The coefficient for stigma is reduced by 38 percent (−.6979 to −.4299) controlling for mastery and 53 percent (−.6979 to −.3257) when self-esteem is controlled. Adjusting for self-esteem and mastery together diminishes the coefficient for stigma by nearly 60 percent. Similar results also obtain for most of the specific quality-of-life areas (not shown).

On the basis of these findings, it appears that perceptions of stigma reduce patients' happiness with life by compromising their basic sense of self-worth and self-efficacy. The lowered sense of self brought about by expectations of stigmatizing social responses severely reduces patients' chances for overall satisfaction and in most specific life areas.

The two aspects of self-concept also reduce the relationships between most of the specific services received and overall quality of life. The coefficients for vocational rehabilitation and financial services each decrease by about 20 percent when self-esteem is held constant. These associations are weakened considerably more, with reductions of 42 percent and 51 percent respectively, after controlling for mastery.

In terms of empowerment services, controlling for mastery or for self-esteem reduces the relationship between perceptions of empowerment and quality of life to nonsignificance (compared to Table 1). Each dimension of self-concept diminishes the relationship of empowerment to life satisfaction by about one-third; controlling for both dimensions reduces the coefficient nearly 40 percent. Further, adjusting for mastery reduces the relationship between attending MICA groups and quality of life by approximately 30 percent, although the relationship remains significant when self-esteem is controlled.

Finally, in terms of structured activities, the coefficient for the amount of time spent in leisure activities in the program is reduced by one-third when both aspects of self-concept are controlled, but remains significant. However, self-concept does not affect the relationship between services for structuring free time and quality of life. Possibly the need for structure is a goal in itself, independent of the need for control or positive self-regard (Rosenfield, 1992).

These findings suggest that perceptions of mastery and self-esteem mediate the association between received services and overall quality of life, and

Table 3 Coefficients for Regressions of Overall Subjective Quality of Life on Perceived Stigma or Received Services, Controlling for Aspects of Self-Concept: Mental Health Patients, 1988–89

Independent Variable	Controlling for Mastery			Controlling for Self-Esteem			Controlling for Self-Esteem and Mastery		
	Coefficient			Coefficient			Coefficient		
	Unstandardized	Standardized	R^2	Unstandardized	Standardized	R^2	Unstandardized	Standardized	R^2
Stigma	−.4299 (.2341)	−.14	.398	−.3257 (.2300)	−.11	.430	−.2857 (.2223)	−.09	.474
Vocational rehabilitation	.1170 (.0739)	.12	.389	.1562* (.0701)	.16	.436	.1257 (.0609)	.13	.471
Financial support	.3915 (.3814)	.11	.390	.6505 (.3599)	.19	.442	.4815 (.3558)	.14	.475
Empowerment	.4960 (.2778)	.13	.392	.4912 (.2694)	.13	.427	.4397 (.2608)	.12	.470
Mental illness/chemical abuse groups	.1388 (.0795)	.14	.401	.2069* (.0753)	.21	.457	.1756* (.0740)	.18	.490
Time in leisure activities	.1694* (.0754)	.21	.413	.1753* (.0732)	.22	.444	.1572 (.0715)	.19	.478
Structure for leisure time	.6820* (.2368)	.22	.431	.6601* (.2322)	.21	.453	.6573* (.2226)	.21	.501

Note: All regressions control for clinical characteristics and demographic characteristics. Numbers in parentheses are standard errors.

*$p < .05$

that their importance varies with the specific service. The influence of both dimensions of self-concept is also supported in the analyses of received services in relation to the specific quality-of-life areas (not shown). Taking the results together, it appears that services promote patients' satisfaction with life by enhancing their confidence in themselves and their sense of control over their lives.

DISCUSSION

I began with a presentation of contrasting views about the consequences of labeling for people with mental illness. Labeling theory predicts that the stigma of being labeled as mentally ill has a significant negative influence on outcomes for mental patients. Opponents think of stigma as inconsequential compared to the positive effects of treatment and receiving high quality services. Integrating these perspectives, I proposed that perceptions of stigma and the receipt of services are related to subjective quality of life through their associations with self-concept, but in opposing ways. Stigma is a problem for most people with chronic mental illness, and perceptions of stigma have a significant negative relationship with patients' quality of life. By contrast, services have a strong positive association with quality of life. Furthermore, the effects of stigma and received services are a result of their relationships with perceptions of self-esteem and self-efficacy.

This study provides a test of the consequences of psychiatric labels, using cross-sectional data. The analyses should be replicated using longitudinal information to disentangle causal direction. Perhaps greater life satisfaction reduces perceptions of stigma and increases the use of services, or use of services enhances quality of life, which in turn reduces perceived stigma. It is also possible that low levels of self-esteem or mastery result in high perceptions of stigma rather than stigma reducing these self-perceptions. Link (1987) found that scores on the perceived devaluation-discrimination scale resemble scores obtained from the general public. However, the self-esteem of patients is lower than that among the general public. If low self-esteem increases perceptions of devaluation-discrimination, patients' devaluation-discrimination scores should be higher than those among the general public. Thus, these relationships do not support this alternative causal explanation. However, such alternative explanations were not formulated by either labeling theorists or their critics before this study. They are therefore of interest only after evidence from the study suggests them. That is, before this research, labeling theorists could assume that received services have little importance in the face of stigma, and critics of labeling theory could assume that stigma matters little compared to received services. Although alternative explanations cannot be completely ruled out without further information, the results of this research cast doubt on both of these assumptions.

In terms of selection effects, it may be possible that the more highly functional patients are selected by staff to receive services that most improve quality of life. However, this possibility is addressed in the analysis by controlling for functioning when examining the relationship of services to quality of life. Another possible alternative explanation is that patients with a greater sense of self-esteem or mastery are better able to obtain services and to have higher life satisfaction. This reasoning assumes, however, that patients with high confidence and self-efficacy must be high-functioning in order to obtain these services. In examining this point of view, aspects of self-concept and level of functioning were not significantly related. Finally, I used a two-stage estimating procedure suggested by Maddala (1987) to check for selection effects in relation to services predicting overall quality of life (Rosenfield, 1992). This procedure estimates the probability of receiving a program service on the basis of symptoms, functioning, and demographics, and enters that probability as an independent variable in the regression analysis predicting quality of life. Results using this technique show that selection effects are not significant in relation to the program services—regressions predicting life satisfaction that include selection effects are similar to those obtained without these effects.

Limitations in generalizability are also an issue in the analysis. The ideal test of this theoretical perspective would be to study populations that include the full range of variation in both stigma and services. Although the sampling problems involved in such a test are difficult, replication of these results is needed in samples with greater variability.

Finally, specific conclusions about the relative importance of the received services versus perceived stigma to quality of life must be made with caution. For example, the importance of stigma may be underestimated because of the measurement of stigma compared to services. Services may have more weight because the measures of services were tailored to the specific services offered by the program, while the measure of stigma assessed general perceptions of devaluation and discrimination. Further development of the stigma measure is needed to more accurately estimate the roles of stigma versus services. Also, I examined high quality services in relation to stigma. Studies of services in other treatment settings would clarify their relative significance. In sum, I conclude that both stigma and received services are important in relation to quality of life, but I do not specify their magnitudes or comparative weights.

CONCLUSION

In spite of its limitations, this research provides a unique combination of data for examining labeling and opposing approaches to the treatment of mental illness. This study is consistent with other attempts to synthesize the labeling and psychiatric approaches. For example, the differences between the original statement of labeling theory and its critics on the causes of chronic mental illness—whether it is the label or the pathology—is reconciled by a modified labeling approach suggesting that the label is a stressor that increases symptoms (Link et al., 1989). Such syntheses provide a basis for a more complex understanding of the social processes underlying the causes and consequences of mental illness.

These results should inform mental health interventions. They suggest that life satisfaction is highest for those who experience little stigma and gain access to high quality services. Life satisfaction is lowest among those perceiving high levels of stigma and lacking such services. A labeling or a psychiatric perspective alone implies different interventions for mental illness. For example, a traditional psychiatric approach without a labeling component suggests that treatment programs for the chronic mentally ill are sufficient, provided the treatment services are good. Indeed, this analysis shows the highly positive effects of high quality care. But this treatment stands as an oasis. Within this oasis, everything is provided—even empowerment as an antidote to stigma. But an oasis implies that a larger, harsher environment surrounds it, and treatment programs exist within communities that for the most part are hostile to people with mental illness (Angermeyer, Link, & Majcher-Angermeyer, 1987). To the extent that stigma exists in this larger environment, the best treatment given by people with the best intentions is not enough, because the treatment has little power to decrease the stigma. The stigmatized constantly refer to the "normal world" (Goffman, 1963). Good adjustment for stigmatized individuals involves acknowledging the differences between themselves and normals, and in this sense, stigma defines the limits of treatment. Combining the insights of labeling theorists and their critics is thus necessary to produce positive patient outcomes. Only interventions that reduce the stigma within communities and provide high quality treatment can truly improve the life chances and quality of life of people living with mental illness.

References

Angermeyer, Matthias C., Bruce G. Link, and Alice Majcher-Angermeyer. 1987. "Stigma Perceived by Patients Attending Modern Treatment Settings: Some Unanticipated Effects of Community Psychiatry Reforms." *The Journal of Nervous and Mental Disease* 175:4–11.

Beard, John H. 1978. "The Rehabilitation Services of Fountain House." Pp. 201–08 in *Alternatives to Mental Hospital Treatment*, edited by L. I. Stein and M. A. Test. New York: Plenum.

Beard, John H., Thomas J. Malamud, and Ellen Rossman. 1978. "Psychiatric Rehabilitation and Long-Term Rehospitalization Rates: The Findings of Two Research Studies." *Schizophrenia Bulletin* 4:622–35.

Becker, Howard. 1963. *Outsiders*. New York: MacMillan.

Bradburn, Norman M. and David Caplovitz. 1965. *Reports on Happiness*. Chicago, IL: Aldine.

Crocetti, Guido, Herzl R. Spiro, and Iradj Siassi. 1974. *Contemporary Attitudes toward Mental Illness*. Pittsburgh, PA: University of Pittsburgh Press.

Farina, Amerigo, Donald Gliha, Louis Boudreau, Jon Allen, and Mark Sherman. 1971. "Mental Illness and the Impact of Believing Others Know About It." *Journal of Abnormal Psychology* 77:1–5.

Frank, Jerome. 1973. *Persuasion and Healing*. Baltimore, MD: Johns Hopkins University Press.

Goffman, Erving. 1963. *Stigma*. New York: Simon and Schuster.

Gove, Walter. 1970. "Societal Reaction as an Explanation of Mental Illness: An Evaluation." *American Sociological Review* 35:873–84.

―――. 1975. *The Labeling of Deviance: Evaluating a Perspective*. New York: Sage.

―――. 1980. "Labeling Mental Illness: A Critique." PP. 53–109 in *Labeling Deviant Behavior*, edited by W. Gove. Beverly Hills, CA: Sage.

―――. 1982. "The Current Status of the Labeling Theory of Mental Illness." Pp. 273–300 in *Deviance and Mental Illness*, edited by W. Gove. Beverly Hills, CA: Sage.

Gove, Walter and Terry Fain. 1973. "The Stigma of Mental Hospitalization: An Attempt to Evaluate Its Consequences." *Archives of General Psychiatry* 29:494–500.

Gurin, Gerald, Joseph Veroff, and Sheila Feld. 1960. *Americans View Their Mental Health*. New York: Basic Books.

Huffine, Carol and John A. Clausen. 1979. "Madness and Work: Short- and Long-Term Effects of Mental Illness on Occupational Careers." *Social Forces* 57:1049–62.

Jones, Edward, Amerigo Farina, Albert Hastorf, Hazel Markus, Dale Miller, and Robert Scott. 1984. *Social Stigma: The Psychology of Marked Relationships*. New York: Freeman.

Killian, Lewis M. and S. Bloomburg. 1975. "Rebirth in a Therapeutic Community: A Case Study." *Psychiatry* 38:39–54.

Kirk, Stuart A. 1974. "The Impact of Labeling on the Rejection of the Mentally Ill: An Experimental Study." *Journal of Health and Social Behavior* 15:108–17.

Lamb, H. Richard. 1982. *Treating the Long-Term Mentally Ill*. San Francisco, CA: Jossey-Bass.

Lehman, Anthony F. 1983. "The Well-Being of Chronic Mental Patients: Assessing Their Quality of Life." *Archives of General Psychiatry* 40:369–73.

Lehman, Anthony F., Susan Possidente, and Fiona Hawker. 1986. "The Quality of Life of Chronic Patients in a State Hospital and in Community Residences." *Hospital and Community Psychiatry* 37:901–7.

Lehman, Anthony F., Nancy Ward, and Lawrence Linn. 1982. "Chronic Mental Patients: The Quality of Life Issue." *American Journal of Psychiatry* 139:1271–6.

Lenoil, Julian. 1982. "An Analysis of the Psychiatric Psycho-Social Rehabilitation Center." *Psychosocial Rehabilitation Journal* 1:55–9.

Link, Bruce G. 1982. "Mental Patient Status, Work, and Income: An Examination of the Effects of a Psychiatric Label." *American Sociological Review* 47:202–15.

―――. 1987. "Understanding Labeling Effects in the Area of Mental Disorders: An Assessment of the Effects of Expectations of Rejection." *American Sociological Review* 52:96–112.

Link, Bruce G. and Francis T. Cullen. 1992. "The Labeling Theory of Mental Disorders: A Review of the Evidence." In *Mental Illness in Social Context*, edited by J. Greenley. Greenwich, CT: JAI.

Link, Bruce G., Francis T. Cullen, James Frank, and John F. Wozniak. 1987. "The Social Rejection of Former Mental Patients: Understanding Why Labels Matter." *American Journal of Sociology* 92:1461–500.

Link, Bruce G., Francis T. Cullen, Elmer Struening, Patrick E. Shrout, and Bruce P. Dohrenwend. 1989. "A Modified Labeling Theory Approach to Mental Disorders: An Empirical Assessment." *American Sociological Review* 54:400–23.

Linn, L. S. 1968. "The Mental Hospital from the Patient Perspective." *Psychiatry* 31:213–23.

Maddala, G. S. 1987. *Limited-Dependent and Qualitative Variables in Econometrics.* Cambridge, England: Cambridge University Press.

Mendel, Werner M. and Robert E. Allen. 1978. "Rescue and Rehabilitation." Pp. 181–200 in *Alternatives to Mental Hospital Treatment,* edited by L. I. Stein and M. A. Test. New York: Plenum.

Mosher, Loren R. and Alma Z. Menn. 1978. "Community Residential Treatment for Schizophrenia: Two-Year Follow-Up." *Hospital and Community Psychiatry* 29:715–23.

New South Wales Department of Health. 1983. *Psychiatric Hospitalization vs. Community Treatment: A Controlled Study.* Wales, UK: New South Wales Department of Health.

Palamara, Frances, Francis Cullen, and Joanne Gersten. 1986. "The Effect of Police and Mental Health Intervention in Juvenile Deviance: Specifying Contingencies in the Impact of Formal Reaction." *Journal of Health and Social Behavior* 27:90–105.

Pearlin, Leonard I., Morton A. Lieberman, Elizabeth G. Menaghan, and Joseph T. Mullan. 1981. "The Stress Process." *Journal of Health and Social Behavior* 22:337–56.

Rosenberg, Morris. 1984. *Society and the Adolescent Self-Image.* Princeton, NJ: Princeton University Press.

Rosenfield, Sarah. 1992. "Factors Contributing to the Quality of Life of the Chronic Mentally Ill." *Journal of Health and Social Behavior* 33:229–315.

Rosenfield, Sarah and Sheree Neese-Todd. 1993. "Why Model Programs Work: Factors Predicting the Subjective Quality of Life of the Chronic Mentally Ill." *Hospital and Community Psychiatry* 44:76–8.

Scheff, Thomas. 1966. *Being Mentally Ill: A Sociological Theory.* Chicago, IL: Aldine.

———. 1974. "The Labeling Theory of Mental Illness." *American Sociological Review* 39:444–52.

Schwartz, Carol C., Jerome K. Myers, and Boris M. Astrachan. 1974. "Psychiatric Labeling and the Rehabilitation of Mental Patients." *Archives of General Psychiatry* 31:329–34.

Stein, Leonard I. and Mary Ann Test. 1976. "Training in Community Living: A Follow-Up Look at a Gold-Award Program." *Hospital and Community Psychiatry* 27:193–4.

———. 1978. "Training in Community Living: Research Design and Results." Pp. 57–74 in *Alternatives to Mental Hospital Treatment,* edited by L. I. Stein and M. A. Test. New York: Plenum.

———. 1980. "Alternative to Mental Hospital Treatment." *Archives of General Psychiatry* 37:392–7.

Stein, Leonard I., Mary Ann Test, and Arnold J. Marx. 1975. "Alternative to the Hospital: A Controlled Study." *American Journal of Psychiatry* 132:517–22.

Sullivan, Harry S. 1941. "Psychiatric Aspects of Morale." *American Journal of Sociology* 47:277–301.

Thoits, Peggy. 1985. "Self-Labeling Processes in Mental Illness: The Role of Emotional Deviance." *American Journal of Sociology* 91:221–49.

Veroff, Joseph, Richard A. Kulka, and Elizabeth Douvan. 1981. *Mental Health in America.* New York: Basic Books.

Wahl, Otto F. and Charles R. Harman. 1989. "Family Views of Stigma." *Schizophrenia Bulletin* 15:137–9.

Weber, Max. 1946. *Max Weber: Essays in Sociology.* Oxford, England: Oxford University Press.

DISCUSSION

1. According to Rosenfield, how do stigma and psychiatric treatment work together to influence the self-concepts and quality of life of people with serious mental illness? What are the implications of her findings for those interested in labeling theory? For those interested in understanding the effectiveness of psychiatric treatment programs?

2. In your opinion, are the stigma-related "costs" worth the potential "benefits" of received services? Given Rosenfield's research, should we do more or less to compel people with mental disorders to seek treatment?

Bernice A. Pescosolido, Eric R. Wright, and William Patrick Sullivan

Communities of Care: A Theoretical Perspective on Case Management Models in Mental Health[†]

Research on social networks has found that social connections are critical for maintaining good mental health. Difficulty relating to others also is a criterion that psychiatrists often view as indicative of psychological problems, and a major emphasis in many modalities of psychiatric treatment is improving the quality of a person's social supports. In this more theoretical paper, Pescosolido and colleagues describe the most common types of "case management"—a special type of care in which providers work with clients to connect them to needed clinical and community resources. They highlight how these different models—to varying degrees and in different ways— help to create or recreate important missing social support systems for people with mental illness.

INTRODUCTION

> I like my case manager. He takes me shopping, he is like a friend (Client calling Indiana Division of Mental Health Hotline Number, 1994).

Case management has emerged as *the* major concept underlying treatment programs for people with chronic illnesses during the past two decades. In the mental health arena, the 1970s found the deinstitutionalization of individuals with severe and persistent mental illness accelerating, while the existing system of community-based services remained inadequately prepared

Pescosolido, Bernice, Eric R. Wright, and William Patrick Sullivan. 1995. "Communities of Care: A Theoretical Perspective on Case Management Models in Mental Health." *Advances in Medical Sociology* 6:37–79.

to deal with the challenge (Brown, 1985; Issac & Armat, 1990). In spite of their well-publicized problems, state psychiatric hospitals were "total institutions" that provided for clients' daily needs under a "one-stop-shopping" model with all services provided "under one roof" (Goffman, 1961; Prior, 1993). Meals, laundry, companionship, recreation, and assistance theoretically were to be found there. With the move to community-based care, this gave way to a system consisting of a number of treatment and social service organizations offering services relevant to the needs of individuals with severe and persistent mental illness.

Early state-based plans for deinstitutionalization were based primarily on the assumption that clients would come for treatment at the newly-established community mental health centers (CMHCs). Few included or implemented a systematic plan to provide assistance for clients' broad-based needs in the community. Quickly, a new group of providers evolved whose job focused on helping former mental patients "survive" in the community by navigating the community mental health and social service systems. By 1977, when the National Institute of Mental Health (NIMH) introduced the Community Support Program (CSP), case management was identified as a critical element of this initiative and later was heralded as the first truly *community*-based form of care (Turner & TenHoor, 1978).

Over the past two decades, case management services have been adopted in a wide variety of forms and across a wide spectrum of practice arenas (Bachrach, 1989). Indeed, so large is the range and scope of activities put under the rubric "case management" that Moore (1990, 444) remarked that it can be viewed "as an undefined set of activities aimed at achieving an undefined set of objectives." And, while a substantial research literature evaluated the greater success of case management over "business as usual" in the early phase, and then "add on" variations as better than "standard case management" in the more recent phases (see e.g., Gans & Horton, 1975; Rubin, 1992; Schwartz, Goldman & Churgin, 1982), we are left with three fundamental questions. First, what are the basic, critical ingredients of case management approaches that produce better outcomes? Second, why do they work? Third, for whom and under what conditions do case management approaches work? These three questions are distinct—the first asks whether a particular set of features are necessary for "success" while the second explores whether there is a common underlying mechanism at work. The third targets the "fit" between characteristics of individuals, their communities, or their illness careers *and* the characteristics of case management programs. Before the first question can be addressed *across* case management approaches or the second and third question addressed even *within* approaches, the gap in our theoretical understandings of these as models of community-based care needs to filled.

In this paper, we take an initial step in this direction. We argue that an essential component of all case management programs, regardless of the treatment remedies offered, lies in the reconstruction and management of social support and networks that may have been damaged, altered due to illness, or be simply inadequate to deal with the new challenges which chronic illness present. Case management models construct social safety nets that differ in the nature of the tie between case manager and consumer, in whether they explicitly target different parts of the lay and treatment community, and in how comprehensive social and treatment interactions are intended to be. In these differences, we argue, lie the success or failure of case management programs because they set the terms in which clients, families, providers, and systems of care adopt or reject treatment modalities.

We do not contend that "more is better" for clinical, cost, or quality of life outcomes. On the one hand, a social safety net may provide welcome support (i.e., individual or community integration for clients) or monitoring (i.e., individual or community regulation). On the other hand, it may provide unwelcome intrusion or coercion (i.e., over-integration or over-regulation). While both integration and regulation are necessary to keep individuals anchored to the societies in which they live, sociologists have long realized that *either* too little or too much of either can produce serious problems and consequences (Duricheim, 1951).

Here, we briefly review dominant approaches to case management in mental health—the "broker" model, clinical case management, Assertive Community Treatment (ACT) and Family-Aided Assertive Community Treatment (FACT). We classify these prominent approaches as four model types where social network ties are specified to be fundamentally differ-ent and, as a result, so are the social functions that they fill. Specifically, we present graphical representations of the underlying relationships among the key individual and community actors—the consumer, the case man-ager or case management team, the larger treatment system, the social service system, and the lay community. Drawing from this conceptual framework, we suggest a series of propositions and hypotheses applica-ble to studies investigating the impact of case management on client out-comes. We conclude with a brief discussion of the implications for policy and evaluation.

APPROACHES AND FUNCTIONS OF CASE MANAGEMENT

Viewed by some as simply old-fashioned social casework, case management in mental health combines a mixture of practical assistance and friendship with elements of the professional helping process (Harris & Bergman, 1988; Moxley, 1989). Moore (1990), for example, sees case management as center-ing on the integration of formal systems of care with family and primary group caretaking responsibilities. Simply put, the case manager functions, in theory, as the human link between the client and community, particu-larly the maze of organizations and providers in the fragmented service system. Over time, a wide variety of case management approaches have been suggested in professional literature and implemented in practice set-tings. But underlying all models are a few basic functions—assessment, care or case planning, linking or brokering, resource acquisition, monitoring, and support.

Classification becomes an important first step in sorting out what critical differences separate case management models and in providing clues to what might be the underlying mechanisms at work. Two previous attempts focus on functions or services. First, Ross (1980) suggests that case management programs exist on one of three levels that relate directly to the *range of functional services* potentially offered by case managers. At the most basic level, only a core of services are offered, specifically outreach, assessment, case planning, and referral. The coordinated approach expands services to include direct casework, advocacy, developing natural support systems, and reassessment. This folds in more therapeutic or direct consumer contact roles and posits a more affective involvement between case managers and consumers. The comprehensive approach adds resource development, quality assurance, crisis intervention, and public education. This approach includes community development activity and emphasizes higher level clinical skills. Second, Ridgely and Willenbring (1992) organize case management approaches based on both functions and specific dimensions of practice. The *characteristics* of case management identified as important discriminators include: duration of contact, intensity or frequency of contact, staff/consumer ratio, focus of service (individual, community, or mixture), availability of the case manager (appointment only vs. 24 hour coverage), degree of consumer input and direction, emphasis on advocacy, level of case managers professional training, the relative authority case managers hold, and team structure.

Our two-step approach combines the strategic advantages of each of these schemes. First, we do not abstract the elements of case management approaches but simply typify them into commonly recognized, ideal models of case management services. By developing and focusing on four district "classes" of case management models, we contact our discussion to real world programs, unlike Ross, and distill our discussion from hundreds of possible variations suggested by the Ridgely and Willenbring multidimensional approach. We review the features that characterize these discrete approaches, recognizing that hybrid models have developed over time as reinvention has appropriately occurred and as practice has matured. Second, *within* the four classes of models, we return to the issue of what particular dimensions separate them. Examining the cluster of ingredients *across* classes of models allows us to construct an underlying mechanism at work. Below, we focus on the first of these steps, describing four classes of case management models. We deal with theoretical mechanisms in the next section.

The Broker Model—Standard Case Management

The classic broker model conceptualizes activities done by case managers that serve to link consumers with services required for successful community living. In practice, the resources that are brokered are usually restricted to areas of basic need and medical/psychiatric services. This model may involve time-limited monitoring and follow-up when resources are secured, and also requires situation specific advocacy. Because the model is conceptualized as a brokering service, case loads can theoretically be heavy and the case manager is reactive, responding to problems or issues when notified by clients. Under these conditions, there is likely to be little affective involvement between the case manager and client. From the treatment organization's point of view, the broker model requires little systemic change, uses few internal resources, and does not require a highly trained professional. In its most pure form, the broker operates in-house and may do the majority of needed work by telephone. In Ross's (1980) terms, this is clearly a minimalist model of case management even though most case management models involve some level of brokering activity.

Given the challenge posed by severe mental illness, including the cognitive difficulties that result from neurobiological dysfunction and the social habilitation that must occur for adequate community functioning, this model has been largely viewed as inadequate. Deitchman (1980) remarks that consumers need a "travel companion" not a "travel agent" and suggests that successful case managers must work directly with consumers as they learn new skills and deal with fears and frustrations in the community. Furthermore, given the nature of severe mental illness and the likelihood of high case loads under this model, case managers are forced into a crisis-management approach with little time to work proactively with consumers. These limitations also suggest that resource acquisition activities may be limited to traditional helping services, to programs host organizations offer, both of which draw from a narrowly defined range of options geared to serve as a social prosthesis for consumer disabilities.

The contours of the broker approach to case management translate into little chance to reduce costs, or most importantly, to integrate consumers into the community and live more normal lives as a result of their contact with case managers. Consequently, we should not be surprised at research which reports case management actually increases costs by diminishing consumer outcomes (Franklin, Solovitz, Mason, Clemons, & Miller, 1987).

The Therapeutic Model—Clinical Case Management

The therapist-case management model, attributed to Richard Lamb (1980), expands the role of the case manager from simple broker to treatment provider. The clinical variant of this model in social work, offered by Harris and Bergman (1987), views the relationship between case manager and consumer as the key to the helping process. Here, case management is seen not only as coordinating care but as "a mode of therapy in itself" constituting "treatment independent of any other treatment in which the patient is involved" (Harris & Bergman, 1987, 296). Case management, described under this model, is inherently integrative, rational, and pro-active. Since the phenomenological conceptualization of mental illness underlying this model sees mental illness as a personally disintegrating experience, the case management model has to deal with a world marked by crisis and chaos. The case manager becomes an auxiliary ego that the consumer can ultimately emulate beginning with simple imitation and leading toward the development of a firm sense of personal competence. Roach (1993), for example, has tied the functions of the clinical case manager to object relations theory. Case managers exert control and establish a protective pace for the consumer as they try to both integrate their personality and strive for independence.

Compared to standard case management, the therapeutic model clearly asserts the importance of the relationship between the case manager and consumer and de-emphasizes managerial and community development roles. This version of clinical case management requires that case managers be highly trained practitioners, knowledgeable in objects relations theory and the therapeutic process. The assessment process and treatment planning are guided by personality and ego theory. By necessity case leads must be smaller and outreach work, advocacy, and resource acquisition activities are reduced as well. The case manager holds a position of control, not geared toward a collaboration between provider and consumer.

Other approaches in this class move away from the hierarchical and somewhat paternalistic approach of classical clinical case management. The Strengths approach, first articulated a decade ago (Rapp & Chamberlain, 1985) has become a widely adopted model of case management and hailed by some as a new paradigm for practice (Saleeby, 1992; Sullivan & Rapp, 1994; Weick, Rapp, Sullivan, & Kisthardt, 1989). This variant is based on two ever-arching assumptions. First, people are successful in daily living when they develop their potential and have access to the necessary resources to do so. Second, following from the first, human behavior is largely a function of the resources available to people in a pluralistic society, which values equal access to resources (Davidson & Rapp, 1976).

The Strengths approach is highly value driven, as is evident in a number of its guiding principles (Freeman & Harris, 1993). These include a focus on individual strengths rather than pathology, the primary of the case manager-client relationship, interventions based on client self-determination, the community viewed as an "oasis of resources" rather than obstacle, aggressive outreach as the preferred model of intervention, and an emphasis on learning, growing, and change for consumers with severe mental illness (Rapp, 1992, 46). The Strengths approach blends features of broker and clinical models but also departs from both in significant ways. The focus on the relationship between the case manager and consumer is consistent with the clinical model of case management. A centerpiece of the care planning function lies in a systematic goal setting strategy that serves an accountability and evaluation function but also models systematic planning and problem solving for consumers. The model departs from most clinical models by affirming client self-determination and collaboration as opposed to the case stranger as expert and pseudo-parent.

Compared even within the class of therapeutic models, the Strengths approach requires that case loads be smaller so that case managers are easily accessible and can be flexible in their job. Successful case manager under the Strengths model are advanced generalists. Advanced degrees are not necessarily required since less emphasis is placed on clinical diagnostic and intervention methods. The focus on resource acquisition as central to the ability of the consumer to thrive in the community is consistent with the standard model of case management. However, it encourages a broad view of social resources, suggesting that natural or normalized resources (i.e., secured from those places where most community members get them rather than from a special program in the mental health sector) be targeted before specialty mental health services (Sullivan, 1992a). Furthermore, by highlighting the importance of outreach services, case managers are encouraged to work directly with consumers to build skills and facilitate opportunities in the community. As such, the Strengths approach requires high affective involvement, which cannot be adequately accomplished in a detached office-based style. Accommodation and support in the community becomes central to success.

Rose's (1992) advocacy/empowerment approach is closely aligned with the Strengths perspective but takes an even bolder stand on the potentialities of consumers and the obligation of case managers to view consumers in context, develop relationships based on honesty and integrity, and facilitate the availability of material, emotional, and social supports. Bebout (1993) recently has suggested a Contextual Case Management Model built on a blending of elements from the individual approaches to assertive case management (see also Moxley, 1989; Gottlieb, 1981for a similar emphasis). The underlying assumptions bear a striking resemblance to the conceptual underpinning of the Strengths approach by highlighting the impress of the social environment on behavior. While recognizing the biophysical nature of severe mental illness, Bebout focuses on the impact of the environment on the course of growth, change, and adaptation in the face of this challenge. From this perspective, change occurs outside-in rather than inside-out, thus, "if you change the system, you change the individual" (Bebout, 1993, 62). To intervene the practitioner must first be astute in assessing social networks. Bebout (1993) offers three ideal types of social networks of concern to those working with those with severe mental illness: integrated, distressed, and fragmented. An understanding of these distinctions helps the practitioner decide how to work with existing network members, recreate or rebuild old patterns of relationships, or to construct networks using social services as a building block.

The Therapeutic Team Approach—Assertive Community Treatment

The growth of Assertive Community Treatment Teams can be dated to the pioneering work of Stein and Test as a part of Wisconsin's Program for

Assertive Community Treatment (PACT) beginning in the early 1970s (Stein & Test, 1980; Test, 1992; see Thompson, Griffith, & Leaf, 1990 for a historical perspective). What makes this approach unique lies in the use of multidisciplinary teams to provide a range of specialty services to consumers, with a clear focus on the prevention of unnecessary hospitalization, and on efforts to build community living skills. While early discussions were less clear on what roles team members might actually perform, recent discussions describe a set of assumptions and values parallel in focus to case management models offered above. In fact, Stein (1990, 649) sees Assertive Continuous Care Teams, one of the many variants of the early PACT model, as "a vehicle for the delivery of treatment, rehabilitation, and case management services."

The emphasis on the team model, reflected in the original PACT model and its later Continuous Treatment Team (CTT) and Assertive Community Treatment (ACT) variants, is based on several assumptions. First, a multidisciplinary team can develop a better assessment of the needs and difficulties of a consumer by drawing from their respective vantage points. Second a team structure prevents burnout among providers by decreasing the range of individual expertise needed and offering support. Third, it improves continuity of care by ensuring that a host of professionals are involved with the consumer so that the departure of any one individual will not cause major disruption. Finally, because of this accountability, consumers are less likely to get list in the system, and team members will be able to quickly spot signs of potential social and psychological difficulty.

Given the extensive exposure of the PACT program in professional literature coupled with years of technical assistance and training offered by Wisconsin-based researchers and practitioners, the Assertive Community Treatment approach has been widely adopted with some states (e.g., Michigan and Delaware) moving toward this approach for treatment of all individuals with severe and persistent mental disorders. The evolution of the basic ACT model has resulted in hybrid programs as well as refinements and modifications from the original. Many variations emphasize outreach, small staff-consumer ratios, frequent consumer contact, the provision of direct service over brokering, and a team approach that in some instances requires highly trained professionals. The focus on direct service provision is emphasized in some variants while the use of community resources is highlighted in others (e.g., rural projects; see Santos et al., 1993). Advocacy is not a centerpiece of most discussions, although it is recognized in some circles. Issues of collaboration and consumer direction have been hotly debated with some expressing the belief that the PACT model is highly directive and authoritarian, and ultimately results in unnecessary dependency (Thompson et al., 1990, for a reply see Stein, 1990). However, across hybrids, the belief in the efficacy of a team versus individual approach to case management stands. And, if case management can be seen as an important aspect and catalyst in the development of a continuum of care, ACT reflects the belief that there must also be continuity in care and caregivers. As Torrey (1986) notes the difficulty that persons with severe mental illness have forming relations and alliances with others, he also observes that as consumers move through the continuum of care they must continually adapt to a new set of providers. The ACT model "implies that the same mental health team will be responsible for a given chronic mentally ill patient no matter where the patient is—hospital, foster home, own apartment—and no matter what the patient's needs" (Torrey, 1986, 1243).

In spite of, or perhaps as a direct response to, the widely varying features of ACT, Witheridge (1991, 51–58) details the essential "active ingredients" of assertive outreach, including the focus on service delivery to those persons who need the most attention in order to prevent hospitalization and homelessness, but focusing first and foremost on improving the quality of people's everyday lives. ACT makes heavy use of staff teamwork, deemphasizing the use of individual caseloads. Staff-to-member ratio are high enough to permit the direct provision of most services (not merely the brokering)—with the staff taking ultimate professional responsibility for client well-being including assertive advocacy on the member's behalf to negotiate troublesome system boundaries and measures to prevent and manage unavoidable crisis outside of the hospital. Finally, ACT involves its members in all aspects of the community support process with most of the program's face-to-face interventions occurring in clients' homes or neighborhoods rather than in staff offices or facilities.

Family-Aided Assertive Community Treatment (FACT)

McFarlane, Stastny, and Deakins (1992) offer "Family-Aided Assertive Community Treatment" (FACT) as an extension of the Wisconsin Training in Community Living (TLC)/Assertive Community Treatment Team models. Specifically, they try to combine the "solidly established" team based treatment programs with "family psychoeducation and multifamily groups" into a more comprehensive model. Family environment has been identified as critical factor in rehospitalization, and this intervention tries to take advantage of the positive influences families can have by integrating willing family members "into the on-going treatment and rehabilitation work conducted by the clinicians" (McFarlane, et al., 1992, 47; Strachen, 1992; Leff & Vaughn, 1984).

Family groups are convened regularly during the course of treatment. These "multi-family groups" are used to educate the family about mental illness, the treatment process, and coping with the stress and burden of caring for someone with a serious mental disorder. These groups also serve as a forum for family members to discuss current problems, to garner support from others facing similar stressors, and to engage in practical problem solving with other family members and clinicians. The presence of clinicians in this process serves to inform family members about the specific treatment efforts and promotes more coordinated responses between the professional and community caregivers. As Bebout (1993) notes, this model facilitates an active and explicit intervention into the social environment as part of case management work.

As the most recent entry into variants of case management, responses to it from providers and consumers as well as evaluations of its effects on treatment and quality of life outcomes have yet to be documented. Preliminary results, as reported by McFarlane and his collegues (1992, 45) are promising. They indicate that "[r]elapse rates after the first twelve months of treatment indicated that the FACT program had fewer relapses (22%) than the TLC-only program (40 percent). "That is, in comparison to ACT approach where a treatment team provided care, the approach that builds a team among professional and family caregivers appears to have made a significant improvement in outcome as measured by the reduction in rehospitalization.

A THEORETICAL VIEW OF THE SOCIAL FUNCTIONS OF CASE MANAGEMENT

Fallot (1993) has argued that various theories and models of case management can be understood as distinct cultures that represent divergent images of the individual person and the world in which people live. They make claims about the "nature of psychological difficulties and strengths, about the processes of human development and change, about the dynamics of the interpersonal world, and about the goals and purposes which animate human life" (Fallot, 1993, 258). When placed in historical context—as approaches that developed in response to one another over the period of deinstitutionalization—they also can be seen to reflect the growing recognition of broader forces that impinge on the ability of individuals with severe and persistent mental problems to live in the community (Prior, 1993).

Coming from the medical sector, it is no surprise that the early approach of the broker model paralleled a narrow medical model approach—as patients come to doctors when they are ill, individuals with mental illnesses living in the community come to see case managers when they have a problem and that provider's job is to take care of it. The movement toward community outreach in clinical case management reacted to that narrow approach by bringing the case manager into the community, out of the office, to promote both medical and nonmedical community integration. ACT reaches one step further by recognizing the advantages of a team over a single provider and by matching the view of broad based medical and psychosocial needs with a complement of providers with expertise across the spectrum of service organizations. Finally, while the community mental health movement in the 1970s included in its coalition the families of individuals with mental illness, it has taken two decades for a systematic approach to case management (i.e., FACT) to be developed ,which explicitly and formally brings them into the basic model underlying the treatment process.

In sum, the "culture" (i.e., the underlying beliefs and norms guiding behavior) for community-based care of individuals with chronic mental illness has changed over time, broadening in its conception of "needs," of "providers," and of "treatment." Case management models operationalize these changing beliefs in their form and function (i.e., their "structure"). Communities, societies, and any social group, then, have two underlying elements—culture and structure. The cultural component is the "content" of the treatment community—the sets of beliefs, norms, and even technology guiding treatment regimens. But the structural component provides the skeleton on which these beliefs and technologies hang and create the links across which information, resources, beliefs, and norms flow. It is no surprise that different cultural ideologies about case management have produced different structures of care.

Under this conceptualization, culture is only half of the underlying image, and perhaps not the most important half. Each of these community-based care models holds a different view of what the important structural elements of "community" are. Central to each class of case management models lies an image and, more importantly, a blueprint of whether and how to link consumers with three structures in the community most relevant to their success—the treatment system, the social service system, and the lay community. These models differ in significant ways with regard to both the extensiveness and types of ties that are created with and around the client in each of these spheres.

In essence, while the case management classes outlined above mark distinctive clinical features (Moxley, 1989; Levine & Fleming, 1985; Schwartz, Goldman, & Churgin, 1982), they also signify important differences in the social nature and context of the consumer-case manager relationship. *Each model attempts to reconstruct the "community" for clients by creating a synthetic, professionally-based set of social network ties for individuals. As a result, each of these classes of these classes of models provides a more or less rich "social support system" [Pescosolido, 1991] in the community.* Case managers' work assists in the creation and maintenance of a variety of social relationships in clients' lives, which in turn helps to create different "communities" in which clients live and cope with their mental health problems.

We argue that social network theory offers a framework for understanding and studying how this social dimension of models of case management matters in direct and indirect ways (see Galaskiewicz & Wasserman, 1993; Scott, 1991; Knoke & Kuklinski, 1982 for general overviews of the perspective). For example, medication compliance is commonly believed to lie at the root of decreases in rehospitalization. Indeed, among the "successful" consumers that Sullivan (1992b) studied, an overwhelming majority (72 percent) cited medication as the "critical element" in their recovery. Our approach does not counter that argument; it complements it. The underlying mechanisms that hinder or encourage the routine taking of medications with sometimes powerful side effects are not well understood. We suggest *why* medication compliance is more likely among successful consumers. Almost as many consumers (67 percent) cite their relationship with their case manager as fundamental to their continued community life (Sullivan, 1992b). We argue that the "working alliance" (Solomon, Draine, & Delaney, 1995) created in case management models are more or less successful regarding medication compliance because they forge the conditions of integration and regulation in the community that promotes support and expedites compliance with prescribed health and illness behaviors. For example, ACT teams with their dense structure and routine contacts creates a set of social conditions, through regular interaction with individuals sharing a "pro-medical" culture, that facilitates the routine taking of psychiatric medications (see Pescosolido, 1991 for detail on a social network model of utilization and compliance).

Here we apply the network perspective to understand how these general models of case management work. We do this by translating the different types of Case Management Models into social networks and use them to highlight the sociological nature of these interventions.

Before we proceed, the scope of our effort needs to be demarcated clearly. Our purpose here is heuristic. In actual practice, treatment will vary from ideal models. Individual cases or programs may not reflect precisely the ideal-typical models presented (see Fisher, Landis, & Clark, 1988; Sullivan, Hartmann, Dillon, & Wolk, 1994; Timney & Graham, 1989). The use of classes of model simply highlights the presentation of basic differences; they do not limit the nature or utility of the propositions and hypotheses that follow from them. In addition, a number of points, some of which have been raised earlier, need to be articulated both as cautions and as clarifications.

First, social networks are not "treatment" per se but may have a dual function. We primarily view them as shaping the likelihood that clients will subscribe to treatment regimens, comply with them, and search for alternative approaches (Pescosolido, 1991, 1992). However, we do not ignore their potential to facilitate community living in and of themselves. According to a wealth of evidence compiled by social support researchers, social network ties of particular configurations and content may have an independent effect on recovery (see Thoits, 1995 for a review). Certainly, ACT "experts" mention community integration as critical to this model and its success (McGrew & Bond, 1995). Second, such a perspective does not suggest that mental health treatment is irrelevant, nor does it necessarily validate current approaches. It is, in fact, detached from the content of therapeutic arguments. It assumes that treatment regimes are more or less likely to be adopted under certain social conditions, allowing us to parcel out the effect of "care" (e.g., the social support component) from "cure" (i.e., the treatment regime). In Rossi and Freeman's (1993) words, the difference between the "net" and "gross" effects of a program lie in how treatments function in the real world environment. If a medical intervention is proven to be *efficacious*, and if community forces coalesce to ensure that the intervention is adopted, then the greatest "success" should be seen for clients under these conditions. Social networks provide the mechanism for understanding the "in situ" conditions that may increase or decrease *effectiveness*. Third, social network ties with treatment personnel cannot be assumed to be helpful, supportive, or harmonious. The simple presence of a link cannot be presumed to increase the adoption and retention of medical regimes. We need to examine the actual structural and substantive flavor of network ties. Fourth, social support is not the only force underlying the operation of social ties. While the integrating effect of ties may be presumed to operate, a regulative effect may be just as powerful. That is, one of the ways that social ties can affect health and illness behaviors is through social control—from low level nagging to take medications to exerting a great deal of pressure to comply with treatment regimes (Horwitz, 1982). Umberson (1987), for example, has found that this type of regulation by wives may explain the salutary of effects of marriage on married men's health. Fifth, following Duricheim (1951), we can expect that more is not necessarily better in relationship to the provision of support or control. That is, either too much or too little integration or regulation can produce deleterious consequences. Neither individuals who are set adrift in a community nor those who feel choked by oppressive monitoring can be expected to participate fully or with motivation in treatment. Sixth, this approach does not assume the absence of conflict nor does it see conflict as unrelated to success or failure. The variants of case management models, classified according to the four groups we presented above, may be the only sources of regular social contact for clients or they may represent a set of ties that exist in conflict with beliefs of other cultures (e.g., ethnic communities, Pescosolido, Wright, Alegria, & Vera, 1995) or the priorities set by other social ties (e.g., drug cultures) with whom they have contact. Clients cannot be seen as embracing the high levels of social interaction that some models require (see Estroff, 1981 on this point). Rather, attempts at contact may be welcomed or rejected by individuals and the pro-mental health system message may be in concert or in contest with others beliefs (Freidson, 1970).

Case Management Models and Community Support Structures

The complex web of factors described above present the real situation that comprises community-based treatment alternatives. Understanding how these factors increase or decrease the likelihood of clients' community success becomes fundamental to unraveling what clinical alternatives work in the community and why. We begin by laying out the basic features of the "community" set within each model of case management.

In the broadest terms, each of these models focuses on the nature of the dyadic relationship between a case manager (CM) and a consumer/client (CL). This relationship is embedded in a larger community characterized by three major institutional structures: the client's lay community (including family, friends, work, church, and other social groups); the medical and mental health treatment system; and the larger social service sector. These institutional structures offer the potential to serve as "anchors" for building an underlying social safety net under consumers living in the community. Each class of case management models differs in the emphasis given to particular types of relationships and the pattern of links created during the course of treatment. Here, we focus on describing the social context which each class of case management models offer. We do this through a series of graphical representations which facilitate uncovering the essential differences among models. In the section that follows, we extend beyond description to examine the implications of these structures, developing hypotheses about how structural components of social network support system affect outcomes.

Throughout the graphs, we use a number of terms and graphical conventions which require some explanation (see "Key" on the graphs). We focus on two classifications of individuals—those attached to the treatment system and those who are served by it. For individuals representing the provider community, we use rectangular symbols; for individuals from the lay community, including clients, we use circles. In the graphs, two kinds of relationships are depicted—dotted lines indicate relationships or network ties that occur only on an "as needed" basis; solid lines indicate network contacts that the case management models expects to be routine. These lines do not indicate the strength of the relationship (see below); rather they simply indicate how and if the case management models specify regularity in the nature of the relationships that should exist. For example, if clients are supposed to contact case managers when they have a problem, the line will be dotted. If case managers are supposed to have daily or weekly contact with clients, the lines will be solid. Each of these lines connect circles (lay individuals) or squares (treatment representatives) with arrows at one or both ends. These arrows indicate the *direction* of the expected relationship. An arrow going only in one direction indicates that the basic responsibility for the relationship ties with the person from whom the lines emanates, a line with arrows at each and places expectations of a reciprocal relationship between the individuals. Again, where a client calls or visits a case manager as needed, the dotted line will have only a one-way arrow that flows from the client to the case manager. Finally, and perhaps the most complicated, is the depiction of direct or indirect connections. We show two possibilities. First, there can be a *direct* relationship—a line goes from one actor to another, for example, when a case manager contacts someone in the social service system to get an appointment for a client (pictured as a line between the case manager and the service system, generally with a one-headed arrow). There can also be *mediated* relationships in the situation where a case manager assists the client in making an appointment by providing information or support to do so. In this case, there is a line between the client and the social service system (indicating that clients take upon themselves the responsibility to make the appointment) but there is also a line from the case manager that touches the line between client and social service system (indicating that it is the job of the case manager to support the client's action, to empower the client, and to assist the client in being successful in the relationship they build or contacts they have with the social service system).

Standard Case Management

In this class of "Broker Models," the case manager serves principally as a central referral source and coordinator of services. Figure 1 depicts graphically the general pattern of relationships in standard case management models. As indicated in this figure, the overall development of regular and routine social ties in this approach is quite weak. The absence of regular or routine ties coupled with the reliance on one person in the treatment system does not produce a picture which resembles a safety net at all. The dominance of dotted lines indicates that the relationship between case manager and client exists only on an "as needed" basis and that no necessary set of links is established by the model regarding any particular sector of the community. The client (circle labeled "CL") is connected to the case manager (square labeled "CM") by a dotted arrow, indicating a weak and/or irregular relationship. The arrow flows from the client to the case manager suggesting that the energy in this system derives from the client's needs or the client's expressed desires. That is, the client goes to their case manager for assistance in order to gain access to or receive assistance in getting services from other providers, typically agencies in the medical/psychiatric treatment system. In this regard, this model is "reactive." Given the typically large case loads and high turnover rates of case managers, the bond forged between client and case manager is not likely to be strong, nor is it likely to persist over time. When clients refuse this service few attempts, beyond phone calls, are made to encourage them to continue in the program. Even the monitoring function

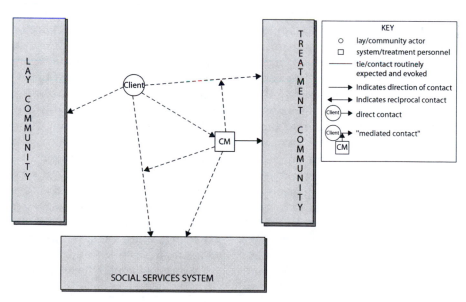

Model Class 1—Standard Case Manager.

of case management rests on clients' willingness to come to the treatment center or clinic.

The "brokering" function is depicted in Figure 1 both by arrows indicating involvement in the client's ties primarily to the treatment system (the lone solid arrow) and the social service system (dotted arrow). Following the path of arrows, when clients come to case managers, this trips action by the case manager in these two systems. The case manager may also facilitate efforts by clients to make these connections themselves (indicated by dotted line from the case managers to the middle of the lines connecting the client to treatment and service systems) and work to "manage" a given client's interactions with other service providers (e.g., with the psychiatrist, Social Security Administration officials). Case managers may also strive to establish relationships with other agencies independent of particular clients (indicated by the dotted and solid lines from the case manager to the treatment and social service sectors respectively). The emphasis of the activity is obtaining services from providers offering medical or psychiatric care or social assistance. Involvement with the lay community members involved with clients is absent or very minimal.

Clinical Case Management

This class of models, as depicted in Figure 2, and varies in distinctive ways from standard case management. Overall, the client's community safety net begins to have some definite shape and stability. Most clearly, the place of the case managers in the web of relationships is quite different. They are both in and out of the treatment system. In this model of therapeutic case management, case managers are responsible for evaluating consumers' needs and for making arrangements for services (hence the much closer proximity of the case manager square to the treatment system and a direct arrow indicating the potential for regular contact with other providers). However, under more recent versions, such as the Strengths Model, case managers are required to forge regular and strong ties with clients (indicated by the solid line between client and case manager). The potential for a meaningful and reciprocal relationship between the two is now possible. The arrow from the client to the case manager is a dotted line because the interaction initiated by the client is still most likely to be problem-focused (Although clearly descriptions of this model portray the consumer-case manager relationship more as a community supporter or friend than in standard case management; Harris & Bergman, 1987). The unbroken line from the case manager to the client also implies that the involvement of the case manager is more systematic and pro-active. Case managers in this class tend to be more heavily and regularly involved with clients, often engaging in "prevention" related treatment, such as insuring compliance with medications and monitoring "early warning signs" of the onset of acute phases (Harris & Bergman, 1987; Lamb, 1980).

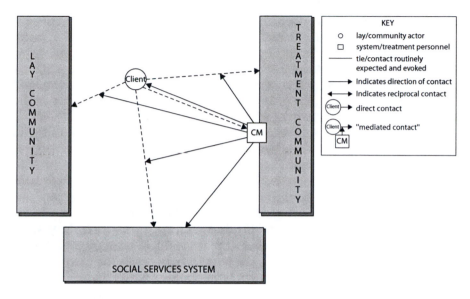

Figure 2 Model Class 2—Clinical Case Management.

The case manager also facilitates the client's active involvement (as depicted by the solid lines, which touch the connections between clients and the three anchors of the community). They are also more involved in their clients' lives and occasionally provide their services in the clients' natural social environments. Whereas in standard case management the treatment focus is principally on treatment and social service needs, here case managers are expected to be more extensively involved in monitoring a number of areas of the client's life, including the client's family and personal relationships, problems with landlords, and even employers or supported employment program personnel (Harris & Bergman, 1987; Lamb, 1980). Case management work itself becomes a vehicle for doing clinical work (Lamb, 1980). For example, when services are unavailable from other facilities, case managers are generally expected to be creative and to develop and provide needed services directly to clients when other community support is unavailable (Rapp & Chamberlain, 1985; Sullivan & Rapp, 1994; Sullivan, 1992a). In short, the responsibility for the consumer-case manager relationship shifts more significantly to the case manager and to a proactive focus on the facilitation of client's community ties.

Assertive Community Treatment

Figure 3 depicts the radically different configuration of social ties required under the TLC, CTT, PACT, and ACT approaches. The qualitative break between this model and the ones described earlier warrants, in our view, the addition of a shaded screen which indicates enough support and regulation under this model to "hang" a real social safety net. The wide-ranging number of proactive ties (indicated by solid lines) and reciprocal relationships (indicated by double-headed arrows) results in a broader and more stable set of anchor points to the treatment community, the social service system, and the lay community. And, the potential density of the ties begins to create the feel of a community safety net (as indicated by the shading).

Specifically, in team approaches, the case manager role is shared by an iinterdisciplinary group of professionals. Although the emphasis on reciprocal relationships between the client and the case manager remains, in ACT, individual team members are expected to develop and maintain their own relationships with their client (see ties between each team member and the client as double-headed arrows). In contrast to the two previous classes, the involvement of the client in their care and with the various case managers is stronger due to the increased contact from multiple team members. Like clinical case management models, the boundary between the case management team and the treatment system is no longer "hard" and much treatment is "in-vivo" (in the community environment). There is also a greater emphasis here on "rehabilitating" clients and enhancing their ability to survive in their natural social environment (indicated by more direct lines from the team into each community anchor and indirect lines intervening with client's relationships to social service system and community).

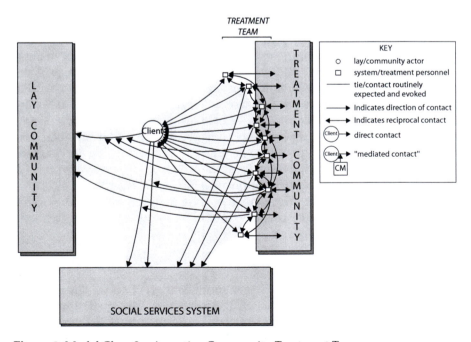

Figure 3 Model Class 3—Assertive Community Treatment Team

As a team, ACT case managers are also responsible for coordinating their treatment efforts and activity with each other (Bond, 1991; Stein, 1990; Thompson et al., 1990). There may be a division of labor in these models where professionals with different backgrounds (e.g., mental health therapists, RNs, occupational or recreational therapists) may "specialize" in providing particular services, but these specialized services are viewed as part of a team process. These specialized roles may further lead to particular patterns of relations with the lay community, providers, and agencies in the treatment and social service sectors. As Figure 3 shows, not all team members have direct or indirect connections to the lay community and social service system. While treatment can occur outside of the team (e.g., hospitalization), the responsibility remains on the team to retain contact with and support comprehensive and continuous care. The involvement of other community members is not an explicit focus of these models. Team members, in the course of their proactive work with and on behalf of the client, are more likely to have routine and regular ties into the social service system and lay community than in other models.

Family-Aided Assertive Community Treatment

Figure 4 presents the network configuration implied under the final class of case management models. Resembling the ACT diagram to a large degree, these models are distinct primarily in the increased stability, range and penetration of contacts into the lay community. And, as a result of this added emphasis, the social safety net, in theory, is more comprehensive, stronger, and more resilient.

In the Family-Aided Assertive Community Treatment (FACT), McFarlane and his colleagues (1992) attempted to combine the rehabilitation focus of ACT with family intervention. Key to this class of models is the explicit focus given to the family and community environment, in our terms, the lay community. In Figure 4, linkages with the family are forged both between clients and with the team of case managers. In addition, the "multi-family groups" have the potential to create support networks among family members, facilitate within group problem solving, and provide emotional support from others facing similar issues. The treatment team's job expands to include enhancing the ability of involved families to become, in essence, a self-help group connected both to the treatment team and clients.

A Comparative Note

Our point is not to advocate for particular treatment modalities. Rather, our presentation of these broad classes is intended to highlight the various patterns of the network ties created with and around the client by one or more case managers. As our presentation of propositions and hypotheses will show, each comes with its own strengths and danger points. We do argue, in general that classes of case management models set the potential for very different configurations of social networks in the community lives of

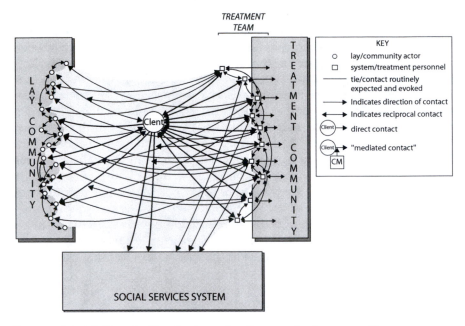

Figure 4 Model Class 4—Family Assertive Community Treatment Team

clients. Further, the nature of this social safety net affects the client outcomes commonly observed in these programs.

Table 1 presents a comparative summary of standard facets of the safety net in terms commonly employed by social network researchers. This table serves to contrast case management models and to introduce and define terms that will be used in the construction of propositions and hypotheses.

At the most global level, the number of ties and the frequency of interaction created increases dramatically across case management models. The focus in both standard and clinical case management ties in the dyad (i.e., two-person relationship) between a single case manager and client. ACT and FACT increase that number dramatically, usually tenfold with the 40 clients for 10 team formula, shifting the focus from the dyad to the network (i.e., the set of ties across a group of individuals). Similarly, the frequency of interaction (i.e., simply how often individuals are in contact) increases across model classes from the "as needed" focus of standard case management to the daily contact anticipated under team models. The directionality of ties targets who initiates contacts between individuals. Across case management models, this differs only in the most basic model where interaction are client initiated (and therefore a unidirectional tie); all other models assume a reciprocal relationship between client and case manager where both are expected to be in contact with the other. Finally, case management models suggest that ties can vary in their multiplicity, that is, the number and types of functions that they serve.

Table 1 Summary of Significant Network Dimensions in the Four General Classes of Case Management Programs

	Type of Case Management Program			
Network Dimensions	Standard Case Management	Clinical Case Management	Assertive Community Treatment/Continuous Treatment Teams	Family-Aided Assertive Community Treatment
Number of case management ties	one	one	many	many
Frequency of interaction	variable as needed	regular	daily in weekly	daily to weekly
Directionality of ties	unidirectional	reciprocal	reciprocal	reciprocal
Multiplexity of ties	limited; referral centered	treatment centered	diffuse/multiplex	diffuse/multiplex
Affective strength of ties	weak	weak to moderate	moderate to strong	moderate to strong
Range of ties				
professionals	low	low	moderate to high	moderate to high
family/community persons	none-low	low to moderate	low to moderate	moderate to high
Density/Interconnections among ties	—	low	high density between client and team high density within team	high density between client and team high density between client and team high density within team high density between team and family/community members high density among members

For example, in standard case management, contacts between case managers and clients tend to be of a limited nature—they offer or are evoked for the limited purpose of brokering formal needs like housing, medical appointments, and so forth. In the other models, network contacts take on a more multiplex character where, for example, the relationship with the case manager can serve a wide variety of functions such as broker, therapist, friend.

To this point, we have discussed the structural dimensions—how the form of the network structure varies under case management models. In addition, the quality or content of the social support system offered under each model is likely to vary. For example, under these structural parameters, the potential for emotional bonds (called "affective strength" in network terms) in form will be variable. With heavy case loads and intermittent contact in standard case management, only weak and formal ties can be expected to form. With increased contact across a wider set of activities and settings, the potential for emotional bonds increases, starting with the Strengths Model in the clinical class through the FACT Model. Similarly, the variety of kinds of people (e.g., medical, client, lay; referred to as "range" of ties) that clients are likely to interact with is also likely to increase across the classes of models, ensured in ACT by the team approach and in FACT with the creation of a lay self-help group.

Finally, the resilience of the net changes across classes. "Density" refers to the degree to which everyone in the caretaking system is connected. For example, how well do case managers know each other, their clients, clients, families, and friends? Under standard case management, that social safety net's density is undefined since there are no interconnections required except between client and case manager. There is no obligation for others surrounding either the case manager or the client to know one another or to act in a concerted manner. This is also the case with the original versions of therapeutic case management, but the proactive and community of focus of the Strengths approach and the social network variants mean that there will be some growing familiarity among some of those involved with the client. The ACT model formalizes this growing familiarity primarily among the professionals involved with a particular client or set of clients through team routine team meetings and frequent contact with clients. Under the ACT model, then, we can expect a dramatic increase in the density of the social networks surrounding clients. Finally, with the formal focus on lay supports, the density among the professional and lay caregivers is greatest leading to the highest potential for information and resource sharing as well as integrated crisis management in the caretaking system. This may also produce the greatest amount of monitoring and social control in the lives of clients.

IMPLICATIONS FOR PLANNING AND RESEARCHING CASE MANAGEMENT PROGRAMS

Conceptualizing case management programs as systemic social networks has both policy and research implications. To date, effects to specify the components of case management programs have been difficult because of the absence of a general analytic framework to talk about what case managers do. Here, we use social network concepts to outline and diagram case managers, linking functions. On the policy and programmatic levels, planners could benefit from using these models to guide planning new case management programs or evaluate existing ones.

An appreciation of the differences between case management models has important implications for researchers attempting to understand the effects of case management and for planners selecting potential programs to introduce in an applied setting. Two issues stand out. First, the particular roles that case managers take on are shaped by social system context. That is, which case management functions are emphasized and which are ignored in applied settings depend on the types of mental health settings in which they operate. Their status within the provider hierarchy can vary greatly depending on the ideology and configuration of "appropriate" cases set by the particular organization in which they work and the place of their organization in the larger public and private systems of care (Austin, 1990; Moore, 1992; Sullivan et al., 1994). Second, the willingness or ability to remain faithful to the conceptual anchors of a chosen model in daily practice also varies. Some aspects of case management, particularly community outreach, resources acquisition, and advocacy, are performed less frequently by case managers than would be anticipated by the models these professional have purportedly adopted (Fisher et al., 1988; Sullivan et al., 1994; Timney & Graham, 1989). This is a function, in part, of a failure to understand or construct the organizational cultures and structures that are needed to support case management. Freeman and Harris (1993) have offered a review of the values and assumptions of popular models of case management and note that some are tied to the logical-positivist tradition while others are more consistent with interpretive paradigms. The values and assumptions that undergird models of case management also impact the relative fit of a model within a host organization.

Our model can also provide concrete guidance for evaluating specific programs and developing larger research agendas, which seek to compare and contrast different models of case management. In many ways, the general classes of case management presented here point to the need to move toward more detailed analysis of the structure of a case manager's or team's relationship with the client and the surrounding institutional environment. Indeed we argue that one of the most effective ways to systematically dismantle the effects of case management programs, including ACT, would be to use social network analysis to identify the critical ingredients (Scott & Sechrest, 1989). Comparing multiple teams in terms of the number or types of ties, or even the nature of ties, would provide an empirical basis on which to link case management service functions with client outcomes. For example, one could test whether ACT reduces hospitalizations by increasing medication compliance or by direct intervention in the admission process to prevent unnecessary hospitalizations.

Even concerns about the efficacy of the models being concerned are misplaced, as the models we present focus attention on not only the *internal* linkages created within the team but on the *external* ties that are created to other institutions in the treatment and social service sectors as well. Two very equivalent ACT programs may be implemented in different cities and may function quite similarly, but because the service environments differ considerably in the available services, the outcomes at the client level may be significantly different.

In sum, understanding how case management provides a community of support for clients provides a first step in understanding both the critical ingredients of community-based care options and the role of the larger social context in shaping the possibilities.

References

Austin, C. D. 1990. "Case management: Myths and Realities." *Families in Society* 71(7): 396–405.

Bachrach, I. I. 1989. "Case Management: Toward a Shared Definition." *Hospital and Community Psychiatry* 40:883–884.

Bebout, R. 1993. "Contexual Case Management: Restructuring the Social Support Networks of Seriously Mentally Adults." Pp. 59–92 in *Case Management for Mentally Ill Patients*, edited by M. Marris and H. Bergman. Langhorne, PA: Harwood Academic Press.

Bond, G. 1991. "Variations in as Amative Outreach Model." Pp. 65–80 in *Psychiatric Outreach to the Mentally Ill*, edited by N. Cohen. San Francisco, CA: Jossey-Bass Publishers.

Brown, P. 1965. *Transfer of Care*. Boston: Rutledge and Kegan Paul.

Deitchman, W. S. 1980. "How Many Case Managers Does it Take to Screw in a Light Bulb?" *Hospital and Community Psychiatry* 31(12):783–789.

Davidson, W. S. and C. A. Rapp. 1976. "Child Advocacy in the Juvenile Justice System." *Social Work* 21:225–232.

Durikheim, E. 1951. *Suicide*. New York: Free Press.

Estroff, S. E. 1981. *Making It Crazy*. Berkeley: University of California Press.

Fallot, R. 1993. "The Cultures of Case Management: An Exploration of Assumptive Worlds." Pp. 257–278 in *Case Management for Mentally Ill Patients*, edited by M. Harris and H. Bergman. Langhorne, PA: Harwood Academic Press.

Fisher, G., D. Landis, and K. Clark. 1988. "Case Management Service Provision and Client Change." *Community Mental Health Journal* 24(2): 134–142.

Franklin, J. L., B. Solovitz, M. Mason, J. R. Clemons, and G. E. Miller. 1987. "An Evaluation of Case Management." *American Journal of Public Health* 77(6):674–678.

Freeman, D. W. and M. Harris. 1993. "The Philosophy of Science and Theories of Case Management: An Investigation into the Values and Assumptions that Underlie Case Management: Theory." Pp. 1–15 in *Case Management for Mentally Ill Patients*, edited by M. Harris and H. Bergman. Langhorne, PA: Harwood Academic Press.

Freidson, E. 1970. *Profession of Medicine*. New York: Dodd Mead.

Galaskiewicz, J. and S. Wasserman. 1993. "Social Network Analysis: Concepts, Methodology, and Directions for the 1990s." *Sociological Methods and Research* 22(1):3–22.

Gans, S. and G. Horton. 1975. *Integration of Human Services: The State and Municipal Levels*. New York: Steger.

Goffman, E. 1961. *Asylums: Essays on the Social Situation of Mental Patients and Other Inmates*. New York: Anchor Books.

Gottlieb, B. H. 1981. "Preventive Interventions Involving Social Networks and Social Support." Pp. 201–232 in *Social Support and Social Networks*, edited by B. H. Gottlieb. Beverly Hills, CA: Sage Publications.

Harris, M. and H. C. Bergman. 1988. "Clinical Case Management for the Chronically Mentally Ill: A Conceptual Analysis." Pp. 5–13 in *New Directions in Mental Health Services*, No. 40, edited by M. Harris and L. L. Bachrach. San Francisco, CA: Jossey-Bass.

Harris, M. and H. C. Bergman. 1987. "Case Management with the Chronically Mentally Ill: A Clinical Perspective." *American Journal of Orthopsychiatry* 57(2):296–302.

Horwitz, A. 1982. *The Social Control of Mental Illness*. New York: Academic Press.

Isaac, R. J. and V. C. Armat. 1990. *Madness in the Streets: How Psychiatry and the Law Abandoned the Mentally Ill*. New York: Free Press.

Knoke, D. and J. H. Kuklinski. 1982. *Network Analysis*. Beverly Hills, CA: Sage.

Lamb, H. R. 1980. "Therapist-Case Managers: Mets than Brokers of Service." *Hospital and Community Psychiatry* 31:762–764.

Leff. J. and C. Vaughn. 1984. *Expressed Emotion in Families: Its Significance for Mental Illness*. New York: Gallford.

Levine, I. and M. Fleming. 1985. *Human Resource Development: Issues in Case Management*. College Park, MD: Center of Rehabilitation and Manpower Services.

McFarlane, W. R., P. Stastny, and S. Duskins. 1992. "Family Aided Assertive Community Treatment: A Comprehensive Rehabilitation and Intentive Case Management Approach for Persons with Schizophrenic Disorders." *New Directors in Mental Health Service* 53:43–54.

McGrew, J. H. and G. R. Bond. 1995. "Critical Ingredients of Assertive Community Treatment: Judgments of the Experts." *The Journal of Mental Health Administration* 22(2):113–121.

Moore, S. 1990. "A Social Work Practice Model of Case Management: the Case Management Grid." *Social Work* 35(1):444–448.

———. 1992. "Case Management and the Integration of Services: How Service Delivery Systems Shape Case Management." *Social Work* 37(5):418–423.

Moxley, D. P. 1989. *The Practice of Case Management*. Newbery Park, CA: Sage.

Pescosolido, B. A. 1992. "Beyond Rational Choice: The Social Dynamics of How People Seek Help." *American Journal of Sociology* 97:1096–1138.

Pescosolido, B. A. 1991. "Illness Careers and Network Ties: A Conceptual Model of Utilization and Compliance." *Advances in Medical Sociology* 2:161–184.

Pescosolido, B. A., E. Wright, M. Alegria, and M. Vera. 1995. "Formal and Informal Utilization Patterns Among the Poor with Mental Health Problems in Puerto Rico." Working Paper Series, Indiana Consortium for Mental Health Services Research.

Prior, L. 1993. *The Social Organization of Mental Illness*. Newbury Park, CA: Sage.

Rapp, C. A. 1992. "The Strengths Perspective of Case Management with Persons Suffering from Severe Mental Illness." Pp. 45–58 in *The Strengths Perspective in Social Work Practice*, edited by D. Saleebey. New York: Longman.

Rapp. C. A. and R. Chamberlain. 1985. "Case Management Services for the Chronically Mentally Ill." *Social Work* 30(5):417–472.

Ridgely, M. S. and M. Willenbring. 1992. "Application of Case Management to Drug Abuse Treatment: Overview of Models and Research Issues." Pp. 12–33 in *Progress and Issues in Case Management*, edited by R. Ashery. Rockville, MD: U.S. Department of Health and Human Services.

Roach, J. 1993. "Clinical Case Management with Severely Mentally Ill Adults." Pp. 17–40 in *Case Management for Mentally Ill Patients: Theory and Practice*, edited by M. Harris and H. Bergman. Langhourne, PA: Harwood Academic Publishers.

Ross, H. 1980. *Proceedings on the Conference on the Evaluation of Case Management Programs*. Los Angeles: Volunteers for Services to Older Persons.

Rossi, P. H. and H. E. Freeman. 1993. *Evaluation: A Systematic Approach. Fifth Edition*. Newbury Park, CA: Sage.

Rubin, A. 1992. "Is Case Management Effective for People with Serious Mental Illness? A Research Review." *Health and Social Work* 17(2):138–150.

Saleeby, D. (Ed.) 1992. *The Strengths Perspective in Social Work Practice*. New York: Longman.

Santos, A. B., P. A. Deci, K. R. Lachance, J. K. Dias, T. Sloop, T. G. Hiers, and J. Bevilacqua. 1993. "Providing Assertive Community Treatment for Severely Mentally Ill Patients in a Rural Area." *Hospital and Community Psychiatry* 44(1):34–39.

Schwartz, S. R., H. H. Goldman, and S. Churgin. 1982. "Case Management for the Chronic Mentally Ill: Models and Dimensions." *Hospital and Community Psychiatry* 33:1006–1069.

Scott, A. G. and I. Sechrest. 1989. "Strength of Theory and Theory of Strength." *Evaluation and Program Planning* 12:329–336.

Scott, J. 1991. *Social Network Analysis: A Handbook*. Newbury Park, CA: Sage.

Stein, I. I. 1990. "Comments by Leonard Stein." *Hospital and Community Psychiatry* 41(6):649–651.

Solomon, P., J. Draine, and M. A. Delaney. 1995. "The Working Alliance and Consumer Case Management." *The Journal of Mental Health Administration* 22(2):126–134.

Stein, I. I. and M. A. Test. 1980. "An Alternative to Mental Hospital Treatment, 1: Conceptual Model, Treatment Program, and Clinical Evaluation." *Archives of General Psychiatry* 37:392–397.

Strachen, A. 1992. "Family Management." Pp. 183–212 in *Handbook of Psychiatric Rehabilitation*, edited by R. P. Lieberman. Elmsford, NY: Pergamon.

Sullivan, W. P. 1992a. "Reclaiming the Community: The Strengths Perspective and Deinstitutionalization." *Social Work* 37(3):204–209.

———. 1992b. "A Long and Winding Road: The Process of Recovery from Severe Mental Illness." *Innovations and Research* 3(3):19–27.

Sullivan, W. P., D. Hartmann, D. Dillon, and J. Wolk. 1994. "Implementing Case Management in Alcohol and Drug Treatment." *Families in Society* 75(2):67–73.

Sullivan, W. P. and C. A. Rapp. 1994. "Breaking Away: The Potential and Promise of a Strengths-based Approach to Social Work Practice." Pp. 83–104 in *Issues in Social Work Practice: A Critical Analysis*, edited by R. Meinert, J. Pardack and W. P. Sullivan. Westport, CT: Auburn House.

Test, M. A. 1992. "Training in Community Living." Pp. 153–170 in *Handbook of Psychiatric Rehabilitation*, edited by R. P. Liberman. New York: MacMillan.

Thoits, P. 1995. "Social Support and Coping Processes: What Do We Know? What Next?" *Journal of Health and Social Behavior* 36:53–79.

Thompson, K. S., E. H. Griffith, and P. J. Leaf. 1990. "A Historical Review of the Madison Model of Community Care." *Hospital and Community Psychiatry* 41(6):625–634.

Timney, C. B. and K. Graham. 1989. "A Survey of Case Management Practice in Addictions Programs." *Alcoholism Treatment Quarterly* 6(34):103–127.

Torrey, E. F. 1986. Continuous Treatment Teams in the Case of the Chronic Mentally Ill." *Hospital and Community Psychiatry* 37(12):1243–1247.

Turner, J. C. and W. J. TenHoor. 1978. "The NIMH Community Support Program: Pilot Approach to a Needed Social Reform." *Schizophrenia Bulletin* 4(3):313–348.

Umberson, D. A. 1987. "Family States and Health Behavior: Social Control as a Dimension of Social Integration." *Journal of Health and Social Behavior* 28:306–315.

Weick, A., C. A. Rapp, W. P. Sullivan, and W. Kisthark. 1989. "A Strengths Perspective for Social Work Practice." *Social Work* 34(4):350–354.

Witheridge, T. F. 1991. "The 'Active Ingredients' of Assertive Outreach." *New Directions in Mental Health Services* 52:47–54.

DISCUSSION

1. What are the most common types of case management? What do you see as the major strengths and weaknesses of each strategy for building social support systems that can help to improve the quality of life of people with serious mental illness?

2. Why is case management such a critical component of contemporary mental health treatment? What better ways can you envision to integrate the many different types of care that people with serious mental illness often require?

Teresa L. Scheid

Reluctant Managers and Ideologies of Care

Parent, Caretaker, Advocate, Best Friend

In her book, Tie a Knot and Hang On, sociologist Teresa Scheid examines mental health services for people with serious mental illness from the providers' point of view. Based on in-depth interviews with providers who work day-to-day "in the trenches" with people who have some of the most serious psychiatric disorders, she explores the varied views providers have of their clients. In this particular chapter, she analyzes the different "ideologies of care" she identified, the types of providers who hold different beliefs, and the implications these views had for the care they provided.

> Ideology is an abstract system of ideas mediated by operational philosophies. Operational philosophies are systems of ideas and procedures for implementing therapeutic ideologies under specific institutional conditions. (Strauss et al., 1964, 360)

Scheid, Teresa L. 2004. "Reluctant Managers" and "Ideologies of Care." Pp. 21–61 in *Tie a Knot and Hang On: Providing Mental Health Care in a Turbulent Environment*. Hawthorne, NY: Aldine de Gruyter.

As Strauss et al. (1964, 361) first articulated, beliefs about care make a difference in the treatment provided and in the structure of organizational roles; ideology is critical to understanding "what is done for patients and who does what kind of work." An analysis of providers' treatment ideologies is also critical to understanding their emotional labor, because it is treatment ideology that identifies the operative feeling rules necessary for performance of the clinical role. Ideologies also help providers reconcile conflicting institutional demands. I begin with a general theoretical discussion of the nature and importance of treatment ideologies and then examine where treatment ideologies are acquired and the different sources of beliefs about mental health work. Treatment ideologies encompass the feeling rules that direct clinical work and specify the appropriate role providers "play" as well as their ideal goals of treatment. Treatment ideologies are also central to the work identity of providers.

Treatment ideologies bind people together. Consequently, different ideologies can be a source of conflict between professional groups. Jurisdictional disputes (see Abbott, 1988) revolve around questions of who has the power to decide which model of care a given group or organization ought to pursue. In the second half of the chapter I look at the specific treatment ideologies exhibited by the providers I interviewed, and examine the prevalence of diverse treatment ideologies in the two public sector organizations I studied in-depth. The primary source of data is the qualitative, in-depth interviews in which providers discuss their treatment practices. While I use some information obtained from private clinicians. I focus on the treatment ideologies of those in the public sector who work with clients with severe, persistent illnesses. Not only do these providers work with similar clients, they also face similar institutional and organizational constraints, and these have a bearing on treatment ideologies and practices.

AN EXPLANATION OF TREATMENT IDEOLOGY

I define treatment ideology as the complex set of beliefs health care providers hold about mental health, illness, and treatment (see Scheid, 1994; for my first definition of treatment ideology). These beliefs consist of specific theories about the etiology (cause) of mental illness, the role of the patient, and the validity of various treatments (many of which were discussed in the previous chapter). This definition of treatment ideology is analogous to that of psychiatric ideology developed by Strauss et al. (1964) in their classic study of psychiatric patients. Strauss et al. (ibid., 8) define a psychiatric ideology as "shared or collective sets of psychiatric ideas" about the etiology and treatment of mental illness.[1] Taking this definition a little further, Eaton et al. (1990) define medical ideology as sets of ideas related to diagnoses that have action consequences. That is, medical ideologies guide the treatment decisions and behaviors of practitioners. They tell the provider what to do and how to do it. Luhrmann (2000) provides an excellent account of the treatment ideologies of psychiatric residents. Ideology, which contains both "is" and "ought" properties, "is a set of ideas with affective overtones that describe both the world that is, and the world that ought to be" (Wilson, 1992, 19). In a discussion of how medical professionals do their work, Abbott (1992) also focuses on diagnosis and treatment as central to constructions of appropriate actions. Thus, treatment ideologies are organized around views about mental health and illness.

However, it is important to bear in mind that treatment ideologies are not an individual's beliefs or opinions. Rather, they are the property of a collectivity or organization (see Berger & Luckmann, 1967), and serve the important function of legitimating existing ways of doing things and structural arrangements. Ideologies are the outcomes of complex processes of intersubjective negotiation between individuals (Fine. 1984), and cannot be reduced to individual beliefs or actions. These negotiations generally occur within organizational frameworks (Levitt & March, 1998). The fact that ideologies are collective in nature does not imply that ideological beliefs are not held by individuals. Negotiations between individuals produce organizational classifications and typifications.

> Ideology is both personal and shared. Simultaneously it is a property of the social actor; it is enacted in a relationship, and is a property of the group or community.... In its cognitive and emotive components we see the importance of the actor; in its enactment we see the role of the community, class, or social network. (Fine & Sandstrom, 1993, 32)

The collective site of treatment ideologies is the organization where providers meet, learn, and work. Ideology is an important reference for action; ideologies can guide and channel the specific behaviors and performances of providers as well as have a direct impact on the formal structure of the organization. Consequently, ideologies overlap both conceptually and empirically with aspects of the organization's culture (Goll & Zeltz, 1991). Ideologies bind people together via common beliefs (Le, culture), and help them enact their roles within the organization (Trice & Beyer, 1993). There is a good bit of literature describing how human service workers and organizations produce the relevant characteristics of their clients, which then legitimate a particular response to these clients (Cicourel, 1968; Holstein, 1992; Pfohl, 1978; Salaman, 1980). That is, organizations do not merely *process* people, they produce them as well (Holstein, 1992; Salaman, 1980).

While ideologies are central features of an organization's culture, they can arise from past experiences and interpretations, prior socialization, training, and concrete work experiences. This is especially true of the treatment ideologies that guide clinical work. Professionals come to a given job or organization with a set of treatment ideologies developed through their training and previous occupational experience. The current organization then plays an important role in shaping, or solidifying, previously held beliefs. In this manner, treatment ideologies are reproduced, and may also be an important source of organizational change.

Imagine it is 1986 and a young clinician, fresh from graduate school and clinical rotation at the University of Madison-Wisconsin, where the model for Assertive Community Treatment (ACT) was developed, has joined the staff at a small rural community mental health center in the South, where the primary form of treatment had been inpatient hospitalization and medication. This clinician might be able to introduce the mental health organization to a new treatment ideology, for example, a new way of dealing with chronically mental ill clients in the community. Or the mental health center and its staff may be too set in its ways (organizational inertia), and may resist efforts to change or innovate. The views of the young clinician may be viewed as "utopian" and completely unworkable. Karl Mannheim (1936) distinguished ideologies (which support the status quo) from utopias (which challenge the status quo). Ideologies not only protect established beliefs and practices (legitimation), they can also provide a shield from the "constant threat of discrepancies arising from individual (or sectional) perceptions, or from new 'external' developments" (Thompson, 1980, 229).

In practical terms, young clinicians (such as the one in my example) will probably have to conform to dominant organizational ideologies and practices because they have little power and little choice (Martin, 1992). The organization is not likely to make a risky change to its practices, unless the "new practices are emotionally laden and ideologically appealing" (D'Aunno et al., 1991. 658) or yield some tangible benefit. As will be shown in discussions of managed care in later chapters, financial benefits have had quite an impact on the treatment practices of clinicians in private practice.

My example of the young clinician raises the question of the relationship between the individual and the organization: Which is the primary source of treatment ideology? Two alternative theories explain the source of organizational beliefs and practices (Findlay et al., 1990). The *importation hypothesis* stipulates that organizational practices result from pre-existing attitudes and behaviors of participants. These practices may originate in professional beliefs about appropriate treatment, which are held by groups external to the organization (professional beliefs are an important institutional constraint to which organizations are expected to conform). The alternative to the importation hypothesis is the *homogenization hypothesis,* which argues that participants are largely shaped by the organization. Critical to this hypothesis is the notion of relative power of the organization, and the power held by professionals who work within the organization, the source of many studies of bureaucratic and professional conflict. Organizations attempt to select employees whose perspectives fit within the overall mission of the organization and individuals also seek employment in organizations that appear "like-minded," although of course such choice is constrained by many different factors, such as availability of jobs and the individual's mobility. One of the critical concerns today is whether managed mental health care will limit the power and autonomy of mental health professionals by imposing organizational constraints on treatment. We will look more closely at this issue in the following chapters.

It is also necessary to examine the source of a given belief system and the relative power and status of the group that promotes it. The external environment plays an important role in shaping both organizational ideologies and individual beliefs. The institutional environment (DiMaggio & Powell, 1991; Meyer & Scott, 1983; Zucker, 1987) consists of the normative beliefs and societal preferences for the treatment of mental illness. A concrete example of the effect of the institutional environment is the societal preference for community-based treatment as opposed to custodial care for individuals with mental illness. Popular books such as Goffman's *Asylums* and Kesey's *One Flew Over the Cuckoo's Nest* helped propel deinstitutionalization and the closing of large state asylums in the 1970s (though other factors, such as fiscal reform and the development of psychotropic drugs were also critical). In order to maintain legitimacy and ultimately to secure resources from the external environment, mental health care organizations must conform to institutional expectations about appropriate mental health care. For example, Ziegenfuss (1983) examined organizational congruence with new environmental pressures that emphasized patient's rights. In the 1970s it was difficult to offer mentally ill people anything more than hospitalization, while currently, it is very difficult to commit an individual to a hospital.

In addition to broad societal normative beliefs, professional norms and practices also constitute an important source of treatment ideology. Hasenfeld (1992) has referred to the beliefs that justify services offered to clients by providers as practice ideologies; obviously, practice and treatment ideologies are analogous concepts. Professional and community standards may converge, diverge, or there may be a lag between the two. There is also likely to be conflict between different professional groups working with the same type of clients or in the same organization. Mental health care providers come from diverse professional backgrounds: psychiatry, psychology, social work, and nursing being the most common fields. Because definitions of mental illness and effective treatment are ambiguous (Mechanic, 1986) different professional groups often hold contradictory ideologies. Meyerson (1991) found that social workers in hospital settings experienced contradictions between medical and psychosocial practices, and between detachment and involvement with clients. Given the diverse sources of treatment ideologies in a given organization, there may well be a "multiplicity of ideologies" that are not "necessarily logically consistent" (Trice & Beyer, 1993, 37). Consequently, Hasenfeld (1992, 14) has described mental health organizations as "rich in ideologies and poor in effective technologies." Psychiatrists and nurses may be more likely to emphasize a biomedical view of mental illness, social workers may accept rehabilitation, and counselors and psychologists may believe psychotherapy is the most effective way to deal with mental illness. Furthermore, as Meyerson (1991) found, contradictory beliefs can be held by individuals of the same profession.

Within the psychiatric and social work literatures, theories about the treatment of mental illness are numerous and reflect different schools of thought about the etiology of mental illness. These theories result in competing counseling models. The concept of a model is more restrictive than that of a treatment ideology and refers to specific procedures or approaches that need not be legitimated by the organization or others with whom one works. MacDonald (1991) describes 18 counseling models in mental health. The larger number of models correspond to existing treatment approaches described in textbooks on psychotherapy or mental health care, and vary from profession to profession. As Benner (1984) has shown with respect to nurses, theoretical belief systems are modified by practical work experiences. In the mental health field a therapist may prefer existential humanism, but may find that this approach does not work well with individuals with chronic mental illnesses and problems with living. It is important to keep in mind that models can be held by individuals and need not be affirmed by coworkers while treatment ideologies are a collective property. Treatment ideologies (as opposed to models or beliefs) consist of a set of beliefs linking evaluations with behavior (Fine & Sandstrom, 1993) and hence have consequences for the prevailing organizational structure.

The literature on treatment practices relies upon constructs based upon established models of care, and does not adequately explore the beliefs about the etiology of illness and treatment underlying these models. An exception is MacDonald (1991), who describes the philosophical orientations that underpin the 18 models of treatment. These philosophies are based upon different domain assumptions about the source of mental illness (the individual or the social environment) and the individual responsible for subsequent changes in the client (self or others).[2] These assumptions about etiology and treatment determine specific treatment ideologies. Heaney and Burke (1995) use data collected from employees at group homes to argue that normalization as a pervasive ideology of care is the guiding ideology for community residential care.

To summarize the discussion thus far, treatment ideologies are shaped by cultural, social, professional, and organizational contexts. Treatment ideologies shape treatment decisions and practices and specify the feeling rules to which providers will attempt to adhere. Consequently treatment ideologies direct the emotional labor of providers and influence the care received by the client. I now turn to the empirical description of the treatment ideologies held by the providers I have interviewed in-depth.

TREATMENT IDEOLOGY SPECIFICATION OF ROLES AND GOALS

In earlier work I developed a typology of treatment ideologies (Scheid, 1994) from in-depth interviews with providers, as well as from the literature on mental health treatment. The typology is based upon two axes, which represent the domain assumptions about two fundamental questions. The first question concerns the appropriate role for the provider. That is, how does the provider behave toward the client? A given role specifies the feeling rules and attitude a provider will assume with their client. Will the provider act as a parent or a friend? A caretaker or an advocate? The second question concerns the goal of treatment. What does the provider work toward? What constitutes success? A provider's treatment role, as well as the goal of treatment, will vary from client to client. However, since the providers I interviewed worked primarily with clients with severe, persistent mental illnesses, some commonality in terms of treatment ideology is to be expected.

There are three possible roles that the mental health provider can take: custodial, supportive, or facilitative. Many providers working in inpatient organizations or institutionalized settings (Goffman, 1961) would describe their role as primarily custodial (though they may not fully embrace this role). The primary function of a custodial role is to meet the client's basic needs and to maintain a sense of order in the institutional environment. A custodial role can also be found in outpatient settings; many providers working in partial hospitalization or clubhouses find themselves playing a custodial role, and treat their clients as young children in need of constant supervision and care. Often such care consists of regulating the clients' behavior.

I am in the role of being the heavy, like no—you have to take your meds in front of us. I'm sorry if they make you tired, if you don't do it I'm going to call your probation office. (Male rehabilitation counselor in a supported employment program)

Providers may also see their role as primarily supportive; they provide ongoing assistance to their clients. Supportive providers help the clients meet their basic social needs, such as finding a job or a place to live. They may help the clients shop for groceries or perform routine housekeeping chores. Often support consists of merely listening, or being there when the clients need someone. The provider's supportive role is central to the case management model, and emphasizes brokerage (or management) functions.

We are the mediators. We do the really hard work. We spend time with these folks, we're the ones that have to negotiate what these people really need, like an apartment. It takes an enormous amount of energy. (Female MSW case manager)

Finally, providers may see their role as facilitating or enabling the clients to meet their treatment goals. Here the client is responsible for achieving a measure of success, but the providers facilitate that process in whatever way they can. Facilitative roles were predominant among providers in private practice; over two-thirds used the word "facilitator" to describe their role. One provider in practice defined this facilitative role as one who is a "motivator to look at options in life and then support the process." Another saw herself as a "cheerleader—I get them to go even when they are too depressed to get themselves out of bed." However, the facilitator role is also common among providers in the public sector.

The second dimension along which treatment ideologies can be arrayed is the appropriate goal of treatment. There are three possible goals: control, adjustment, or autonomy. Treatment may be oriented toward control of the client, such as involuntary commitment, use of restraints, or use of medications to tranquilize a client. Generally the goal of such treatment is to prevent the client from being "a nuisance to the community" or to "help them to stay out of trouble with the law" or, more seriously, to keep them from harming themselves or others.

More often the intended outcome of treatment is to adjust the client to the social world of the mental health organization or the larger community. Providers want their clients to achieve stability in the community, to conform to wider expectations, or to at least appear normal. The term *stabilization* was used by a majority of providers in public practice when asked to describe their treatment goals. They used this term to mean keeping the client "out of the hospital, stabilized on medications, able to function in a more independent living environment, and to have more effective social interactions."

The third treatment goal is autonomy, Providers want clients to gain increasing control over their lives and thus have greater opportunities for independent choice. Rather than maintaining the clients, the provider prefers that clients no longer need mental health care, or that they will be "able to live in a place of their own choice and [be] comfortable with the mental and physical resources" available to him or her. Often this means that clients will have some tolerance of, or insight into, their illnesses as a means of controlling the illness and their lives. Once again, providers in private practice were more likely to stress autonomy as the goal of treatment, and they generally said that only the client could determine the appropriate goal of treatment. As one provider said, "It depends on the goal of the client."

Both dimensions can be seen as stages in a continuum of treatments, and a given provider can serve different roles with different clients, or may assume these different roles with the same client. Clients may begin their treatment career needing to be controlled; hence the providers must play a custodial role. The clients may then "progress" to the point where they are working toward greater community adjustment, and the providers begin to play a supportive role. Finally, the client may move to a stage at which they can assume greater autonomy, and then the providers may become facilitators, or advisors, no longer providing support, but offering a different type of guidance. However, while the goal of treatment may change with each client, or as a given client makes "progress," providers likely feel most comfortable in one type of role regardless of the treatment goal. Facilitators are not likely to enjoy having to pay a more supportive or custodial role, and a supportive provider may lack the skills to become a facilitator. While social roles are acquired via social interaction, a provider's personal inclination makes some roles difficult to assume, raising the question of the relationship of emotional labor and identity.

Figure 1 shows the underlying dimensions of treatment ideologies (treatment roles and goals) arrayed in a typology, with the corresponding treatment

	ROLE OF THE PROVIDER		
TREATMENT GOALS			
	CUSTODIAL	SUPPORTIVE	FACILITATIVE
CONTROL	Coercive	Guardianship	Authorization
ADJUSTMENT	Supervisory	Caretaking	Reparenting
AUTONOMY	Enforcement	Normalization	Empowerment

Figure 1 Typology of Treatment Ideologies

ideology identified. (An earlier version of this typology was presented in Scheid, 1994.) Some custodial providers act as agents of social control, and adhere to a coercive treatment ideology. They are likely to be found in inpatient settings, jails, or other institutions based on overt social control. Many of the providers interviewed had previously worked on inpatient units, and described the coercive ideologies prevalent in "asylums,"

> We put them in straps and leathers, we shot them up, and not just thorazine and haldol, but sodium phenithol... you're talking about a fifty-bed unit with six staff. It was like a jail. No treatment, no behavior problems, just march them in and march them out. (Female nurse case manager)

However, coercive treatment ideologies can also be found in outpatient settings (Estroff, 1981; Goldin, 1990; Teram, 1991). Many of the providers in my research on outpatient commitment liked the law because it gave them more "control" over clients, it was a way to "twist their arm" and provided needed "leverage" in therapy (Scheid-Cook, 1991; Scheid, 1993). Providers who were critical of outpatient commitment felt that it didn't provide them with enough control over their clients; they "wished there were more teeth to enforce compliance." Case managers interviewed in the 1990s also sometimes took on more coercive ideologies, even though they saw their role as caring. "You have this caring relationship with them, and you just say. 'You have to do this'."

Alternatively, custodial providers may also work toward greater adjustment of the client, and hence adhere to a treatment ideology that is coercive rather than supervisory. These providers work to ensure that their clients do not get into trouble whether in the hospital, in the community, or at work, and view their clients as in need of a good deal of supervision. Many of the providers I interviewed about outpatient commitment felt that the law "worked" because it helped them to supervise their clients in the community more closely. More recently, some providers interviewed in the 1990s found they had to assume a supervisory role with their substance abuse clients, though generally they were not comfortable with this role.[3] A supervisory role was especially likely where the provider also functioned as a payee, or worked closely with the client's payee. A payee is the individual who controls the clients' financial resources, primarily because the clients have not acted responsibly with their money, or are likely to spend it on drugs or alcohol.

Custodial providers may also seek greater autonomy for their clients, within the confines of a given institutional space. These providers act as enforcers, giving the clients all possible freedom within a given set of organizational constraints and rules. For example, some providers work with clients who are so severely disabled, either physically, emotionally, or cognitively, that they need ongoing custodial support, yet the clients are still able to exercise autonomous choice within that institutional space once their basic daily needs are met. In this case, providers act as agents of enforcement and ensure that clients do not stray too far afield. One case manager described the situation of being "an enforcer" in the following way:

> We are more willing to take chances with people...okay...you want to take your meds a little less often in front of us...okay...we'll give you a chance to do that, it's your life, not our life, but bear in mind, if you get sick and start acting weird, we are going to go to court against you, or call your probation officer. (Male MA case manager)

The client is granted autonomy, but the provider must enforce the boundaries around that sphere of autonomy.

Looking at the second column of the typology we have provider roles that entail a more supportive stance toward their clients. When dealing with clients who need control, these providers adhere to a treatment ideology described as guardianship. Such providers attempt to watch over their clients to help them eliminate the types of behavior that calls forth a coercive response such as forced medication, restraints, or commitment. Under a guardianship ideology, such responses would be used reluctantly, but would be viewed as necessary for the client. However, the provider tries to watch over the client and protect them from such harsh measures. Accordingly, the provider acts in a kind and benevolent manner. The following example comes from a provider's previous experience in an inpatient unit:

> I knew very soon I wasn't going to help anybody, I mean, we had someone who was on 2400 milligrams of thorazine a day...I wasn't going to change them, or help them. But I decided if I could be kind to them that's really something for them. Because the staff was abusive, and power hungry. To be in a supportive role is so much nicer. (Female nurse case manager)

Supportive providers are more comfortable seeking greater adjustment for their clients, and describe their treatment ideology as one of caretaking. Caretakers monitor medications and behavior, work to stabilize their clients in the community, and provide needed supports. Caretakers want to provide a haven for their clients either as an inpatient or outpatient, and will work within their organization to offer a variety of programs such as drop-in centers or clubhouses, that give clients a sense of belonging.

> This is the only place where some of them get physically touched—this is a place to get love—we're not going to put all these people back to work, back into the community. (Female rehab worker in a clubhouse)

A caretaking ideology seeks to develop settings where clients can be accepted for who they are. "We don't try to make them do things they don't want to, here they get what they need without a lot of stress." Caretakers see treatment as involving "a lot of support, encouragement, listening, and trust building." Their clients

> need the security of knowing somebody's there. I don't put a lot of energy into trying to change people. Often I don't say anything, just listening is needed. (Female MSW case manager)

Caretakers spend a lot of time ensuring that their clients' needs are met. Their goal is to "help them [the clients] become more functional in the community, deal with their hygiene, make sure they have food, that sort of thing, helping them to stay out of trouble with the law, find them places to live" (Female case manager).

Normalization refers to treatment techniques that result in behaviors characterized as socially normative. Under a normalization ideology the ultimate goal of treatment is community adjustment; clients are expected to resume normal lives in the community. Hence, much of the work of the provider oriented toward helping the client obtain income and housing that would enable them to live independently.

> I see how far people can go if they have a roof over their heads and their basic needs are cared for, then they can go and think about other things, like volunteer work. (Female rehab counselor)

Treatment often consists of socialization, or teaching clients social norms, needed skills, and ultimately the social control needed to fit into existing social roles. While supportive, the provider respects the client's autonomy.

> Just because you have a mental illness you don't lose the right to self-determination…We try to be as non-directive as possible in terms of making some life decisions…we would rather assist people in developing skills rather than force people to do what we want…we write plans for the client. (Male MSW supervisor and case manager)

Furthermore, providers adhering to a normalization ideology want their clients' "level of involvement with the mental health system to be less and less." In contrast, caretakers are more likely to see themselves playing a long-term role in their clients' lives; they "don't close charts anymore," since their clients are not expected to move on: "We're not going to put all these people back into the community."

The facilitative provider is most likely to see clients as partners in the treatment process. If the goal is control, the treatment ideology may be one of authorization. The provider works with the clients to teach them how the system works, to enlighten them as to the nature of their predicament and why others in society perceive them as needing social control. Facilitative providers are very likely to be uncomfortable with clients who need overt social control, but may find themselves in treatment settings where social control is an issue. Adolescent units and residential treatment settings often have clients who need to learn more social control, yet the role of the provider is more facilitative than supportive or coercive. Authorizers develop a trusting relationship with their clients, "so that they will do what they need." They may see medication as a means to control the symptoms of mental illness, but will work with their clients to educate them about their illness and need for medication.

If the goal of treatment is adjustment, facilitative providers often take on the role of quasiparents. Reparenting ideologies can be difficult to distinguish from caretaking ones, largely because of the wide variety of parenting styles. While "parents" do provide care, caretaking is viewed as a necessary evil and as only a temporary stage in the treatment process. They want the client to grow up and move out, and are critical of caretakers:

> Many people get into this field as caretakers. We do too much caretaking—we don't do enough to make them independent—teach them skills and appropriate behaviors, such as not picking your nose in public. (Female case manager)

Quasiparents argue that clients need fewer supportive services and more skills training; clients need to be taught to do things on their own. Rather than being walked through the system, clients need to be "pointed in the right direction" and if necessary given "a push." They need to learn certain behaviors that are necessary to functioning successfully or to adjust to the community.

> Reparenting is...we are going to teach you to clean your body, when you can do that you can go on a pass. Oops! You got drunk—you lose your privileges for a month. I'm sorry, you still have to brush your teeth and clear your room. You learn a new skill, you can go out again...You learn ten new skills and you can move up a level. (Male MA case manager)

As this quote illustrates, quasiparents do not generally grant their clients as much autonomy as providers who advocate normalization or empowerment. The quasiparent knows what is best for the client, or what the client needs, and tries to get the client "to move in the *right* direction."

> I try to work with that person...working toward what they see as their goals...sometimes pushing them to feel what that is, influencing them in a direction that I think is best...and sometimes I think that's a little invasive, but I try to use my relationship with them to facilitate growth. (Male MSW case manager)

Reparenting does not engender the long-term dependency that the other treatment ideologies do; the client is expected to make progress and move on.

> I see us becoming more of a teaching model than a case management model. We are not going to get people very far in life without teaching them skills. (Female MA case manager)

This quote also illustrates the conflict between the ideals of care versus cure; providers want to see their clients' progress toward greater independence and less reliance on the mental health system. The ideologies of caretaking and reparenting reflect the conflict between the mandates to care for clients or to cure them. While both caretakers and parents adhere to the biopsychosocial model of mental health, they hold different views about their roles and the goals of treatment (reflecting the contradictions inherent in the model of community-based care) and were often critical of one another.

An empowerment treatment ideology seeks greater client control over mental health services, if not complete independence from the mental health system. Empowerment explicitly rejects the idea of clinical intervention (Paulson, 1992). Instead it strives to enable clients to obtain those resources that give them control over their environments (Hasenfeld & Chesler, 1989).

> I believe in being equal to clients. I mean they are the professionals in their lives, not me...and I think you need to empower clients, and if you (the client) are less of a person than I am, I'm not doing anybody any good. (Female MA case manager)

With the advent of empowerment ideologies, empowered clients are now called by the politically correct term *consumers*.

> As a team we need to find ways to help the consumer participate in treatment, to take more responsibility and authority, with us as consultants rather than treatment that is *done* to them. (Male MSW case manager)

Rather than being socialized, or re-socialized, consumers are entrusted and authorized to assume control for their own lives and providers trust them to do so. Consumers set their own goals, and are encouraged to have a role in making decisions about service offerings and other critical organizational areas. As one provider described,

> I figure out what I can do for them, not to do it for them, but trying to get them to take responsibility for themselves. My background is really strong on

consumer rights and responsibilities. I agree that people have a "right to fail" so you learn from your mistakes. We don't need to encourage dependence, but independence. I have been shocked at the lack of consumer involvement here in decision making. (Female MA case manager)

Ultimately, empowerment has the potential to challenge the status quo of mental health treatment and lead to radically new ways of understanding and approaching the treatment of mental illness. However, while much lip service has been paid to empowerment, most mental health organizations have not really involved consumers as autonomous agents in the organizational decision making processes. As one treatment team supervisor noted:

I've seen a shift in talking about consumer involvement and client choice, and I'm not exactly sure how—but hopefully we can integrate that a little more by getting staff to value that more.

Providers who grant their clients autonomy are more likely to adhere to a normalization ideology. One provider who referred to himself as a "Shepherd" notes that

it's my job to help persons think through what they want to accomplish, and how they might go about that, and so I see myself as herding now and then to help them maintain independent living. (Male MA case manager)

While such providers grant some autonomy, the client is not fully empowered or entitled to self-determination.

TREATMENT IDEOLOGIES IN PRACTICE

Having delineated the different treatment ideologies at the theoretical level, I will examine empirically the prevalence of these ideologies among providers and within specific organizational contexts, focusing on data obtained from in-depth interviews with providers in the two public sector mental health programs. Specific organizational practices and service interventions are "an enactment of the organization's practice ideology" (Hasenfeld, 1992, 13). Different treatment ideologies will result in distinct treatment technologies and service interventions, and these have a direct impact on both client level outcomes and providers' evaluations of an organization's effectiveness. Diverse treatment ideologies point to considerable disagreement about organizational goals (referred to as goal incongruence) as well as to potential conflict between different groups of providers.

It is important to keep in mind that the treatment ideologies identified by the typology are ideal types (Weber, 1946), that is, they are analytical constructs that help us to conceptualize empirical reality. Individuals will espouse elements of different ideologies, although it is possible to determine what kind of ideology a provider is most comfortable with, or has utilized in the past. In-depth interviews give a heightened sense of a provider's preferred, or actualized, treatment ideology. Often the critical incidents provide important clues as to how the provider prefers to act.

Table 1 presents the predominant treatment ideologies of the providers interviewed at the CARE ($n = 21$) and SUPPORT ($n = 14$). I eliminated one psychiatric technician from this analysis who worked on the crisis stabilization unit at CARE. Not surprisingly, this individual expressed a treatment ideology consistent with the need for social control even though she saw herself in a facilitative role. The majority of the providers are case managers, although some perform more psychosocial rehabilitation services such as housing or employment than case management per se. In addition to noting the organization in which the provider worked I also examine treatment ideology in terms of gender and professional role. All eight African Americans worked with CARE and hence it would be difficult to protect their identity if race were also a factor.

Given that the research was collected in outpatient settings, very few providers adhered to primarily custodial roles, or sought control of their clients. Those that articulated some elements of these ideologies ($n = 3$) were all male, over 45, and worked in a position where control, or a custodial role, was necessary (i.e., partial hospitalization—which is a day program—or a jail diversion program). Given that treatment ideologies are properties of a collectivity, these two mental health organizations exhibit cohesion around those treatment ideologies that are consistent with outpatient, community-based treatment, which is an important institutional demand. Community-based care postulates both adjustment and autonomy for clients' care as well as cure. Furthermore, providers can be both supportive and facilitative in their relations with clients. Often the role and the specific goal depend on the client.

> The endpoint is the best possible functioning and independence...symptom free, or at least have a level of symptoms that will let them get on with their life...there are times when we have to take control, but I think that is painful for staff, so we avoid taking too much control and try to give it back when that's possible. (Male MSW supervisor)

Generally, the first treatment goal for a client is adjustment. Most providers hope that clients will move to greater autonomy and self-determination, although some never talk about clients gaining control over their lives. While the ideologies can be thought of as a continuum (with greater freedom at the ends of the axis) providers do not view all ideologies as equally valid. Thus there is potential for interorganizational conflict.

In both mental health organizations, more providers adhered to a normalization treatment ideology (36 percent at SUPPORT and 38 percent at CARE); followed by 29 percent of those at SUPPORT being more likely to articulate a reparenting ideology and 33.3 percent of those at CARE holding a caretaking

Table 1 Analysis of Treatment Ideologies (percentages: $n = 35$ providers)

Treatment Ideology	Organization		Gender		Occupation			
	Care (14)	Support (21)	Male (14)	Female (21)	Case-Mgr (22)	Nurse (7)	Rehab (4)	Other (2)
Custodial								
Coercive (0)								
Supervisory (0)								
Enforcement (0)								
Supportive								
Guardianship (0)								
Care-taking (9)	14%	33%	7%	38%	14%	71%	—	50%
Normalization (14)	36	38	43	33	27	29	100	50
Facilitative								
Authorization (1)	0	5.0	7.0		5.0			
Reparenting (7)	29	14	29	14	32			
Empowerment (5)	21	10	14	14	23			

ideology. This difference may be due to gender as opposed to organizational philosophy. Twenty-eight percent of the providers interviewed at CARE were male, and 57 percent of the providers at SUPPORT were male (which matches the overall demographic distribution at these sites); overall 60 percent of the providers were female and 40 percent were male. Male providers were more likely to espouse a normalization ideology (43 percent), followed by reparenting (29 percent). Female providers were most likely to adhere to a caretaking ideology (38 percent) followed by normalization (33 percent).

In terms of professional backgrounds, all of the providers who saw their roles as facilitators were case managers, which is not surprising given their role duties. Providers who adhered to normalization were more likely to be case managers (27 percent), or rehabilitation workers (28 percent). In large part due to their professional training and holistic orientation, nurses were more likely to adhere to a caretaking model (71 percent); the one male caretaker was also a nurse—the only male nurse in the sample. This supports much of the literature on the caregiving orientation of the nursing profession (Chambliss, 1996).

Although the data are merely exploratory, they demonstrate the ways in which providers have "enacted" the broader institutional demands for community-based care. The majority of the providers adhere to treatment ideologies that are consistent with the principles of community-based cater caretaking, reparenting, normalization, and empowerment. There is evidence of conflict between institutional demands for care as opposed to cure, normalization as opposed to empowerment. Case managers were far more likely to assume a facilitative role, nurses a supportive role. We might therefore expect case managers and therapists to be more frustrated by the caretaking needs of their clients, and some evidence of this was found in the quote cited above.

We can also expect treatment ideologies to change over time within specific organizational settings in response to the changing institutional demands for care described in the previous chapter. The surveys at CARE used two open-ended questions I used in prior research to determine the treatment ideology of providers. First, I asked providers to identify their treatment objectives or goals: "In your opinion, given your existing caseload, what constitutes successful care or treatment of a client?" Second, I asked them to describe their role with clients: "I must assume the role of a (please provide a descriptor for how you see your role in the relationship with your clients)." From the responses to these two questions I categorized provider's treatment ideologies. Unfortunately, not all providers answered both questions, and many providers described their role in terms of their occupational role (i.e., nurse or social worker) so the data are limited. Although the providers' brief responses to these two questions do not reflect the complexity of their treatment ideologies, this analysis does give us some insight into changes in treatment ideologies over time.

I first look at changes from 1998 to 2000 in providers' descriptions of successful care or treatment because they were more developed than their descriptions of their role. The responses were easily classified into the three categories described earlier: control, adjustment, and autonomy. In 1998, 26 providers completed well-developed answers describing their role, and in 2000, 27 providers did. Control goals emphasized stability: providers wanted their clients "stabilized on medications, educated about illness and medications" (1998, #62). Several providers mentioned "management in a facility." Other providers talked more directly about "client compliance" as a treatment goal (2000, #54). Adjustment meant:

> Linking clients with all possible services, the ability to ensure follow through and satisfaction with services, the client is able to live in a place on their own and have their basic needs met. (1998, #30)

Autonomy was achieved if the client moved to greater independence:

> If they demonstrate less dependence on the system and move to a more independent living environment, or become an active participant in their treatment. (2000, #69)

The number of providers indicating their treatment goal was client adjustment remained stable at 17 in 1998 and 16 in 2000. However, the number of providers indicating coercive treatment goals dropped from 7 to 2, while the number of providers seeking greater autonomy for their clients increased from 2 to 9.

Table 2 compares changes in the treatment objectives of providers at CARE between 1990 and 2000. In 1990, normalization was the most prevalent treatment ideology at CARE (36 percent), in 2000 caretaking (28 percent) and reparenting (28 percent) are slightly more prevalent than normalization (24 percent). Providers were somewhat less likely to articulate empowerment in 2000, although they did seek greater autonomy for their clients. This may be a reflection of an increasingly bureaucratic system of care that has disempowered providers.

Table 2 Changes in Treatment Objectives at CARE (%).

Treatment Ideology	1990 (N=14)	2000 (N=25)
Caretaking	14%	28%
Normalization	36	24
Authorization	0	4
Reparenting	29	28
Empowerment	21	16

CONCLUDING POINTS

I begin with the caveat that the typology of treatment ideologies developed in this chapter is not fixed and is not intended to represent all potential ideologies about the treatment of those with serious mental illness. It is historically framed by the institutional expectations and demands (rational myths) about the treatment and care of individuals with serious mental illness that prevailed in the 1980s and 1990s, (when the data were collected). As with ideal types in general (Weber, 1946), when the institutional environment changes, the range of potential ideologies may change as well to reflect new conditions and demands. (See Scott et al., 2000; for an excellent discussion of the effects of changing institutional environments on health care.)

Given that the institutional environment dictates psychosocial rehabilitation, and case management is viewed as the best means to achieve community integration for clients with severe mental illness, it is not surprising that the two mental health organizations studied exhibited treatment ideologies largely consistent with these institutional demands. Yet within the spacious framework of psychosocial rehabilitation, providers did enact more specific ideologies with differing emphasis on the degree of autonomy granted to the clients, and the type of assistance the provider offered to help clients meet these goals. Furthermore, treatment ideologies were clearly properties of the treatment team, or organizational unit in which providers worked. They were generally described in terms of the way "we do things" around here, and "different agencies do have different perspectives on what their obligations are to clients." Thus, providers articulated instances when their own preferences conflicted with those of the wider group or organization.

There was not much evidence of homogenization. At neither site did providers receive much informal indoctrination; instead most "imported" their models of care. This was particularly evident at SUPPORT, where the majority of providers had MSWs from a nearby university. However, there is as much variability in specific treatment ideologies at SUPPORT as there is at CARE, where many providers lacked a master's degree and came from different educational and occupational backgrounds. This similarity in the type and variability of treatment ideology underscores the importance of the institutional environment, the two organizations' commitment to providing innovative, community-based care, and the degree of autonomy granted to mental health workers in these two sites.

While the treatment ideologies espoused at SUPPORT and CARE are consistent with broad institutional mandates for community-based care, the potential for conflict over the best means to achieve such care remains. In particular, providers who advocate empowerment and greater consumer control are in conflict with those providers who see clients as needing greater direction and guidance (or even control). Evidence showed the dilemma faced by providers who must choose between merely managing the care provided to a client and moving clients along in their development. Few of the providers felt their clients needed therapy; instead they viewed their clients' needs from within the framework of community-based care. Case management was viewed as the primary means to provide necessary care, and was not seen as merely a means to manage care. Individuals with serious mental illnesses need a broad array of community supports, and providers recognized the critical role they played coordinating those services. Many had also been socialized to believe (or had learned from experience) that therapy by itself simply did not work with clients with severe mental illnesses. One MSW provider stated quite bluntly that her previous counseling sessions with schizophrenics "were one hour of torture." However, some providers felt that they relied on medication too heavily and that more therapy was needed.

There was some diversity of treatment ideologies within each organization, indicating the potential for conflict over service offerings and treatment technologies. At both organizations providers disagreed over the need for supported employment versus day treatment programs, extended community outreach versus specialized programs for particular client groups, medication compliance versus the right to refuse medications, and the feasibility of consumer-run services. These choices are necessitated by restricted resources. With managed care, the restriction of services forces providers to make hard choices about different service offerings. (In the words of one provider. "Taxpayers aren't willing to support more programs such as this.") Furthermore, those services that demonstrate proven outcomes are given the greatest preference. The outcome of debates over the type of community mental health care that works best will be determined in part by the salience and support for the different treatment ideologies described in this chapter, as well as the new ones that may arise.

ENDNOTES

1. In their study of two psychiatric hospitals, Strauss et al. (1964) identified three philosophies: soma to the rapeutic (or organic), psychotherapeutic, and millen or sociotherapeutic (environmental). It is clear these philosophies correspond to the biomedical, psychosocial, and social models described in the previous chapter. Strauss et al. (1964) also described a polarity between ideologies that emphasized treatment, as opposed to custodial care, arguing that the problems of chronic illness required moral (as opposed to merely medical) considerations. In a later work Strauss et al. (1985) focus on how chronic illness changes the practice of medicine and care Kleinman (1988) has also argued that the medical model is inappropriate for chronic illness.

2. McDonald (1991) also argues that in order for treatment to be effective there must be a match between a client and his/her provider in terms of their domain assumptions. As noted by Broman et al. (1994) a mismatch between the goals and expectations of the provider and the client may well lead to poor outcomes.

3. It is interesting that both CARE and SUPPORT used outpatient commitment for clients with substance abuse problems.

References

Abbott, Andrew. 1988. *The System of Professions*. Chicago: University of Chicago Press.

———. 1992. "Professional Work." Pp. 145–162 in *Human Services as Complex Organizations*, edited by Y. Hasenfeld. Newbury Park, CA: Sage.

Benner, Patricia. 1984. *From Notice to Expert: Excellence and Power in Clinical Nursing Practice*. Menlo Park, CA: Addison–Wesley.

Berger, Peter and Thomas Luckman. 1967. *The Social Construction of Reality*. New York: Anchor Books.

Chambliss, Daniel. 1996. *Beyond Caring: Hospitals, Nurses, and the Social Organization of Ethics*. Chicago: University of Chicago Press.

Cicourel, Aaron V. 1968. *Method and Measurement in Sociology*. New York: The Free Press.

D'Aunno, Thomas. 1992. "The Effectiveness of Human Service Organizations: A Comparison of Models." Pp. 341–361 in *Human Services as Complex Organizations*, edited by Y. Hasenfeld. Newbury Park, CA: Sage.

Eaton, William, Christian Ritter, and Diane Brown. 1990. "Psychiatric Epidemiology and Psychiatric Sociology: Influences on the Recognition of Bizarre Behaviors as Social Problems." Pp. 41–68 in *Research in Community Mental Health* (Vol 6), edited by James R. Greenley. Greenwich, CT: JAI Press.

Estroff, Sue E. 1981. *Making it Crazy: An Ethnography of Psychiatric Patients in an American Community*. Berkeley, CA: University of California Press.

Findlay, William, Elizabeth Mutran, Redney Zeitler, and Christina Randall. 1990. "Queues and Care: How Medical Residents Organize Their Work in a Busy Clinic." *Journal of Health and Social Behavior* 31: 292–305.

Fine, Gary A. 1984. "Negotiated Orders and Organizational Cultures." *Annual Review of Sociology* 19: 239–262.

———, and Kent L. Sandstrom. 1993. "Ideology in Action: A Pragmatic Approach to a Contested Concept." *Sociological Theory* 11: 21–38.

Goffman, Irving. 1961. *Asylums*. New York: Anchor Books.

Goldin, Carol S. 1990. "Stigma, Biomedical Efficacy and Institutional Control." *Social Science and Medicine* 30: 895–900.

Goll, Irene and Gerald Zeitz. 1991. "Conceptualizing and Measuring Corporate Ideology." *Organization Studies* 12: 191–207.

Hasenfeld, Yeheskel (ed.). 1992. *Human Services as Complex Organizations*. Newbury Park, CA: Sage.

——— and Mark A. Chesler. 1989. "Client Empowerment and the Human Services: Personal and Professional Agendas." *Human Relations* 25: 499–521.

Heaney, C. A. and A. C. Burke. 1995. "Ideologies of Care in Community Residential Services: What Do Caregivers Believe?" *Community Mental Health Journal* 31: 449–462.

Holstein, James A. 1992. "Producing People: Descriptive Practice in Social Work." *Current Research in Occupations and Professions* 7: 23–39.

Levitt, Brian and James G. March. 1998. "Organizational Learning." *Annual Review of Sociology* 14: 319–340.

Luhrmann, T. M. 2000. *Of Two Minds: The Growing Disorder in American Psychiatry*. New York: Alfred Knopf.

MacDonald, Don. 1991. "Philosophies that Underlie Models of Mental Health Counseling More Than Meets the Eye." *Journal of Mental Health Counseling* 13: 379–392.

Mannhein, Karl. 1936. *Ideology and <ill/> An Introduction to the Sociology of Knowledge.* New York: Harcourt Brace Publishers.

Martin, Joanne. 1992. *Cultures in Organizations: Three Perspectives.* New York: Oxford.

John W. Meyer and W. Richard Scott. 1983. *Organizational Environments: Ritual and Rationality.* Beverly Hills: Sage.

Mechanic D. 1986. "The Challenge of Chronic Mental Illness: A Retrospective and Prospective View." *Hospital and Community Psychiatry* 37: 891–896.

Meyerson, Debra E. 1991. "Normal Ambiguity: A Glimpse of an Occupational Culture." Pp. 131–156 in *Reframing Organizational Culture,* edited by P. J. Frost, L. F. Moore, M. R. Louis, C. Lundenberg, and J. Martin. Newbury Park, CA: Sage.

Paulson, R. 1992. "Advocacy and Empowerment: Mental Health Care in the Community." *Community Mental Health Journal* 28: 70–71.

Pfohl, Stephan, J. 1978. *Predicting Dangerousness: The Social Construction of Psychiatric Reality.* Lexington, MA: Lexington Books.

Powell, Walter W. and Paul J. DiMaggio. 1991. "Introduction." Pp. 1–38 in *The New Institutionalism in Organizational Analysis.* Chicago: University of Chicago Press.

Salaman, Graerne. 1980. "Organizations as Constructors of Social Reality." Pp. 237–256 in *Control and Ideology in Organizations,* edited by G. Salaman and K. Thompson. Cambridge, MA: MIT Press.

Scheid, Teresa. 1993. "Controller and Controlled: An Analysis of Participant Constructions of Outpatient Commitment." *Sociology of Health and Illness* 15: 179–193.

———. 1994. "An Explication of Treatment Ideology Among Mental Health Care Providers." *Sociology of Health and Illness* 16: 668–693.

Scheid-Cook, Teresa L. 1991. "Outpatient Commitment as Both Social Control and Least Restrictive Alternative." *Sociological Quarterly* 32:433–460.

Scott, W. Richard, Martin Ruef, Peter Mendel, and Carol A. Caroneer. 2000. *Institutional Change and Organizational Transformation of the Healthcare Field.* Chicago: University of Chicago Press.

Strauss, Anselm, Leonard Schatzman, Rue Burcher, Danuta Ehrlich, and Melvin Sabshin. 1964. *Psychiatric Ideologies and Institutions.* London: The Free Press.

Teram, Eli. 1991. "Interdisciplinary Teams and the Control of Clients: A Socio-Technical Perspective." *Human Relations* 44: 343–356.

Thompson, Kenneth. 1980. "Organizations as Constructors of Social Reality." Pp. 216–236 in *Control and Ideology in Organizations,* edited by G. Salamon and K. Thompson. Cambridge, MA: MIT Press.

Trice, Harrison M. and Janice M. Beyer. 1993. *The Cultures of Work Organizations.* Engelwood Cliffs, NJ: Prentice-Hall.

Weber, Max. 1946. *From Max Weber: Essays in Sociology,* edited and translated by H. H. Gerth and C. W. Mills. Oxford University Press.

Wilson, Richard. 1992. *Compliance Ideologies: Rethinking Political Culture.* Cambridge, MA: Cambridge University Press.

Wilson, Mitchell. 1993. "DSM-III and the Transformation of American Psychiatry." *American Journal of Psychiatry* 150: 399–410.

Zucker, Lynne G. 1987. "Institutional Theories of Organization." *Annual Review of Sociology* 13: 443–464.

DISCUSSION

1. What is a treatment ideology? What were the different ideologies that Scheid identified among the clinicians she interviewed? How do these different ideologies reflect different views about the goals of psychiatric treatment and the role of providers?

2. What types of providers were most likely to hold the different ideologies Scheid identified? What do these patterns tell you about different types of providers? Where and how do you think these providers developed these ideologies? To what extent, and in what ways, do you think these ideologies may be reflected among other psychiatric provider groups and treatment settings?

3. What are the implications of the different ideologies for the quality of care provided to clients? In what ways are these beliefs likely to impact providers' behavior toward their clients? How might these different ideologies influence the clinical outcomes of psychiatric treatment?

MENTAL ILLNESS, THE FAMILY, AND SOCIETY

W hile not generally recognized as a significant societal challenge by the public in the United States, the impact of mental illness on the family and society is extensive and complicated. Many of the early selections in this reader have documented a wide array of psychosocial consequences for individuals labeled with and directly affected by mental disorder. Mental illness, however, can also have a profound impact on the person's family by increasing stress, imposing new caregiving responsibilities, and requiring families to change their behavior and expectations. At the same time, mental illness and the mental health system are deeply intertwined with many of our most significant social problems, especially crime, poverty, and homelessness. The nature of these connections is not always clear and frequently very complicated, and much sociological theory and research has tried in recent years to clarify and disentangle the many complex mechanisms linking mental illness and various social problems. This type of work is critical for informing the development of more effective social programs and policies to address mental illness in society.

Despite the significant challenges mental illness presents for families and society, there are many who see new ways for society to respond to mental illness and address the many-related social challenges. Indeed, over the past three decades, we have witnessed the emergence of both the consumer-survivor and family movements that have challenged us to confront the societal stigma of mental illness and to create a different and more companionate system for addressing mental health problems. Responding to the needs of people with mental illness and their families, however, will require concerted social and political action. The final selections in this reader offer some recent alternative visions for the future of our mental health care system and suggest specific ways we should change how our society responds to those directly and indirectly affected by mental illness.

Mental Illness and the Family

Harriet Lefley

Caregiver Stress and Dimensions of Family Burden[†]

In this selection, Lefley reviews research on the impact of mental illness on the family. Drawing heavily on stress theory, she argues that caregivers experience a wide-variety of stressors. Specifically, she differentiates between the objective and subjective dimensions of burden as well as the gratifications of caregiving and how they factor into how families respond when someone they love develops a mental illness. Her review highlights the many varied forces that shape the families' experience of mental illness.

Hatfield (1987) has pointed out that the effect of mental illness on the family is affected by three major variables:

> (1) where the ill person lives and who is charged for responsibility for his or her care; (2) the meaning of the illness to the family and especially the way in which that meaning is influenced by prevailing theories of etiology; and (3) the degree of understanding, compassion, and support given to affected families and the skill and appropriateness of help offered by the community. (p. 3)

In this chapter, we deal with the multiple sources of stress for family caregivers. To date, the effect of mental illness on caregivers has primarily been viewed in terms of a narrow definition of family burden. This concept has typically been restricted to interactions with the mentally ill relative. There are multiple sources of stress that create a burden for the caregivers of mentally ill individuals—situational, societal, and iatrogenic. Caregiver burden derives not only from the experiential aspects of living with severe mental illness in the family but also from the caregiver's interactions and frustrations with the treatment system, the welfare and legal systems, and an indifferent or stigmatizing society. Conversely, burden can be mitigated, as

Lefley, Harriet. 1996. "Caregiver Stress and Dimensions of Family Burden." Pp. 65–80 in *Family Caregiving in Mental Illness*. Thousand Oaks, CA: Sage.

Hatfield (1987) suggests, by understanding and appropriate help offered by the treatment system and the community at large.

We begin with a discussion of the conceptualization and measurement of family burden as it applies in the case of mental illness. The original distinction between objective and subjective family burden referred respectively to the reality demands of the illness and to the caregivers' distress in reacting to or fulfilling these specific demands. Many researchers, however, consider global emotional distress, whether evidenced somatically or psychologically, as indicative of subjective burden. Emotional distress is manifest as we discuss the experiential aspects of living with someone with severe mental illness, especially within the same household. Various clinical indicators and effects on physical health are discussed and two extremes of the caregiving experience are presented. On the one hand is empirical research on violence in the household, with suggested precipitants and some possible remedies. At the other extreme are a few studies suggesting that some caregivers experience gratifications in this role and the relation of gratification to the clients' behaviors as well as to cultural differences in perceptions of burden. The data presented suggest that psychodynamic aspects of burden seem related to (a) perception of caregiving as normative, (b) the caregivers' mastery of the task, and (c) the level of dysfunction of the mentally ill relative.

Attitudes of the larger society, treatment by mental health professionals, and deficits in the service delivery system can be discrete sources of stress for caregivers. We end this chapter with a current empirically based assessment of caregiver needs before going on to explore the current array of services for families.

CONCEPTUALIZING AND MEASURING FAMILY OR CAREGIVER BURDEN

Schene, Tessler, and Gamache (in press) identified 21 instruments developed to measure caregiver burden in severe mental illness. Almost all researchers made a theoretical distinction between objective and subjective burden. In developing instruments, objective burden has typically been viewed as the number and type of tasks involved in caregiving, with subjective burden the perceived difficulty or distress connected with each task. Some investigators consider symptoms and dysfunction as objective and assess the caregiver's subjective burden in relation to each particular problem associated with the illness. Other researchers also include general measures of subjective burden, such as anger, depression, embarrassment, worrying, and tension, that are not necessarily anchored to measures of objective caregiving.

The analysis by Schene et al. (in press) found that some dimensions are included in almost all instruments. Worrying, the effect of the patient's disorder on family routine, and effects on leisure, distress, and financial consequences are typical. Other dimensions include cognitive preoccupation, feeling threatened, having to change personal plans, and feelings of loss and grief.

Numerous studies have indicated high levels of psychological distress among caregivers of persons with major mental illnesses. Some well-designed studies show figures as high as 75 percent suffering adverse emotional reactions (Scottish Schizophrenia Research Group, 1985). Research on a clinic sample of caregivers in England indicated that both objective and subjective burden measures on a family burden scale were significantly correlated with anxiety, insomnia, and depression scores on clinical scales (Oldridge & Hughes, 1992). Cook (1988) found a high level of emotional distress among both mothers and fathers residing with a mentally ill adult child, with mothers manifesting significantly higher degrees of anxiety, depression, fear, and emotional drain. In an Australian study, Winefield and Harvey (1993) found that caregiver psychological distress was high compared with norms on various standardized measures of adjustment. The level of behavioral disturbance of the mentally ill relative predicted caregiver distress after controlling for the caregiver's age, sex, and social supports. An unexpected finding was that caregivers of female relatives reported greater distress than those caring for male relatives.

Grieving and loss are an often unacknowledged feature of caregiver burden. Miller, Dworkin, Ward, and Barone (1990) found that families of the mentally ill experience a syndrome of grief and mourning very similar to that experienced by others suffering from real or psychic loss. Atkinson (1994) studied grief among parents who had adult children with schizophrenia, parents who had lost an adult child through death, and parents whose child had sustained a head injury that resulted in organic personality disorder. Mean age at first episode or death in all three groups was 21 to 22 years. The research found significant differences in grieving reactions and substance abuse: Parents of schizophrenic adults had more ongoing grieving, whereas parents of adults with head injuries had more substance abuse.

The authors found an inverse grieving pattern for parents of schizophrenic children vis à vis the other parents. The latter had a greater initial grief reaction—because the child either died or was expected to die through head injury. In both cases, the grieving diminished over time. In contrast, parents of schizophrenic children had low initial levels of grieving that rose over time. The researchers found that most of these parents were not told the diagnosis and prognosis but learned it piecemeal over a period of years. The authors concluded that once learned, parental loss of a child through schizophrenia leads to a pattern of chronic grief. They also suggest that the characteristic pattern of exacerbations and remissions in schizophrenia may play a unique role in shaping the parents' reactions.

FAMILIES' EXPERIENCE OF LIVING WITH MENTAL ILLNESS

It is evident that objective burden refers to the reality demands of coping with mental illness and subjective burden to family members' personal suffering as a result of the disorder. Yet years of experience in working with families of mentally ill persons suggest that the existing instruments often fail to capture the extent and psychological effect of either of these dimensions. Examples of objective burden go far beyond mere caregiving responsibilities. They include (a) the mentally ill person's economic dependency and inability to fulfill expected role functions, (b) disruption of household routines, (c) caregivers' investments of time and energy in help-seeking and negotiating the mental health system, (d) confusing and often humiliating interactions with service providers, (e) financial costs of the illness, (f) deprivation of needs of other family members, (g) curtailment of social activities, (h) impaired relations with the outside world, and (i) inability to find appropriate alternatives to hospitalization or facilities for residential placement outside the home.

Subjective burden includes mourning for the premorbld personality, perhaps once bright with promise. In many cases, there is a feeling of dual loss—loss of the person who was and of the person who might have been. There are stressful effects on one's own mental and physical health, feelings of stigmatization, inability to make or fulfill personal plans, empathic suffering for the pain of a loved one, and worries of aging parents about the future of a disabled child who will surely outlive them.

Economic strain, real and attributed stigma, isolation, burnout, and need for respite are widely prevalent aspects of the burden of mental illness in the family. Negative effect on other family members, particularly the young, is an ongoing concern and may result in a need for ancillary interventions and a new generation of psychotherapists' bills.

Behavior management issues are ongoing tensions between mentally ill persons and their family members. Caregivers frequently have to contend with abusive or assaultive behaviors; mood swings and unpredictability; socially offensive or embarrassing situations; negative symptoms of amotivation, apathy, or anhedonia; and conflicts over money likely to be ill managed, squandered, or lost.

Conflicts often arise regarding behaviors disturbing to household living. These include poor personal hygiene and offensive odors in the home, excessive smoking and fire hazards, indifference or actual damage to household property, and sleep reversal patterns that may result in pacing or loud music at odd hours of the night. Relatives' refusal to take their medications is a common area of contention, particularly when there is a known pattern of relapse.

Passive withdrawal and excessive inactivity may be as burdensome to families as acting-out behaviors. A study by Cook (1988) of families of severely mentally ill adults enrolled in a psychosocial rehabilitation agency found chronic worrying among mothers. She states the following:

> A look at their offspring's situations leads to the conclusion that these worries were, well-founded. These were mothers whose children had histories of medication noncompliance and recurrent psychotic episodes accompanied by repeated hospitalizations. They were mothers whose children led socially

impoverished lives, spending large amounts of time alone in their rooms sleeping, being depressed, or living in a fantasy world. (p. 46)

Attentional and information-processing deficits, such as the prolonged silences and delayed reactions of schizophrenia, are frustrating and may be perceived as a lack of human relatedness by family members. Although they may recognize that these are not purposive distancing mechanisms, this interference with normal communication tends to further deprive caregivers of the rewards of human interaction and reciprocity that most people expect from those they love.

Perhaps the most devastating stressor for caregivers of persons with mental illness is learning how to cope with their relative's own suffering over an impoverished life. Persons with long-term mental illness are often acutely aware of their lack of skills, impaired productivity, and poor future prospects. They can see that others of their own age are married, starting families, and finalizing career plans. Typically, they both desire and fear the demands of these roles. For persons who were previously hospitalized, community reintegration poses the threatening need to acquire or relearn vocational or psychosocial coping skills in a competitive environment. Mentally ill persons' own mourning for lost developmental stages of learning, failed aspirations, and restricted lives can be uniquely stressful for those who love them and can feel their pain.

Feelings of helplessness to make things better for their children generate acute suffering in parents of long-term patients. The suffering is compounded by guilt if sympathy alternates with frustration and rage at aversive behavior. Guilt is a theme that often arises in family support groups. With changes in views of psychogenesis, many families have finally learned that they do not have to feel guilty for having caused these devastating disorders in a loved one. Yet there is frequent speculation over whether they are doing the right thing, making the right treatment decisions, or behaving in ways that are most likely to be helpful for their relative, regardless of its cost to themselves.

There is an analogue of survivor guilt among families of the mentally ill—the guilt of normal living. There are frequent expressions of remorse about living in decent surroundings when the patient does not and about enjoying family gatherings or milestones such as graduations, weddings, births, or holiday gatherings in which the mentally ill relative cannot participate because of his or her situation or condition. The relatives may even be exempted from family rituals, sometimes because their presence is too difficult or potentially disruptive, and sometimes because they themselves reject the stimulation. Yet their absence is an accusation and a deprivation, and the family wishes they could be there.

Among caregivers, there is almost ubiquitous guilt about hospitalizing a mentally ill relative, even under conditions of assault, florid symptomatology, or flagrant self-neglect. And indeed, when patients recover, there is a strong likelihood of anger and recrimination toward caregivers for having done that which was necessary and even potentially lifesaving at the time. Caregivers also suffer impossible dilemmas when they must choose between keeping a highly disruptive dependent offspring at home and risk the cause of psychological damage to other siblings or children (Backlar, 1994; Deveson, 1991).

Caregivers must learn to deal both with the patient's behaviors and with their own reactions, to distinguish between volitional and nonvolitional behavior, to recognize and deal with manipulation, and to know how and when to set limits. In controlling their own behavior, they must learn to effect a balance between the criticalness and over involvement of high expressed emotion and the dangers of affect-suppression, withdrawal, helplessness, and susceptibility to exploitation that sometimes are associated with low expressed emotion (see Hatfield, Spaniol, & Zipple, 1987). They must deal with their own legitimate anger and unjustified guilt. They must also learn to tolerate the suffering of people they love, avoid being overwhelmed by empathic pain, and come to terms with their own rescue fantasies.

PHYSICAL HEALTH OF CAREGIVERS

Family burden may also affect the caregivers' physical health. In a study of mental illness in families of mental health professionals, Lefley (1987b) found that 38 percent of the sample reported an effect on the physical health of caregivers, with mothers and siblings being most affected. Research on maternal caregivers by Greenberg, Greenley, McKee, Brown, and Griffin-Francell (1993) reported that subjective burdens related to stigma and worry were significant predictors of negative health status after controlling for multiple variables that might affect these relationships. These included mother's age, education, and marital status; adult child's gender, residence, and psychiatric symptoms; other life stressors; and objective burdens of care. The authors note that family members may seek treatment for health problems exacerbated by the stress of caregiving. They suggest that primary health care professionals should be encouraged to maintain fact sheets on mental illness in their waiting rooms. This may be a mechanism for enabling families to talk to their health provider about their caregiving stress and about coping with a mentally ill family member.

VIOLENCE IN THE HOUSEHOLD

The research indicates that a small group of patients living in the household may pose a serious risk of bodily harm to caregivers. Torrey's (1994) analysis of recent studies and media accounts of violent behavior by persons with serious mental illness led him to conclude that (a) the vast majority of mentally ill persons are not more dangerous than others in the general population but (b) a small subgroup of patients may indeed be more dangerous. This subgroup undermines the efforts of advocates to reduce stigma by denying an association between serious mental illness and violence. Rigorous studies in the United States (Link, Andrews, & Cullen, 1992) and in the United Kingdom (Wesseley et al., in press) have found an association of violent behavior not with mental illness per se but with psychotic symptoms; the sicker the patient, the more prone he or she is to violence.

The implications for family caregiving are profound. In a study by Tulane researchers Swan and Lavitt (1986) of 1,156 members of the National Alliance for the Mentally Ill (NAMI), 38 percent of the sample reported that their ill relative was assaultive or destructive in the home either sometimes or frequently. The strategy most commonly used by family members to prevent violence was to restrict their own behavior. Parents described patterns of avoiding confrontation, criticism, or even disagreement as "walking on eggshells." Their most adaptive way of dealing with violence was by calming and soothing the patient rather than asserting limits. Parents who were able to separate themselves emotionally from the violent activity and view the patient as ill showed the highest level of positive adjustment. Yet these families paid a heavy price. Their social and recreational activities were restricted, and friends and relatives no longer visited the home.

Personal in-depth home interviews by Gubman and Tessler (1987) with a sample of 30 Alliance for the Mentally Ill (AMI) families indicated that nearly 50 percent had to cope with violent behavior one or more times and 33 percent reported having to call the police. A later study of a stratified sample of 1,401 NAMI families by a Johns Hopkins team (Skinner, Steinwachs, & Kasper, 1992) found lower percentages: 20 percent of the relatives with a serious mental illness had threatened to harm and 11 percent had physically harmed another person. Torrey (1994) notes considerably higher percentages in studies of hospital admissions. Among patients admitted to psychiatric hospitals who had physically attacked someone within the past 2 weeks, Straznickas, McNiel, and Binder (1993) found that family members had been the target 56 percent of the time, and a similar study by Tardiff (1984) reported that families had been the object 65 percent of the time.

Estroff et al. (1994), studying a comparable sample of seriously mentally ill inpatients, reported that more than half the targets of violence were relatives, particularly mothers living with a respondent. This pattern of directing violence toward mothers, the primary and often the only caregiver, was found in all of the cited studies. A number of maternal deaths through violence have also been reported anecdotally in NAMI circles as well as in print (Richardson, 1990).

The research team of Estroff et al. (1994) found significant differences in the characteristics of the social networks of persons with various diagnoses. In Estroff et al.'s research, which distinguished between threats and acts, respondents with a diagnosis of schizophrenia were more likely than persons with other diagnoses to commit violent acts but not more likely to threaten violence. Financial dependence on family was associated with more violent threats and acts. Confused thinking was not associated with violence, but denial and perhaps delusional thinking seemed to be operative.

Respondents who were violent perceived their significant others as threatening but did not perceive themselves as being threatening in return. "The respondents who were violent felt malice and danger from significant others and perceived and experienced hostility in their interpersonal networks" (677). The authors concluded that the interpersonal and social contexts of mentally ill persons and their perceptions of these contexts are important considerations in assessing the risk for violence.

In the study by Straznickas et al. (1993), patients who attacked parents, children, and siblings were most likely to live with their victims in the same household. Similar proportions of patients who attacked family members and of those who attacked nonrelatives lived with other people rather than alone. Compared with other assaultive patients, those who attacked parents were significantly younger (33.4 + 11 years) and those who attacked their children were significantly older (65.3 + 19 years). This suggests two types of bi-generational living arrangements: In one case, aging parents were caring for younger, assaultive mentally ill adult children and, in the other; "sandwich generation" adults were caring for aging mentally ill parents. Married patients were significantly more likely to attack their spouses. Patients who attacked their parents or nonrelatives were likely to be single. These researchers make the following points:

> Why might the primary caregiver be the family member at most risk? This finding may be due partly to the fact that family members who live with aggressive patients are more frequently in contact with the patients. Therefore, they are more readily available as potential targets when the patients become assaultive. In addition, our results suggest that attempts by caretakers to place limits on patients often precede assaults. Also, psychotic symptoms such as paranoid delusions involving the family caregiver are common in patient assaults on family members, as is concurrent drug or alcohol abuse by the patient. (Straznickas et al., 1993, 387)

Suggested solutions are referrals to peer support groups to help families learn how to react to aggressive escalation. Straznickas et al. also suggest that family therapy may be helpful in cases in which a patient's violence is related to difficulties with communication, problem-solving, and conflict resolution. Mentally ill family members with substance abuse problems should be referred to relevant treatment programs and support groups. They make a final suggestion that involvement of the criminal justice system is a viable option for managing violence.

ONGOING ISSUES IN ASSESSING BURDEN

Cultural Perceptions of Burden

Guarnaccia et al. (in press) have pointed out that there are cultural differences in perceptions of burden and that the more family members see caregiving as part of what one ordinarily does for an ill member of the family (or for an adult child still living at home), the less likely they are to provide accurate information on caregiving tasks and burdens. Phenomenologically, these are not viewed as extraordinary responsibilities.

This finding highlights the need to distinguish respondents' perceptions of both objective and subjective indicators of burden. Distress may be manifested in multiple ways, physiological as well as psychological (Greenberg et al., 1993), and caregiving stress is likely to be a function of individual response styles as well as cultural norms. Thus some caregivers who consider it part of their role to care for chronically ill adults may report no subjective burden, unaware, for example, that their tiredness, dysthymia, and susceptibility to colds are related manifestations of distress. Yet as Noh and Turner (1987) have demonstrated, the family's perception of mastery and control of the situation seems to result in minimal subjective burden. When caregiving is viewed as a natural function and there is no perception of inordinate stress, mastery may be an implicit component of the caregiver's task.

Gratifications in Caregiving

Recent reports in the literature suggest that family caregiving is not invariably burdensome and that there are certain gratifications and rewards in caregiving, both practical and psychological. Elderly adults may suffer from the burdens of taking care of dependent adult children (Lefley, 1987a), but these adult children may also be supports to older parents who benefit from their companionship and physical help in running their households (Bulgar, Wandersman, & Goldman, 1993).

In a study of 725 clients with serious mental illness in rural Wisconsin, Greenberg, Greenley, and Benedict (1994) found that 24 percent of the clients lived with their families and these clients tended to provide substantial help. Of this number, between 50 percent and 80 percent helped by doing household chores, shopping, listening to problems, providing companionship, and sharing news about family and friends. For the total sample, family respondents reported that 59 percent of the clients provided companionship. The researchers point out that recognition of clients' contributions could help reduce stigma and expand community opportunities for persons with serious mental illness. They also caution, however, that not all clients can make contributions to their families. Indeed, they note that in some instances, the help a client provides may be an additional source of family burden because of the poor quality of performance or the effort needed to structure the client's activity.

Relation of Gratification and Burden to Relatives' Dysfunction

Caregiving gratification does not necessarily translate into acceptance of the caregiving role. In a study of Australian family caregivers by Winefield and Harvey (1994), caregiving gratification was contingent on whether and when the patient was symptomatic or relatively well. Almost one third of the caregivers reported no gratifications at all and this figure rose to 96 percent when the patient was ill. When caregivers could describe some positive aspects, 64 percent of their comments referred to enjoying the patient as a person and 27 percent to the practical advantages of their presence, such as sharing the housework. Another 9 percent felt that caregiving satisfied the sense of obligation inherent in their role. Despite these expressions of gratification, 78 percent of the sample preferred that the patient live outside the home.

D. Johnson (1994) analyzed the family burden literature, including the findings of 9 surveys and 12 intervention studies, to determine whether and in what ways burden can be relieved, in examining the research, he concluded that (a) there were no differences between affective disorders and schizophrenia in the amount of burden experienced and (b) there was one common feature that transcended diagnostic categories. The extent and degree of family burden appeared to be related to the level of dysfunction of the mentally ill relative. Johnson felt that although there was some evidence that interventions could be helpful, the evidence was sparse and the research too variable in quality. He suggested a number of program components that had demonstrated success in easing family burden and urged incorporation of these components in prevention programs. This, of course, revives the issue of the willingness of mental health systems to provide education and help to family caregivers.

SOCIETAL AND IATROGENIC STRESS

Societal stress derives from cultural attitudes that tend to stigmatize both mentally ill persons and their families. Cultural attitudes devalue persons with psychiatric disorders, with concordant neglect of their needs. The massive underfunding of services and research and negative expectations of recovery clearly affect the resources available to caregivers.

Cultural attitudes toward families often reflect older myths of parental causation. The popular media still talk about "crazymaking" families, and a substantial number of clinicians and media talk show hosts still perpetuate these ideas. For families of persons with mental illness, there is both the shame of attribution and shame by association. In his foreword to the book *Hidden Victims*, which deals with the healing process of families of the mentally ill, E. F. Torrey describes some of these societal pressures:

> Imagine what it would be like to have a member of your family afflicted with a condition whose sufferers, whenever the condition is depicted on television, are portrayed as violent 73 percent of the time....Imagine what it would be like to have your neighbors afraid to come to your house, and your children ashamed to bring their closest friends home to visit. Imagine having your relatives obliquely talking about your ill family member, unmistakably implying

that your side of the family is guilty of something akin to original sin. No wonder Eugene O'Neill in *Strange Interlude* had the family hide their mentally ill
aunt in the attic so that the family will not be disgraced. (Torrey, 1988a, xi–xii)

Fortunately, mentally ill people are no longer hidden in the attic, but
generalization of stigma persists. Objective burdens of stigma may include
caregivers being held responsible for not being able to control the patient's
aberrant behavior, reluctance of acquaintances to come to the house, or social
ostracism of individual family members. Children with a parent or sibling
who is mentally ill may be teased, maligned, or rejected by peers. In many
cases, mental illness in the family jeopardizes relationships with friends,
neighbors, and other relatives (Lefley, 1992).

THE MENTAL HEALTH SYSTEM AS STRESSOR

Major sources of stress reported by families include (a) reluctant, ambiguous,
and contradictory communications froth professionals; (b) failure of the provider system to offer training or involvement in treatment planning to caregivers; (c) increasing financial drain, with inability of families to predict cost-benefit
ratios of investments in treatment, often at considerable sacrifice to other family
members; (d) difficulty in finding legitimate alternatives to hospitalization or
adequate services in the community support system; and (e) stressors in dealing with the legal and criminal justice systems. These last are particularly acute
when police are poorly trained in recognizing and dealing with psychotic disorders. Legal constraints on crisis intervention or involuntary hospitalization
of persons showing florid symptoms but unproven dangerousness are extraordinarily stressful for the families who have to live with these individuals. In
the current era of managed care, a further stress on families is generated by
fiscal policies of limited inpatient treatment. This often results in premature
discharge, with patients returning home still in a psychotic state.

IATROGENIC BURDEN

Many of today's caregivers have endured 15 to 30 years of major mental illness. During this period in history, experiences with professionals frequently
have been frustrating and double-binding. For the most part, inconsistent and
often contradictory patterns of help and information have persisted throughout the course of the illness. Many of these conditions are still reported today,
particularly by families with members who have had multiple exposures to
various parts of the service delivery system. In one type of situation, there
is tacit rejection of communication with the family, save as respondents to
questions on the patient's history. If caregivers attempt to learn more, they
encounter deflection of questions, reluctance to provide diagnosis on the

grounds of labeling, protestations of confidentiality, and sometimes implications that the family's concern is pathological or self-serving.

In some situations, family members have been catapulted into family therapy regardless of their desires, with the implicit or explicit message that the patient's illness is symptomatic of a family problem. But caregivers' requests for information and education continue to be ignored. There are reports of families who deeply resent what is perceived as enforced family therapy, particularly when they, as reluctant participants, are exposed to the observations of multiple therapists and students. But they are afraid the mentally ill person will suffer or be denied other needed treatment if they reject treatment for themselves. The validity of informed consent under these conditions, the ethics of denying necessary information to caregivers, and parameters of the confidentiality issue are discussed by McElroy and McElroy (1994).

A main problem seems to arise from residual negative attitudes and from professionals' attributions that somehow the patients' symptomatic behaviors must reflect something wrong going on in their families. Cook (1988), who has done considerable research on family burden, is particularly disturbed by persistent clinical attitudes toward mothers, as noted in the following passage.

> Clinicians should be aware of the degree to which the disciplines of psychology and psychiatry have engaged in documented scapegoating of mothers in explaining the origins of pathological behavior in their children. More importantly, they should both acknowledge and attempt to correct for the *effects upon their own clinical understanding* of being taught and socialized in this professional context of maternal scapegoating. (Cook, 1988, 48, original emphasis)

MENTAL HEALTH SYSTEM DEFICITS

A related source of family burden derives from deficits in the mental health system. Research indicates that families suffer both because of inadequate services for clients and because an almost total lack of services for themselves. In a scientific survey of 1,401 NAMI members (Skinner et al., 1992), respondents indicated a strong concern with finding adequate community programs for their relatives. The respondents reported that 45 percent of the ill relatives had no productive activity at all. Less than one-half of the clients were involved in rehabilitative activities, such as employment, volunteer work, school, or day treatment programs.

Caregivers' problems stem both from a lack of services and from being ignored by the mental health professionals with whom they come in contact. A focus group study of caregivers found the following:

> Families experienced profound burdens as a result of their interactions with the mental health care system, particularly in negotiating crisis situations; acting as patient advocates and case managers; obtaining adequate community

resources, continuity of care, and information; dealing with legal barriers; and communicating with mental health professionals. (Francell, Conn. & Gray, 1988, 1296)

More current research indicates that a substantial number of families continue to be dissatisfied with their contacts with mental health professionals (Biegel, Li-yu, & Milligan, 1995).

Despite some progress, in many areas there have been few substantive changes since a decade ago when Holden and Lewine (1982) reported on families' frustrations about lack of employment and adequate living arrangements for their ill members and professionals' failure to direct them to community resources. Hanson and Rapp (1992), studying family members' perceptions of how well community mental health programs and services met their needs, found that few facilities offered families any information about the illness or practical advice on how to cope. There was little in the way of emotional support or communication on the client's treatment and progress. Family members also reported that less than one-third of the programs offered the client follow-up contact after hospitalization, preparation for independent living, or case management outside the office.

The latter is an extremely important point because a study by Grella and Grusky (1989), which similarly found widespread dissatisfaction with services, nevertheless found that family members' satisfaction with specific services seemed to depend on their contact with a case manager.

> The role played by case managers in providing information and support to families even surpassed the impact of overall system coverage and quality in determining family satisfaction. In particular, case managers' role in increasing family members' support of their mentally ill relative was crucial to families. This finding is consistent with the assertions of advocates for the families of seriously mentally ill clients, who stress the need to increase services for families in the form of supportive interactions with system representatives. (835)

This conclusion was strengthened in a study of families' concerns regarding community placement of their relative following hospitalization. Solomon and Marcenko (1992b) found a pronounced need for case managers to be trained in social skills, behavioral techniques, coping strategies for families, and problem-solving techniques. These families indicated they were more satisfied with services for their relatives than for themselves. They indicated a need for family education about medications and about how to motivate their mentally ill relatives. As we shall see, these educational needs form the basis of most of the new interventions.

References

Atkinson, S. D. (1994). Grieving and loss in parents with a schizophrenic child. *American Journal of Psychiatry, 151,* 1137–1139.

Backlar, P. (1994). *The family face of schizophrenic.* New York: Tarcher/Putnam.

Biegel, D. E., Li-Yu, S., & Milligan, S. E. (1995). A comparative analysis of family caregivers' perceived relationships with mental health professionals. *Psychiatric Services, 46*, 477–482.

Bulgar, M. W., Wandersman, A., & Goldman, C. R. (1993). Burdens and gratifications of caregiving: Appraisal of parental care of adults with schizophrenia. *American Journal of Orthopsychiatry, 63*, 255–265.

Cook, J. A. (1988). Who "Mothers" the Chronically mentally ill? *Family Relations, 37*, 42–49.

Deveson, A. (1991). *Tell me I'm here*. New York: Penguin.

Estroff, S. E,. Zimmer, C., Lachicotte, W. S., & Benoit, J. (1994). The influence of social networks and social support on violence by persons with serious mental illness. *Hospital & Community Psychiatry, 45*, 669–679.

Francell, C. G., Conn, V. S., & Gray, D. P. (1988). Families' perceptions of burden of care for chronic mentally ill relatives. *Hospital & Community Psychiatry, 39*, 1296–1300.

Greenberg, J. S., Greenley, J. R., & Benedict, P. (1994). Contributions of persons with serious mental illness to their families. *Hospital & Community Psychiatry, 45*, 475–480.

Greenberg, J. S., Greenley, J. R., McKee, D., Brown, R., & Griffin-Francell, C. (1993). Mothers caring for an adult child with schizophrenia: The effects of subjective burden on maternal health. *Family Relations, 42*, 205–211.

Grella, C. E., & Grusky O. (1989). Families of the seriously mentally ill and their satisfaction with services. *Hospital & Community Psychiatry, 40*, 831–835.

Guarnaccia, P. J., Parra, P., Deschamps, A., Milstein, G., & Argiles, N. (1992). Si dios quiere: Hispanic families' experiences of caring for a seriously mentally ill family member. *Culture, Medicine, and Psychiatry, 16*(2), 187–215.

Gubman, G. D., & Tessler, R. C. (1987). The impact of mental illness on families: Concepts and priorities. *Journal of Family Issues, 8*, 226–245.

Hanson, J. G., & Rapp, C. A. (1992). Families' perception of community mental health programs for their relatives with a severe mental illness. *Community Mental Health Journal, 28*, 181–197.

Hatfield, A. E. (1987). Families as caregivers: A historical perspective. In AB Hatfield & HP Lefley (Eds.), *Families of the mentally ill: Coping and adaptation* (pp. 3–29). New York: Guilford.

Hatfield, A. B., Spaniol, L., & Zipple, A. M. (1987). Expressed emotion: A family perspective. *Schizophrenia Bulletin, 13*, 221–226.

Holden, D. F., & Lewing, R. R. J. (1982). How families evaluate mental health professionals, resources, and effects of illness. *Schizophrenia Bulletin, 8*, 626–633.

Johnson, D. L. (1994). Current issues in family research: Can the burden of mental illness be believed? In H. P. Lefley & M. Wascow (Eds.), *Helping families cope with mental illness* (pp. 309–328). Newark, NJ: Harwood Academic.

Lefley, H. P. (1987a). Aging parents as caregivers of mentally ill adult children: An emerging social problem. *Hospital & Community Psychiatry, 38*, 1063–1070.

Lefley, H. P. (1987b). The family's response to mental illness in a relative. In A. B. Hatfield (Ed.), *Families of the mentally ill: Meeting the challenges* (New Directions for Mental Health Services No. 34, pp. 3–21). San Francisco: Jossey-Bass.

Lefley, H. P. (1992). The stigmatized family. In P. J. Fink & A. Tasman (Eds.), *Stigma and mental illness* (pp. 127–138). Washington, DC: American Psychiatric Press.

Link, B. G., Andrews, H., & Cullen, F. T. (1992). The violent and illegal behavior of mental patients reconsidered. *American Sociological Review, 57*, 275–292.

McElroy, E. M., & McElroy, P. D. (1994). Family concerns about confidentiality and the seriously mentally ill: Ethical implications. In H. P. Lefley & M. Wascow

(Eds.), *Helping families cope with mental illness* (pp. 243–257), Newark, NJ: Harwood Academic.

Miller, F., Dworkin, J., Ward, M., & Barone, D. 1990. A preliminary study of unresolved grief in families of seriously mentally ill patients. *Hospital & Community Psychiatry, 41,* 1321–1325.

Noh, S., & Turner, R. J. (1987). Living with psychiatric patients: Implications for the mental health of family members. *Social Science & Medicine, 25,* 263–272.

Oldridge, M. L., & Hughes, I. C. T. (1992). Psychological well-being in families with a member suffering from schizophrenia. *British Journal of Psychiatry, 161,* 249–251.

Richardson, D. (1990). Dangerousness and forgiveness. *Journal of the California Alliance for the Mentally Ill, 2*(1), 4–5.

Schene, A. H., Tessler, R. C., & Gamache, G. M. (in press). *Caregiving in severe mental illness:* Conceptualisation and measurement. In H. C. Kundsen & G. Thornicroft, (Eds.), *Mental health service evaluation.* New York: Cambridge University Press.

Scottish Schizophrenia Research Group. (1985). First episode schizophrenia: IV. Psychiatric and social impact on the family. *British Journal of Psychiatry, 150,* 340–344.

Skinner, E. A., Steinwachs, D. M., & Kasper, J. D. (1992). Family perspectives on the service needs of people with serious and persistent mental illness. *Innovations & Research, 1*(3), 23–30.

Solomon, P., & Marcenko, M. O. (1992b). Family members' concerns regarding community placement of their mentally disabled relative: Comparisons one month after release and a year later. *Family Relations, 41,* 341–347.

Straznickas, K. A., McNiel, D. E., & Binder, R. L. (1993). Violence toward family caregivers by mentally ill relatives. *Hospital & Community Psychiatry, 44,* 385–387.

Swan, R. W., & Lavitt, M. R. (1986). *Patterns of adjustment to violence in families of the mentally ill.* New Orleans, LA: Tulane University, School of Social Work, Elizabeth Wisner Research Center.

Torrey, E. F. (1988a). Foreward. In J. T. Johnson (Ed.), *Hidden victims: An eight-stage healing process for families and friends of the mentally ill* (pp. xi–xiii). New York: Doubleday.

Torrey, E. F. (1994). Violent behavior by persons with serious mental illness. *Hospital & Community Psychiatry, 45,* 653–662.

Wesseley, S. C., Castle, D., Douglas, A. J., et al. (in press). The criminal careers of incident cases of schizophrenia. *Psychological Medicine.*

Winefield, H. R., & Harvey, E. J. (1994). Needs of family caregivers in chronic schizophrenics. *Schizophrenic Bulletin, 20,* 557–566.

DISCUSSION

1. What is the difference between objective and subjective burden? Which is more significant in terms of understanding the impact of mental illness on family members? What are the primary sources of stress associated with the two types of caregiver burden?

2. How does the mental health system contribute to the burden and stress families experience when trying to cope with a loved one's mental illness? How could we improve our mental health system to be more supportive of caregivers?

Susan A. Muhlbauer

Navigating the Storm of Mental Illness: Phases in the Family's Journey[†]

Much like people who are directly affected by psychiatric disorders, family members often go through a social adaptation process that affects many aspects of their lives. In this reading, sociologist Susan Muhlbauer describes the phases that families go through as they respond to the development of a mental illness in a close relative.

One in five Americans, approximately 60 million people, has a mental illness (U.S. Department of Health and Human Services [DHHS], 1999). For between 4 and 5 million of these individuals, mental illness is severe and persistent (Lefley, 1996; Stuart & Laraia, 1998). At least 25 percent of this population lives at home with family. At a minimum, 1.25 million families live with members who have a severe and persistent mental illness (Rose, 1996). For these families, the struggle with mental illness can become, metaphorically, an ongoing journey through a storm of hurricane proportions. Families often have difficulty navigating. The storm's topography is ambiguous, experienced guides are rare, and safety beacons are dim or absent. Families can flounder, and mentally ill members can be abandoned (Yarrow, Schwartz, Murphy, & Deasy, 1987).

Although aspects of this journey have been explored, information is dated. The experience has been substantially altered by recent social, political, economic, and technological changes (Rose, 1996). Reexamination of mental illness as a holistic family process has been suggested as a means of expanding understanding (Tuck, du Mont, Evans, & Shupe, 1997).

The purpose of this study was to examine the development and process of severe and persistent mental illness from a family member's/caregiver's perspective. Goals were (a) to examine the experience in a holistic manner that explored recent changes and permitted understanding of possible patterns or phases, and (b) to determine family issues or themes characteristic of particular phases. The study was designed as a step in the process of developing needed interventions enhancing family services.

BACKGROUND: ROUTES ALREADY SURVEYED

Severe and Persistent Mental Illness and the Family

Initial research was dominated by belief that families had a powerful etiological role in the mental illness of their member (Maurin & Boyd, 1990). Focus

---

Muhlbauer, Susan. 2002. "Navigating the Storm of Mental Illness: Phases in the Family's Journey." *Qualitative Health Research* 12:1076–1092.

on parenting issues as causative factors for psychotic illness was instrumental in developing the belief among professionals that the etiology of major mental disorders, particularly schizophrenia, was rooted in family dysfunction. Current evidence suggests that professionals acting on that belief added to the trauma experienced by families (Torrey, 1995). Family emotional tone, termed *expressed emotion*, was correlated to relapse by the ill member (Brown, Carstairs, & Topping, 1958).

Researchers, however, reversed perspective and examined the effect of mental illness on the family, and they discovered that the impact reverberated across the entire spectrum of family life (Maurin & Boyd, 1990). Consequences of stigma were noted and addressed (Clausen & Yarrow, 1955; Rose, 1996). Mental illness was recognized as creating a significant burden for caretakers and was explored in increasing depth (Yarrow et al., 1987). Behaviors, typically threats and unrealistic demands, that most distressed caregivers, were investigated (Grad & Sainsbury, 1963). Negative feelings experienced by caregivers, including concern for the future, fear, tension, and difficulty sleeping, were explored (Herz, Endicott, & Spitzer, 1976). Connections between a family's burden of care and a mentally ill individual's level of functioning, symptoms, and behavior became increasingly evident (Loukissa, 1995).

Study on the effect of psychiatric illnesses such as schizophrenia and bipolar disorder on the family continued (Miklowitz, 1994). Chronic mental illness and burden of care was examined (Francell, Conn, & Gray, 1988). However, although researchers examined expressed emotion in families with schizophrenic members extensively, minimal investigation of the phenomenon was done in families with other severe and persistent mental illnesses (de Cangas, 1990). Family burden and stress received continued examination (Reinhard & Horwitz, 1995). Focused primarily on the negative aspects of the experience, research indicated that caregiving family members had significant problems with anxiety, depression, and resource issues (Hobbs, 1997). Minimal examination of the experience as a whole occurred.

Phases in Living with Mental Illness in the Family

Current discussion is primarily anecdotally based and supports the concept of phase- or stage-like development. Tessler, Killian, and Gubman (1987) empirically identified nine stages, from initial awareness of problem without recognition of symptoms through ever-present worry about the future. Terkelsen (1987), noting a lack of longitudinal investigations, described an empirically based process involving 10 phases. Spaniol and Zipple (1994), acknowledging a lack of information, maintained that general characteristics could be recognized, including recovery as a growth process divided into four phases: discovery/denial, recognition/acceptance, coping, and personal/ political advocacy. Tuck et al. (1997), investigating the experience of caring for an adult child with schizophrenia, proposed the following eight-phased process: struggling to frame events as normal, seeking help, transformation of a loved child, living with constantly changing levels of hope, endless caring, gathering personal meaning, preserving identity, and knowing. Although interesting, Tuck's qualitative study was based on interviews with only nine family members and focused solely on the process experienced by families whose members had schizophrenia. Another qualitative study, based on 50 in-depth interviews with relatives of individuals with mood disorders or schizophrenia, identified a four phased pattern of emotional unfolding: experiencing emotional anomie, getting a diagnosis, perceiving illness permanency, and acceptance (Karp & Tanarugsachock, 2000).

Although researchers have begun to address the process that families experience, studies concentrating on this area are few, the number of respondents is generally small, and the focus is usually on families experiencing schizophrenia. A need exists for research with larger numbers of respondents across a broader spectrum of diagnoses and experiences.

METHOD

I developed a qualitative research design using semistructured interviewing within a framework of symbolic interaction through its paradigm of dramaturgical interviewing.

Data Collection Procedures

Data were obtained from participants' responses to questioning guided by a semistructured interview outline. Adherence to the outline facilitated a systematic exploration of the participant's experience. In this study, I interviewed participants until no new themes or phases emerged, and 26 interviews were conducted.

Sample

Following Institutional Review Board approval, interviewees were recruited by letter from a list of 49 family members who had participated in psychoeducational groups sponsored by the College of Nursing. Twenty-eight individuals responded. Two of the women were eventually unable to participate because of personal or health reasons, and 26 individuals were interviewed. These 18 women and 8 men met the following inclusion criteria: (a) past participation in the 36-hour psychoeducational course, (b) existence of a family member with a severe and persistent mental illness, (c) involvement within the past several years in assisting their family member with management of the mental illness, and (d) willingness to participate in a 1½- to 2-hour audiotaped interview. Individuals with severe and persistent mental illnesses (who did not participate in the interviews) were defined as functionally impaired adults who (a) met the criteria for a mental illness including the schizophrenias, major depressive disorders, bipolar disorders, disabling obsessive compulsive disorders, or others; (b) experienced recurrent relapses and a need for periodic restabilization and possible rehospitalization; and (c) typically had been ill for over a year and were disabled in major areas of living (Lefley, 1996).

The participants, a self-selected and highly motivated group of Midwestern Caucasian individuals, ranged in age between 40 and 76 years, with a mean age of 56. Twenty-one participants, 15 women and 6 men, were parents; 4 couples participated but were interviewed separately. Four participants, 2 male and 2 female, were spouses or significant others. The remaining participant, a female, was a sibling. Twenty participants were in their first marriage, 3 were in a second marriage, 2 were divorced, and 1 was separated. As a whole, the group was well-educated. All participants were high school graduates; 21 had additional education. Seven participants had community college or technical training, 8 had baccalaureate degrees, and 6 had graduate degrees. In relationship to occupation, 18 participants were in, or before retirement had held, white-collar jobs, and 6 held blue-collar jobs. Five participants were retired.

Data Collection and Analysis Procedures

Data collected from the audiotaped interviews and from notes recording verbal, contextual, and affective material were combined to create an integrated record of each interview.

I submitted data to a content analysis process containing both quantitative and qualitative components (Berg, 1998). In the quantitative component, I used tally sheets to measure data frequencies. I organized the sheets into an information matrix that contained the following demographic data about each study participant: age, gender, martial status, family role, education, and occupational background. The matrix also contained the following information about the mentally ill family member: age, sex, age when illness diagnosed, diagnoses, length of illness, current living situation, work status, insurance, and disability status. The readily accessible quantitative data contained in the information matrix served as base or anchor for the qualitative analysis.

Development of the qualitative analysis required additional structure. Analysis was developed from questions on process and human agency (Lofland & Lofland, 1995). I examined data through parameters specific to three process types: cycles, spirals, and sequences.

- *Cycles* are events that reoccur in a repeating pattern when the last act in one series precedes the recurrence of the first in a new series.
- *Spirals* are less stable patterns involving escalation and de-escalation intervals.
- *Sequences* are time-ordered series of steps or phases that differ from cycles or spirals in that the sequences show neither the connection of the first and last steps as in cycles nor the accelerated movement from a stronger to a weaker level, as in spirals.

In the analysis of human agency, I emphasized the view of humans as creatures actively trying to influence their environment through maneuvering, striving, and struggling. Analysis focused on strategies—the means by which an individual interacts with a situation—that participants used as they struggled to deal with mental illness in a family member.

Analysis of data involved recording, coding, organizing, and synthesizing (Lofland & Lofland, 1995).

FINDINGS

Characteristics of the Mentally Ill Population

Participants provided the following data about family members. Mentally ill individuals ranged in age from 18 to 73 years, with a mean of 33 years. Seventeen were adult children, four were spouses or significant others, and one (a female) was a sibling. Thirteen had never married, three were currently married, and five were divorced or separated. A majority had some education beyond high school, but most had been unable to complete their education. The typical individual was diagnosed in late teens (19.5 years), had been ill for nearly a decade, had a minimum of two or three diagnoses, a history of multiple hospitalizations, and had a positive family history for mental illness. I was surprised to discover that many had part-time involvement in either work or school. Some lived, with family support, in their own apartments.

To understand the experience, it was essential to understand the problems and behaviors involved. Per participant description, most mentally ill family members had substantial difficulty with memory and concentration. Many had problems with hallucinations, delusions, and violent behaviors. Other significant issues were substance abuse, social skills, social relationship problems, and difficulty managing money, coupled with difficulty in coping with stress and change. Other less frequently reported problem areas included self-care deficits, fatigue, and grandiose behaviors. The majority had substantial problems in multiple areas.

Phases of Experience in Navigating the Storm

Analysis of data revealed a spiraling and cycling of events, consistent with previous reports, that eventually developed into a sequential progression of phases through which the majority of participants journeyed (Spaniol & Zipple, 1994; Terkelsen, 1987; Tessler et al., 1987; Tuck et al., 1997). Movement was reported through the following phases: (a) development of awareness, (b) crisis, (c) cycle of instability and recurrent crises, (d) movement toward stability, (e) continuum of stability, and (f) growth and advocacy. Each phase had specific characteristics.

Phase 1—Development of Awareness: Storm Warnings

Phase 1 of the journey, the awareness spiral, was characterized by (a) recognition of a problem coupled with increasing concern and (b) escalating but ineffective efforts to seek assistance. Duration varied from days to years, depending on the progression of symptoms and problems. Participants readily recalled early concerns, help-seeking behaviors, and frustration with health care providers. The comments of one elderly woman whose daughter had a psychotic disorder demonstrated themes reported by a majority of participants.

> From the time she was in preschool, we began to feel that there were things that were more than just unique to her. Perhaps there were some abnormalities. She cried so many times, "Don't leave me! You won't die before I do, will you?" We discussed it with the pediatrician, he said, "Mothers worry too much." We talked to our rabbi....We took her to two counselors and a psychiatric social worker. We took her to a psychiatrist....We were told, "You are overprotective. Let her be more independent."

In contrast to denial, which research generally portrays as a fairly common response to the emergence of a family member's mental illness, the majority of participants reported a pattern of recognizing a problem, seeking assistance, and having concerns negated (Yarrow et al., 1987).

Whether problem behaviors increased slowly or happened within hours or days, most participants acknowledged knowing that something was wrong, but they were unable to define that "wrongness." One mother said, "We knew something was terribly wrong, we didn't have a name for it." Families typically and unsuccessfully tried to manage increasing difficulties until their inability to control the situation became evident in the form of a crisis precipitated by their family member's bizarre behavior. That crisis marked the beginning of phase 2.

Phase 2—Crisis: Confronting the Storm

Phase 2 of the journey was the crisis culmination of the awareness spiral. It was characterized by (a) an exacerbation of problems beyond the family's ability to control; (b) an abrupt confrontation with the mental health care system, usually via an emergency room admission resulting in a mental illness diagnosis; (c) tremendous emotional distress; (d) problems communicating with health care providers; and (e) financial concerns.

The participants consistently reported confronting their family members' psychotic and relatively frequent violent behavior during the crisis phase. One participant shared the following:

> It was totally out of reality. It was very frightening. I watched him change from the kid that you saw, the normal child, to a totally different child, a child

you couldn't recognize. His total body, his facial affect, everything was gone. It was like he had disappeared. It was very frightening....I didn't have a clue what to do.

Crisis episodes, even nonviolent ones, were terrifying and traumatic. Consistent with earlier research, the crisis usually resulted in formal entrance of the ill family member into the mental health system with a concurrent mental illness diagnosis. Participant reaction to the labeling of the relative as mentally ill alternated between concern over the long-term consequences and relief over having an explanation for previously inexplicable behavior (Karp & Tanarugsachock, 2000). Participants reported that learning their family member had a mental illness offered them a way to deal with negative feelings toward the person. One participant said, "Information made me hold her less accountable. She wasn't a horrible, evil person, this woman I was so afraid of, she was ill." Participants reported feeling that having a diagnosis offered the potential for a means of treatment.

In relationship to interactions with mental health care providers, the majority of participants stated that they had problems communicating and noted that providers often did not listen or provide important information. This theme intensified over time. Regarding financial and insurance issues, participants focused on difficulty paying for needed mental health services. They reported either substantial or complete depletion of their mental health insurance coverage during the initial crisis. One participant, a husband, displayed both themes as he described trying to tell the unit social worker about the effect of his wife's severe depression on their children.

She said, "I cannot talk to you without a release of information from your wife." Then she walked away and left me standing, embarrassed, in the hallway...I'm still frustrated at not being able, at least, to express myself...I had to pay a $28,000 hospital bill [his insurance had only covered about $25,000 of the $50,000-plus bill] but nobody would talk to me.

As time went on, problems intensified. Resolutions were poor, and the family's initial relief and optimism declined.

Phase 3—Cycle of Instability and Recurrent Crises: Adrift on Perilous Seas

The journey continued in a third phase. Typically years in length, it was characterized by the following themes: (a) instability and recurrent crises; (b) anger, grief, and loss; (c) searching for explanations, treatment, and increased knowledge; (d) intensifying financial concerns and problems with insurance; (e) occasional acknowledgment of assistance from newer treatments and technologies; (f) frequently expressed dissatisfaction with mental health care services and providers; and (g) issues related to stigma.

Participants described becoming painfully aware of the chronic trajectory of the journey. Relapses or exacerbations were the norm. The mother of a young woman with bipolar disorder stated, "Once we knew what was wrong and the medications started to work, I thought. 'We can handle this. All she has to do is take her lithium. 'I never dreamed she wouldn't." The daughter's inability to comply with treatment resulted in years of crisis, turbulence, and tremendous strain for her family. Another participant recalled her feelings.

> The anger was just in every direction. The anger was at myself, at not being able to just get up and get going with some kind of a plan. It was at the rest of the family, because I thought they should be doing more to help. I didn't know what, but I felt everybody should be doing something. And very angry at him. (son with paranoid schizophrenia)

This mother's intense anger was a fairly representative response, as was her sense of helplessness. Participants also described their sense of grief and loss. The father of a middle-aged man with schizophrenia poignantly articulated his loss and grief.

> Essentially you lost a child and all the hopes and dreams you had for that child. I've thought about this at various times, if Justin had been well, I would have had grand-children. I would have him helping me instead of me helping him. He would have a family. That won't happen. It's a long-term loss, a future loss. It's like having a child die, but the difference is that when the child dies, you mourn that child and then move on. With this, the mentally ill child, that mourning never really quits.

The sense of loss and grieving, previously documented in research describing parental grief in response to mental illness in a child (Karp & Tanarugsachock, 2000; MacGregor, 1994), was a clearly articulated theme that consistently ran through participant interviews.

As phase 3 progressed, participants searched for explanations for the constant or recurring symptoms. Explanations typically involved either family deficits or physiological abnormalities. One mother reported that her other son blamed his brother's illness (paranoid schizophrenia) on the family's inability "to love him enough." Searching for information, families reported becoming disillusioned by the difficulties encountered with the mental health care system. Unhappy with responses and concerned about adequacy of information, participants then reported seeking knowledge from self-help groups.

Phase 3, consistent with research emphasizing the cost of mental illness (Clark & Drake, 1994), was also characterized by a continuing theme of financial concern. Most participants reported losing access to insurance coverage either through disqualification or depletion of lifetime limits for mental health services. Families turned to governmental entitlement programs. These programs were often difficult to access, and their use created additional issues. Positive results from the use of new treatments occasionally further complicated financial issues and resulted in ethical dilemmas involving work and entitlement systems. The mother of a young man with schizophrenia described her experience.

> After three times and hiring a lawyer [was able to get approved for SSI and Medicaid]. The lawyer didn't say anything I hadn't said in the last appeal, but they don't get serious until you are on your third appeal and have someone representing you. It was very frustrating. But if he didn't get Medicaid, how could he have medication [costs between $500 and $800 per month]? There's no way he could start working now and lose his Medicaid or he would not have his medication [and would not be able to work because he would again become psychotic].

The majority of participants reported confronting similar issues and indicated plainly that management of financial concerns was a tremendous stressor and burden.

Significant problems in interactions with the mental health care system also continued. Concerns reported in earlier phases intensified. One participant, after describing his unsuccessful attempts to communicate with his wife's psychiatrist, stated, "I have to accept that. I know he is good. If everyone respects him, I guess I'd better too [pause]...I don't think the good man knows how to listen." Another man stated, "I've felt like an outcast at the hospital...just a necessary evil." Participants described learning to "work the system." One mother described her technique in a matter-of-fact manner: "Of course they wouldn't tell me anything. I learned to work the system, I called the social worker and said, 'Just give me information about schizophrenia.' Well, inadvertently they would tell me about him." Needing to learn methods to get desperately needed information was a prominent theme in this phase.

Although concerns related to stigma had been apparent earlier, the theme now intensified. Participants reported having to share at least some information with others. Several reported traumatic encounters with negative stereotypes, but the majority acknowledged being surprised by how well they were treated when involved in face-to-face interactions. One mother said, "If someone would ask me, I'm not going to say, 'No, she isn't. I would say, 'Yeah.' But, you know, people don't come around and ask you either, don't even pay much attention to it anymore." Although unexpected, this response was consistent with earlier research that also denied direct, face-to-face stigma experiences (Wahl & Harman, 1989).

Participants did report confronting an institutionalized type of stigma, comparable to institutionalized racism, embedded in governmental and corporate regulations that were more problematic and profound than any face-to-face encounter (Murphy & Choi, 1997). One father, whose daughter was doing well in treatment, explained:

> Where the problem comes is the employment and insurance. If she gets there [able to be employed full-time], then she will face it. I'm sure it will be difficult

for her to get a good job or full coverage insurance [because of discriminatory employment and insurance regulations]....This is where the stigma part will be hard for her.

Eventually, participants reported, a measure of control was painfully gained. This control correlated with changes in expectations and interactions. As changes coalesced, families progressed into the fourth phase, movement toward stability.

CLINIC TREATS MENTAL ILLNESS BY ENLISTING THE FAMILY

By *ANEMONA HARTOCOLLIS*

It was hard to tell just who was the patient, as the Cunanan siblings—Jennifer, Adrian, and Anthony—sat in a row on three chairs in a sparsely decorated therapist's office at *Beth Israel Medical Center* in Manhattan.

It was Jennifer Cunanan, 27, who did most of the talking, describing life with Adrian, 30, a computer consultant who has bipolar disorder and who went through a severe manic episode in March. He would go two days without sleeping, she said, then become so frazzled that he depended on his family to carry out life's daily chores, like shopping and cleaning.

"All of us would like someone to sweep up after us," Ms. Cunanan said, half understanding, half resentful, as her brother listened, his eyelids drooping from exhaustion.

Adrian's brother and sister, as well as the woman he is dating, are critical components of his therapy at Beth Israel, where a fledgling clinic aggressively treats people with bipolar disorder by involving their family members. The clinic, the Family Center for Bipolar Disorder, was set to be formally dedicated on Wednesday, though it has evaluated some 60 families since 2006, in a program that doctors say is unique in the city and based on a model developed at the *University of Colorado*.

Family-focused therapy, as it is called, breaks the image of the psychiatrist sitting in his chair, alone in a room with the patient, as well as the traditional wisdom that patient confidentiality is sacrosanct. In family therapy, the family might be treated as part of the problem; in contrast, in family-focused therapy the point is not to treat relatives, but to enlist their help in managing the patient's illness.

"We've tested it in a number of different trials against different types of therapy, and consistently find that if you combine medication and family-focused therapy, you get quicker recoveries from episodes and longer intervals of wellness," said David J. Miklowitz, a professor of psychology and psychiatry at the University of Colorado, whose pioneering research on the topic inspired the Beth Israel clinic. "So the relapses are less common, and their functioning improves, including relationship and family functioning."

For many years, Dr. Miklowitz said, the extreme mood swings of bipolar disorder had been thought of "as sort of an exclusively genetic, biologically treated illness," to be managed primarily with medication. But his most recent study, reported a year ago in the *Archives of General Psychiatry*, showed that long-term therapy of 30 50-minute sessions over 9 months, with medication, cut median recovery time to 169 days, compared to 279 days for those receiving short-term therapy of 3 sessions over 6 weeks.

The study also showed that family therapy had slightly better results than other types of psychotherapy, Dr. Miklowitz said, though the difference was found to be statistically insignificant.

Nonetheless, he and the founder of Beth Israel's clinic, Dr. Igor Galynker, said their experiences with patients showed that families are in the best position to catch early warning signs of a manic or depressive episode.

"It can be something as subtle as a change in lipstick shade," Dr. Galynker said. "Only a person who knows them very, very well would know."

Patients often do not recognize the symptoms. "Because the mania feels so good, there's no way for me to know that I'm doing it," Mr. Cunanan explained. "That's why it's so important to have the family involved."

Dr. Galynker and his patients agreed to open therapy sessions to a reporter with the hope of dispelling the stigma that surrounds mental illness, which can sometimes make patients ashamed to confide in those close to them.

Because there is data that shows bipolar illness to be hereditary, Dr. Galynker said that being open about the disease could help the children of people with bipolar disorder to understand the risks of inheriting it. People with bipolar disorder can cycle between depression and mania. The manic highs, with attendant feelings of excitement, elation, grandiosity, and obsession, can be so gratifying that patients fail to realize they are part of an illness and prelude to a breakdown.

It was a depressive swing that brought Helen Kraljic Fama and her husband to Beth Israel's clinic, on 17th Street near First Avenue, nearly 30 years after Ms. Fama suffered her first bout with the disease.

Ms. Fama, 50, who was once a bookkeeper and a cashier, said her manic episodes include an obsession with numbers, which she feels are friendly to her. ("I always brag that she scored a perfect 800 on her math SAT," said her husband, Anthony P. Fama, 60.) In her last bout, in March, she was watching a John Travolta movie, *Swordfish*, when her fingers began working an imaginary keyboard as she communicated with the numbered codes on the screen.

The subsequent depression, coupled with the guilt she feels about her inability to work, or even to make dinner, has left her sometimes feeling like "ending it all," she said.

Ms. Fama recently walked from her home in Queens to the 59th Street Bridge, thinking of jumping off, but changed her mind when she saw a lot of construction workers on the bridge. So she had breakfast at a restaurant, then called her brother to take her home.

In a therapy session on Monday, Dr. Galynker suggested enlisting Ms. Fama's brother to keep her company at home while Mr. Fama was at his job as a supermarket manager in Manhattan.

"Can I rely on your brother?" Dr. Galynker asked Ms. Fama.

"Oh, yes," she replied, clutching her purse as if it were her anchor in a storm. "He's telling me to look in the mirror, see how pretty I am."

Mr. Cunanan said that both of his manic episodes came at times that he later recognized as being particularly stressful. The first was after the September 11 terrorist attacks, shortly after his graduation from the University of California in Irvine. He was overcome by feelings that he had to save the world by setting up some sort of charity, and eventually was hospitalized, while his family had little understanding of what was wrong.

Seven years later, the second manic episode came amid the stress of starting a relationship with a woman he had been infatuated with for 10 years, and a job promotion; he said he had felt as if he needed to prove himself worthy of both.

One night in March, Mr. Cunanan woke the woman he was seeing, Michelle Camaya, at 4 a.m., asking, "Do you trust me?" When she said that she did, he persuaded her to come with him to Kennedy Airport and fly to Los Angeles, where he wanted to deliver 16 e-mail messages of support to his former college dance team, which was about to perform in a nationally televised competition.

Mr. Cunanan had been convinced, he now recalls, that hand-delivering those messages would have somehow changed the fate of the dance team, and perhaps even the world.

"Hey, life is fragile," he remembers thinking. "There was a sense of urgency."

He returned to New York the next day and the warning signs mounted. He remembers thinking, "If I could do this in 24 hours, what could I do in a week?" Within three days, he imagined, he could create a nonprofit corporation that would help people fulfill their passions. "I felt enlightened," he said. "This would be the best Easter present for the world."

In an effort to calm him down, Ms. Camaya took him to a Bikram yoga class, where he began doing the poses in what he described as a "militant, superfocused" way, with robotic intensity. When Ms. Camaya told him to change his clothes, he took that as a command and began taking his clothes off and putting them back on.

Ms. Camaya called his brother, who got him home. Mr. Cunanan persuaded them to go to the roof to watch the sunrise, but once there, he announced that he felt like jumping off. His brother Anthony, 25, called 911, and the police talked Adrian into going peacefully to Bellevue, but Adrian persuaded doctors there to let him go. Eventually, his brother and sister tricked him into going back to the hospital and into signing the paperwork to be admitted.

Mr. Cunanan and his siblings say that after three months of family therapy, he is functioning at a level that took him two years to reach the last time.

"I think a huge part of it is really just gaining back my self-confidence, after going through a pretty traumatic experience that's pretty hard on the soul," Mr. Cunanan said. "Having their support has been great."

Source: Anemona Hartocollis. "Clinic Treats Mental Illness by Enlisting the Family." *New York Times*, June 4, 2008. Retrieved July 27, 2008, http://www.nytimes.com/2008/06/04/nyregion/04clinic.html#

Phase 4—Movement toward Stability: Realigning the Internal Compass

Substantial alterations in participant thoughts, values, and behaviors were the hallmarks of the journey in the fourth phase. Themes included (a) finding ways to regain control, (b) managing feelings of guilt and helplessness, (c) changing perceptions and expectations, (d) struggling with ethical and limit-setting issues related to control, and (e) developing workable symptom management techniques. Participants described struggling to regain control of their lives while accepting limits in managing the lives of their ill relatives. One woman, the wife of a man who experienced recurrent severe depressions, described her experience as a "sorting through" process that allowed her to make choices. She noted, "You can make a decision to continue on doing the same thing over and over again or stop it." With this statement, she acknowledged her ability to control her response to her husband's behavior even though she was unable to control his behavior.

Another participant talked about how he dealt with similar issues and the comfort and support he found in his religious and spiritual beliefs.

That [belief] helps my peace of mind, if you will, a little bit. It doesn't take it [the feelings] away. It just alleviates it to the extent that we know we can no longer really control this, and that's the big thing, really...I can't control the situation, there's not a cure for the situation, and I didn't cause it. And this helps me a lot.

Participants, acknowledging increased understanding, reported changes in their perception of behaviors initially perceived as selfish, indulgent, provocative, or willful. Many participants, for example, considered excessive sleeping an indication of laziness. The husband of a middle-aged woman with severe depression shared his experience: "I just thought she wouldn't work. I thought she was lazy. I didn't know it was a symptom of depression." Objectionable actions were reframed as symptoms of an illness, thus providing a feasible and acceptable explanation for behavior that was often bizarre and occasionally threatening. The result was usually decreased anger, increased tolerance, and clearer understanding. This shift in emotions lessened the tension and hostility in the home. The resulting drop in ambient anxiety made it easier for the mentally ill individual to function. Modifying expectations to make them realistic was cited as helpful by a majority of participants. Knowledge that allowed participants to make interactional changes also led to a decrease in feelings of self-blame and guilt. Energy could then be directed into more useful responses.

Participants discussed struggling with ethical dilemmas related to control, autonomy, independence, privacy, and freedom. Issues focused on balancing those rights against their relative's intermittent inability to comprehend the consequences—often the danger—of their behavior. The mother of a man with paranoid schizophrenia shared her family's experience when faced with the potentially violent behavior of a son returning home after hospitalization.

> We all talked among ourselves that if he was totally out of control and made an attempt to hit us, to hurt us, we'd just have to call 911. And, if necessary, literally run out of the door...or lock him in his room...I reversed the locks before he came home so that it could not be locked from the inside [so he couldn't lock himself in the bedroom but they could lock him in if needed]. I know that's against human rights and dignity, but sometimes you do what you have to do. That did not last long. Eventually we took the lock off, no lock at all. And we try to respect that privacy. You knock on the door before you just barge in because that is his space.

Concerns about ethical issues and limits of responsibility were consistent themes in this phase. Arriving at some manner of resolution allowed participants to progress in their ability to cope.

With changes in perspective, decreased guilt feelings, and clarification of concerns about independence and autonomy, participants reported increased decision-making ability. They noted recognizing the need to provide clear limits on problem behaviors, particularly noncompliance with treatment and substance abuse, which magnified psychotic or violent activities. One participant described an episode with her son.

> He was still self-medicating with drugs and alcohol. There was one experience where he hallucinated, evidently visually, along with what he was hearing. We just more or less told him he would have to leave the house [after he had hit his father]. He would just have to go. You know, if he wouldn't seek help and if he was going to continue to use alcohol and drugs, then he could not live in our house.

As indicated, this phase occasionally saw the exodus of the ill family member, a fairly common finding in research literature (Karp & Tanarugsachock, 2000; Yarrow et al., 1987). In this circumstance, it was typically the choice of the mentally ill relative in response to limits set by participants on behaviors perceived as being under the relative's control. In variance with previous reports, this exodus typically was temporary, with some contact, often erratic, being maintained. The primary focus of this phase was the beginning of restabilization of family life through a process by which the participant became able to act rather than simply react to inappropriate behaviors. Actions resulted from a struggle to balance the needs of their families and themselves with the needs of the ill member.

Participants also discussed their increasing ability, typically from integrating information and experience, to assist with symptom management. One mother recalled aids she used to help her severely depressed adolescent son concentrate and organize his thoughts.

> He always loved art and painting. We'd get paint-by-number sets [to help him organize his thoughts]. He was really into that for about a month. The puzzles helped when he was having trouble putting his thinking together...he knew he had to focus on this 50- or that 500-piece puzzle. I'd see him many times downstairs working, I'd say, "Oh, you're working on..." He'd say, "Yeah, this helps me think because I know I've got to think to find all of the blue pieces together for the sky."

Participants noted that over time, they became more skilled at techniques that helped family members manage symptoms and make decisions. Elaboration of these skills resulted in the development of care patterns.

Phase 5—Continuum of Stability: Mastering Navigational Skills

As a majority of participants discussed increasing successes with symptom management and decision making, a fifth phase of the journey, the continuum of stability, became evident. Themes of this phase included (a) further development of the participant's expertise in managing symptoms and creating workable care patterns; and (b) the use of a variety of support systems, including the mental health care system/professionals, friends, and support/psychoeducational groups.

Participant symptom management expertise tended to develop in the areas of cognitive deficits and anxiety. One participant described a fairly typical pattern of assisting a family member to manage cognitive deficits that distorted decision making:

> When a decision comes up, I do not say, "You need to do this." I will very carefully lay out paths that she could take and the consequences. I will ask her, and I don't just lay it out, I ask her....So I lay out her different options and the consequences, or I help her discover them.

The participant was aware that the relative dealt more capably with information that was laid out concretely and explained how that knowledge was incorporated into problem solving.

> We talk about it; we write it down. It has gotten to the point where we draw pictures out or like a chart...a flow chart. This is where the goal you want is. This is how.

Demonstrating in a concrete way how the relative could be successfully involved in the intricacies of a complex and abstract decision-making process, the participant also discussed learning to deal concretely with abstract difficulties in the area of boundary management.

> She had a hard time with that [managing boundaries] until I came up with the Image that you are blue and I am red. And sometimes you need to make blue decisions and I need to make red decisions. And in our relationship and our house, we make purple decisions...I don't know what it was about the terminology that wasn't clicking. But as soon as I put it in color [she understood].... I tell her that her mother is yellow and her relationship with her mother is green. And my relationship with her mother is orange, and we shouldn't get the green in with the orange. And, by God, we don't want any of that yellow in with our purple. And as soon as I made those color analogies, this light bulb came on.

As this participant indicated, many consumers were able to process abstract ideas if those ideas could be introduced and interpreted concretely. Visualization was often helpful.

Participants consistently described how they attempt to provide aid by sharing their own experiences. Through self-disclosure, they offered ideas about how others would perceive and respond to the situation their family member found perplexing and difficult. One mother noted, "I tell him how I'd feel about it so he has some idea what normal feelings would be."

Management of anxiety was also an important issue. Participants varied in awareness of their relative's vulnerability, but many noted its crippling effect. A primary goal for these families became rapid management of escalating anxiety.

Because increases in anxiety often occurred around episodes of over-stimulation, participants worked to maintain control as a containment measure. One woman discussed helping her son contain anxiety and psychotic symptoms in the over-stimulation of a holiday family gathering. Anxiety escalating, he began hearing voices calling him names. Inaccurately attributing the name-calling to his brother, he became convinced that he was being insulted. His agitation increasing, he incorporated a visitor into his delusional system and prepared to attack. At that point, the mother, preoccupied with food preparation, realized what was occurring and intervened.

> I went out there and said, "No, you cannot do this." And he says, "I don't care. That is [individual from his delusional system], and I am going to get him." And I said, "No, you're not." "You know," I says "I've really got a lot to do here. I've got to get dinner on and by you doing this, it really hurts me. It really hurts me by your doing this." And he says, "Okay, Mom."

She then directed him to go to a quiet place in the house where he could calm down. She knew if the overstimulation was stopped, his symptoms would subside. She had learned that her son could not tolerate extended periods in a stimulating environment, even an environment with his brothers and sisters, and had created a quiet room in the basement to which he could retreat. Knowing her son had lost awareness and insight, she quietly intervened and gave needed direction that permitted him the quiet time needed to regain control. As this example indicates, participants found that managing the environment through choices limiting exposure to overstimulation helped to prevent or de-escalate erratic responses.

Consistent with information derived from research an expressed emotion, participants talked about the need to keep their home atmosphere calm and quiet, noting their relative was more functional in that environment (Lefley, 1996). They offered reassurance and calm messages. One mother summarized succinctly: "I try to give him positive thoughts."

A final anxiety-producing concern involved accessing and using complex social service systems. Anxiety on receiving a letter from a social service agency was so overwhelming that recipients were often unable to open the envelope. Participants reported that, anxious and unable to manage, relatives depended on them for help. One stated, "I have to navigate the system for her. I am the gateway for her."

Despite the positive effect of continual and unconditional support, participants admitted to eventually recognizing their limitations. Several reported becoming depressed and seeking therapy. Acknowledging the need for assistance, many emphasized the value of support from families dealing with similar issues; community self-help groups and psychoeducational groups provided access to others with similar experiences. One participant, the father of a young woman with multiple psychotic symptoms, noted,

It was helpful to listen to people that have the diseases and had it under control....I can't emphasize enough learning about is so very helpful... don't worry about where it came from, whether it is hereditary in your family. Learn to accept it. Don't be ashamed because it is nothing you did.

As the family's expertise grew, longer interludes of respite resulted, although chaos could recur with illness exacerbation. Families developed strategies to help their mentally ill members manage symptoms, handle money, control anxiety, and adapt to change. Insisting that ill members comply with treatment became an increasingly effective strategy, as was access to new treatments and medications, which usually became available because of successful enrollment in Medicaid.

Phase 6—Growth and Advocacy: Sailing Existential Seas

As participants recalled experiences and talked about personal change, a number described development of their journey into a sixth phase characterized by subjective awareness of personal growth and substantial fears about their loved one's future. The sense of personal growth developed, at times, into a sense of empowerment with concurrent advocacy behaviors. Although apprehensive about relapses, participants described deriving meaning, value, and personal growth from their experiences. One man considered his experience a source of value clarification.

I can look back and I can see that my attitude has changed. I think it's probably made my wife's relationship and mine much stronger. It causes you to take a look at yourself and see what changes you need to make....When something like this happens, it brings you back down to square one in reality. In that respect, it hasn't been all bad. I think I've grown because of it...little things don't upset me as much as they used to. Should everybody go through this? [laughs] No!

Some, obviously not all, participants talked about their increasing ability to effect change. One man talked about a growing sense of competency and capability: "One of the things that has come out of this is self-empowerment. You find out that you can do stuff that you never thought you would be able to do previously." Active in his community, this participant had been able to provide a voice for the needs of his son and others who could not speak as dearly. Despite the burdens experienced, participants were able to articulate areas of strength and growth. A number reported finding meaning and purpose that reshaped their perceptions and values. In essence, they described satisfaction and comfort in the development of meaning from an existential nightmare and validated research that emphasized the health and strength of families functioning successfully in overwhelming circumstances (Doornbos, 1996).

Despite growth, however, tremendous issues and problems remained. All participants expressed concern about the future centered on how their relative would survive after they were unable to provide care. One mother asked,

> But what happens when we are gone and when we can't monitor her? Are people like her supposed to be just thrown to the wolves? Which right now is what I see happening. And, somehow, the general public does not seem to be interested enough and the politicians in making some kind of provisions for people like this.

Consistent with earlier research (Tuck et al., 1997), some participants acknowledged feeling helpless. The elderly mother of a middle-aged man with paranoid schizophrenia stated dearly, "I can't plan for the future." All participants expressed concern about their relative's future. Most participants identified this as their greatest worry.

CONCLUSIONS AND RESEARCH IMPLICATIONS

Consistent with past anecdotal and research information, data from the study supported a sequential progression of phases inherent in the process of mental illness. The following six phases were identified: (a) cycle of awareness, (b) crisis, (c) cycle of instability and recurrent crisis, (d) movement toward stability, (e) continuum of stability, and (f) growth and advocacy. Although each phase was characterized by a number of specific and important themes, the following topics were consistent across phases: (a) significant problems communicating with providers within the mental health care system; (b) substantial financial/resource issues, including the effect of institutionalized stigma, which limited resources; (c) strongly felt needs on the part of the participants for access to information; and (d) the use of knowledge as the basis of the participant's development of symptom management care patterns. In contrast to abandonment reported in earlier research, data from this study acknowledged the exodus of some mentally ill members from the family system but also indicated eventual reintegration of the mentally ill family member in later phases of the process.

Information from this study must be considered within the scope of its generalizability and limitations. Data were drawn from a stable, well-educated, self-selected and highly-motivated group of middle-aged to elderly Caucasian Midwesterners. Information can probably be extrapolated to similar groups, but obvious limitations exist in further generalization.

Results suggest the need for replication of this study in other ethnic and socioeconomic groups and in groups who have not experienced a similar psycho-educational intervention. If additional research supports the existence of similar phases in a variety of groups, the possibility exists to further define specific phases and determine concurrent family needs, thus allowing for the development of more specifically and appropriately tailored interventions.

References

Berg, B. L. (1998). *Qualitative research methods for the social sciences* (3rd ed.). Boston: Allyn & Bacon.

Brown, G. W., Carstairs G. M., & Topping, G. (1958). Post hospital adjustment of chronic mental patients. *The Lancet, 2,* 685–689.

Clark, E., & Drake, R. (1994). Expenditures of time and money by families of people with severe mental illness and substance use disorders. *Community Mental Health Journal, 30,* 145–163.

Clausen, J., & Yarrow M. R. (1955). The impact of mental illness on the family. *Journal of Social Sciences, 11,* 4.

de Cangas, J. (1990). Exploring expressed emotion: Does it contribute to chronic mental illness? *Journal of Psychosocial Nursing, 28*(2), 31–34.

Doornbos, M. (1996). The strengths of families coping with serious mental illness. *Archives of Psychiatric Nursing, 10,* 214–220.

Francell, C. G., Conn V. S., & Gray, P. D. (1988). Families' perceptions of burden of care for chronically mentally ill relatives. *Hospital and Community Psychiatry, 39,* 296–300.

Grad, J., & Sainsbury, P. (1963). Mental illness and the family. *The Lancet, 1,* 544–547.

Herz, M. L., Endicott J., & Spitzer R. L. (1976). Brief versus standard hospitalization: The families. *American Journal of Psychiatry, 133,* 795–801.

Hobbs, T. (1997). Depression in the caregiving mothers of adult schizophrenics: A test of the resource deterioration model. *Community Mental Health Journal, 33,* 387–399.

Karp, D., & Tanarugsachock, V., (2000). Mental illness, caregiving, and emotional management. *Qualitative Health Research 10*(1), 6–25.

Lefley, H. (1996). *Family caregiving in mental illness.* Thousand Oaks, CA: Sage.

Lofland, J., & Lofland, L. (1995). *Analyzing social settings: A guide to qualitative observation and analysis* (3rd ed.). Boston: Wadsworth.

Loukissa, D. (1995). Family burden in chronic mental illness. A review of research studies. *Journal of Advanced Nursing, 21,* 248–255.

MacGregor, P. (1994). Grief: The unrecognized parental response to mental illness in a child. *Social Work, 39,* 160–166.

Maurin, J. T., & Boyd, C. B. (1990). Burden of mental illness on the family: A critical review. *Archives of Psychiatric Nursing, 4*(2), 99–107.

Miklowitz, D. J. (1994). Family risk indicators in schizophrenia. *Schizophrenia Bulletin, 20,* 137–149.

Murphy, J. W., & Choi, J. M. (1997). *Postmodernism, unraveling racism and democratic institutions.* Westport, CT: Praeger.

Reinhard, S., & Horwitz, A. (1995). Caregiver burden: Differentiating the content and consequence of family caregiving. *Journal of Marriage and the Family, 57,* 741–750.

Rose, L. (1996). Families of psychiatric patients: A critical review and future research directions. *Archives of Psychiatric Nursing, 10*(2), 67–76.

Spaniol, L., & Zipple, A. (1994). Coping strategics for families of people who have a mental illness. In H. Lefley & M. Wasow (Eds.), *Helping Families Cope With Mental Illness* (pp. 131–146). New York: Harwood Academic.

Stuart, G. W., & Laraia, M. T. (1998). *Principles and practices of psychiatric nursing* (6th ed.). New York: Mosby.

Terkelsen, K. (1987). The evolution of family reposes to mental illness through time. In A. B. Hatfield & H. Lefley (Eds.). *Families of the mentally ill: Coping and adaptation* (pp. 151–166). New York: Guilford.

Tessler, R. C., Killian, L. M., & Gubman, G. D. (1987). Stages in family response to mental illness: An ideal type. *Psychosocial Rehabilitation Journal, 10,* 3–16.

Torrey, E. F. (1995). *Surviving schizophrenia* (3rd ed.). New York: HarperCollins.

Tuck, I., du Mont, P., Evans G., & Shupe, J. (1997). The experience of caring for an adult child with schizophrenia. *Archives of Psychiatric Nursing, 11,* 118–125.

US. Department of Health and Human Services. (1999). *Mental health: A report of the surgeon general-executive summary.* Rockville, MD: U.S. Department of Health and Human Services Administration, Center for Mental Health Services, National Institutes of Health, National Institute of Mental Health.

Wahl, O. & Harman, C. R. (1989). Family views of stigma. *Schizophrenia Bulletin, 15*(1), 131–139.

Yarrow, M., Schwartz, C., Murphy, H., and Deasy, L. (1987). The psychological meaning of mental illness in the family. In E. Rubington & M. Weinberg (Eds.) *Deviance: The interactionist perspective* (5th ed.) (pp. 25–32). New York: Macmillan.

DISCUSSION

1. What are the major phases that family members go through in adapting to a close relative's mental illness? What social factors influence this process and how individual caregivers experience the different phases? How are these phases similar to and different from the identity changes that people coping with depression go through, which you read about earlier in this book?

2. In what ways does the mental health system—with its array of services intended to ameliorate the suffering of mental illness—actually contribute to family burden or help family members "navigate the storm of mental illness"? What changes do you think are necessary to make our current mental health system more effective in responding to the needs of family members of people with mental illness?

Mental Illness and Social Problems

Linda A. Teplin and Nancy S. Pruett

Police as Streetcorner Psychiatrist: Managing the Mentally Ill

In this now classic paper, Linda Teplin and Nancy Pruett summarize findings from an early qualitative study that examined how police respond to mentally disordered individuals in the community. They focus our attention on how police make field decisions, and the personal and situational factors that influence them, when they encounter someone they know or suspect may have a mental illness.

M anaging mentally disordered people in the community historically has been a part of police work (Bittner, 1967). Police play a major role in referring persons for psychiatric treatment, particularly within the lower socioeconomic strata (Cobb, 1972; Gilboy & Schmidt, 1971; Hollingshead & Redlich, 1958; Liberman, 1969; Sheridan & Teplin, 1981; Sims & Symonds, 1975; Teplin, Filstead, Hefter, & Sheridan, 1980; Warren, 1977; Wilkinson, 1975). Over the years, police handling of the mentally ill has been complicated by public policy modifications, for example, deinstitutionalization, more stringent commitment criteria, and cutbacks in treatment programs. As a result, the numbers of mentally ill persons involved with police have increased while, at the same time, the police officer's dispositional options have decreased (Teplin, 1983, 1984a, 1984b).

This paper examines police handling of the mentally ill within the current public policy structure. Based on data from an observational study of 1,396 police–citizen encounters, this paper will describe the decision-making normative framework police use to manage the mentally ill within the community.

Teplin, Linda A., and Nancy S. Pruett. 1992. "Police as Streetcorner Psychiatrist: Managing the Mentally Ill." *International Journal of Law and Psychiatry* 15:139–156.

BACKGROUND

Involvement of police with the mentally ill is based on two legal principles: (1) the police power function, that is, to protect the safety and welfare of the public; and (2) *parens patrie*, which involves protection for the disabled citizen (Fox & Erickson, 1972; Shah, 1975). Most mental health codes specify the parameters of police involvement with the mentally ill and instruct police to initiate an emergency psychiatric apprehension whenever the person is either "dangerous to self or others" or, "because of his illness is unable to provide for his basic physical needs so as to guard himself from serious harm" (cf. California Welfare and Institutional Code, 1980; Illinois Revised Statutes, 1981). Thus, police involvement with the mentally ill is mandated by the law. However, the actual disposition of a mentally disordered person is inherently a complex social process. While the law provides the legal structure and decrees the police officer's power to intervene, it cannot dictate the police officer's response to that situation (Bittner, 1967, 1970). Unlike other professionals, the police do not have a body of technical knowledge with respect to psychiatry which they use as formulae in the performance of their role (Rumbaut & Bittner, 1979). As with all law enforcement decisions, the police must exercise discretion in choosing the most "appropriate" disposition in a given situation (Goldstein, 1979; Gottfredson & Gottfredson, 1980; Manning, 1977, 1984; Smith, 1986; Smith & Visher, 1981; Wilson, 1968).

In mental health cases, the situation is further complicated by the nebulous definition of "mental disorder." There is a large gray area of behavior, which depending upon cultural values, community context, and administrative practice, might be labelled criminal, psychiatric (Stone, 1975), or merely "odd" (Monahan & Monahan, 1986). In short, dispositional decisions vis-à-vis the mentally ill are an inherently problematic social judgement. As a consequence, police have developed a shared understanding of how things "should" be done (i.e., an informal operative code) in order to "manage" the mentally disordered citizen.

Bittner's (1967) study is considered to be the seminal work in this area. He found that police made psychiatric referrals reluctantly; police initiated hospitalizations only when the situation had the potential to escalate into a "serious problem" (e.g., danger to life, physical health, property, and/or order). Bittner found that there needed to be indications of external risk accompanied by signs of serious psychological disorder (e.g., suicide, distortions in appearance, violent acts, bizarre behavior, public nuisances) for the police to justify a psychiatric referral. He concluded that, except for cases of suicide attempts, the decision to take someone to the hospital was based on overwhelming conclusive evidence of illness.

Several other investigators have confirmed police reluctance to initiate an emergency psychiatric apprehension (cf. Matthews, 1970; Rock, Jacobson, & Janepaul, 1968; Schag, 1977; Urmer, 1973). Schag (1977) reported that most police-initiated commitments to mental hospitals were precipitated by an overt act or threat of self-harm. Like Bittner, he found that an act of self-injury was a *prima facie* justification for commitment. In those cases in which an overt act or threat was not present, the presence of a psychiatric history, creation of a public disturbance, and/or bizarre conduct were considered in initiating a commitment.

The probability of the police initiating a hospitalization was also affected by the structural constraints governing hospitalization versus other dispositional alternatives. Rock and associates (1968) found that the more procedural steps there were between the street and hospital, the less likely that police would make an emergency apprehension. Similarly, Matthews (1970) noted that the police officer must calculate how much time alternative courses of action would consume as compared to hospitalization. In sum, the literature documents the pivotal role the police have played historically with regard to the mentally ill.

Police involvement with the mentally ill has become further complicated by several major public policy modifications vis-à-vis mental health delivery. First, the deinstitutionalization of mental patients over the last 30 years has increased the sheer number of mentally ill persons (both deinstitutionalized and "never institutionalized") who may potentially become involved with police.

Second, recent cutbacks in mental health services across the United States have meant that outpatient care often means "no care." Fiscal reductions in mental health programs have resulted in an increasing number of mentally ill persons who are denied treatment because of a lack of available programs and/or a paucity of financial resources (Kiesler, 1982; National Institute of Mental Health [NIMH], 1985). Reductions in mental health funding have also reduced the available number of inpatient beds in public hospitals (NIMH, 1985) as well as the breadth of treatment alternatives (Kiesler & Sibulkin, 1987). These reductions in service are all the more critical when we take into account the changing demographic characteristics. Because of the "coming of age" of post-World War II babies, the absolute number of young persons at risk for developing psychotic disorders is overrepresented in the population (Bachrach, 1982).

Third, the recent, more rigorous legal standards for involuntary mental hospitalization have meant that the simple presence of mental illness and need for service are insufficient to warrant commitment. Rather, the individual must be seriously mentally ill and dangerous to self or others. Many mentally ill persons who would have been committed in years past may now choose to live in the community without treatment.

In sum, the juxtaposition of demographic changes and deinstitutionalization have increased the burden of the mentally ill on police. At the same time, more stringent mental health codes and the diminished treatment options have reduced the police officer's available referral alternatives. Clearly, police now operate in a very different community context than in years past.

This paper will examine the police officer's role as streetcorner psychiatrist within the current sociopolitical milieu. Specifically, we will explore the basic decision rules governing the three major dispositional alternatives available to the police: (1) hospitalization; (2) arrest; and (3) informal disposition. In so doing, it will be demonstrated that the disposition of a mentally disordered citizen is based less on the degree of apparent psychiatric symptomatology than on a complex array of contextual and situational variables.

METHOD

A large-scale observational study of police activity was conducted to observe firsthand how police officers manage mentally ill persons. Police officers in a Midwestern city in the United States (Standard Metropolitan Area over 1,000,000) were observed in their routine interactions with citizens for 2,200 hours over a 14-month period during 1980–81; 283 randomly selected officers were included. Observers included the first author as well as five clinical psychology PhD students (three male, two female).

Observations were conducted during all hours of the day; evenings and weekends were oversampled to obtain a maximum of data in a minimum of time. Data were collected in two busy urban police districts; these districts were chosen because of their socioeconomic and racial/ethnic diversity, as well as because they were fairly typical of this particular city. All types of police–citizen interactions were observed, irrespective of any involvement with mentally disordered persons. This procedure was necessary to obtain data on situations unrelated to mental disorder to use for baseline comparisons.

While a standardized mode of assessment to test for the presence of mental disorder would have been preferable, the naturalistic setting of the research obviously precluded making in-depth psychological assessments. In view of the limitations posed by the naturalistic setting, the presence of severe mental disorder was ascertained by the field-worker via a symptom checklist, which listed the major characteristics of severe mental illness, for example, confusion/disorientation, withdrawal/unresponsiveness, paranoia, inappropriate or bizarre speech and/or behavior, self-destructive behaviors.

The observed citizen was defined to be mentally ill if he or she possessed at least one of the symptoms on the checklist *and* was given a global rating of "mentally disordered" by the field-worker. Both indications were necessary to avoid categorizing persons as mentally ill when they were merely exhibiting bizarre or unusual behavior. Thus, the environmental context as well as a number of psychiatric clues were taken into account.

To insure that this assessment method accurately discriminated between persons who did and did not exhibit signs of serious mental disorder, a separate validity study was undertaken. Using a sample of 61 randomly selected jail detainees, the results of the method used in the present investigation were compared with those generated via a standardized psychiatric assessment instrument, the NIMH Diagnostic Interview Schedule (Robins, Helzer, Croughan, Williams, & Spitzer, 1981). There was a 93.4 percent agreement between the two measures as to the presence/absence of severe mental disorder.

To maintain the natural ambience of the data collection procedure, neither tape recording devices nor extensive note taking were permitted during the observations. The apparent lack of an obvious formal data-collection procedure appeared to enhance cooperation between police officers and field-workers. To ease recollection of the data for subsequent transcription, field-workers were allowed to make a list of all police–citizen encounters that occurred during the observational period. The data were later recorded in two ways.

Quantitative Data

The objective characteristics of the encounter were coded according to an instrument developed expressly for this purpose, the "Incident Coding Form" (ICF). This instrument was designed to record the concrete behaviors and descriptive categories central to the police officers' handling of all police–citizen interactions. An ICF was completed for every encounter between a police officer and a citizen, which involved at least three verbal exchanges. Tests of interrater reliability exceeded 97 percent.

Qualitative Data

Each field-worker was given a dictaphone for home use so that a narrative of the shift could be reconstructed within 24 hours of the observation period. These qualitative data were recorded according to a specified format, which included general shift information, impressionistic data concerning the officer, and most importantly, a complete narrative of each police–citizen encounter. This last data component included the reasoning underlying police officers' discretionary judgements in relation to their management of the mentally ill.

Overall, 1,396 police–citizen encounters involving 2,555 citizens were observed and coded. This is a rate of approximately one citizen for every observational hour. Excluding traffic-related incidents, the database included 1,072 police–citizen encounters involving 2,122 citizens.

FINDINGS

Tables 1 and 2 show that of the 2,122 citizens observed, 85 persons (30 suspects and 55 nonsuspects) were judged by the field-worker to be mentally disordered. The marginals indicate that police tend to resolve situations informally, irrespective of the person's state of mental health. However, Table 1 illustrates that, for suspects, the presence or absence of mental disorder significantly determined the type of disposition; chi-square = 13.66, $p < .001$. Mentally ill suspects had an arrest rate nearly double that of non-ill suspects (46.7 percent vs. 27.9 percent). Perhaps what is most striking about both Tables 1 and 2 is the relative rarity of hospitalization; hospitalization was initiated for only 13.3 percent of the mentally ill suspects (Table 1) and 10.9

Table 1 Presence/Absence of Severe Mental Disorder by Disposition: Suspects Only

Suspects	Disposition, % and (N)			
	Hospitalized	Arrested	Informal Disposition	Total
Ill	13.3(4)	46.7(14)	40.0(12)	5.9(30)
Non-ill	0.0(0)	27.9(133)	72.1(343)	94.1(476)
Total	0.8(4)	29.1(147)	70.2(355)	100.0(506)

*Fisher's Exact Test, $p < .0001$, $df = 1$. Since the expected values were too small to perform a chi-square statistic, we used an analogy to Fisher's Exact Test for a three by two table (Mehta & Patel, 1983).

Table 2 Presence/Absence of Severe Mental Disorder by Disposition: Nonsuspects Only[a]

Nonsuspects	Disposition, % and (N)[b]		
	Hospitalized	Informal Disposition	Total
Ill	10.9(6)	89.1(49)	3.4(55)
Non-ill	0.0(0)	100.0(1561)	96.6(1561)
Total	0.4(6)	99.6(1610)	100.0(1616)

[a]Includes victims, witnesses, complainants, objects of concern, and subjects of assistance.
[b]The category, "Arrested," does not appear in this table because, by definition, nonsuspects cannot be arrested. The police officer's definition of citizen role was used.
*Fisher's Exact Test, $p < .0001$, $df = 1$.

percent of the nonsuspects (Table 2). Not surprisingly, police never sought to hospitalize any citizen who was defined by the field-worker as "nonmentally disordered."

Given the disruptive nature of many symptoms of severe mental disorder, it is interesting that police rarely resort to hospitalization. The data presented in Tables 1 and 2 suggest a number of questions. Under what circumstances are hospitalizations initiated? Is the type of disposition (hospitalization, arrest, or informal) determined largely by the degree of apparent disorder? What extrapsychiatric factors affect the police officer's choice of disposition? To explore these questions the following section presents qualitative data relevant to each of the three major dispositions shown in Table 1. Two types of data are presented: (1) information ascertained via direct observation of the 85 mentally disordered citizens, and (2) anecdotes communicated to the field-worker by the officers about their prior experience in handling mentally disordered persons.

Hospitalization

Our finding concerning the rarity of emergency hospitalization is strikingly similar to Bittner's (1967) finding of more than 2 decades ago. However, the infrequent utilization of the hospital in the present investigation was a result of a number of structural characteristics peculiar to the current postdeinstitutionalization milieu.

Police were acutely aware of the reduced number of psychiatric placements available to them. While state hospitals were once the primary treatment facility, they have been replaced by community-based mental health centers. Unfortunately, these mental health centers (many housed within private hospitals) often have very strict admission criteria. We found that virtually every police officer was aware of the stringent requirements for admission into the local psychiatric hospital: the person must be either actively delusional or suicidal. Police knew that persons who were alcoholics, narcotic addicts, or defined by hospital staff to be "dangerous" were *persona non grata* at the hospitals, even if they also exhibited signs of serious mental disorder. Persons with criminal charges pending, no matter how minor, were deemed unacceptable. It was common knowledge among officers that if a citizen met the above-mentioned exclusionary criteria, hospitalization was not an available disposition.

The following vignette illustrates one of the few situations that met the criteria for hospitalization. Hospitalization was initiated because the citizen was seriously delusional and too public in her deviance to be ignored by the police:

At 22:00 a radio call came on saying there was a white female, age 28, who was taking off her clothes in front of the ———— building. She was dressed in dirty clothes and was very disheveled. She was repeatedly pulling up her T-shirt and exposing herself and making obscene gestures at the crowd that had gathered. Several officers helped her into the wagon. She kept saying, "Fuck [the mayor]." She said she had walked from [the suburbs] to make some statements to the mayor...she continued yelling things [profanities] out of the back [of the wagon]....There was no evidence of alcohol or drugs, so it looked like a straight psychiatric case...the woman said she had been in a psychiatric hospital and that she was manic-depressive....(Shift #171, Encounter 2)

Even those mentally disordered individuals who meet admission criteria and seek voluntary admission are rarely hospitalized without bureaucratic impediments. The following vignette illustrates the structural constraints, which often impede police when initiating even a voluntary hospitalization. This case is notable because it illustrates the frequent situation in which the services offered do not match those that are required:

Between 22:00 and 23:00, call for suicide risk. Dispatcher said this was the third call...Citizen, male, age 73...approached the officers and said other officers had been there several times that night. He said he had talked with the Human Service people, but was still feeling suicidal....Human Service people had gotten him an appointment for Monday morning to see if they could get him in a nursing home. Citizen had agreed, but now said he could not handle the situation so he had gone out and started drinking. On one of the earlier calls that evening, the police had confiscated several knives and other items Citizen had planned to use to commit suicide....He had tried to commit suicide twice before. He had old scars on his wrists...after one suicide attempt he was hospitalized....It was clear that Citizen was not getting the help he felt he needed...he said he'd been drinking this night in order to get up the courage to kill himself...asked to go to [hospital]...so officers drove to [local hospital]...the psychiatric unit at the hospital was full so they could not take him and said we should try another hospital...police called the wagon...Officer I said Citizen needed to go to [state mental hospital]. The wagon officers looked at each other disgustedly and one asked why the man needed to go....The wagon officers then reluctantly had Citizen climb in the back [of the wagon]...Officers I and II felt they really didn't have any means of handling the situation and that there were no resources in the community to help them out...mental health system...is only geared for people who have already made a suicide attempt and can be taken to the hospital, or who represent a definite danger to others....(Shift #326, Encounter 11)

While suicidal risk may be insufficient for hospitalization, persons who have already attempted suicide are readily admitted by the hospital, as indicated in the following vignettes:

Radio call for an injured person at a nursing home. Citizen 1...a double amputee in a wheelchair...was sitting holding his head between his knees...he had broken a bottle and cut part of what was left of his leg with the bottle...Officer I took Citizen 2 [a nurse] aside and asked her what [amputee's] problem was and whether he had done this before. He asked her if she thought [man] was suicidal...[and if he] had been referred for psychiatric help. He said obviously the man needs some kind of help and the nurse said, "Well, if he needs it he'll be referred for it." Officer I said no, "I'm asking you if he has been referred for psychiatric help?"...Officer I said that he obviously had some deep problems...he needs help. [Nurse] had recontacted the doctor and was making arrangements for [amputee] to go to ———— hospital for a psychiatric evaluation. She was going to call the ambulance and have him transported tonight....In sum...Officer I took the time to talk things over and find out about the situation. He was instrumental in getting the patient transferred to the [psychiatric] hospital. (Shift #397, Encounter 2)

Three months ago, Officer I was working the midnight shift [with a partner]. It was about 2:30 a.m. [They]...happened to notice a man standing on a corner wearing a sweatshirt, parka and slacks. He was about thirty-years-old, white. As they drove by, they noticed him wave. They said it was the kind of reaction where he probably didn't really need the police until he saw them, and decided to stop them. They...came back, and pulled up, with the passenger-side officer rolling down his window and asking what he wanted. The man responded that he wanted to go to the ———— hospital. They asked him why. Before anyone could do anything, he pulled out a knife and plunged it into his chest. The man was admitted to the hospital. (Shift #38)

Despite the importance of the police in aiding the mentally ill, "managing mentals" was not regarded by the officers as a "good pinch." Since the officer's activity index and criminal arrest quota excluded psychiatric dispositions, involvement with the mentally ill was unrecognized and unrewarded by the police department. Coupled with the scarcity of placements and the hospitals' strict admission criteria, the lack of rewards tended to inhibit the police from making psychiatric referrals.

An added complication was that the current philosophy of community-based treatment apparently discouraged police from using the hospital as a resource. Police did not understand the policy of community care. They perceived rapid release of "their mentals" to be a personal slight on their judgement, a waste of their time, and an unwillingness by the mental health profession to "do something." Police frequently lamented that "no place will take them" or "how nuts does someone have to be?" In short, the current normative structure discourages police from initiating hospitalizations. Without the aid of the mental health system, police of necessity incorporate streetcorner psychiatry to maintain the mentally ill in the community.

ACTIONS CONSIDERED INSANE OFTEN DON'T MEET THE STANDARDS OF NEW YORK'S LEGAL SYSTEM

By *ANEMONA HARTOCOLLIS*

A diagnosis of schizophrenia and repeated commitments to mental institutions might seem like obvious qualifications for an insanity defense—or maybe not.

Experts say the legal standard for insanity is very different from what most laymen and even psychiatrists would consider crazy behavior.

The case of David Tarloff, 39, who is charged with second-degree murder in the slashing death of *Kathryn Faughey*, an Upper East Side therapist, is the latest to raise questions about when a defendant is too mentally ill to be responsible for his behavior.

Mr. Tarloff's family has said he has a history of schizophrenia, going back to young adulthood. Others with similar histories, like *Andrew Goldstein*, who pushed a woman in front of a subway, and Kevin McKiever, who stabbed a former Rockette in the back, have been convicted of the crimes.

"The truth is in the State of New York, you can be extremely crazy without being legally insane," *Ronald L. Kuby*, a criminal defense lawyer who has handled cases of mentally ill defendants, said Tuesday. "You can hear voices, you can operate under intermittent delusions, you can see rabbits in the road that aren't there and still be legally sane."

What matters to the justice system is whether the defendant is capable of telling the difference between right and wrong, and of understanding the consequences of acts, in spite of mental illness.

With those legal standards in mind, investigators were looking for signs that Mr. Tarloff was acting rationally before Dr. Faughey's death, law enforcement officials said Tuesday.

Investigators said they were considering, for instance, whether Mr. Tarloff had looked for an escape route or had consciously concealed the weapons that he used.

A textbook example of such behavior, said *Robert Gottlieb*, a defense lawyer, would be, "If you buy a ticket under a false name, so you're already planning to flee using an alias."

Mr. Gottlieb represented *Peter Braunstein*, a former magazine writer who was convicted in May of dressing as a firefighter in a ruse to get into a former colleague's apartment, where he sexually abused her.

Mr. Braunstein's writings, his orders from eBay and his rental of a storage locker became focuses of the trial, as the prosecutor tried to show that Mr. Braunstein knew what he was doing because he had planned every step of the crime.

The first step in a case like Mr. Tarloff's is to determine whether he is fit to stand trial, which requires an evaluation of his mental state. Prosecution experts may find that even though he is competent to stand trial, he was insane when police say he committed the crime. And then the district attorney could work out a plea that would send him to a psychiatric institution.

Such a plea can often mean that a defendant will spend more time in a psychiatric facility than if he were found guilty at trial, N. G. Berrill, a psychologist and the executive director of the New York Center for Neuropsychology and Forensic Behavioral Science, said Tuesday.

"It's not the cakewalk that people fantasize," Dr. Berrill said.

If Mr. Tarloff went to trial and a jury found him not responsible for his behavior because of mental illness, he would be sent to a mental institution where he would be re-evaluated at least every two years, Dr. Berrill said Tuesday. But, he said, doctors tend to be very conservative about ending treatment.

Daniel Rakowitz, who killed a girlfriend in 1989, was found not guilty by reason of insanity and remains in a maximum-security psychiatric center.

But insanity defenses rarely work during trials, Dr. Berrill said, because juries are wary of being tricked by a defendant who is faking insanity, and because they are afraid of letting a violent person back out on the streets.

He cited the case of Mr. Goldstein, a schizophrenic accused of pushing *Kendra Webdale*, 32, in front of a subway train in 1999. He was tried twice for murder and convicted in the second trial. After that conviction was overturned because of hearsay evidence, Mr. Goldstein pleaded guilty to manslaughter.

Mr. Goldstein might have seemed a perfect candidate for an insanity defense, Dr. Berrill said. "He's got the history, he's off his meds, he's hearing voices, and why in the world would you push a complete stranger onto the subway tracks?" he said.

Mr. Kuby recalled one of his clients, Mr. McKiever, a schizophrenic who had bounced in and out of mental institutions. He was accused of killing a former Rockette, Alexis Ficks Welsh, in 1991 by stabbing her as she walked her dogs near Central Park.

Mr. McKiever was twice declared incompetent to stand trial. But after being medicated, he was able to stand trial; he was convicted and sentenced to 25 years to life.

Source: Anemona Hartocollis. "Actions Considered Insane Often Don't Meet the Standards of New York's Legal System." *New York Times*, February 20, 2008. Retrieved July 27, 2008, http://www.nytimes.com/2008/02/20/nyregion/20prosecute.html

Arrest

Although there is a stereotype that police spend the bulk of their time making arrests, our data show that arrest occurs relatively rarely. However, the arrest rate for the mentally ill is significantly greater than for non-ill persons (see also Teplin, 1984b) because arrest is often the only disposition available that will bring the situation under control. For example, arrests would take place when persons were not sufficiently mentally disordered to be admitted by the hospital, but were too public in their deviance to be ignored. In such situations, the probability of arrest was increased whenever it was thought that the mentally ill person would continue to annoy "decent people," and therefore result in a subsequent call for police service.

Our data indicate that it was common practice for the police to obtain a signed complaint from a third party (thus facilitating arrest) even in situations where psychiatric hospitalization was thought to be the more appropriate disposition. The police officer's rationale for this procedure was to ensure the ready availability of an alternative disposition (arrest) in the event that the hospital found the individual unacceptable for admission. The police officer's ingenuity was apparently born out of necessity since, as noted above, the hospitals had very specific criteria for admission. The following vignette illustrates a situation in which the person was apparently mentally ill, but was thought to be insufficiently ill to be admitted to the hospital and was subsequently arrested:

The officer indicated that this man had been on the street calling women names, calling them whores, and shouting at black people, calling them "niggers" and chasing them. The officer said he thought the guy was crazy, "you know paranoid"....A woman had signed a complaint and asked that he be arrested because he was bothering her....The man sounded like a paranoid schizophrenic...both from my observation of him and his response to questions the officer put to him in the station. He was very vague about himself and who he was, and felt that people were out to get him. He couldn't understand why he was in the police station. When he was taken to his cell he began shouting to be let out, and kept shouting the rest of the time he was there. The officer said the man denied having any psychiatric treatment or being under psychiatric care. In this situation he was charged with disorderly conduct. The officer said that there wasn't enough to take him into the mental health center, because his behavior wasn't that severe for the hospital to accept him. (Shift #119)

Arrest is also the only disposition available to the officer in cases where the person is defined as "too dangerous" by the hospital or has any type of pending criminal charge, as indicated by the following two vignettes:

A young man was banging on his mother's door with a meat cleaver....He was threatening to kill someone else and was trying to get into this mother's home for a gun. She wouldn't let him in, and had called the police to get rid of him and/or calm him down. When the police got there, Officer II decided that the man needed to be hospitalized as he was dangerous to himself and others. So they called for a wagon to take the man to [state mental hospital]...but they also wanted a complaint signed by the mother for disorderly [conduct] in case [the hospital] wouldn't take him. It turned out that [the hospital] would indeed not take the man so he ended up being locked up for disorderly conduct. (Shift #180)

Citizen I was the victim of the knifing assault by Citizen 2 and had suffered some minor cuts on her face, arms, and hands....They were drinking beer and [victim] decided that she would go to the store to buy more beer. Upon her return she found [the other woman] beating her [own] children....A quick look at the kids showed they had been severely beaten. [The victim] stated that, upon finding [other woman] beating the children, she attempted to restrain [her] and the latter woman grabbed a knife blade from a kitchen drawer and attacked [the victim who] called the police...demanding the officers arrest [the other woman]. She stated that [the assailant] had beaten her children before, was on some sort of probation for this and has a history of psychiatric treatment....There was evidence in her behavior of a psychiatric problem. Officer I had to restrain [the assailant] a number of times as she tried to bolt from the apartment and return to...reclaim her children...[She] was verbally abusive, resistant....At the station, [she] was charged with assault...Officer I stated that [this] was clearly a psychiatric case, should probably go to [psychiatric hospital]. However, because she had [criminal] charges against her, [hospital] won't accept her. It's hospital policy not to accept police referrals with charges pending against them. (Shift #148, Encounter 2)

These vignettes illustrate the inconsistency between the legal structure and streetcorner implementation of the law. Although "dangerousness to self or others" is one of the major criteria for commitment in most mental health codes, this characteristic renders citizens undesirable by many hospitals. Once rejected for hospitalization, the only available disposition is often arrest.

Mentally ill persons who have additional problems (e.g., substance abuse) are also likely candidates for arrest. For example, mental health programs find that people who have been drinking are disruptive to the patient milieu and often will not accept them for treatment. Conversely, detoxification programs feel that they are not equipped to deal with persons suffering from a psychiatric impairment. The following narrative is illustrative of a rather typical situation in which the jail was the last stop of several in an attempt to find a placement for a person who was both mentally ill and intoxicated.

At 8:00 p.m. we...saw that an ambulance was stopping in back of a parked bus....They [ambulance personnel] ran inside the bus and brought out a large burly black man. The officers exclaimed, "Charlie, what are you doing?" Charlie greeted them with equal friendliness. Evidently, Charlie was the neighborhood character....The bus driver, not realizing Charlie was drunk, was afraid he was ill and had called for an ambulance. The paramedics, seeing that Charlie was only drunk, left him in our charge. The officers asked Charlie if he wanted to go to detox and he said "sure"....The people [at detox] took one look at Charlie and would not accept him. Evidently, he was potentially violent and disruptive....The officers asked if they would sign a complaint. They said yes. Evidently he had been [to the jail] so often that they already had a sheet on him so it was easy to get him into a cell. The officer explained to me that Charlie was a problem because he wasn't crazy enough to go to the mental hospital. The people at [the mental hospital] wouldn't accept him because he was potentially violent and often drunk. The detox people didn't want him, even though he was an alcoholic, because he was potentially violent and bothered other patients with his crazy ways. So that left the jail. They would put him in lock-up overnight; he would go to court in the morning and then would be released. In the meantime, they would get him off the street. Charlie was booked for disorderly conduct. The detox facility was the complainant, although he had done nothing disorderly. (Shift #81, Encounter 3)

The qualitative data indicate that multiply impaired persons (such as those described above) are more likely to be arrested because of the overall organization of the mental health care delivery system. Although our public health system is composed of a complex array of services, each subsystem designs its programs to fit a specific need. Thus, the majority of programs are designed as if clients are "pure types," for example, they are *either* alcoholic or mentally ill. Because of the narrowly defined parameters of each of the various subsystems, a number of multiply impaired persons are deemed unacceptable for treatment in each of the service delivery facilities. In this way, many potential users "fall through the cracks" of the various caregiving subsystems into the criminal justice net. As illustrated in the above vignette, police would often make the rounds of the various service agencies before resorting to arrest.

"Serious" incidents were also more likely to culminate in an arrest. However, unlike Bittner's (1967) study, the definition of "seriousness" in the present investigation was not always correlated with the severity of the offense. A number of sociopsychological contingencies determined whether or not the serious criterion would be invoked. For example, situations in which the citizen was disrespectful of the police officer were nearly always thought to be serious as illustrated by the following two vignettes:

> Radio call for a disturbance at a bar....The bartender...stated to the officer that a lady sitting at the bar...had been trying to get people to buy her drinks and had been bothering the other customers and creating a disruption....The officers asked her if she would leave. The lady said no. The officer then radioed for a wagon....The officer then asked her if she wanted to leave or would she rather go to jail. She said she didn't care....When the wagon arrived, he told her, "Let's go"...her behavior had been rather strange but, as Officer I stated later, there was no reason to take her to the hospital because she was just causing a disturbance and was not endangering herself or anyone else....The sergeant commented that...even though he suspected that she had some sort of mental problem, the fact that she wouldn't leave the area made a legal disposition necessary. (Shift #125, Encounter 2)
>
> We received a call to investigate a disturbance at the el [elevated train] station....When we arrived at the scene we were met by a female newspaper dealer who said earlier...a woman was in the el station, screaming and trying to take some of the newspapers....As we were walking out, the woman who caused the original problem came back into the station...she ran amuck. She jumped on the police officer and started hitting him with closed fists and she was really landing blows. He was taken by surprise, but after a brief struggle...he led her out of the el station to the car....During this time she began screaming at him that he was an agent of the devil and that she was a messenger from God; that she would see to it that he was punished by God for having her arrested. Nevertheless...he arrested her on a disorderly conduct charge. (Shift #291, Encounter 2)

Similarly, situations that were public, which offended "decent people," and those with a willing complainant were nearly always defined by police to be serious:

> Batman is seriously syphillitic, a street person well known to the officers. He used to be entirely painted green, but has stopped doing that. He is bug-infested. There is a hole in the side of his face where the spirochyte has caused his face to become disfigured. He goes into [expensive department stores] and scares the customers because he's so unsightly, but sometimes will steal petty things....Officer I said that [hospital] had gotten tired of taking Batman, they felt he was a hopeless case and had given up on him. So now, the only thing to do with him was send him to lock-up. He said, "Police don't give up on patients the way doctors, psychiatrists or psychologists do. They keep locking people up and the court system doesn't give up on people. The recidivism rate is extremely high." (Shift #170, Encounter 4)
>
> We...were met by an elderly woman who said there was a man sleeping in a car behind the apartment building. She said that the night before, this man had been acting real crazy and had thrown rocks at the building....We saw the suspect sleeping in the back seat of a rather old Dodge. The suspect presented a very bizarre sight....Most of his hair was off, but there were ridges of hair all over his head...actual gouges in his scalp. There were also numerous

slash marks up and down his wrists, extending up to the elbows. [He] looked disoriented, was very filthy, but looked physically fit, perhaps a body builder at one time. He was quite acquiescent.... They [officers] put cuffs on him and told him they were going to take him in for damage to property and, probably, disorderly conduct. At this point, the woman who called the police made the general comment that this man didn't belong in jail, but in a hospital as he was sick...[However,] the man was taken away...to the station and booked. (Shift #284, Encounter 1)

In sum, arrest was used as a disposition in three types of situations: (1) when the police officer's first choice would have been hospitalization, but the officer felt that there was a strong probability that the potential patient would be judged unacceptable by the hospital; most often, they were rejected because they fell into the cracks between the narrowly defined parameters of the various service subsystems; (2) in encounters which that were character-ized by their publicness and visibility, which at the same time exceeded the tolerance for deviant behavior within the community and offended "decent people;" and (3) in situations in which the police felt there was a high likeli-hood that the person would continue to "cause a problem" (and thus result in a "callback"). In such encounters, police resorted to arrest as a way of manag-ing the person by removing him or her from the scene.

Overall, formal dispositions were made (either hospitalization or arrest) when police felt that the situation was likely to escalate and require subse-quent police assistance. Clearly, the large gray area between behavior that is mentally disordered and that which is merely disorderly allows a great deal of discretion in choosing the final disposition. It is frequently unclear whether the individual is "bad" and should be arrested, "mad" and should be hospitalized, or simply "odd" and would be tolerated within the com-munity. Nevertheless, the data indicate that the degree of psychiatric symp-tomatology is only one of many predictive variables determining the police disposition of the case.

Informal Dispositions

Our finding that informal dispositions were the predominant resolution is consistent with prior studies (Bittner, 1967; Schag, 1977). Police handled over 70 percent of all mentally ill persons via informal means. Requiring neither paperwork nor unwanted "downtime" (time off the street), informal disposi-tions are the police officer's resolution of choice.

There are three major categories of mentally disordered persons who are likely to be handled by informal means: (1) neighborhood characters, (2) "troublemakers," and (3) quiet "crazies."

Neighborhood Characters. Police are familiar with "neighborhood characters," that is, persons who reside within the community and whose idiosyncratic behavior(s) and/or appearance set them apart from "decent people." Virtually any officer can tell you about "Crazy Mary," "Mailbox Mollie," "Dirty Dean," and "Ziggy." These are neighborhood characters who are defined by the police as "mentals" but who are not hospitalized because the familiarity, predictability, and consistency of their eccentricities enable the police and local community to tolerate their deviant behavior. Interestingly, familiarity with the citizen's particular psychiatric symptomatology enables the officers to act as a streetcorner psychiatrist. In this way, police play a major role in maintaining the mentally ill within the community. The following vignettes depict common encounters of this type in which the neighborhood character is greatly comforted by the police officer's apparent concern:

> A man called the police to inform them that he was being monitored by another man. He said the man had planted a microdot in his apartment and kept track of his every action. The complainant had a lot of electronic equipment in his apartment....He claimed the man who was monitoring him was able to jam his CB radio and call the man obscenities over the radio. He asked the officers to listen....The man said he's also called the FBI and wanted to file a report with the police. Officer I said he went along with the man, letting him think the officers would take such a report, but he didn't do anything....The man seemed appreciative of their efforts and they told him to let them know if he got any more information on the threatening man. The man was clearly disturbed, but as he was not dangerous to himself or others, he was not taken to [hospital]. The police just humored him. Officer II agreed that there's a necessity for deception in some cases. (Shift #213)
>
> A lady in the area claims she has neighbors who are beaming rays up into her apartment. Usually...the officer handles the situation by telling the person, "we'll go downstairs and tell the people downstairs to stop beaming the rays," and she's happy. Officer II seemed quite happy about this method of handling the problem. (Shift #220)

Troublemakers. Troublemakers, like neighborhood characters, are known to the police and are most likely to be managed by informal means; in other words, they are unlikely to be arrested or hospitalized. However, unlike the neighborhood character, the police officer's use of informal dispositions with troublemakers is not dictated by their predictability. Rather, informal dispositions are the resolution of choice because troublemakers are thought to be too difficult to handle via either arrest or hospitalization. The symptoms of their mental disorder are such that they cause disorder and disrupt the routine of the police. Police related the following vignettes:

> Whenever she came into the [police] station she caused an absolute disruption. She would take off her clothes, run around the station nude, and urinate on the sergeant's desk. They felt it was such a hassle to have her in the station, and in lock-up, that they simply stopped arresting her. (Shift #036)
>
> I think Harry is paranoid. Whenever the police go near him for any reason, even if it had nothing to do with him, he would get very upset and begin calling downtown, causing all kinds of flak in the department. So they leave him completely alone, even though they feel he is a certified cashew nut. (Shift #036)

These vignettes indicate that being labelled a troublemaker allows the individual to act in ways that would otherwise tend to result in either arrest or hospitalization. Police feel that although formal intervention may be periodically warranted in such cases, such persons are usually not worth the hassle and disruption.

Quiet "Crazies." Persons whose symptoms of mental disorder are relatively unobtrusive are also likely to be handled informally. Such persons offend neither the populace nor the police with vocal or visual manifestations of their illness. Their symptoms are not seen as being serious enough to warrant hospitalization. Moreover, quiet crazies are seen as more disordered than disorderly and are unlikely to provoke arrest, as the following vignettes illustrate:

She [complainant] said the man down the block…had been trying…the door next to her restaurant….Both officers recognized the man as a street person….This was clearly a mental health case not going to [the hospital] based on discretion used by the officers…the man was wearing several stocking caps underneath the helmet, a pair of hexagonal shaped glasses, over safety goggles, several scarfs around his neck…4–5 layers of shirts, sweaters, jackets topped by an overcoat…carrying a brown shopping bag…and a cardboard box….Officer I searched him…as Officer I was talking information…the man kept saying "thank you" after he found out he was not going to be arrested…The man said he'd seen a psychiatrist in Kentucky and Indiana. The man said he'd never been to [local hospitals]….Officer II said, "[hospital] probably wouldn't have wanted that man anyway." He said they would have let him go when they saw he was coherent and they don't care about the street or shopping bag person….It was clear that Officer II saw [hospital] making clear discriminations about who were likely prospects for being kept there. (Shift #213, Encounter 1)

As [a citizen] waved to us, Officer I identified her as a "crazy lady," stating he had seen her in the neighborhood, gesturing at passers by….by appearance, [she] was fairly identifiable as a mental health case…dressed bizarrely, wearing many layers of clothing. She spoke in a hyperactive, excited way….She told a story about having friends who were afraid to come back to [city]…They went out of town and had left their car on the streets…the car had picked up a lot of parking tickets…her friends were afraid to come back because they thought something terrible would happen to them because they had all these tickets. It became clear very quickly that [her] story didn't make any sense….In response to [her] distress, [officer] became quite placating, sympathetic and reassuring. Rather than arguing that there was no reason for her friends' fear, he told her what to tell her friend to do about these tickets…Officer I gave up after she wasn't placated, ending by saying, "okay it will be alright dear. We have to go now." She remained as revved up as in the beginning….Afterwards, Officer I expressed feelings of resignation about such situations. He said…either they are victims of crime or just in need of something which the police are not able to provide. (Shift #278, Encounter 5)

In both vignettes, the citizens were judged neither sufficiently disordered to warrant a mental health referral nor sufficiently disruptive to warrant an arrest.

CONCLUSION

Managing mentally disordered persons in the community has always been a necessary part of police work. In recent years, the police officer's role as streetcorner psychiatrist has expanded as a result of deinstitutionalization and other public policy modifications. However, the legal structure does not dictate the resolution of encounters with the mentally ill. Whether the disordered individual is defined by police to be "bad" (and should be arrested), "mad" (and therefore hospitalized), or merely "eccentric" is decided by discretion rather than by rules of law. Of necessity, police have developed an informal operative code to implement the legal structure.

This paper has demonstrated the importance of extrapsychiatric variables in determining the informal operative code. The police officers' decision to hospitalize, arrest, or manage a mentally ill citizen informally is based less on the degree of psychiatric symptomatology than on the sociopsychological and structural factors pertinent to each situation. By and large, the police do not rely on conventional mental health resources; arrest, too, is a relatively infrequent disposition. Rather, informal dispositions are the resolution of choice.

Further investigations of police decision making are needed to determine the extent to which the present findings can be generalized. Studies of rural areas are of particular importance to determine if and how the exigencies of rural life alter the police officer's choice of management strategies. Multijurisdictional studies are also needed to investigate the impact of the legal structure on police management of the mentally ill. For example, how do commitment criteria, whether restrictive or liberalized, affect the police officer's choice of disposition? The extent of mental health services and the availability of outpatient commitment as a treatment alternative are also likely to affect police decision-making (Mulvey, Blumstein, & Cohen, 1987), and warrant further study.

Police departments must be made aware of their pivotal role as a mental health resource. Programs to educate and train police about extralegal dispositions for mentally ill citizens have been advocated by a number of mental health professionals (cf. Finn & Sullivan, 1987; Monahan & Monahan, 1986; Teplin, 1984a, 1984b, 1991) and in the Criminal Justice Mental Health Standards adopted by the American Bar Association. Accordingly, police departments in the United States have begun to include mental health training in their programs (Finn & Sullivan, 1987). In this way, law enforcement agencies are acknowledging and preparing police for their legitimate role as "streetcorner psychiatrist."

References

Bachrach, L. L. (1982). Young adult chronic patients: An analytical review of the literature. *Hospital and Community Psychiatry, 33,* 189–197.

Bittner, E. (1967). Police discretion in emergency apprehension of mentally ill persons. *Social Problems, 14,* 278–292.

Bittner, E. (1970). *The function of police in modern society.* Washington, DC: National Institute of Mental Health.

California Welfare and Institutional Code 5150 (West 1980).

Cobb, C. W. (1972). Community mental health services and the lower socioeconomic classes. *American Journal of Orthopsychiatry, 43,* 404–414.

Finn, P., & Sullivan, M. (1987). *Police response to special populations.* Washington, DC: U.S. Department of Justice, National Institute of Justice, Office of Communication and Research Utilization.

Fox, R. G., & Erickson, P. G. (1972). *Apparently suffering from mental disorder.* Toronto, Canada: University of Toronto Centre of Criminology.

Gilboy, J. A., & Schmidt, J. R. (1971). "Voluntary" hospitalization of the mentally ill. *Northwestern University Law Review, 66,* 429–453.

Goldstein, P. J. (1979). *Prostitution and drugs.* Lexington, MA: Lexington Books.

Gottfredson, M., & Gottfredson, D. (1980). *Decision making in criminal justice: Toward the rational exercise of discretion.* Cambridge, MA: Ballinger Publishing Co.

Hollingshead, A. B., & Redlich, F. C. (1958). *Social class and mental illness.* New York: John Wiley & Sons.

Illinois Revised Statutes. chap. 91 1/2 3-606 (1981).

Kiesler, C. A. (1982). Public and professional myths about mental hospitalization: An empirical reassessment of policy-related beliefs. *American Psychologist, 37,* 1323–1339.

Kiesler, C. A., & Sibulkin, A. E. (1987). *Mental hospitalization: Myths and facts about a national crisis.* Beverly Hills: Sage Publications.

Liberman, R. (1969). Police as a community mental health resource. *Community Mental Health Journal, 5,* 111–120.

Manning, P. (1977). *Police work: The social organization of policing.* Cambridge, MA: MIT Press.

Manning, P. (1984). Police classification and the mentally ill. In L. Teplin (Ed.), *Mental health and criminal Justice* (pp. 177–198). Beverly Hills: Sage Publications.

Matthews, A. (1970). Observations on police policy and procedures for emergency detention of the mentally ill. *Journal of Criminal Law, Criminology, and Police Science, 61,* 283–295.

Mehta, C. R., & Patel, N. R. (1983). A network algorithm for performing Fischer's Exact Test in R x C contingency tables. *Journal of the American Statistical Association,* June, 427–434.

Monahan, J., & Monahan, B. (1986). Police and the mentally disordered. In J. Yuille (Ed.), *Police Selection and Training* (pp. 175–186). The Hague, The Netherlands: Martinus Nijhoff.

Mulvey, E. P., Blumstein, A., & Cohen, J. (1987). Reframing the research question of mental patient criminality. *International Journal of Law and Psychiatry, 9,* 57–65.

National Institute of Mental Health. (1985). *Mental health, United States, 1985* (DHHS Publication No. ADM 85–1378). Washington, DC: U.S. Government Printing Office.

Robins, L., Helzer, J., Croughan, J., Williams, J., & Spitzer, R. (1981). *NIMH Diagnostic Interview Schedule: Version III.* Rockville, MD: NIMH, Division of Biometry and Epidemiology.

Rock, R., Jacobson, M., & Janepaul, R. (1968). *Hospitalization and discharge of the mentally ill.* Chicago: University of Chicago Press.

Rumbaut, R. G., & Bittner, E. (1979). Changing conceptions of the police role. In N. Morris & M. Tonry (Eds.), *Crime and justice: An annual review of research* (Vol. 1) (pp. 239–288). Chicago, IL: University of Chicago Press.

Schag, D. (1977). *Predicting dangerousness: An analysis of procedures in a mental center.* Unpublished doctoral dissertation, University of California, Santa Cruz.

Shah, S. (1975). Dangerousness and civil commitment of the mentally ill: Some public policy considerations. *American Journal of Psychiatry, 132,* 501–505.

Sheridan, E. P., & Teplin, L. A. (1981). Police-referred psychiatric emergencies: Advantages of community treatment. *Journal of Community Psychology, 9,* 140–147.

Sims, A., & Symonds, R. (1975). Psychiatric referrals from the police. *British Journal of Psychiatry, 127,* 171–178.

Smith, D. A. (1986). The neighborhood context of police behavior. In M. Tonry & N. Morris (Eds.). *Crime and justice: An annual review of research* (Vol. 8). Chicago, IL: University of Chicago Press.

Smith, D. A., & Visher, C. A. (1981). Street-level justice: Situational determinants of police arrest decisions. *Social Problems, 29,* 167–177.

Stone, A. (1975). *Mental health and law: A system in transition.* Washington, DC: U.S. Government Printing Office.

Teplin, L. A. (1983). The criminalization of the mentally ill: Speculation in search of data. *Psychological Bulletin, 94,* 54–67.

Teplin, L. A. (1984a). Managing disorder: Police handling of the mentally ill. In L. A. Teplin (Ed.), *Mental health and criminal justice* (pp. 157–176). Beverly Hills, CA: Sage Publications.

Teplin, L. A. (1984b). Criminalizing mental disorder: The comparative arrest rate of the mentally ill. *American Psychologist, 39,* 794–803.

Teplin, L. A. (1991). The criminalization hypothesis: Myth, misnomer or management strategy. In S. Shah & B. Sales (Eds.), *Law and mental health: Major developments and research needs* (DHHS Publication No. ADM 91–1875). Washington, DC: U.S. Government Printing Office.

Teplin, L. A., Filstead, W., Hefter, G., & Sheridan, E. (1980). Police involvement with the psychiatric emergency patient. *Psychiatric Annals, 10,* 202–207.

Urmer, A. (1973). *The burden of the mentally disordered on law enforcement.* Sacramento, CA: ENKI Research Institute.

Warren, C. A. (1977). *The social construction of dangerousness.* Los Angeles, CA: University of Southern California.

Wilkinson, G. S. (1975). Patient-audience social status and the social construction of psychiatric disorders: Toward a differential frame of reference hypothesis. *Journal of Health and Social Behavior, 16,* 28–38.

Wilson, J. Q. (1968). The police and the delinquent in two cities. In S. Wheeler (Ed.), *Controlling delinquents* (pp. 9–30). New York: John Wiley & Sons.

DISCUSSION

1. What did Teplin and Pruett find to be the most common disposition when police confronted a mentally disordered person? Did the response of police officers differ when they encountered someone with and without a mental illness? What was the preferred disposition of police officers when dealing with apparently mentally disordered persons?

2. What factors influenced how police officers responded to mentally disordered persons? To what extent did the manifest appearance or knowledge

of psychiatric disorder plan in the police officers' decision making? What was the nature of the impact of other "extra-psychiatric" factors on how police responded to mentally disordered individuals?

Eric Silver and Brent Teasdale

Mental Disorder and Violence: An Examination of Stressful Life Events and Impaired Social Support

Prior research suggests that people with mental illnesses are significantly more likely to engage in violence than those without mental illness; however, this research has focused almost exclusively on clinical factors, namely the presence or absence of a psychiatric disorder. In this paper, sociologists Silver and Teasdale reframe our understanding of violence among those with mental illness by exploring the social context within which violent behaviors occur.

After over a decade of research, considerable evidence has accrued suggesting that people with mental disorders are significantly more likely to engage in violence than people without mental disorders (Arseneault et al., 2000; Monahan, 1992; Swanson et al., 1990), particularly when their disorders involve paranoid psychotic symptoms (Link, Andrews & Cullen, 1992; Link, Monahan, Stueve & Cullen, 1999; Swanson et al., 1996) or when they co-occur with substance abuse (Steadman et al., 1998). The link between mental disorder and violence has been observed across a variety of sampling strategies, outcome measures, and mental disorder measures, and with controls for a wide range of sociodemographic characteristics (for reviews, see Link & Stueve, 1995; Monahan et al., 2002; Mulvey, 1994). However, despite the robustness of this association, little is understood about why mental disorder and violence are linked (Hiday, 1995, 1997; Mulvey, 1994; Silver, 2000).

Most prior explanations of the relationship between mental disorder and violence emphasize clinical characteristics, such as paranoid psychotic symptoms (Link, Monahan, Stueve & Cullen, 1999; Link & Stueve, 1994), substance abuse disorders (Steadman et al., 1998), and treatment nonadherence (Swanson et al., 1996; Swartz et al., 1998). These explanations are rooted in the assumption that the causes of violence by mentally disordered people are linked fundamentally to the mental disorder itself (Monahan, 1992). The most prominent example of such theorizing is found in the work of Bruce Link and Ann Stueve (1994) and Bruce Link, John Monahan, Ann Stueve, and

Silver, Eric, and Brent Teasdale. 2005. "Mental Disorder and Violence: An Examination of Stressful Life Events and Social Support." *Social Problems* 52:62–78.

Francis T. Cullen (1999). Using epidemiological data from the United States and Israel, Link and Stueve (1994) and Link, Monahan, Stueve, and Cullen (1999) found that the relationship between mental disorder and violence was due primarily to the presence of paranoid psychotic symptoms (or what they termed "threat/control-override [TCO] symptoms"), symptoms most commonly observed among patients with schizophrenia. According to Link and Stueve (1994) and Link, Monahan, Stueve, and Cullen (1999), TCO symptoms consist of delusional beliefs that produce feelings of personal threat and involve intrusion of thoughts that override self-control. Link and Stueve (1994) and Link, Monahan, Stueve, and Cullen (1999) argued that whether or not these beliefs are grounded in reality, they influence the individual's definition of the situation in such a way as to increase the likelihood of violence. In other words, Link and Stueve's (1994) and Link, Monahan, Stueve, and Cullen's (1999) research suggests that mentally disordered people engage in violence because violence is a reasonable response to the distorted realities they perceive as a result of their mental disorders.

Although theories that focus on clinical characteristics, such as delusions, may be of practical value to clinicians with responsibility for managing their patients' behavior in the community, such theories fall short of addressing the more basic question of what causes such symptoms to emerge in the first place and what relationship those causal factors have to the occurrence of violent behavior. In short, the association between a particular set of clinical symptoms and violence does not preclude the possibility that both may be rooted in social factors originating external to the individual's mental state. To address this possibility, research in this area must move beyond a narrow focus on clinical characteristics toward a perspective that takes into account the social and interpersonal contexts within which both mental disorder and violence occur. The current study attempts to develop and test such a perspective.

Specifically, we test a model of the relationship between mental disorder and violence that draws on the social stress literatures in mental health and criminology (Agnew, 1992; Aneshensel, 1992; Cullen, 1994; Pearlin, 1999; Thoits, 1995). These literatures focus on the role that stressful life events and social support play in producing emotional and behavioral outcomes for individuals. Social stress researchers in mental health have long observed that stressful life events and social support contribute to the onset and course of mental disorder (Aneshensel, 1992; Lin, Ye, & Ensel, 1999; Thoits, 1995; Turner & Lloyd, 1999), and a substantial body of criminological research and theory suggests that stressful life events and social support are important links in the causal pathways that produce violence (Agnew, 1992; Capowich, Mazerolle, & Piquero, 2001; Colvin, Cullen, & Vander Ven, 2002; Cullen, 1994; Hirschi, 1969). Together, these literatures suggest that mental disorder and violence may each be rooted in the stress and support contexts within which individuals live.

Against this backdrop, the current study examines what happens to the relationship between mental disorder and violence when stressful life events and impaired social support are taken into account, using cross-sectional data from the Durham site of the National Institute of Mental Health's Epidemiological Catchment Area Surveys ($N = 3{,}438$). We hypothesize that the relationship between mental disorder and violence will be reduced when stressful life events and social support are taken into account because of the influence that stressful life events and social support have on the occurrence of both violence and mental disorder.

STRESS, SUPPORT, AND MENTAL DISORDER

Sociologists of mental health consistently have found that stressful life events raise the risk of mental disorder (for reviews, see Aneshensel, 1992; Dohrenwend, 2000; Pearlin, 1989, 1999; Thoits, 1995). According to Bruce P. Dohrenwend (2000), "the greater the uncontrollable negative changes in the ongoing situation...following the occurrence of a negative event, the greater the likelihood that disorder will develop" (12). While mental health problems can cause life stress, the causal link can also operate in the opposite direction, from life stress to mental health problems (Turner, Wheaton, & Lloyd, 1995; for a detailed discussion, see Thoits, 1983). The reverse causal relationship of stressful events leading to mental disorder becomes particularly apparent when life stress is measured using acute life events. Acute life events are not typically affected by individual behavior or psychological functioning (for reviews, see Aneshensel, 1992; Thoits, 1995). In contrast to acute life events, chronic stressors are persistent experiences that require readjustments over a prolonged period of time (e.g., ongoing marital or legal problems). Chronic stressors, thus, are more likely than acute events to be affected by an individual's psychological functioning or behavior (for a detailed discussion, see Aneshensel, 1992).

Therefore, in examining the contribution of stress to the association between mental disorder and violence, the current study uses an acute life events approach. Methodologically, this approach increases our confidence that any observed association between life stress and mental disorder is due to the effect of life stress on mental disorder, rather than the reverse (the effect of mental disorder on life stress). However, focusing on acute life events is not without its limits. According to Carol S. Aneshensel (1992), "the expedient solution of restricting measures to acute events appears methodologically rigorous, but sacrifices many interesting social elements within the universe of stress," (22) a point we return to later in the discussion.

In addition to stressful life events, sociologists of mental health have also found a consistent relationship between *social support* and mental disorder (for reviews, see Aneshensel, 1992; Thoits, 1995). Nan Lin, Alfred Dean, and Walter Enzel (1986) define social support as the "perceived or actual instrumental and/or expressive provisions supplied by the community, social networks, and confiding partners" (18). This definition suggests two major aspects of social support. First, the objective delivery of support is distinct from the perception of support. People do not receive support mechanically, but interpret, appraise, and anticipate support in the context of social situations (House, 1981; Matsueda, 1992; Turner & Lloyd, 1999; Vaux, 1988). Second, social support consists of two broad types: instrumental and expressive. Instrumental support involves the relationship as a means to an end in which the individuals involved seek out information, advice, guidance, material aid, or financial assistance. Expressive support involves the relationship as an end in itself, in which the individuals involved seek out intimacy by sharing love and affection, venting frustrations, and mutually affirming each other's worth and dignity (Cullen, 1994; Turner & Lloyd, 1999). Although various dimensions of social support have been studied, the bulk of the evidence suggests that *perceived emotional support* is most important in relation to psychological well-being (Cohen & Wills, 1985; Turner & Lloyd, 1999; for reviews, see Aneshensel, 1992; Thoits, 1995). Thus, the current study measures social support based on individual perceptions of, and satisfaction with, the degree of support received from family, friends, and other known persons.

STRESS, SUPPORT, AND VIOLENCE

The social stress model in mental health conceives of stressful life events and social support as exogenous factors: stressful life events increase psychological disorder, social support decreases it. In this section, we review recent literature from the field of criminology that provides a sociological basis for expecting a similar relationship among stress, support, and violent behavior (Agnew, 1992; Colvin et al, 2002; Cullen, 1994; Hirschi, 1969).

The assertion that stressful life events increase the likelihood of violence corresponds to arguments put forth by Robert Agnew (1992). In his theory of general strain, Agnew (1992) argues that individuals who are stressed (i.e., those who experience events or situations in which positive or valued stimuli are removed or threatened, or negative stimuli are presented) are more likely to experience negative affective states such as anger, fear, and frustration. These affective states, in turn, create an internal pressure for what Agnew (1992) calls "corrective action." This pressure is most likely to lead to violent behavior when violence is viewed as an alternative means to goal achievement, or as a form of retribution aimed at punishing those believed responsible for the strained situation. Consistent with Agnew's perspective, Catalano and associates (1993), using data from the Epidemiological Catchment Area (ECA) survey, found economic hardship in the form of job loss to be an important cause of interpersonal violence among the general public. Moreover, a substantial amount of literature in sociology and psychology suggests that stressful life events affect a range of negative outcomes, including drug use, juvenile delinquency, and aggressiveness (for a review, see Colvin et al., 2002). To date, however, no study has examined whether stressful life events contribute to the association between mental disorder and violence.

Although it is difficult to pinpoint the causal direction between life stress and violence using cross-sectional data, our reliance on an inventory of acute life events to measure life stress helps to minimize the risk that our measure of stress is an outgrowth of respondents' violent behavior. Nonetheless, to further minimize the risk of confounding our violence and stress measures, stress items measuring whether the respondent had been "divorced" or "separated" from a spouse or partner, or whether the respondent or a family member had "any legal problems," were eliminated from our life stress scale because of the reasonable possibility that such experiences may have been brought on by respondent violence.

In addition to stressful life events, the literature on social stress and crime emphasizes the importance of *social support* as a key variable. Drawing on Travis Hirschi's (1969) social bond theory, Francis T. Cullen (1994) argues that "the more social support in a person's social network, the less crime will occur" (p. 540). This is because social support is an important precondition for the provision of effective social controls. According to Cullen (1994), socially supportive relationships foster social control by functioning as a stock of social capital (Coleman, 1988) that the individual must protect in order to retain. Specifically, having a stake in supportive relationships may decrease the likelihood that disputes with others will escalate to violence. To behave violently is to risk the loss of valued support. This conceptualization of the relationship between social support and social control is directly related to Hirschi's (1969) bond of attachment and is consistent with Albert J. Hunter's (1985) notion of "private" control, in which the allocation or threatened withdrawal of sentiment, support, and mutual esteem are key elements influencing the likelihood of deviant behavior (for a detailed discussion, see Bursik & Grasmick, 1993).

Individuals involved in supportive relationships are likely to experience a greater degree of social control over their behavior than those who are not involved in such relationships (Cullen, 1994; Hirschi, 1969; Hunter, 1985). Relatedly, individuals with weak attachments to others are expected to experience fewer social controls over their behavior, thereby enabling them to engage in greater amounts of deviance, including violence. To the extent that a lack of social support raises the risk of both mental disorder and violence, we expect that controlling for social support will reduce the observed association between mental disorder and violence.

In sum, this study tests whether the relationship between mental disorder and violence is affected by exposure to stressful life events and impaired social support. Stressful life events are hypothesized to lead to violence by increasing the prevalence of blocked goals and thereby producing corrective actions that may include violence (Agnew, 1992). Social support is hypothesized to reduce violence by facilitating informal social control and stakes in social capital (Cullen, 1994; Hirschi, 1969; Hunter, 1985). These hypotheses are tested in a series of logistic regression equations in which we examine the magnitude of the association between mental disorder and violence before and after controlling for stressful life events and social support. Our expectation is that the relationship between mental disorder and violence will be substantially reduced when stressful life events and social support are taken into account, indicating that both mental disorder and violence are rooted in the stress and support contexts within which individuals live.

DATA, METHODS, AND STATISTICAL PROCEDURES

Sample

Between 1980 and 1983, the National Institute of Mental Health sponsored a series of representative, adult household surveys in New Haven, Baltimore, St. Louis, Los Angeles, and Durham to examine the prevalence and demographic distribution of diagnosable psychiatric disorders (treated and untreated) in the general population (Robins & Regier, 1991). At each site, between 3,000 and 5,000 household residents were interviewed. All interviews were conducted in the field by trained lay-interviewers. Interviews took approximately 60 to 90 minutes to complete. Although not intended for this purpose, the ECA data were subsequently used by Jeffrey Swanson (1994) and Swanson and associates (1990) to provide the first-ever large sample estimates of the prevalence of violent behavior among people with and without diagnosable mental disorders in the general population.

The current study uses data from the Durham site of the ECA project ($N = 3,438$), where, in addition to measures of mental disorder and violence, measures of stressful life events and social support also were gathered (Landerman et al., 1989). This study focuses on the Durham site because Durham was the only ECA site in which stressful life events and social support data were gathered in addition to the standard research protocol that measured mental disorders. The addition of the stress and support data provides us with the unique opportunity to examine the contribution of stressful life events and social support to the association between mental disorder and violence. The Durham site encompassed a five-county area of north central North Carolina consisting of one urban county (Durham) and four contiguous rural counties (Vance, Franklin, Granville, & Warren). The Durham Catchment Area had a population of 269,863 in 1980, and contained a diverse population, including some very poor communities as well as communities inhabited largely by individuals working in major research institutions in the Research Triangle area. The response rate at the Durham site was 79 percent. The sex and age distributions of the Durham sample were highly comparable to that of the United States general population in 1980; however, the Durham sample contained a higher proportion of African Americans than the United States general population in 1980 (36.4 percent versus 10.4 percent) and a lower proportion of whites (63.0 percent versus 84.1 percent). Thus, all of our multivariate analyses are conducted with statistical controls for race (and other demographic variables).

Measures

Violence. Five items from the ECA survey instrument were used to measure violent behavior within the past year:

1. Have you been in more than one fight that came to swapping blows, other than fights with your husband/wife/partner?
2. Have you used a weapon like a stick, knife, or gun in a fight?
3. Have you gotten into physical fights while drinking?
4. Did you hit or throw things at your wife/husband/partner? If so, were you the one who threw things first, regardless of who started the argument?
5. Have you spanked or hit a child, (yours or anyone else's) hard enough so that he or she had bruises or had to stay in bed or see a doctor?

Although the selected items cover a wide range of assaultive behavior, they overlap considerably and do not enable the severity or frequency of specific violent acts to be coded. Moreover, because only 3.2 percent of the sample answered affirmatively to at least one of these questions (the most frequent type of violence was fighting, followed by partner violence and use of a weapon), the *violence* measure was coded as a dichotomy where "1" includes subjects who committed at least one violent act in the past year and "0" includes those who committed no violent acts in the past year (Swanson et al., 1994; Swanson et al., 1996; Swanson et al., 1990).

Mental Disorder: Diagnostic Groupings. The core interview used in the ECA project was the Diagnostic Interview Schedule (DIS) (Helzer & Robbins, 1988; Robins et al., 1981), a structured, self-report instrument consisting of a lengthy series of preset questions with structured follow-up probing to assess the presence of psychiatric symptoms among adult respondents. The DIS was designed to enable trained lay-interviewers to assess *DSM-III* diagnostic criteria among the general population. Following Swanson and associates (1990), respondents were counted as possessing a major mental disorder if they met the lifetime criteria for a given disorder and reported that symptoms of the disorder were present during the one-year period preceding the research interview. Individuals with major mental disorders were grouped into two broad categories: those with a *major mental disorder only,* including schizophrenia or major affective disorders, who did not also have a substance abuse disorder ($n = 97$, 2.8 percent of the total sample; hereafter referred to as major mental disorder); and those with a *substance abuse disorder,* regardless of whether they also had a major mental disorder ($n = 193$, 5.6 percent of the total sample). The Durham data contained too few cases with both a major mental disorder and a substance abuse disorder ($n = 31$, less than 0.9 percent of the total sample) to justify analyzing them separately.

In addition to major mental disorders, the current study also identifies cases with *less severe disorders,* including phobias and somatic, panic, and eating disorders. Although prior research has not found these disorders to be associated with violence, separating out these cases allows us to make more valid comparisons between groups with major mental disorders and those with no mental disorder. A total of 461 cases (13.4 percent of the sample) scored as having at least one of these less severe forms of mental disorder.

Stressful Life Events. Respondents were asked to report on 19 different *stressful life events* that may have occurred during the year prior to the interview. The questions focused on changes in respondents' health, family and living situations, work, and finances. Respondents also were asked whether each event had a positive, negative, or neutral effect on their lives. The social stress literature suggests that stress is less related to the mere occurrence of life events than to the degree to which those events are experienced as unwanted or negative (Aneshensel, 1992; Pearlin, 1999). Thus, the stressful life events measure used here consists of a sum of the number of life events that respondents experienced as negative. As mentioned earlier, items measuring whether the respondent had been "divorced" or "separated" from a spouse or partner, or whether the respondent or a family member had "any legal problems," were omitted from the scale so as not to confound the violence measure.

Social Support. Social support was measured using the Duke Social Support Scale, a 35-item instrument developed and standardized by the Duke Epidemiological Catchment Area project (Landerman et al., 1989). Because most subjects reported adequate to high levels of social support and because of the high correlation between the two indices (Pearson $r = .68$), the indices were combined into a scale coded "1" for individuals with extremely low scores (i.e., in the lowest quartile) on one of the indices (16.9 percent of the total sample), and 2 for individuals with extremely low scores (i.e., lowest quartile) on both indices (11.7 percent of sample). All other cases were scored as "0". This measure is interpreted as an indicator of *impaired social support*.

Demographic Controls. Demographic characteristics were measured as follows: *gender* is a dichotomous variable (1 = male; 0 = female); *age* is the number of years since birth; *race* is a dichotomous variable coded "1" for African Americans, with white and other race/ethnicities (i.e., mostly Asian and Native American) as the reference category. Marital status is a dichotomous variable coded "1" for respondents *living with a spouse or partner* at the time of the interview. Following a procedure developed by Charles B. Nam and Mary G. Powers (1965), *socioeconomic status* was measured using a census-based ranking that combined a respondent's education, occupational status, and household income. Using data from the Public Use Sample of the 1980 census, occupations were ranked according to mean percentiles on educational level and income for all incumbents to a given occupational title. In addition to these occupational ranks, percentile scores also were formed for each respondent's education and for household income (and personal income when available), using data from the 1980 United States Census *Characteristics of the Population*. The socioeconomic status measure was then

Table 1 Descriptive Statistics ($N = 3{,}438$)

	Range	Mean	Standard Deviation
Violence	0.00–1.00	0.032	0.177
Major mental disorder only	0.00–1.00	0.028	0.165
Any substance abuse disorder	0.00–1.00	0.056	0.230
Any less serious disorders	0.00–1.00	0.134	0.341
Stressful life events	0.00–4.00	0.554	0.874
Impaired social support	0.00–2.00	0.404	0.689
Gender (1 = male)	0.00–1.00	0.461	0.499
Age (in years)	18.00–95.00	41.954	17.574
Race (1 = African American)	0.00–1.00	0.356	0.479
SES	0.40–97.75	48.886	23.994
Living with spouse or partner	0.00–1.00	0.608	0.488

formed by averaging education, occupation, and household income percentiles (Holzer et al., 1986). Table 1 provides descriptive statistics for all of the variables included in this study.

Our analysis proceeds in two stages. First, we examine bivariate relationships between the key constructs of our model, violence, stressful life events, impaired social support, and mental disorder. Second, we use multivariate logistic regression to examine what happens to the relationship between mental disorder and violence after we control for stressful life events and impaired social support.

RESULTS

Bivariate Analyses

Table 2 shows a breakdown of violence, life stress, and social support impairment for each category of mental disorder. Consistent with prior research (Swanson et al., 1990), individuals with a substance abuse disorder showed the highest rates of violence (19.2 percent), followed by individuals with a major mental disorder (8.3 percent), followed in turn by individuals with less serious disorders (2.2 percent) and no disorders (2.1 percent). Also consistent with prior research, individuals with mental disorders were significantly more likely to have experienced stressful life events in the past year than those with no mental disorders, and significantly more likely to have experienced impaired social support (Aneshensel, 1992).

Multivariate Analyses

What happens to the association between mental disorder and violence when stressful life events and impaired social support are statistically controlled?

Table 2 Violence, Life Stress, and Social Support by Mental Disorder

Diagnostic Groupings	No Mental Disorders ($n = 2,687$)	Less Serious Mental Disorders ($n = 461$)	Major Mental Disorder Only ($n = 97$)	Any Substance Abuse Disorder ($n = 193$)	Total Sample ($N = 3,438$)
Percent violent[†]	2.1	2.2	8.3	19.2	3.2
Percent with two or more stressful life events[†]	11.3	17.6	28.9	32.1	13.8
Percent with impaired social support[a†]	9.1	18.5	25.0	24.9	11.7

[a]Includes subjects who scored in the lowest quartile on both the satisfaction and perceived support indices.
[†]$p < .001$ (χ^2 test, $df = 3$).

This question is addressed in Table 3, which shows unstandardized coefficients and odds ratios from a series of logistic regression equations predicting violence. (The unstandardized coefficients indicate the change in the log odds of violence that is associated with a one-unit increase in an independent variable. The odds ratios indicate the multiplicative change in the odds of violence that is associated with a one unit increase an independent variable.)

As shown in Model 1 of Table 3, mental disorder and violence are significantly related, a result that was shown previously in Table 2. Specifically, the odds of engaging in violence was 4.41 times greater for people with major mental disorder than for those without mental disorder, and the odds of engaging in violence was 11.16 times greater for people with any substance abuse disorder than for those without mental disorder. Model 2 introduces demographic controls to the equation. Not surprisingly, older people and those of higher SES were significantly less likely to engage in violence. Although being male and being African American were significantly related to violence at the bivariate level (data not shown), they were not significantly related to violence when the other demographic characteristics and mental disorder variables were controlled. The nonsignificant result for males is due primarily to the association in these data between being male and having a substance abuse disorder. Specifically, 10.2 percent of males were rated as having a substance abuse disorder compared to only 1.7 percent of females and, as shown in Models 1 and 2, having a substance abuse disorder was significantly related to violence. The nonsignificant result for African Americans is due primarily to the association that exists in these

Table 3 Results of Logistic Regression Predicting Past Year Violence (N = 3,438)

	Model 1		Model 2		Model 3		Model 4		Model 5	
	UC	OR	UC	OR	UC	OR	UC	OR	UC	OR
Major mental disorder only[a]	1.48	4.41***	1.29	3.63**	1.09	2.97*	1.07	2.92*	0.91	2.48*
Any substance abuse disorder[a]	2.41	11.16***	1.99	7.35***	1.76	5.81***	1.77	5.87***	1.56	4.76***
Less serious mental disorders[a]	0.05	1.05	−0.04	0.96	−0.12	0.89	−0.20	0.82	−0.26	0.77
Gender	—	—	0.20	1.22	0.25	1.28	0.29	1.34	0.34	1.40
Age	—	—	−0.07	0.93***	−0.07	0.93***	−0.07	0.93***	−0.07	0.93***
Race	—	—	0.32	1.38	0.28	1.32	0.17	1.19	0.14	1.15
SES	—	—	−0.02	0.98**	−0.02	0.99*	−0.02	0.98*	−0.01	0.99
Living with spouse or partner	—	—	0.49	1.63	0.48	1.62	0.69	1.99	0.66	1.93
Stressful life events	—	—	—	—	0.38	1.49**	—	—	0.33	1.39*
Impaired social support	—	—	—	—	—	—	0.62	1.86**	0.57	1.77**

[a]Compared to no mental disorder. UC = Unstandardized Coefficient; OR = Odds Ratio.
*$p < .05$
**$p < .01$
***$p < .001$

data between being African American and having low socioeconomic status. Specifically, 30.3 percent of African Americans scored in the lowest quartile of the SES measure, compared to 12.6 percent of whites (and other race and ethnic groups), and, as shown in Model 2, having low SES was significantly related to violence.

Together, demographic characteristics reduced the odds ratio for major mental disorder by 18 percent, from 4.41 to 3.63, and reduced the odds ratio for substance abuse disorder by 34 percent, from 11.16 to 7.35. These results indicate that a substantial portion of the relationship between mental disorder and violence is due to the associations of these variables with demographic factors. However, the increased risk of violence associated with major mental disorders and substance abuse disorders remained significant after controlling for demographics.

Model 3 of Table 3 adds stressful life events to the equation. As shown, stressful life events were positively associated with violence (OR = 1.49, $p < .01$). In addition, adding stressful life events to the equation produced an additional 18 percent reduction in the odds ratio for major mental disorder, from 3.63 to 2.97, and an additional 21 percent reduction in the odds ratio for substance abuse disorder, from 7.35 to 5.81.

In order to determine the effect of impaired social support on violence, Model 4 of Table 3 removes stressful life events and adds impaired social support to the equation. As shown, impaired social support was positively associated with violence (OR = 1.86, $p < .01$). Moreover, adding impaired support to the equation produced a 20 percent reduction in the odds ratio for major mental disorder, from 3.63 to 2.92, and a 20 percent reduction in the odds ratio for substance abuse disorder, from 7.35 to 5.87.

Model 5 of Table 3 includes both stressful life events and impaired social support in the equation. As shown, controlling for stressful life events and impaired social support resulted in a 32 percent total reduction in the odds ratio for major mental disorder, from 3.63 to 2.48, and a 35 percent total reduction in the odds ratio for substance abuse disorder, from 7.35 to 4.76. In addition, the odds ratio for SES was rendered nonsignificant when stressful life events and impaired social support were added to the equation, indicating that some of the increased risk for violence associated with low SES is due to the disproportionate exposure of persons with low SES to stressful life events and impaired social support. Together, these results are consistent with the hypothesis that the relationship between mental disorder and violence is due, in part, to the higher levels of stress and support impairment experienced by people with mental disorder. However, although substantially reduced in magnitude, the relationship between mental disorder and violence remained significant after controlling for impaired social support and stressful life events.[1]

Discussion

Research on the relationship between mental disorder and violence has focused largely on the effects of clinical characteristics (Link, Monahan, Stueve, & Cullen, 1999; Link & Stueve, 1994; Swanson et al., 1996; Swanson et al., 1990), with little attention to the potentially important contribution that social factors, such as stressful life events and impaired social support, might make to this association. To address this gap we formulated and tested a model of the association between mental disorder and violence in which both were hypothesized to be rooted in the stress and support experiences of individuals. Consistent with this model, we found significantly higher levels of stress and impaired social support among mentally disordered people

---

[1] An examination of interaction terms between mental disorder and stressful life events, mental disorder and impaired support measure, and the three-way interaction among mental disorder, life stress, and impaired support produced null results. This suggests that the effect of stressful life events and impaired social support on violence are not contingent on the presence of mental disorder but rather operate similarly across mentally disordered and non-mentally disordered respondents.

who engaged in violence. More importantly, we found that the relationship between mental disorder and violence was substantially reduced when we controlled for stressful life events and impaired social support. Specifically, the relationship between major mental disorder (including schizophrenia and major affective disorder) and violence was attenuated by 32 percent, and the relationship between substance abuse disorder and violence was attenuated by 34 percent when stressful life events and impaired social support were controlled statistically.

These results are consistent with the hypothesis that the relationship between mental disorder and violence is due, in part, to the stress and support contexts to which individuals are exposed. In addition, we found a considerable portion of the relationship between mental disorder and violence to be rooted in demographic characteristics. These findings suggest that future studies of the relationship between mental disorder and violence should include stress and support measures in their analyses, in addition to the demographic variables typically included in such studies, in order to avoid problems of model misspecification. Specifically, studies that do not include such measures are likely to overstate the magnitude of the association between mental disorder and violence, leading to erroneous conclusions regarding the extent to which they are related. In addition to slowing theoretical progress in this area, ignoring the stress and support contexts of individuals may unnecessarily limit the focus of treatment interventions aimed at reducing violence to clinical factors alone (Steadman & Ribner, 1982).

This study is part of a growing body of research and theory applying stress and support concepts to the study of criminal violence (Agnew, 1992; Aseltine, Gore, & Gordon, 2000; Capowich et al., 2001; Cullen, 1994; Hoffman & Cerbone, 1999; Sigfusdottir, Farkas, & Silver, 2004). In support of this approach, we found strong evidence that stressful life events and impaired social support are key factors affecting the social distribution of violence in the general population. The finding that life stress and impaired social support had significant independent effects on violence after controlling for demographic characteristics and mental disorder provides considerable empirical support for the further exploration of a social stress approach to explaining violent behavior. Moreover, by focusing on the relationship between mental disorder and violence, and by showing that this relationship is due in part to contextual experiences related to stress and social support, this study provides an important empirical foundation to guide future studies of mental disorder and violence toward a greater focus on factors that go beyond the individual's clinical characteristics to include their stress and support experiences.

It is important to keep in mind, however, that our analyses were based on cross-sectional data. Because of this, we were unable to distinguish empirically between alternative causal orderings that may exist among our independent measures (mental disorder, stressful life events, and impaired social support). Lacking longitudinal data, we built our model around the assumption suggested by the social stress literatures in criminology and mental health: life stress and social support are exogenous to mental disorder and violence. Nonetheless, a plausible alternative to this model is one that would posit the *stress-inducing* and *support-inhibiting* effects of mental disorder in a causal sequence leading to violence. Such a model might be written as follows:

mental disorder → *stressful life events and impaired social support* → *violence*

Consistent with the stress literature in criminology, this alternative model suggests that stressful life events and impaired social support influence the likelihood of violence. However, in contrast to the stress literature in mental health, this model suggests that mental disorder may *contribute to* the higher levels of stress and support impairment found among mentally disordered people.

One way that this may occur is through involvement in conflicted social relationships (Felson, 1992; Hiday, 1997; Silver, 2002). Elsewhere the first author (Silver, 2002) has argued, "people with serious mental disorders, particularly those experiencing delusional beliefs or hallucinations, or those with substance abuse disorders, may introduce a variety of negative stimuli into their relationships with others" (206). Such negative stimuli may result in conflicts as others attempt to exert social control by persuading the mentally disordered person to desist from disturbing or annoying behavior or to comply with treatment (Hiday, 1997). For example, a recent study of the perceptions of coercion among hospitalized psychiatric patients found that approximately two thirds of patients who felt coerced into being hospitalized also reported feeling angry and fearful as a result (Monahan et al., 1999). This suggests that conflict associated with efforts at informal social control by caretakers may inadvertently contribute to violence among mentally disordered people by eliciting negative emotions. This may be particularly true when social control efforts include *involuntary* treatment interventions, such as forced hospitalization or forced medications. Thus, mental disorder may contribute to stress exposure by eliciting others' social control behaviors that the mentally disordered person experiences as unwanted (and therefore stressful), thereby increasing the likelihood that violence will occur.

Mental disorder may also inhibit social support. A central aspect of the stereotype of mental disorder is dangerousness, which is strongly associated with attitudinal rejection and social distancing by the general public (Link et al., 1999). Based on an analysis of General Social Survey data gathered in 1996, Bruce Link, Jo C. Phelan, Michaeline Bresnahan, Ann Stueve, and Bernice A. Pescosolido (1999) concluded that "if the symptoms of mental illnesses continue to be linked to fears of violence, people with mental illnesses will be negatively affected through rejection" (1332–33). Such rejection may contribute to the lower levels of social support typically observed among mentally disordered people by limiting the pool of supportive others with whom they may form social bonds. In short, to the extent that mental disorder leads to decreased support and increased stress, the alternative causal sequence shown above remains a plausible alternative to the one described at the outset of this article. Distinguishing between these alternative causal models remains an important task for future research.

In the end, we were unable to fully explain the relationship between substance abuse disorder and violence. This relationship remained significant after controlling for demographic characteristics, stressful life events, and impaired social support, suggesting that substance abuse may exert a direct effect on the likelihood of violence independent of the stress and support contexts of individuals. For example, substance abuse may disinhibit aggressive impulses leading to an association between substance abuse disorders and violence that is not mediated by other factors (Swanson et al., 2002). Alternatively, we may have failed to measure appropriately the specific types of stress that may lead to both substance abuse and violence.

For example, the current study examined only acute life events that occurred within the past year and thus did not address the potentially important role of enduring or chronic life stress as a mediator of the mental disorder-violence relationship. However, it remains plausible that the effects of stress on both mental disorder and violence operate in a cumulative fashion over the life course. This may be particularly true for mentally disordered people who attempt to manage stress by using substances to "self-medicate." Although the concept of chronic stress has not been tested in a study of mental disorder and violence, it has received a good deal of attention in the mental health literature (Aneshensel, 1992; Pearlin, 1989; Turner et al., 1995) and some attention in the criminology literature (Hoffman & Cerbone, 1999). For example, recent and chronic life stress have been shown to contribute to the occurrence of depressive symptoms among community residents, helping to explain variation in depressive symptoms across key social variables, including race, gender, and social class (for a review, see Aneshensel, 1992). In addition, stressful life events have been shown to have a cumulative effect on delinquency over the life course, suggesting that early and persistent exposure to stress may be an important link between social demographics and delinquency (Hoffman & Cerbone, 1999). Thus, the hypothesis that chronic stress may also contribute to the relationship between substance abuse and violence remains plausible and should be examined in future research.

Given that most prior studies of the relationship between mental disorder and violence have been based on cross-sectional data, future studies would benefit greatly from adopting a longitudinal perspective. Longitudinal data would enable researchers to identify the processes by which social and clinical factors produce violence over time and to distinguish between the causal models discussed above. Although detailed longitudinal data recently have been gathered on samples of discharged psychiatric patients (Silver, 2000; Steadman et al., 1998), no comparable data exist for the general population. Looking to the future, a cost-effective way to generate such data might be to use life event-calendars on a general population sample (Horney, Osgood, & Marshall, 1995). In addition, future studies should seek out more detailed information on the types, frequency, and seriousness of violence committed by individuals with and without mental disorder. Although significant advances have been made in measuring violence among discharged psychiatric patients (Silver, 2000; Silver, Mulvey, & Monahan 1999; Steadman et al., 1998), mental health surveys of the general population remain rare. Those that have been performed lack detailed data on violence, stressful life events, and impaired social support. If gathered together, such data would enable researchers to better understand the contributions of stressful life events and impaired social support to the association between mental disorder and violence, as well as to the occurrence of violence more generally.

References

Agnew, Robert. 1992. "Foundation for a General Strain Theory of Crime and Delinquency." *Criminology* 30:47–87.

Aneshensel, Carol S. 1992. "Social Stress: Theory and Research." *Annual Review of Sociology* 18:15–38.

Arseneault, Louise, Terrie Moffitt, Avshalom Caspi, Pamela J. Taylor, and Phil A. Silva. 2000. "Mental Disorder and Violence in a Total Birth Cohort." *Archives of General Psychiatry* 57:979–86.

Aseltine, Robert H., Susan Gore, and Jennifer Gordon. 2000. "Life Stress, Anger and Anxiety, and Delinquency: An Empirical Test of General Strain Theory." *Health and Social Behavior* 41:256–75.

Bursik, Robert J. and Harold G. Grasmick. 1993. *Neighborhoods and Crime: The Dimensions of Effective Community Control.* New York: Lexington Books.

Capowich, George, Paul Mazerolle, and Alex Piquero. 2001. "The Role of Interpersonal Networks in Response to Strain: Testing and Extending General Strain Theory." *Journal of Criminal Justice* 29:445–62.

Catalano, Ralph, David Dooly, Raymond W. Novaco, Georjeanna Wilson, and Richard Hough. 1993. "Using ECA Survey Data to Examine the Effect of Job Layoffs on Violent Behavior." *Hospital and Community Psychiatry* 44:874–79.

Cohen, Sheldon and Thomas A. Wills. 1985. "Stress, Social Support, and the Buffering Hypothesis." *Psychological Bulletin* 98:310–57.

Coleman, James S. 1988. "Social Capital in the Creation of Human Capital." *American Journal of Sociology* 94:95–120.

Colvin, Mark., Fracis T. Cullen, and Thomas Vander Ven. 2002. "Coercion, Social Support, and Crime: An Emerging Theoretical Consensus." *Criminology* 40:19–42.

Cullen, Francis T. 1994. "Social Support as an Organizing Concept for Criminology: Presidential Address to the Academy of Criminal Justice Sciences." *Justice Quarterly* 11:527–59.

Dohrenwend, Bruce P. 2000. "The Role of Adversity and Stress in Psychopathology: Some Evidence and Its Implications for Theory and Research." *Journal of Health and Social Behavior* 41:1–19.

Felson, Richard B. 1992. "'Kick 'em When They're Down': Explanations of the Relationship between Stress and Interpersonal Aggression and Violence." *The Sociological Quarterly* 33:1–16.

Helzer, John E. and Lee N. Robins. 1988. "The Diagnostic Interview Schedule: Its Development, Evolution, and Use." *Social Psychiatry and Psychiatric Epidemiology* 23:6–16.

Hiday, Virginia A. 1995. "The Social Context of Mental Illness and Violence." *Journal of Health and Social Behavior* 36:122–37.

———. 1997. "Understanding the Connection between Mental Illness and Violence." *International Journal of Law and Psychiatry* 20:399–417.

Hirschi, Travis. 1969. *Causes of Delinquency*. Berkeley: University of California Press.

Hoffman, John P. and Felicia Gray Cerbone. 1999. "Stressful Life Events and Delinquency Escalation in Early Adolescence." *Criminology* 37:343–73.

Holzer, Charles B., B. M. Shea, Jeffrey W. Swanson, Phillip J. Leaf, J. K. Myers, Linda K. George, and P. M. Bednarski. 1986. "The Increased Risk for Specific Psychiatric Disorders among Persons of Low Socioeconomic Status: Evidence from the NIMH Epidemiological Catchment Area Study." *American Journal of Social Psychiatry* 6:259–71.

Horney, Julie, D. Wayne Osgood, and Ineke Haen Marshall. 1995. "Criminal Careers in the Short-Term: Intra-Individual Variability in Crime and Its Relation to Local Life Circumstances." *American Sociological Review* 60:655–73.

House, James S. 1981. *Work, Stress, and Social Support*. Reading, MA: Addison-Wesley.

Hunter, Albert J. 1985. "Private, Parochial and Public Social Orders: The Problem of Crime and Incivility in Urban Communities." Pp. 230–42 in *The Challenge of Social Control: Citizenship and Institution Building in Modern Society*, edited by G. D. Suttles and M. N. Zald. Norwood, NJ: Aldex Publishing.

Landerman, Richard, Linda K. George, Richard T. Campbell, and Dan G. Blazer. 1989. "Alternative Models of the Stress Buffering Hypothesis." *American Journal of Community Psychology* 17:625–42.

Lin, Nan, Alfred Dean, and Walter Enzel. 1986. *Social Support, Life Events, and Depression*. Orlando, FL: Academic Press.

Lin, Nan, Xiaolan Ye, and Walter M. Ensel. 1999. "Social Support and Depressed Mood: A Structural Analysis." *Journal of Health and Social Behavior* 40:344–59.

Link, Bruce G., Howard Andrews, and Francis T. Cullen. 1992. "The Violent and Illegal Behavior of Mental Patients Reconsidered." *American Sociological Review* 57:275–92.

Link, Bruce G., John Monahan, Ann Stueve, and Francis T. Cullen. 1999. "Real in Their Consequences: A Sociological Approach to Understanding the Association between Psychotic Symptoms and Violence." *American Sociological Review* 64:316–32.

Link, Bruce G., Jo C. Phelan, Michaeline Bresnahan, Anne Stueve, and Bernice A. Pescosolido. 1999. "Public Conceptions of Mental Illness: Labels, Causes, Dangerousness, and Social Distance." American *Journal of Public Health* 89:1328–33.

Link, Bruce G. and Ann Stueve. 1994. "Psychotic Symptoms and the Violent/Illegal Behavior of Mental Patients Compared to Community Controls." Pp. 137–60 in *Violence and Mental Disorder: Developments in Risk Assessment*, edited by J. Monahan and H. J. Steadman. Chicago, IL: University of Chicago Press.

———. 1995. "Evidence Bearing on Mental Disorder as a Possible Cause of Violent Behavior." *Epidemiological Reviews* 17:1–10.

Matsueda, Ross L. 1992. "Reflected Appraisals, Parental Labeling, and Delinquency: Specifying a Symbolic Interactionist Theory." *American Journal of Sociology* 6:1577–611.

Monahan, John. 1992. "Mental Disorder and Violent Behavior Perceptions and Evidence." *American Psychologist* 47:511–21.

Monahan, John, Charles W. Lidz, Stephen K. Hoge, Edward P. Mulvey, M. M. Eisenberg, Loren H. Roth, William P. Gardner, and N. Bennett 1999. "Coercion in the Provision of Mental Health Services: The MacArthur Studies." Pp. 13–30 in *Research in Community and Mental Health, Vol. 10: Coercion in Mental Health Services—International Perspectives*, edited by J. Morrissey and J. Monahan. Stamford, Connecticut: JAI Press.

———. 2002. "The Scientific Status of Research on Clinical and Actuarial Predictions of Violence." Pp. 423–45 in *Modern Scientific Evidence: The Law and Science of Expert Testimony*, 2d ed., edited by D. Faigman, D. Kaye, M. Saks, and J. Sanders. St. Paul, MN: West Publishing Company.

Mulvey, Edward P. 1994. "Assessing the Evidence for a Link between Mental Illness and Violence." *Hospital and Community Psychiatry* 45:663–68.

Nam, Charles B. and Mary G. Powers. 1965. "Variation in Socioeconomic Structure by Race, Residence, and Life Cycle." *American Sociological Review* 30:97–103.

Pearlin, Leonard I. 1989. "The Sociological Study of Stress." *Journal of Health and Social Behavior* 30:241–56.

———. 1999. "The Stress Process Revisited: Reflections on Concepts and Their Interrelationships." Pp. 395–416 in *Handbook of the Sociology of Mental Health* edited by C. S. Aneshensel and J. C. Phelan. New York: Kluwer Academic/Plenum Publishers.

Robins, Lee N., John E. Helzer, Jack Croughan, and Kathryn Ratcliff. 1981. "National Institute of Mental Health Diagnostic Interview Schedule: Its History, Characteristics, and Validity." *Archives of General Psychiatry* 38:381–89.

Robins, Lee N. and Darrel A. Regier. 1991. *Psychiatric Disorders in America*. New York: Free Press.

Sigfusdottir, Inga Dora, George Farkas, and Eric Silver. 2004. "The Role of Depressed Mood and Anger in the Relationship between Family Conflict and Delinquent Behavior." *Journal of Youth and Adolescence* 33:509–22.

Silver, Eric. 2000. "Extending Social Disorganization Theory: A Multilevel Approach to the Study of Violence among Persons with Mental Illnesses." *Criminology* 38:301–32.

———. 2002. "Mental Disorder and Violent Victimization: The Mediating Role of Involvement in Conflicted Social Relationships." *Criminology* 40:191–212.

Silver, Eric, Edward P. Mulvey, and John Monahan. 1999. "Assessing Violence Risk among Discharged Psychiatric Patients: Toward an Ecological Approach." *Law and Human Behavior* 23:235–53.

Steadman, Henry J., Edward P. Mulvey, John Monahan, Pamela C. Robbins, Paul S. Appelbaum, Thomas Grisso, Loren H. Roth, and Eric Silver. 1998. "Violence by People Discharged from Acute Psychiatric Inpatient Facilities and by Others in the Same Neighborhoods." *Archives of General Psychiatry* 55:393–401.

Steadman, Henry J. and Stephen A. Ribner. 1982. "Life Stress and Violence among Ex-Mental Patients." *Social Science and Medicine* 16:1641–47.

Swanson, Jeffrey. W. 1994. "Mental Disorder, Substance Abuse, and Community Violence: An Epidemiological Approach." Pp. 101–36 in *Violence and Mental Disorder: Developments in Risk Assessment*, edited by J. Monahan and H. J. Steadman. Chicago, IL: University of Chicago Press.

Swanson, Jeffrey W., Sue Estroff, Marvin Swartz, Randy Borum, William Lachicotte, Catherine Zimmer, and Ryan Wagner. 1996. "Violence and Severe Mental Disorder in Clinical and Community Populations: The Effects of Psychotic Symptoms, Comorbidity, and Lack of Treatment." *Psychiatry* 60:1–22.

Swanson, Jeffrey W., Charles E. Holzer, Vijay K. Ganju, and Robert T. Jono. 1990. "Violence and Psychiatric Disorders in the Community: Evidence from the Epidemiologic Catchment Area Surveys." *Hospital and Community Psychiatry* 41:761–70.

Swanson, Jeffrey W., Marvin S. Swartz, Susan M. Essock, Fred C. Osher, Ryan Wagner, Lisa A. Goodman, Stanley D. Rosenberg, and Keith G. Meador. 2002. "The Social-Environmental Context of Violent Behavior in Persons Treated for Severe Mental Illness." *American Journal of Public Health* 92:1523–31.

Swartz, Marvin S., Jeffrey W. Swanson, Virginia A. Hiday, Randy Borum, Ryan Wagner, and Barbara J. Burns. 1998. "Violence and Severe Mental Illness: The Effects of Substance Abuse and Nonadherence to Medication." *American Journal of Psychiatry* 155:226–31.

Thoits, Peggy A. 1983. "Dimensions of Life Events that Influence Psychological Distress: An Evaluation and Synthesis of the Literature." Pp. 33–103 in *Psychosocial Stress: Trends in Theory and Research,* edited by H. Kaplan. New York: Academic Press.

———. 1995. "Stress, Coping, and Social Support Processes: Where are We? What Next?" *Journal of Health and Social Behavior* 36(extra issue):53–79.

Turner, R. Jay and Donald A. Lloyd. 1999. "The Stress Process and the Social Distribution of Depression." *Journal of Health and Social Behavior* 40:374–404.

Turner, R. Jay, Blair Wheaton, and Donald A. Lloyd. 1995. "The Epidemiology of Social Stress." *American Sociological Review* 60:104–25.

Vaux, Alan. 1988. *Social Support: Theory, Research, and Intervention.* New York: Praeger.

DISCUSSION

1. How do stressful life events and social support influence the likelihood that a person with mental illness will engage in violent behavior? How is this process similar to and different from the violent behavior that people in the general population might exhibit?

2. What are the clinical and policy implications of their findings for reducing violence among people with serious mental illness? How much control can mental health professionals or policy makers exert over the factors that Silver and Teasdale identify as having an impact on the likelihood of violent behavior among people with mental illness?

Thomas R. Insel

Assessing the Economic Costs of Serious Mental Illness

Sociological interest in the relationship between socioeconomic status and mental ill-ness reflects primarily a concern about the individual-level impact of mental illness on a person's ability to make a living and support her/himself in society. The economic impact of mental illness, however, extends beyond this individual level. As Insel sug-gests in this brief editorial, there are a variety of economic costs of mental illness for the nation. While many of the economic costs are direct, such as that on an individ-ual or group of people's abilities to earn an income or pay for mental health care, most of the costs to society, Insel argues, are indirect and more difficult to estimate.

> It goes without saying that the excess costs of untreated or poorly treated mental illness in the disability system, in prisons, and on the streets are part of the mental health care crisis. We are spending too much on mental illness in all the wrong places. And the consequences for consumers are worse than the costs for taxpayers.
>
> —Michael F. Hogan (1)

What do mental disorders cost the nation? The costs of health care are con-sidered one of the greatest challenges in U.S. public policy (2). In 2006, health care costs reached 16 percent of the nation's gross domestic product, on a path to reach 20 percent by 2016 (3). While mental disorders contribute to these costs at an estimated 6.2 percent of the nation's spending on health care (4), the full economic costs of mental disorders are not captured by an analysis of health care costs. Unlike other medical disorders, the costs of mental dis-orders are more "indirect" than "direct." The costs of care (e.g., medication, clinic visits, or hospitalization) are direct costs. Indirect costs are incurred through reduced labor supply, public income support payments, reduced educational attainment, and costs associated with other consequences such as incarceration or homelessness. Another kind of indirect cost results from the high rate of medical complications associated with serious mental illness, leading to high rates of emergency room care, high prevalence of pulmonary disease (persons with serious mental illness smoke 44 percent of all ciga-rettes in the United States), and early mortality (a loss of 13 to 32 years) (5). While indirect costs have been challenging to quantify, they are critical for informing public policy. Once we assess the key components of the economic burden of mental disorders, we can have a more informed discussion about what should be invested to prevent and treat these illnesses.

Insel, Thomas R. 2008. "Assessing the Economic Costs of Serious Mental Illness." *American Journal of Psychiatry* 165:663–665.

Kessler et al. (6) focus on one source of indirect costs: the costs from loss of earnings. The analysis is based on the National Comorbidity Survey Replication (NCS-R), a population-based epidemiological study of mental disorders. In this survey, data from nearly 5,000 individuals were used to estimate loss of earnings by comparing earnings in the previous 12 months of persons with mental disorders with 12-month earnings of persons without mental disorders. The analysis focused on individuals with serious mental illness. The results, based on a generalized linear model analysis, demonstrate a mean reduction in earnings of $16,306 in persons with serious mental illness (both with and without any earnings) and also that about 75 percent of the total reduction in earnings came from individuals who had some earnings in the prior year (versus those who did not have any earnings at all). By extrapolating these individual results to the general population, the authors estimated that serious mental illness is associated with an annual loss of earnings totaling $193.2 billion.

There are several surprises in this report. One is the gender difference in earnings: even when the earnings of men with serious mental illness dropped to $28,070 (compared with men without serious mental illness), these earnings were still higher than earnings in women without serious mental illness. This result cannot be explained by a large number of women outside of the workforce, because analysis of those subjects with positive earnings

THE ECONOMIC IMPACT OF DEPRESSION

As employers become increasingly concerned about health care costs, there is a growing interest on the economic impact of various health conditions. Druss, Rosenheck, and Sledge, in a study published in 2000 in the *American Journal of Psychiatry*, used medical claims data and corporate records to compare the health and disability costs of depression with four other common health conditions incurred in one large corporation with more than 15,000 employees in 1995. They found that the annual per capita health and disability costs for a person treated for depression was $5,415, a figure that is very comparable to the annual per capita health and disability expenditures for employees with diabetes ($5,472), heart disease ($5,523), hypertension ($3,732), and back problems ($4,388). This estimate included the cost of both mental and non-mental health care as well as the cost of the loss of productivity as measured by sick days taken. In total, the authors estimated that the cost of depression for this single large employer was between $2 and $3 million in 1995.

Source: Benjamin Druss, Robert A. Rosenheck, and William Sledge. 2000. "Health and Disability Costs of Depressive Illness in a Major US Corporation." *American Journal of Psychiatry* 157(8):1274–1278.

only demonstrated the same profound difference in earnings based on gender. A second unexpected finding is that the loss of earnings is not mainly a function of chronic unemployment. Finally, when one extends these findings to the general population, the financial loss is considerably larger than previous estimates (7, 8), which seems only partly explained by inflationary considerations.

While $193.2 billion seems enormous, it is important to recognize that the NCS-R yields a conservative sample for estimating economic impact. As a door-to-door survey, NCS-R did not assess individuals hospitalized in institutions, incarcerated in prisons or jails, or who are homeless. Indeed, NCS-R had so few subjects with schizophrenia or autism that these diagnoses were not part of the original epidemiological analysis, even though both are associated with chronic disability and lifelong loss of income on a far greater per capita basis than mood or anxiety disorders.

Accepting this conservative estimate of a loss of $193.2 billion in earnings each year from serious mental illness, can we estimate the total economic impact of serious mental illness? In Table 1 we begin to answer this question, adding the new estimates of income loss to data from 2002 on the direct costs of health care and disability benefits, including Social Security Disability Insurance (SSDI) and Supplemental Security Income (SSI) cash assistance, food stamps, and public housing financed by federal and state revenues. Missing are the costs of health care for comorbid conditions. Missing are estimates for the loss of productivity due to premature death and the loss of productivity of those with serious mental illness who are institutionalized, incarcerated, or homeless. Missing is the cost of incarceration, although as many as 22 percent of individuals in jails and prisons have been diagnosed with mental illness (9). Missing is the cost of homelessness, although approximately one-third of adult homelessness is associated with

Table 1 Components of the Economic Burden of Serious Mental Illness, Excluding Incarceration, Homelessness, Comorbid Conditions, and Early Mortality (in Billions)

Type of Cost	1992[a]	2002[b]
Health care expenditures	$62.9	$100.1[c]
Loss of earnings	$76.7[d]	$193.2[e]
Disability benefits (SSI and SSDI)	$16.4[d]	$24.3[f]
Total	$156.0	$317.6

[a]Nominal 1992 dollars based on general Consumer Price Index data; $1 in 1992=$1.28 in 2002 (www.bls.gov/cpi).
[b]Nominal 2002 dollars.
[c]Source: Mark et al. (4).
[d]Source: Rice et al. (7).
[e]Source: Kessler et al. (6).
[f]Author's calculations based on data from the Social Security Administration (www.ssa.gov/policy/docs/stat-comps).

serious mental illness (8). And, of course, missing from any such tabulation is the cost to family members who bear much of the emotional and financial burden of these illnesses. The $317 billion estimated economic burden of serious mental illness in Table 1 excludes costs associated with comorbid conditions, incarceration, homelessness, and early mortality, yet this sum is equivalent to more than $1,000/year for every man, woman, and child in the United States.

A little more than 5 years ago, Dr. Michael Hogan, chair of the President's New Freedom Commission on Mental Health, noted that "we are spending too much on mental illness in all the wrong places" (1). This is even more true in 2008 than in 2002. The costs of social services for persons with these chronic, disabling illnesses will likely continue to climb. The questions we must ask ourselves are not new, but they remain urgent: How can we ensure that mental health care is cost-efficient as well as effective for patients? How will we reduce homelessness, job loss, and incarceration? And perhaps most importantly, how much should we invest in disseminating effective treatments and finding better treatments in order to reduce these costs?

References

1. Hogan MF: Spending too much on mental illness in all the wrong places. *Psychiatr Serv* 2002; 53:1251–1252
2. Catlin A, Cowan C, Hartman M, Heffler S: National Health Expenditure Accounts Team: National health spending in 2006: a year of change for prescription drugs. *Health Aff (Millwood)* 2008; 27:14–29
3. Poisal JA, Truffer C. Smith S, Sisko A, Cowan C. Keehan S, Dickensheets B: Health spending projections through 2016: modest changes obscure Part D's impact. *Health Aff (Millwood)* 2007; 26:w242–w253
4. Mark TL, Levit KR, Coffey RM, McKusick DR, Harwood HJ, King EC, Bouchery E, Genuardi JS, Vandivort-Warren R, Buck JA. Ryan K: National Expenditures for Mental Health Services and Substance Abuse Treatment, 1993–2003: SAMHSA Publication SMA 07–4227. Rockville, Md, Substance Abuse and Mental Health Services Administration, 2007
5. Colton CW, Manderscheid RW: Congruencies in increased mortality rates, years of potential life lost, and causes of death among public mental health clients in eight states. *Prev Chronic Dis* 2006; 3:A42
6. Kessler RC, Heeringa S, Lakoma MD, Petukhova M, Rupp AE, Schoenbaum M, Wang PS, Zaslavsky AM: Individual and societal effects of mental disorders on earnings in the United States: results from the National Comorbidity Survey Replication. *Am J Psychiatry* 2008; 165:703–711
7. Rice DP, Kelman S, Miller IS: Estimates of economic costs of alcohol and drug abuse and mental illness, 1985 and 1988. *Public Health Rep* 1991; 106:280–292
8. Harwood H, Ameen A, Denmead G, Englert E, Fountain D, Livermore G: The Economic Cost of Mental Illness, 1992. Rockville, Md, National Institute of Mental Health, 2000
9. James DJ, Glaze LE: Bureau of Justice Statistics Special Report: Mental Health Problems of Prison and Jail Inmates. Washington, DC, U.S. Department of Justice, Office of Justice Programs, 2006

DISCUSSION

1. Describe the direct and indirect costs of mental illness to U.S. society. What is the total economic burden of serious mental illness on our society? Do direct or indirect costs contribute more to the overall economic burden on our society? How does the economic burden of mental illness compare to that of other health conditions?

2. What do you think the implications of these data are for federal and state mental health policy? What changes would you recommend in the ways we currently fund mental health services or pay for health care in the private health insurance market?

Deborah K. Padgett

There's No Place Like (a) Home: Ontological Security Among Persons with Serious Mental illness in the United States

In this study, Padgett examines the experience of becoming housed using qualitative data gathered from a small sample of formerly homeless individuals with mental illness. In addition to providing an overview of policies and services for the homeless mentally ill and an innovative "housing first" approach to engaging homeless mentally ill adults into care in New York City, Padgett offers insights into the world views of people who are homeless and suffer from a mental illness and what their concerns are in making the transition from being homeless to being housed.

A sense of déjà vu accompanied the July 2006 announcement by New York City Mayor Michael Bloomberg that homeless encampments in the city would be cleared out and their occupants placed in supportive housing. Mayor Bloomberg's announcement was part of a keynote address delivered at the annual meeting of the National Alliance to End Homelessness, an organization that had earlier announced a plan to end homelessness by the year 2010 (National Alliance to End Homelessness, 2000). Dating back to the early 1980s, the "crisis" of urban homelessness in the United States has endured despite many millions of dollars directed to its demise.

As the homelessness crisis enters a third decade, few individuals are as adversely affected as persons with serious mental illness. Persons with schizophrenia and other major psychiatric disorders have a much higher risk of homelessness and housing instability (Caton & Goldstein, 1984; Link et al., 1994; Phelan & Link, 1999). Whether seen on city streets or hidden from

Padgett, Deborah K. 2007. "There's No Place Like (a) Home: Ontological Security Among Persons with Serious Mental Illness in the United States." *Social Science and Medicine* 64:1925–1936.

public view, homeless mentally ill adults traverse an "institutional circuit" (Hopper, Jost, Hay, Welber, & Haugland, 1997) in which the streets and shelters alternate with exhausted family support and various transitional housing programs that exist as way stations on a continuum leading to the final destination of having one's own apartment. Difficulties in reaching this endpoint are many and setbacks are common (Allen, 2003; Hopper, 2002).

Studies of the relationships between housing, health and psychological well-being can be classified as dealing with three interrelated dimensions: (1) the material benefits of housing as shelter from the elements (Shaw, 2004); (2) health threats associated with substandard housing and neighborhoods (Bashir, 2002; Dovey, 1985; Marsh, Gordon, Heslop, & Pantazis, 2000) and, (3) the psychosocial benefits of housing as "home" (Dupuis & Thorns, 1998; Jackson, 1995; Low & Lawrence-Zuniga, 2003; Shaw, 2004; Somerville, 1992; Wu, 1993). Perhaps understandably, public health officials have been primarily concerned with the second of these, although interest in the positive *and* negative consequences of housing has increased in recent years (Bashir, 2002; Dunn, 2000; Howden-Chapman, 2004; Wilkinson, 1996).

It is a well-known axiom that possession of housing, that is, a roof over one's head, is necessary but never sufficient for having a "home" (Rykwert, 1991). Shaw (2004) distinguishes between the "hard" aspects of housing, that is, the material conditions of a dwelling, and its "soft" dimensions. that is, a subjective sense of being "at home." The latter connotes "ontological security," the feeling of well-being that arises from a sense of constancy in one's social and material environment which, in turn, provides a secure platform for identity development and self-actualization (Giddens 1990; Laing 1965).

It has been argued that one way to acquire ontological security is from having a place, such as a home, where one carries out daily routines and gains a sense of mastery and control away from the outside world's scrutiny (Dupuis & Thorns, 1998). Ontological security, or the lack of it, was first used by Laing (1965) to describe the experience of those with serious mental illness. It is ironic that those people whose ontological security is most threatened due to mental illness are also those least likely to be in housing circumstances that would promote ontological security.

Thus far, ontological security in the housing and health literature has been studied in the context of home ownership (Cairney & Boyle, 2004; Dupuis & Thorns, 1998; Easterlow, Smith, & Mallinson, 2000, Hiscock, Macintyre, Kearns, & Ellaway, 2003, Hiscock, Kearns, Macintyre, & Ellaway, 2001; Nettleton & Burrows, 1998; Saunders, 1989) and type of housing (Evans, Wells, & Moch, 2003). Viewed as "satisfying some innate desire of human beings in Western societies" (Kearns, Hiscock, Ellaway, & Macintyre, 2000, 387), home ownership seems far removed from the realities of life for urban homeless adults.

Studies of ontological security and home ownership have often had difficulties in ascertaining the presence of such an amorphous concept (Kearns et al., 2000; Vigilant, 2005). However, this may be because previous studies have not concentrated on situations in which ontological security is most affected. In this study, the focus is on the transition between homelessness and having a home, presumably a key period for changes in ontological security that may make it more readily identifiable. Previous work has suggested that the concept of "home" comes into sharpest relief in the context of "homelessness" (Gurney, 1997; Wardaugh, 1999).

This phenomenological experience of getting a home after losing it is rarely reported on in the literature. The tendency in previous research has been to make static comparisons between "housed vs. unhoused" or "owners vs. renters," thereby failing to capture the dynamic experience of housing deprivation among the destitute poor, which can range from doubling up with family to sleeping on a park bench (Hopper et al., 1997; Takahashi & Wolch, 1994; Tomas & Dittmar, 1995; Vigilant, 2005). This dynamic experience is difficult to capture given the transient states of homelessness and being housed, particularly among those with serious mental illness (Hopper et al., 1997; Wardaugh, 1999).

This qualitative descriptive study examines the subjective meaning of 'home' among 39 persons who were part of a unique urban experiment that provided homeless mentally ill adults in New York City with immediate access to independent housing in the late 1990s (Tsemberis, Gulcur, & Nakae, 2004). The following questions were addressed using grounded theory analyses of life history interviews:

1. How do study participants who obtained independent housing experience, enact and describe having a home?
2. To what extent do these experiences reflect "markers" of ontological security?

Findings will be presented on the housing status and living arrangements of these individuals two years after the experiment ended to ascertain changes both over time and between those who had obtained their own housing during the experiment and those who had not.

POLICIES AND SERVICES FOR THE HOMELESS MENTALLY ILL IN THE UNITED STATES

The United Nations has ordained housing as a basic human right that should be secure, habitable, and affordable but this goal remains elusive for much of the world's population (United Nations, 1991). In the United States, the severe shortage of low-cost housing that began in the 1980s and continues to the present day set the stage for the ongoing homelessness crisis (Lovell & Cohn, 1998).

Yet the fate of homeless mentally ill adults is also affected by policies designed to ensure that they are "housing ready" before approval is given for them to have a home (Tsemberis, 1999). This dominant "treatment first" approach provides temporary quarters in transitional housing, that is, group homes, crisis centers, half-way houses, supervised single-room occupancy hotels (SROs), and psychiatric rehabilitation facilities.

For most homeless persons in the United States, the status of being without housing is temporary and relatively short-lived (Phelan & Link, 1999). Indeed, recent research has focused on the small subset of "chronically homeless" who are responsible for a disproportionate share of the costs of care in terms of hospital beds, emergency rooms visits, and incarceration. (Culhane, Metraux, & Hadley, 2001; Gladwell, 2006; Mangano, 2003). This group, afflicted by substance abuse and/or mental illness, is considered among the hardest-to-reach and engage into services (Aidala, Cross, Stall, Harre, & Sumartojo, 2005; Rowe, Fisk, Frey, & Davidson, 2002; Ware, Tugenberg, & Dickey, 2004).

Epidemiological research on the mentally ill homeless in the United States has focused largely on the "demand side" rather than the "supply side," thus giving priority to studies of characteristics of homeless individuals rather than systems of care (Hopper et al., 1997). Homeless advocates take a broader view, focusing upon government policies that underfund the building of low-cost housing in favor of interim solutions such as public shelters and residential programs (Mangano, 2003). The federally funded Section 8 program (recently renamed the Housing Choice Voucher Program) offers recipients a subsidy to rent from private landlords, but is limited both in availability and by landlords' willingness to accept the vouchers (Allen, 2003).

Services for the homeless mentally ill in the United States represent several overlapping systems of care: (1) homeless services (shelters, food pantries, soup kitchens, and drop-in centers); (2) the public mental health system (hospitals, residential treatment programs, and outpatient clinics); (3) substance abuse programs (therapeutic communities, inpatient programs, and 12-step groups) for the estimated 50–70 percent who abuse substances (Drake et al., 2001); and, (4) social services and health care programs serving the poor.

Different funding streams, staff expertise, and service philosophies distinguish these systems, yet they all share a requirement of clients: gaining access to valued services—especially housing—requires complying with a set of rules and restrictions (Allen, 2003). From the perspective of the homeless service consumer, these contingencies of care can seem daunting. Accepting them is also a high-stakes gamble since rule breaking usually leads to expulsion and a return to the streets.

This treatment first approach, which dominates the landscape of services for the homeless mentally ill in the United States, can be viewed as rungs on a ladder beginning with a shelter or a drop-in center where persons sleep on cots or chairs and usually have access to meals, bathing facilities and lockers. The next steps up the ladder are a supervised dormitory-type facility—usually a bed plus locker—followed by a shared bedroom in a supervised SRO hotel or group home.

Individuals may enter the system on a higher rung, and those less impaired and more compliant may skip rungs, but reaching the top of the ladder, that is, getting an apartment, requires one to give evidence over a period of weeks or months of: (1) adhering to the psychiatric treatment regimen (including taking medications); (2) "clean time," or abstaining completely from substance use; (3) agreeing to have a "representative payee" (usually the program) control the client's disability and other income while in treatment; and, (4) conforming to behavioral requirements such as curfews, random urine testing, and maintaining personal hygiene (Tsemberis, 1999; Allen, 2003).

Persons may sidestep the ladder altogether if they have family help or financial resources to pay for housing or if they are fortunate enough to obtain a Section 8 voucher and accommodating landlord. But a bout of homelessness usually reflects the exhaustion of personal resources, resulting in dependency upon the system.

FROM A RANDOMIZED EXPERIMENT TO A "NATURAL" EXPERIMENT: THE NEW YORK HOUSING STUDY (NYHS) AND ITS SUCCESSOR, THE NEW YORK SERVICES STUDY (NYSS)

In the early 1990s, a consumer-centered approach emerged that fundamentally challenged the status quo. The "housing first" approach separated treatment from housing, considering the former voluntary and the latter a fundamental human right (Carling, 1990; Ridgway & Zipple, 1990). As such, it removed the ladder continuum and made access to housing the first step and subsequent steps subject to consumer choice rather than coercion (Tsemberis, 1999).

The first implementation of a housing first approach in the United States took place in New York City with the founding of Pathways to Housing, Inc. in 1992 (Tsemberis, 1999). Pathways to Housing ("Pathways") departed from the treatment first approach by offering: (1) immediate access to independent permanent housing not contingent on treatment compliance and retained regardless of the client's temporary departure for inpatient treatment or incarceration; (2) choice and harm reduction with respect to mental health treatment and substance use; and, (3) integrated case management services that work in conjunction with housing staff and a nurse practitioner to address ongoing housing and health needs. It resembles treatment first in requiring money management or "rep payee" status by the program for most tenants to ensure that the rent is paid.

In 1997, Pathways to Housing became part of a federally funded randomized experiment, the NYHS. The NYHS was a 4-year trial in which homeless mentally ill adults received immediate housing through Pathways (the experimental condition) or "usual care" (treatment first) and were assessed for an array of outcomes (Tsemberis et al., 2004). Quantitative findings from the NYHS revealed significantly greater housing stability among the experimental group members enrolled in Pathways (Padgett, Gulcur, & Tsemberis, 2006; Tsemberis et al., 2004).

The present analyses capitalize upon a natural experiment in examining housing outcomes following the end of the randomized experiment of the NYHS. The NYSS began in 2004 (2 years after the NYHS ended) and its Phase 1 relied upon a sample drawn from previous NYHS participants. As such, it represents a community-based (rather than treatment setting-based) sample whose housing status after 2002 remained an open question.

ONTOLOGICAL SECURITY AND THE TREATMENT FIRST VS. HOUSING FIRST PHILOSOPHIES

Conceptual fuzziness continues to surround terms such as "ontological security" and "home" in large part due to their contextual and subjective nature (Hiscock et al., 2003; Kearns et al, 2000; Mallett, 2004; Shaw, 2004). According to Dupuis and Thorns, the four 'markers' or conditions of ontological security are met when: (1) home is a place of *constancy* in the material and social environment; (2) home is a place in which the *day-to-day routines of human existence* are performed; (3) home is where people feel *in control* of their lives because they feel *free from the surveillance* that characterizes life elsewhere; and, (4) home is a *secure base around which identities are constructed* (1998, 29, italics added for emphasis).

Transitional housing for the homeless mentally ill offers little to sustain these conditions. Stays are intended to last days and weeks (although they can extend into years) and turnover is high due to dropout, referrals elsewhere, and/or graduation to the next step up the ladder. Nor are most day-today routines of normal life possible, since occupants share meals and bathroom facilities and are assigned chores such as kitchen help and cleanup. Also apparent is the constant surveillance and lack of privacy in these settings, where congregate living, staff supervision, medication administration, and random drug tests are common prerequisites to staying housed and in the program.

Dupuis and Thorns' last condition for ontological security (related to identity construction) taps into one of the deepest divides between treatment first and housing first philosophies; With the former emphasizing acceptance of one's identity as mentally ill and (if appropriate) as an addict or alcoholic before treatment can be engaged and effective (Estroff, Lachicotte, Illingworth, & Johnston, 1991; (Koekkoek, Van miejel, & Hutschemaekers, 2006). Interestingly, while addiction-related identities are viewed as mutable and capable of being cast aside or put under control; acceptance of one's mental illness identity is considered an ongoing prerequisite for treatment success (Olfson, Marcus, Wilk, & West, 2006).

The housing first program exemplified by Pathways does not make treatment engagement and effectiveness dependent upon acceptance of these identifying labels. Other markers of ontological security—constancy, control, daily routine, and privacy—are implied by the 'housing first' philosophy of choice and autonomy (Tsemberis, 1999), yet little is known about if or how allegiance to these precepts affects making a home and the subjective sense of ontological security.

METHODS

Sampling and Recruitment

Purposive sampling was used to select study participants (SPs) from the roster of subjects from the NYHS with the goal of selecting 40 for Phase 1 in-depth interviews. Persons in the earlier study had a documented *DSM* Axis 1 disorder and were referred for housing and services either from the streets or from hospitals; 90 percent also had substance abuse problems (Tsemberis et al., 2004).

As part of their final interview in the NYHS, SPs had been asked for contact information and permission to be recruited for future studies. Only individuals who gave permission to be contacted were considered for recruitment. Inclusion was based upon nominations criteria developed to include persons drawn from both the experimental and control groups and who had both "positive" and "negative" outcomes in the earlier study (defined in terms of success in psychiatric rehabilitation, controlling substance use and maintaining stable housing). Two members of the NYSS team, who had been senior interviewers in the earlier study and had first-hand knowledge of the study population, independently identified, with 100 percent agreement, a roster of 60 eligible participants who met sampling inclusion criteria for the NYSS. Of these, 39 were located and contacted; all of those reached agreed to participate in the study. Of the 39, 21 had been members of the experimental group and 18 were from the control group. The slight imbalance was due to greater ease in locating participants from the experimental group.

Study Design and Data Collection

The study design included two life history interviews, the first an open-ended query eliciting life stories with probes when relevant for experiences related to mental illness and substance abuse, homeless experiences, and other life events deemed relevant by the study participant. The second interview, which was individually tailored, elicited further detail or accuracy checks. Although we occasionally sought factual information, we maintained a strong emphasis upon respecting participants' own "narrativizing: of what had happened to them.

Interviews, which lasted from 45 minutes to 3 hours, were scheduled at a private location of choice to the participant (usually their current residence or the NYSS offices). Each interview was audiotaped and transcribed verbatim for entry into ATLAS/ti software. Interviewers met weekly to discuss any follow-up actions needed and debrief about their own feelings and reactions regarding the participants and their difficult life stories. All study protocols were approved by the author's university Institutional Review Board (IRB).

Coding and Grounded Theory Analysis

Procedures for coding the transcripts followed grounded theory and constant comparative analyses (Charmaz, 2006; Strauss & Corbin, 1990). First, members of the staff independently coded a single transcript and met to discuss their findings and develop a preliminary list of codes. Second, two members of the team independently coded three more transcripts, thereby adding codes and refining the list. The set of focused codes was complete (saturated) by the tenth transcript. Third, all transcripts were co-coded separately by two members of the team—any discrepancies were discussed and consensus reached. Two study participants and a psychiatric consumer advocate consulted with the team on the findings to provide feedback and "member checking."

Constant comparative analysis (Strauss & Corbin, 1990) was used to identify key themes related to living arrangements, housing and the making of a home. Sensitizing concepts representing domains of ontological security, for example, privacy, guided these analyses but emergent (unanticipated) themes were also pursued.

RESULTS

Characteristics of the Sample

Study participants had a mean age of 48 years and were predominantly male (67%). In terms of race/ethnic composition, they were 41 percent African American, 41 percent white, and 15 percent Hispanic; one person was of Arab descent. The most common psychiatric diagnosis was schizophrenia (56 percent) followed by bipolar disorder (22 percent), and major depression (22 percent). A history of co-occurring substance abuse was common, with 33 of 39 reporting lifetime substance abuse. At the time of the interviews, none reported heavy use of any substances, although 10 participants reported occasional use of alcohol and/or marijuana.

Housing Status and Living Arrangements

As might be expected, housing status had changed for several of the participants since their involvement in the NYHS. Sampling was based on an intent-to-treat strategy, and 5 of 18 control group members subsequently crossed over to Pathways when given the opportunity (this offer was made as an ethical compromise for those who remained homeless at the end of the NYHS). As shown in Table 1, 7 of the 21 persons originally in the experimental group were not residing in Pathways apartments, having entered more intensive treatment settings (from which 2 subsequently returned to their Pathways apartments shortly after the interviews were completed) or other transient housing. Of the 13 persons remaining in the control group after the departure of the 5 crossovers, 11 were living in supervised facilities and 2 had obtained apartments through Section 8 vouchers (see Table 1). Given the unstable housing arrangements and other life problems of NYHS participants, these outcomes are best viewed as a snapshot rather than fixed over time.

In terms of living arrangements, none of the study participants lived with a partner, family member or close friend. Instead, they lived alone in their apartments or in rooms located in transitional treatment housing. Although

Table 1 Housing Arrangements of Study Participants at the Time of the Interviews ($N = 39$)

| | Housing Status | | | |
Original Study Group	Pathways apartment	Other apartment	Supervised settings/treatment	Other transient housing
Pathways ($N = 21$)	14	0	5	2[a]
Controls ($N = 18$)	5[b]	2	11	0

[a]One shelter resident was receiving Pathways case management services.
[b]Crossovers to Pathways after earlier study completion.

many participants maintained contact with family and were acquainted with housemates or neighbors, social isolation characterized the descriptions they gave of their lives.

THEMES

Themes that address the research questions as well as emergent or unanticipated themes are presented below. Participant identification numbers (NYSS ID numbers) follow each quote, along with the participant's previous status and any change in status by the time of the interview.

CONTROL AND SELF-DETERMINATION

Having one's own apartment offered both 'freedom from' and "freedom to" opportunities (Kearns et al., 2000). One man noted:

Int: What did you like about it being your own apartment? 108: Just having it...Stay over anytime you wanted to. You know, things like that. Go shopping. You don't have to....People can't tell you what to do in your own place. You have your own say-so. What goes on in your own apartment. Things like that. #108 (Pathways group, who had moved to supervised treatment setting at time of interview)

A young woman valued her freedom to stay away from an abusive boyfriend.

And now I'm here I got my space. I got the balls to be like, yo I'm not taking that shit no more. Get up and just go. If I wanna see him I go see him but he gotta know...I gotta place to live. And I got to go home eventually and you can't hold me down and stuff like that. You can't do that. #121 (Control group, who had crossed over to Pathways by time of interview)

Two other women quoted below were blunt about having "freedom from" having to trade sex for money or a night's lodging.

I want it to be my home. I don't want no dirty motherfuckers in there with their dicks hanging or jerking off, or fucking around. I don't want it...As much as I need money, I said no. [He said] '"Come on, 10 or 12 bucks." I Said, "No, it ain't worth it. I'm sorry. I will starve. I'll drink water. I'll make it, somehow. You know, you can live on water for a day or two. #137 (Control group, who had crossed over to Pathways by time of interview)

Int: Why was it so important for you to have your own apartment...? #118: Because I would have my privacy. I would be able to fix it up the way I like it. And I won't have to put up with a man. #118 (Pathways Group)

Women were especially vocal about the protective benefits of having their own apartment. Given higher rates of sexual and physical assault among homeless women compared to homeless men (Padgett & Struening, 1992), control and self-determination also meant having a safe harbor.

ROUTINES OF DAILY LIFE: "THE SIMPLE THINGS"

Study participants spoke with pride of the seemingly minor but deeply gratifying aspects of having a home, whether it was doing the laundry or taking a walk in the park.

...that's what makes me feel good at times, the simple things. To be able to get up and know that I got two new shirts, a clean pair of jeans, clean socks and I can feel good about myself. I explain that to my peers too. That's what part of recovery's about. #144 (Pathways Group)

You get your own room, you mind your business, you live by yourself, you know. You go down to the park, you look at the birds. Look at the dogs. What the hell. You say hello to normal people. #137 (Control group, who had crossed over to Pathways by time of interview)

Participants' appreciation of these rather mundane aspects of daily life is set against a backdrop of (and their own extensive experience with) the constrained routines of residential treatment settings, including early wake-up calls and early bedtimes, congregate dining, dormitory-style sleeping arrangements and restrictions on movement beyond the circuit of day treatment, medical appointments, and other approved outings.

PRIVACY AND FREEDOM FROM SUPERVISION

Participants viewed their apartments as havens from the noise and stress of urban life, particularly after spending months or years on the streets or in shelters where privacy was not possible. As one older woman commented:

Sometimes it gets stressful. But I manage because I got a home to come home to and relax. #118 (Pathways group)

This contrasted with earlier experiences in transitional housing where monitoring of residents was part of daily life. One man noted:

> I don't think I ever really needed all that supervision. Plus I was already in my late fifties and I feel like, oh my god, I really don't need this. But...you know, but it was a necessary evil because I had to go through what everybody else went through. But I'm glad I'm out of that...I'm glad I'm living on my own. #128 (Control group, who had moved to other apartment by time of interview)

Emergency living arrangements such as doubling up could also bring infringements on privacy and freedom. A middle-aged woman related such an experience.

> I stayed with my girlfriend and her mother. I had to sleep in the living room. I couldn't watch TV after eleven. I couldn't give out the phone number. I couldn't touch anything in the refrigerator. Meanwhile, I put all my food stamps in the house. I gave her three hundred a month. I had no privacy...And they treated me like crap. #140 (Control group)

As illustrated in the above quotes, monitoring by others was a fact of life for participants. Its manifestations ranged from the overtly intrusive, unannounced searches and mandatory urine tests—to passive surveillance intended to prevent rules infractions such as fighting or substance use.

IDENTITY CONSTRUCTION (AND REPAIR)

As mentioned earlier, ontological security is enhanced by having a 'home' as a secure base around which identities can be constructed. For study participants, this meant self-reflection and repairing identities damaged along the way. A woman recalled a childhood very different from her adult years.

> It wasn't until I got with Pathways that I started straightening up, like, learning how to stop using, you know, taking a good look at me, and realizing who I really am. You knowy I grew up in a church. I had good discipline when I was growing up. My mother wouldn't even let us say curses. We wasn't even allowed to say the word 'behind'. #118 (Pathways group)

A man in his 40s reflected upon his earlier success as a musician before mental illness and homelessness took their toll:

> Int: It sounds like getting this apartment was a turning point. 139: Well yeah,...definitely one of the big turning points because it simply allowed me to um, reevaluate things, you know, and just, and get my life together from there. Int: When you say reevaluate things, what kinds of things did you think about? 139: Direction, just where was I heading...what was my purpose, you know......I've always been a musician, an artist of some sort but things were

kind of confusing at that point. I needed just to sit back and just see what was happening. #139 (Pathways group)

As illustrated above, study participants with previous work experience used it as a basis for identity reconstruction (additional examples include nurse, bank clerk, taxi driver, and computer programmer). Others sought out new work identities drawing upon their life experience, e.g., becoming a peer counselor.

Perhaps not surprisingly, the restoration and repair of social roles and identities was a goal. Being or becoming a parent, reaching out to estranged family members, and seeking out new relationships were all part of the pursuit of a 'normal' life. However, as discussed in the following section, having a home base also opened the door to thoughts about an uncertain future.

THE 'WHAT'S NEXT' OF HAVING A HOME

One of the more salient themes in this study was the existential 'what's next?' question that can emerge after leaving the survival mode of the streets and having the 'luxury' to contemplate a future.

> I have to either get myself a job, a volunteer position, or something...I have to be doing something constructive. In other words, go back into society, you know what I mean. I just got this apartment...the goal is to reintegrate you back into society. Int: What does that mean? 128: Kind of like, you know, don't rely on mental health services as much. Try to be a lot more independent...Which I try to do right now only...you know what, actually, I'm very stable here. As soon as I get my money, the rent's paid, all my bills are paid. #128 (Control group, who had moved to other apartment by time of interview)

Some participants were concerned that they could maintain their sobriety when their program did not require abstinence in order to stay in one's apartment.

> I haven't had like a stable you know, uh, life like in an apartment for a long time. So this is all new to me...I'm just getting adjusted to like, you know, get sober and clean. And doing a lot of things sober. And it's like, I'm learning how to live. #128 (Control group, who had moved to other apartment by time of interview)

It is noteworthy that complete independence from any program involvement was not yet a reality for any of the study participants, and some voiced this with regret.

> I wanted like, to pay for my own apartment...do it on my own...it's mostly like a charity case or something in my eyes, you know. I wish I could just get a job and pay for my own things and yeah, be my own person. #111 (Pathways group)

Finally, participants were keenly aware of their own mortality, having lost many peers to drugs, violence and the cumulative health problems of life on the streets. As one middle-aged man said:

> I didn't expect to live to be 40. So every time I say, when it hits 4 more years, I'll ask thank God, can you give me 4 more? I'm on my medications. I'm doing great having my own apartment. The only problem is the future. #103 (Pathways group)

Addressing the 'what's next' questions carries a degree of urgency born of the risk of premature mortality and it also points to the difficulties of overcoming years of adversity and disablement.

STAYING IN TRANSITIONAL HOUSING

Some study participants reluctantly accepted the need for residential treatment, even if it was not their optimal situation.

> ... I miss it. I wish that I can get my apartment back and start all over again. It'd be nice. But, I told my social worker that I'd rather stay here, just in case I get sick again. Then I don't have to go through all the trouble again. Of going through the hospital and-starting all over again, and have to work from the bottom. #108 (Pathways group, who had moved to supervised treatment setting at time of interview)

For others, the abstinence requirement was a barrier to reaching the top of the ladder. An older man described this dilemma.

> So my case manager he said that I had relapses. And that I have to be sober for a year or two...Then they can apply for an apartment...And I have to get a reference or I have to be referred by someone...I'm not a pretentious guy...But I need an apartment. You understand? It doesn't matter distance. We have a subway system so great, you see? #131 (Control group)

For some, the yearning for a 'home' was tangible even as they began to give up hope.

> Int: What do you think would help you to feel better? 140: Something that'll never happen. Int: And what's that? 140: To have my own place...not associated with [adult home] at all. 'Cause you know even when you get your own place, they still check up on you once a month and they've got a key to your place. You can't have any animals. I really want two or three cats. To tell you the truth, I wouldn't mind a dog either. I can never have pets. I'll never truly be on my own. #140 (Control group)

The above quote was from a woman who had lived in a group home for 3 years since leaving the streets and shelters. In this brief quote, several previous themes are touched on as being absent from her life—self-determination, privacy, and enjoyment of 'the simple things' such as having a pet.

DISCUSSION

Findings from this and previous studies affirm that formerly homeless individuals with serious mental illness can live on their own without the need for on-site supervision and monitoring (Tsemberis et al., 2004; Greenwood, Shaefer-McDaniel, Winkle, & Tsemberis, 2005). Findings specific to this report demonstrate that they can also enjoy the benefits of a 'home'. Markers of ontological security were clearly in evidence for those living in their own apartments—a sense of control, reassuring daily routines, privacy, and the capacity to embark upon identity construction and repair. Participants' ability to maintain the 'rhythms of life' (Jenkins & Carpenter-Song, 2005, p. 407) may seem unsurprising to some, but must be viewed in juxtaposition to an entrenched view among mental health providers that most persons with schizophrenia or bipolar disorder are too unstable to live on their own or experience the psychological benefits of solitude and personal agency (Koekkoek et al., 2006; Lamb & Weinberger, 2005).

Study participants' engagement in everyday activities, e.g., grocery shopping, cooking meals and entertaining friends, is the behavioral counterpart of 'normalizing talk' (Estroff et al., 1991) offered by persons with serious mental illness as a means of gaining parity with their nonmentally ill peers. At the same time, having a secure base after years of struggle affords the 'freedom to' reflect on past losses, ongoing dependencies and future prospects. Regardless of their housing status, all study participants were reliant upon disability income and case management services from programs serving persons with psychiatric disabilities. They were also well aware that they faced an uncertain future, having witnessed the premature deaths of many of their family members and peers.

Demonstrating that persons with serious mental illness can make a home for themselves when offered housing attests to the rather low threshold of expectations set for them after two decades of homelessness in the United States. International replications of the Pathways model for the homeless mentally ill are being planned in Japan and elsewhere, but their development is still in the early stages (Dr. Sam Tsemberis, personal communication). National and local differences in housing policies, service systems, provider attitudes and housing availability point to the need for adjustments without sacrificing fidelity to the model's core values.

Achieving this minimal first step toward normalcy points to the thorny issue of social exclusion that confronts the seriously mentally ill regardless of where and how they live. The 'what's next' questions raised by study participants reflect an awareness of the challenges they face in seeking full independence and social acceptance. In addition to the disabling effects of cumulative trauma and adversity, societal stigma and discrimination undermine such efforts (Hopper, 2002). The recent growth in support for 'recovery-driven' services emphasizing self-determination and hope (Deegan, 1988; Davidson, 2003; Jenkins & Carpenter-Song, 2005) highlights the legitimacy of calls for system change as well as the difficulties attending such change.

This study is potentially limited by its location in New York City, which may not be representative of other urban areas in the size of its homeless population and the scope of services designed to assist them. Yet it could also be argued that the attainment of a 'home' after a harsh life on the city's streets and amidst its extremely tight housing market is that much more meaningful. Another potential limitation is the lack of full induction in applying the grounded theory analyses, i.e., the use of sensitizing concepts related to ontological security. Although several of these concepts "earned their way" (Charmaz, 2006, p. 68) into the findings and the analyses were structured to remain open to fresh insights (e.g., the 'what's next' dilemma), it is plausible that others were overlooked.

The study has a number of strengths including its deployment of strategies for rigor (Padgett, 1998) such as debriefing, interviewer supervision, member checking and two interviews per participant. A strong emphasis on rapport and trust made it unlikely that the participants misled us, although social desirability bias is still possible. Every attempt was made to stay closely grounded to the data in making interpretations.

CONCLUSION

Ontological security was originally developed within the mental health field where the emphasis was on the breakdown in ontological security experienced by those with schizophrenia. The treatment approach for such persons reflects the belief that ontological security cannot be regained until the mental illness is addressed. Research in the housing and health field, including this study, suggests that housing can provide a fundamental building block for ontological security, thus lending support to a housing first approach. This study shows the benefits of cross-disciplinary work for policy and theoretical development.

This study capitalized upon a unique experiment in which homeless mentally ill adults were provided immediate access to independent housing without prior restrictions or proof of readiness. Contrary to the dominant policies and practices in the United States, housing first makes an offer that few individuals will (or did) refuse and from which most benefited, both materially and psychologically. Yet the fate of the homeless mentally ill in the United States is heavily influenced by programs and policies favoring transitional over permanent housing in the mistaken belief that such persons are not capable of stable, independent living in the community.

Finally, this study has shown that the subjective experience of ontological security can now be extended from home-owners to newly housed persons with serious mental illness. Yet, just as a house (or apartment) does not make a home, a home does not make a life. Other core elements of psychiatric recovery such as hope for the future, having a job, enjoying the company and support of others, and being involved in society (Davidson, 2003; Deegan, 1988; Jacobson & Greenley, 2001) have only been partially attained by this study's participants. Having a 'home' may not guarantee recovery in the future, but it does afford a stable platform for re-creating a less stigmatized, normalized life in the present.

REFERENCES

Aidala, A., Cross, J. E., Stall, R., Harre, D., & Sumartojo, E. (2005). Housing status and HIV risk behaviors: Implications for prevention and policy. *AIDS and Behavior, 9*(3), 251–259.

Allen, M. (2003). Waking Rip van Winkle: Why developments in the last 20 years should teach the mental health system not to use housing as a tool of coercion. *Behavioral Sciences and the Law, 21,* 503–521.

Bashir, S. A. (2002). Home is where the harm is: Inadequate housing as a public health crisis. *American Journal of Public Health, 92*(5), 733–738.

Cairney, J., & Boyle, M. H. (2004). Home ownership, mortgages and psychological distress. *Housing Studies, 19*(2),161–174.

Carling, P. J. (1990). Major mental illness, housing and supports: The promise of community integration. *American Psychologist, 45,* 961–975.

Caton, C., & Goldstein, J. (1984). Housing change of chronic schizophrenic patients: A consequence of the revolving door. *Social Science & Medicine, 19*(7), 759–764.

Charmaz, K. (2006). *Constructing grounded theory: A practical guide through qualitative analysis.* Thousand Oaks, CA: Sage.

Culhane, D. P., Metraux, S., & Hadley, T. (2001). The impact of supportive housing for homeless people with severe mental illness on the utilization of the public health, corrections and emergency shelter systems: The New York-New York Initiative. *Housing Policy Debate, 5,* 107–140.

Davidson, L. (2003). *Living outside mental illness: Qualitative studies of recovery in schizophrenia.* New York: New York University Press.

Deegan, P. E. (1988). Recovery: The lived experience of rehabilitation. *Psychosocial Rehabilitation Journal, 11,* 11–19.

Dovey, K. (1985). Home and homelessness. In I. Altman, & C. Werner (Eds.), *Home environments* (pp. 35–52). New York: Plenum Press.

Drake, R. M., Essock, S. M., Shaner, A., Carey, K. B., Minkoff, K., Kola, L., et al. (2001). Implementing dual diagnosis services for clients with severe mental illness. *Psychiatric Services, 52*(4), 469–476.

Dunn, J. R. (2000). Housing and health inequalities: Review and prospects for research. *Housing Studies, 15*(3), 341–366.

Dupuis, A., & Thorns, D. C. (1998). Home, home ownership, and the search for ontological security. *The Sociological Review, 46*(1),24–47.

Easterlow, D., Smith, S. J., & Mallinson, S. (2000). Housing for health: The role of owner occupation. *Housing Studies, 15*(3), 367–386.

Estroff, S. E., Lachicotte, W. S., Illingworth, L. C., & Johnston, A. (1991). Everybody's got a little mental illness: Accounts of illness and self among people with severe persistent mental illnesses. *Medical Anthropology Quarterly, 5,* 331–369.

Evans, G. W., Wells, N. M., & Moch, A. (2003). Housing and mental health: A review of the evidence and a methodological and conceptual critique. *Journal of Social Issues, 59*(3), 475–500.

Giddens, A. (1990). *Consequences of modernity.* Oxford: Polity Press.

Gladwell, M., (2006). Million-dollar Murray: Why problems like homelessness may be easier to solve than to manage. The New Yorker, February 13 and 20, 2006.

Greenwood, R. M., Shaefer-McDaniel, N. J., Winkle, G., & Tsemberis, S. J. (2005). Decreasing psychiatric symptoms by increasing choice in services for adults with histories of homelessness. *American Journal of Community Psychology, 36*(3–4), 226–238.

Gurney, C. M. (1997). "Half of me was satisfied": Making sense of home through episodic ethnographies. *Women's Studies International Forum, 20*(3), 373–386.

Hiscock, R., Kearns, A., Macintyre, S., & Ellaway, A. (2001). Ontological security and psychosocial benefits from the home: Qualitative evidence on issues of tenure. *Housing Theory and Society, 18*(1–2), 50–66.

Hiscock, R., Macintyre, S., Kearns, A., & Ellaway, A. (2003). Residents and residence: Factors predicting the health disadvantage of social renters compared to owner-occupiers. *Journal of Social Issues, 59*(3), 527–546.

Hopper, K. (2002). Returning to the community-again. *Psychiatric Services, 53*(11), 1355.

Hopper, K., Jost, J., Hay, T., Welber, S., & Haugland, G. (1997). Homelessness, severe mental illness and the institutional circuit. *Psychiatric Services, 48*(10), 659–665.

Howden-Chapman, P. (2004). Housing standards: A glossary of housing and health. *Journal of Epidemiology and Community Health, 58,* 162–168.

Jackson, M. (1995). *At home in the world.* Durham, NC: Duke University Press.

Jacobson, N., & Greenley, D. (2001). What is recovery? A conceptual model and explication. *Psychiatric Services, 52*(4), 482–485.

Jenkins, J., & Carpenter-Song, N. (2005). The new paradigm of recovery from schizophrenia: Cultural conundrums of improvement without cure. *Culture, Medicine and Psychiatry, 29,* 379–413.

Kearns, A., Hiscock, R., Ellaway, A., & Macintyre, S. (2000). 'Beyond four walls'. The psychosocial benefits of home: Evidence from West Central Scotland. *Housing Studies, 15*(3), 387–410.

Koekkoek, B., Van meijel, B., & Hutschemaekers, G. (2006). "Difficult patients" in mental health care: A review. *Psychiatric Services, 57*(8), 795–802.

Laing, R. D. (1965). *The divided self: An existential study in sanity and madness.* London: Pelican Press.

Lamb, H., & Weinberger, L. E. (2005). One-year follow-up of persons discharged from a locked intermediate care facility. *Psychiatric Services, 56*(4), 198–201.

Link, B. G., Susser, E., Stueve, A., Phelan, J., Moore, R. E., & Struening, E. L. (1994). Lifetime and five-year prevalence of homelessness in the United States. American *Journal of Public Health, 84*(12), 1907–1912.

Lovell, A. M., & Cohn, S. (1998). The elaboration of "choice" in a program for homeless persons labeled psychiatrically disabled. *Human Organization, 57,* 8–20.

Low, S., & Lawrence-Zuniga, D. (Eds.). (2003). *The anthropology of space and place: Locating culture.* Malden, MA: Blackwell.

Mallett, S. (2004). Understanding home: A critical review of the literature. *The Sociological Review, 52*(1), 62–89.

Mangano, P. (2003). Plenary remarks. In *Proceedings of the US Conference of Mayors.* Boston, Massachusetts, January 23, 2003.

Marsh, A., Gordon, D., Heslop, P., & Pantazis, C. (2000). Housing deprivation and health: A longitudinal analysis. *Housing Studies, 15*(3), 411–428.

National Alliance to End Homelessness. (2000). A plan not a dream: How to end homelessness in ten years. Washington, DC. Available from: /www.naeh.orgS, accessed July 12, 2006.

Nettleton, S., & Burrows, R. (1998). Mortgage debt, insecure home ownership and health: An exploratory analysis. *Sociology of Health and Illness, 20*(5), 731–753.

Olfson, M., Marcus, S., Wilk, J., & West, J. C. (2006). Awareness of illness and non-adherence to antipsychotic medications among persons with schizophrenia. *Psychiatric Services, 57*(2),205–211.

Padgett, D. K. (1998). *Qualitative methods in social work research.* Thousand Oaks, CA: Sage.

Padgett, D., & Struening, E. L. (1992). Victimization and traumatic injuries among the homeless: Associations with alcohol, drug, and mental problems. American *Journal of Orthopsychiatry, 62,* 525–534.

Padgett, D. K., Gulcur, L., & Tsemberis, S. J. (2006). Housing first services for people who are homeless with co-occurring serious mental illness and substance abuse. *Research on Social Work Practice, 16,* 74–83.

Phelan, J., & Link, B. G. (1999). Who are 'the homeless'? Reconsidering the stability and composition of the homeless population. *American Journal of Public Health, 89* (9), 1334–1338.

Ridgway, P., & Zipple, A. (1990). The paradigm shift in residential services: From the linear continuum to supported housing services. *Psychiatric Rehabilitation Journal, 13,* 11–31.

Rowe, M., Fisk, D., Frey, J., & Davidson, L. (2002). Engaging persons with substance use disorders: Lessons from homeless outreach. *Administration and Policy in Mental Health, 29*(3), 263–273.

Rykwert, J. (1991). House and home. *Social Research, 58*(1), 51–62.

Saunders, P. (1989). The meaning of 'home' in contemporary English culture. *Housing Studies, 4*(3), 177–192.

Shaw, M. (2004). Housing and public health. *Annual Review of Public Health, 25,* 397–418.

Somerville, P. (1992). Homelessness and the meaning of home: Rooflessness and rootlessness? *International Journal of Urban and Regional Research, 16*(4), 539.

Strauss, A., & Corbin, J. (1990). *Basics of grounded theory.* Newbury Park, CA: Sage.

Takahashi, L. M., & Wolch, J. R. (1994). Differences in health and welfare between homeless and housed welfare applicants in Los Angeles County. *Social Science & Medicine, 38*(10), 1401–1413.

Tomas, A., & Dittmar, H. (1995). The experience of homeless women: An exploration of housing histories and the meaning of home. *Housing Studies, 10*(4), 493–495.

Tsemberis, S. (1999). From streets to homes: An innovative approach to supported housing for homeless adults with psychiatric disabilities. *Journal of Community Psychology, 27,* 225–241.

Tsemberis, S., Gulcur, L., & Nakae, M. (2004). Housing first, consumer choice, and harm reduction for homeless individuals with a dual diagnosis. *American Journal of Public Health, 94,* 651–656.

United Nations. (1991). The right to adequate housing. UN Commission on Economic, Social and Cultural Rights. Available from: /http://www.unhchr.ch/housing/S, accessed July 28, 2006.

Vigilant, L. G. (2005). "I don't have another run left with it": Ontological security in illness narratives of recovering on methadone maintenance. *Deviant Behavior, 26,* 399–416.

Wardaugh, J. (1999). The unaccommodated woman: Home, homelessness and identity. *The Sociological Review, 47*(1), 91–109.

Ware, N. C., Tugenberg, T., & Dickey, B. (2004). Practitioner relationships and quality of care for low-income persons with serious mental illness. *Psychiatric Services, 55*(9), 555–559.

Wilkinson, R. (1996). *Unhealthy societies: The afflictions of inequality.* London: Routledge.

Wu, K-M. (1993). The other is my hell; the other is my home. *Human Studies, 16*(1–2), 193–202.

DISCUSSION

1. What are the key values or needs of formerly homeless individuals who have a mental illness? How do these values and needs reflect the social dimensions of the experience of mental illness or mental health care?

2. Given Padgett's findings, how can we improve services for homeless people with mental illness? What changes should we make in current homeless shelter and other social service programs designed to respond to the needs of homeless people with mental illness?

The Consumer and Family Movements

Athena Helen McLean

From Ex-patient Alternatives to Consumer Options: Consequences of Consumerism for Psychiatric Consumers and the Ex-patient Movement

Beginning in the 1970s, a diverse social movement developed in response to the poor societal treatment of people with mental illness. In this paper, sociologist Athena McLean traces the history of this movement, the social and economic factors that gave rise to it, and the many groups that comprise it, including several very different primary consumer groups as well as family and professional organizations. Her analysis highlights the varied motivations and goals of the various organizations that comprise this movement and examines the impact these organizations have had on changes in the mental health system.

S ince the early 1970s in the United States, diverse groups of recipients and former recipients of mental health services have mobilized for change in the nation's mental health system. The movement was started by a small group of antipsychiatry political activists who called themselves "ex-inmates" or "ex-patients." Today, it includes members of that group, now called "survivors," and of another group, who call themselves "consumers" and accept the medical model of mental illness (1, pp. 1053–54). Advocates from both groups, although retaining their ideological differences, have now come to negotiate within the mental health system, as part of a more general "consumer movement."

Drawing from ethnographic and historical research I conducted between 1991 and 1996, this article reviews the way in which the psychiatric ex-patient

McLean, Athena Helen. 2000. "From Ex-Patient Alternatives to Consumer Options: Consequences of Consumerism for Psychiatric Consumers and the Ex-Patient Movement." *International Journal of Health Services* 30:821–847.

movement developed in the United States from a political antipsychiatry emancipatory movement in the early 1970s to a consumer movement by the mid-1980s. In tracing this shift, I first explain ex-patient activists' earlier refusals to negotiate for government reform, their varied alliances with professional groups (e.g., radical therapists and rights protection and advocacy groups), and their eventual efforts at government reform. I then examine how two major forces in the mental health system during this period—the Community Support Program of the National Institute of Mental Health and the family consumer movement (the National Alliance for the Mentally Ill)—along with state Mental Health Associations, helped promote the shift to consumerism. After evaluating the consequences of the reconfigured movement for consumers and ex-patients by the early 1990s and into the present, I discuss these developments in terms of the unique nature of consumerism in the United States and the more recent turn to a managed care restructuring of mental health services.

EVOLUTION OF THE EX-PATIENT/CONSUMER MOVEMENT IN THE UNITED STATES

The ex-patients who mobilized for change in the early 1970s were loosely organized into the Psychiatric Inmates Liberation Movement, one of many emancipatory civil and human rights liberation movements of the 1960s (2, 3). The movement was overwhelmingly antipsychiatry, anti–medical model, and opposed to forced treatment and involuntary commitment. Participants located mental illness not in individual impairments but in oppressive social conditions. Having been institutionalized as "mental patients" during the early part of deinstitutionalization in the United States, they experienced outrage at the indignities of prolonged hospitalization, forced treatment, and abuse by service providers, and they felt betrayed by psychiatrists who fostered their dependence and offered little hope (3).

The debilitating consequences of these experiences—damaged self-esteem, motivation, and confidence and a profound sense of hopelessness—destroyed their trust in institutions and in authoritative control by experts. They came to see psychiatry as an oppressive, harmful institution and were cautious about organizing their movement nationally for fear of creating similar oppressive conditions. They also opposed accepting government funding, for fear their goals would be co-opted and depoliticized.

A large number of spokespersons for this movement were well-educated, bright, articulate persons who grew up in middle- and upper-middle-class families (2). Many had been institutionalized during their young adult years and discovered that, as their personal situation improved, they no longer depended on psychiatry. Others tried to free themselves from their dependency on a mental health system they found more debilitating than helpful.

As ex-patients came together informally for mutual support, and heard others' stories, their own feelings of injustice became validated. Many found they were beginning to regain self-esteem, which initiated their own progression toward recovery. Thus empowerment—gaining control and self-determination over their lives—became a personal and political goal of many ex-patients (1, 4).

Political and Ideological Background and Alliances

Even before the coalescence of the ex-patient movement, individual advocates initiated patients' rights litigation during the civil liberties consciousness of the early 1960s; it was in this context that ex-patients' rights groups developed (5, p. 527). Intellectually, the movement was nurtured by the consciousness raising of the feminist movement, the societal critiques of the radical therapists, the labeling arguments of the gay liberation movement, and the philosophies of self-help movements (5, pp. 524–525; 6). The major vehicle for communicating among the ex-patients was *Madness Network News.* The National (and later, International) Conference on Human Rights and Psychiatric Oppression, which convened annually from 1973 to 1985, also served as a forum for meeting and for exchanging ideas.

The Radical Therapists. During the 1960s and early 1970s, a diverse array of mental health professionals, who called themselves "radical therapists," voiced dissatisfaction with traditional therapy. Their reasons included the following: its ineffectiveness (7, p. 7); the power relations and social oppressiveness inherent both in traditional forms of therapy (7, pp. 15–17) and in the medical model of mental illness (8, p. 122); the class and racial determinants of available services (7, p. 7); the alienation of therapists from those they treat (7, p. 8); and the role of the traditional therapist in promoting adjustment to oppressive social and economic conditions rather than liberation from them (7, pp. 16–17). Radical therapists offered some alternative combination of radical therapeutics and/or radical politics (7, pp. 15–16; 8, p. 21).

Although allied with the radical therapists, who shared their criticism of psychiatry and the social basis of madness, the ex-patients later parted ways in order to preserve their independence (2). *The Radical Therapist*, a journal published between 1970 and 1972, contained several articles by ex-patients (7, pp. 107–10). Many ex-patients thought the radical therapists' critiques were largely intellectual exercises (3, p. 324), in contrast to their own active confrontations with psychiatry's use of physical restraints and invasive treatments (2, p. 11). The radical bases of the radical therapists' critiques also varied in their political understandings and therapeutic solutions. Some accepted a Marxian social structural critique, while others were more concerned with developing radical intrapsychic or interpersonal therapeutic interventions (8, pp. 122–123). The continued use of psychiatric medications by some radical therapists and their devotion to trendy new treatments led many ex-patients to question what they and the radical therapists had in common (2, p. 21; 5); by the mid-1970s, active collaboration had ended (2).

The Conference on Human Rights and Against Psychiatric Oppression also began as a joint effort between radical therapists and ex-patients, but by 1976 radical therapists no longer attended (3). Similarly, *Madness Network News*, which covered the ex-patient movement in the United States between 1973 and 1986, began as a joint effort with radical therapists, but within a few years, after struggles for control, the radical therapists dropped out (3). Ex-patients and radical therapists often engaged in civil disobedience during the early 1970s, disrupting professional psychiatric meetings. One group of ex-patients who demonstrated against an American Psychiatric Association meeting during this period found themselves preempted by another group of radical therapists, and quickly removed them (9). Thus, despite considerable overlap in ideology and interests, the experience of psychiatric oppression suffered by the ex-patients made them wary of collaborations with even radical professionals, who could threaten their autonomy and divert their mission.

Advocates for Patients' Rights. During the 1970s, programs advocating for the civil and treatment rights of institutionalized patients were being established in various states, and the national Mental Health Law Project (later renamed the Bazelon Center) engaged lawyers in individual and class-action suits (10). In 1980, several members of the Mental Health Law Project formed the National Association for Rights Protection and Advocacy (NARPA), the only independent advocacy organization in the United States. NARPA is the one organization in which collaboration among ex-patients, attorneys, sympathetic professionals, and nonlegal advocates has persisted (10). According to NARPA's bylaws, at least one-third of its board of directors must be ex-patients, and its board members have often exceeded that proportion.

Although earlier advocates had worked to regain the civil rights of incarcerated psychiatric patients and the right to *gain* treatment while committed, the more radical advocates also fought for the right of hospitalized and ex-patients to *refuse* treatment (5, pp. 530–31; 11, p. 295). Whereas many groups (e.g., mental health planners and administrators, mental health providers, states Mental Health Associations, civil rights advocates, and ex-patients) had converged on the issue of the right to treatment, ex-patients found themselves alone with the more radical legal advocates on the right to refuse treatment (11, pp. 295–96). NARPA has provided one source of support for this right as it has advocated both the right to choose specific treatments and protection from forced treatment of any kind (12).

A Reformist Turn

By 1980, some ex-patients felt that the movement had become disorganized, weak, and limited in its reach. Attendance at the International Conference had sharply declined, and new social concerns were capturing participants' attention. Many ex-patients thought a national organization was needed to provide national exposure (2, p. 22) and to address the problems of homelessness and the pressing social and economic conditions to which patients and ex-patients were subject when discharged into the community. They began to advocate for change through lobbying, litigation, their own ex-patient alternatives, and statewide conferences. They were also beginning to engage in dialogue with psychiatrists and other mental health professionals at national mental health meetings. Ex-patients who had picketed the annual meetings of the American Psychiatric Association in one year debated its members in the next.

This reformist turn by some of their members was the beginning of a profound split among the ex-patients. When the Community Support Program of the National Institute of Mental Health offered to fund the first annual Alternatives Conference for consumers and ex-patients in order to establish a national consumer organization, an intense debate ensued exposing the anarchistic, radical reformist, and conservative ideological differences and the class differences in the movement (2, p. 12). These differences were revealed in comments articulated in *Madness Network News* throughout 1985 and 1986.

One goal of the first Alternatives Conference, held in 1985, was to begin establishing a national ex-patient/consumer organization. The National Mental Health Consumers' Association was founded, but its refusal to take a position against forced treatment—a central human rights issue for ex-patients—led to the formation of a separate national organization, the National Alliance of Mental Patients, later renamed the National Association of Psychiatric Survivors. While the National Mental Health Consumers' Association was more conservative and accepted the medical model of mental illness (4), the ex-patients fought against the medical model and treatments that stemmed from it. The ex-patients' adamant opposition to all forced treatment laws contrasted with the indifference on this topic of the consumers—many of whom were advocating for more treatments and greater access to them. These different stances on forced treatment highlighted the fundamental philosophical difference between the two groups and the irreconcilable division this created in the movement. Despite their differences however, both organizations welcomed ex-patients and consumers. The National Mental Health Consumers' Association was more familiar to consumers, but it had not established a clear membership. The National Alliance of Mental Patients, with its 300 members, served as the intellectual lifeblood of the movement and maintained a seasonal newsletter to encourage dialogue among its members.

The founding of these two organizations struck a final blow to the anarchist element of the ex-inmate movement. The last International Conference on Human Rights and Psychiatric Oppression was held later in 1985. The next year, *Madness Network News,* under financial duress and amidst internal ideological strife, ceased publication. Its last issue blamed the Community Support Program for successfully co-opting the antipsychiatry movement. With the death of the International Conference and *Madness Network News,* those opposing national organizing efforts lost connection to the movement.

The ex-inmate/ex-patient movement became transformed into a more organized, though politically more divergent, "consumer/ex-patient" movement (more recently called "consumer/survivor") (1), whose ideologically diverse members were willing to work with the mental health system and government agencies. This reconfigured movement and its consequences for consumers and ex-patients can be understood only in the context of larger social, political, and economic developments in the mental health scene in the United States during this time. One such development was the founding of the Community Support Program; the other, the burgeoning family consumer movement.

LARGER SOCIAL AND POLITICAL DEVELOPMENTS

The Community Support Program

The Community Support Program (CSP) was initiated in 1977 by the National Institute of Mental Health (NIMH) as a corrective to problems resulting from deinstitutionalization of psychiatric patients from long-term institutions (13). In 1963, federal legislation mandated the release of institutionalized patients into the community, without establishing structures to provide for their multiple clinical and material needs. Services were fragmented, and no clear lines of responsibility had been established among federal, state, and local agencies to organize and finance them (14, 15). The CSP staff intended to provide national leadership to integrate the services at the state level.

The CSP was driven by a recognition of the inadequacy of the medical model's individual orientation for dealing with the multiple needs of seriously ill persons in the community. It sought to produce a comprehensive model of community care founded on a rehabilitative approach to treatment, sensitive to client needs (13).

Involving Families. In a period when biomedicine was gaining momentum within psychiatry, NIMH staff recognized the controversial nature of their approach. To gain congressional support to fund the CSP, they knew they would need a strong constituency to back it—a voting public that would let its wishes be known. Steven Sharfstein, the psychiatrist heading the CSP effort, turned to families of seriously mentally ill adults for that backing (16).

Some of these families had been involved in citizen boards established by the 1963 Community Mental Health Restoration Act. Many had previously contacted NIMH out of frustration with costly, unproductive mental health treatment. Given the conventional wisdom of the time, which pointed to parents as the cause of schizophrenia, some families had not yet "come out of the closet." Sharfstein (16) realized they needed to gain power before they could give their support, and he encouraged his staff to involve families in an empowered position, face to face with providers in national conferences and policy-making committees. Other families, very wealthy and secure and unthreatened by "going public," had already begun to mobilize changes in their communities (17) and to recognize their political clout (18, p. 158). This incipient family movement achieved a national level of organization as the National Alliance for the Mentally Ill (NAMI), and the CSP helped fund many of its new chapters.

Support to Ex-Patients and Consumers. The Community Support Program was slower to bring in ex-patients and primary consumers (the direct recipients of mental health treatment) because they were not seen as a legitimate and significant constituency to help push its programs. The very idea of enlisting their input was quite novel in the late 1970s (19). No precedent had yet existed for handling the legal and financial details of bringing in a group of persons still regarded as fragile. Under encouragement from Bill TenHoor, a progressive CSP staffer, Judi Chamberlin, author of a book that became known as the bible of the ex-patient liberation movement (20), was invited to early national CSP learning conferences. Her contributions opened doors to ex-patients at future conferences.

The CSP was nurtured by many progressive thinkers, both within and outside NIMH, whose purview extended beyond mental health to broader issues encompassing human rights. Its intellectual fervor for new ideas rendered it receptive to the thoughts of ex-patients themselves. Its social orientation for providing services and sustenance in the community was compatible with the general approaches ex-patients supported. Its rehabilitative orientation, defined by its sensitivity to client-defined needs, was also philosophically compatible with their perspectives.

Given the CSP's commitment to a consumerism driven by the power of its constituency (the families of primary consumers) and the satisfaction of client-defined needs (those of the primary consumers), its staff established structures to enable recipients' participation in making policy for mental health services. They did this through federal laws that defined state obligations for involving recipients and by promoting consumer-run alternative services (1, p. 1054). Unfortunately, the CSP, like the community mental health movement of which it was a part, was never sufficiently funded to fulfill its intentions.

The Family Movement

During the 1970s, while the CSP was promoting family consumerism, many families were already seeing themselves as consumers as they searched for new treatment options (21). Many had exhausted their insurance benefits and were forced to delve into the family estate to pay for ineffective, and often indicting, hospital treatment. Families eventually came to see that it was they who had the greatest vested interest in treatment since they would be living with its consequences. Thus the early family advocates insisted that they should be in control or, at the very least, "full partners" (18, p. 159) in treatment, and demanded direct accountability from professionals.

Birth of the National Alliance for the Mentally Ill. With increasing opportunities to meet through CSP meetings and congressionally mandated Community Mental Health Center boards, families began to compare their disappointments in available treatments and in the demeaning approaches of professionals. They eventually came to doubt the dominant psychogenic theories and the stigmatizing and ineffective treatments they often faced as part of their adult children's family therapy (21). They began to organize local advocacy and support groups, and by September 1979, the National Alliance for the Mentally Ill (NAMI) was founded. Within one decade, with funding support from the CSP, it grew from 284 to 80,000 members.

Fueled by indignation about being wrongfully blamed and economically exploited for treatments that failed them and their family members, families directed their energies to forcefully creating change (21). Recent developments in biomedical technology, enabling direct exploration of the brain, encouraged them that science could discover the organic source of madness in the diseased brain. They became committed to promoting a biomedical psychiatry that freed them of blame and offered an explanation that conformed to their own understanding of their relatives' developmental history (22, 23).

Having come from the professions, academia, or high military posts, some of the most active NAMI leaders were experienced in negotiating power, were well connected professionally and socially, and knew how to enlist support and use muscle. By their very first NAMI conference, they had already received support from the heads of NIMH and had developed influential and strategically placed contacts throughout the nation's capital.

NAMI's Activities. The National Alliance for the Mentally Ill worked to improve mental health services for severely ill persons, to increase research, and to advance training, albeit in directions restricted by the biomedical perspective. NAMI did not simply lobby for funding. Its advocates sought direct control of the processes of knowledge production by becoming actively engaged in the professional discourses on mental illness and research and by strategically positioning themselves in ways to alter these discourses. They achieved this through educational and legislative efforts directed at remedicalizing psychiatry (22). At the *national* organizational level, NAMI focused more on changing psychiatric ideologies than on improving and extending services, which may be why they failed to attract minority and lower-class families. As NAMI grew stronger, its allegiance to biomedical psychiatry eventually outweighed its support for the CSP, which was devoted to community services. NAMI withdrew yet more support after the CSP staff forged alliances with ex-patients, whose positions against forced treatment and biomedicine stood in direct opposition to their own.

Consequences of the Family Movement for Consumers/Ex-Patients

Promotion of Consumer Choice in the Market. NAMI's influence within NIMH succeeded in moving the Institute in a biomedical direction (21, pp. 974–77) and eventually in moving it out of the Alcohol, Drug and Mental Health Administration and into the National Institutes of Health. This move represented a symbolic and political victory reaffirming NAMI's position that mental illness was a brain disease. This shift bode poorly for the CSP, with its community orientation. By 1993 the CSP had moved out of NIMH and into the Center for Mental Health Services of the Substance Abuse and Mental Health Services Administration. In its less prestigious location in what had become a heavily scientistic environment, the CSP's capacity as an agent of change was further restricted. The consumer/ex-patient movement thus became limited in achieving gains because its key proponent at the federal level had become further marginalized within an administration now dominated by the biomedical model.

While elevating biomedical psychiatry, NAMI at the same time appreciated the need to empower patients in their relationships with their doctors by encouraging a partnership ethos—one they had acquired by working with providers on citizen boards and policy-making committees (14, p. 168). This reinforced the position of primary consumers that patients must actively participate in optimizing their treatment. Privately paying consumers who were already empowered to "shop for" a good psychiatrist were now more likely to seek one who would listen to their concerns and welcome their input.[1] Thus NAMI helped foster consumer choice in the marketplace.

Even before the development of this partnership ethos, improved institutional conditions, promoted by consumer advocacy, and shorter stays, stimulated by the deinstitutionalization movement (25), had created a new kind of consumer. This new consumer did not experience the same extremes of helplessness and oppression as did the founders of the ex-patient movement. Many in fact valued the provider-consumer relation and wanted to support it, not challenge it, in their work as consumer advocates (1, p. 1067). Such persons, who could be called true "consumers," reinforced the more conservative strain of the consumer/ex-patient movement.

Intensifying a Two-Tiered Mental Health System. While succeeding in heightening the private consumer's control over treatment, NAMI's efforts only exaggerated preexisting differences in a two-tiered treatment system (5, pp. 533–34). In the public sector, where inadequate funding resulted in long waits for only a few minutes with a psychiatrist at monthly visits, clinics served as treatment mills for renewing prescriptions, and little more. Under pressure to "process" huge caseloads, the psychiatrists employed part-time to manage these cases lacked adequate time to observe a patient and to discuss symptoms and side effects of treatment. At one drop-in center I studied, several consumers complained that they would wait for hours to meet with a psychiatrist just to have him or her brusquely dismiss their concerns about symptoms or side effects with accusations of treatment noncompliance. This situation produced consumers who "consumed" treatment without exercising any choice in clinician or control over treatment.

The opportunity for a public-sector consumer to participate in treatment, let alone be an "equal partner" in it, has been unimaginable in such understaffed

---

[1] Despite the inroads made for many private-sector consumers in participating in treatment, this is far from reality for more seriously impaired patients (24).

clinics. In addition, the realities of long waiting lists for limited services have restricted both the amount of service and treatment available (such as expensive medications, available only through a lottery in some states) and the extent to which public-sector clients have been able to exercise genuine consumer choice. Under profit-driven managed care, which has controlled mental health services in recent years, the situation in public-sector mental health has only worsened (26, 27). The rupture between the private and public systems has further widened as social programs in the public sector are being closed and increasing numbers of persons are going without any treatment (28, p. 110).

Thus, in a two-tiered system of mental health services, opportunities to exercise choice and control over treatment have varied significantly between the private and public sectors. Gains acquired from consumerism became manifest in an *uneven empowerment* by class (29), representative of the broader social structure, that served to reproduce—and perhaps exaggerate—pre-existing inequalities. These differences in class produced different kinds of consumers with different experiences of psychiatric oppression and expert control, different understandings about "consumer empowerment," and different expectations from a consumer movement (1, 4).

NAMI's promotion of consumerism thus yielded markedly different opportunities for public- and private-sector consumers to gain control over their treatment. Furthermore, its endorsement of biomedical treatment over community support promoted the dependence of public-sector consumers on chemotherapeutic management by the clinic while offering them minimal opportunities to gain control over other aspects of their lives. Biomedicine was ill equipped to handle the personal and social processes of recovery that can occur while living with a disability. Although the privately paying consumer gained some control over treatment, the isolation of the brain as the sole locus of concern at the same time extracted or diminished the importance of the individual's control over recovery (30, 31). It was in reaction to the neglect of mind, or person, by biomedical treatment and to the continued control by experts in the public sector that consumer and ex-patient activists looked to user-controlled alternatives.

Mental Health Associations

Although a far less significant player than the family movement, the national Mental Health Association and its state chapters were working to promote mental health and consumerism well before the term *consumer* "became part of the public consciousness" (32, p. 610). While not providing advocacy services (33, p. 2036), Mental Health Associations have nonetheless advocated for the rights of mental health patients (32), generally testifying on the side of plaintiffs in patients' rights suits (33, p. 2036). Early in the 1960s, the National Mental Health Association worked to reform the mental health system by promoting passage of legislation for community mental health centers and their services and by fighting to eliminate unpaid patient labor (32, pp. 612–13). It has also worked to secure services and promote accountability of providers in the mental health system, but always *within* that system.

Clifford Beers, an ex-patient who founded the Mental Health Association in 1909, was forced to modulate his intense criticism of the mental health system in order to gain public support for his reform movement, particularly among those who could provide economic support (2, pp. 9–10). In the process, he was diverted from his original goal of bringing ex-patients and their families into the movement, and it took many years to correct this. As recently as 1980, some state Mental Health Associations had still chosen to exclude consumers and their families from their boards (9).

In promoting his movement, Beers had garnered support from sympathetic professionals such as psychologist William James. The Mental Health Associations have remained supportive of professionals, while never forfeiting their loyalties to consumers. Thus, on reform, they have tended to take moderate positions between providers and ex-patients, arguably weakening their position on particular issues (33, pp. 2036–37). Because of the association's history of involvement with professionals, ex-patients and related patients' rights advocacy groups have tended to avoid collaboration with them (33, p. 2036). Their preference for service-oriented advocacy, however, has made Mental Health Associations ideal collaborators with *consumers* (both primary organizations and family organizations) with whom they have co-sponsored numerous projects since the 1980s. In their various consumer collaborations supported through the Consumer Support Program since the 1980s, the Mental Health Associations have worked to foster consumerism in the United States. However, because they have not taken extreme oppositional stands on such issues as forced treatment as advocated by NAMI and other organizations, their power as a national player has somewhat diminished in recent years. Economic support from sponsors such as drug companies has also been diverted to NAMI. In order to survive, the Mental Health Association is considering merging with NAMI (9).

The Consumer–Survivor Movement, Recovery, and Consumer Professionals

Frederick J. Frese and Wendy Walker Davis

Consumers' voices about what is needed and what is valuable are increasingly being heard. For instance, in 1992, the National Mental Health Consumers' Association adopted a mission statement that included six areas critical for consumers to lead meaningful and productive lives: employment, housing, benefits, mental health systems, self-help, and lack of discrimination. Federal law now requires that states receiving funds for mental health services must have consumers on all mental health boards. More recently, the Mental Health

Statistics Improvement Program Task Force of the Center for Mental Health Services developed with consumers a report card that reflects a consumer perspective on the measures and indicators needed to adequately assess the quality and outcomes of services. There is increasing research into the views and needs of consumers, including research by consumer researchers (e.g., Campbell, 1989). In a number of studies, service recipients attributed more importance to services that improve quality of life than to treatments designed to reduce symptoms (e.g., Felton, Carpinello, Massaro, & Evants, 1996).

RECOVERY

Because of the presence of pervasive stigmatization, the concept of recovery (Anthony, 1993) is especially important in working with individuals who have serious mental illness. Internalizing the negative attitudes of the larger society, people who have been newly diagnosed often feel hopeless about their future. In fact, one of the most common messages they receive from others—professionals as well as loved ones—is to downsize their expectations. In response, they may assume that a full life is now out of reach, and that satisfying relationships and educational and occupational achievements will be impossible. Hopes for the future may be dashed further by the course of mental illness, which is often characterized by alternating periods of remission and exacerbation.

A key element in recovery is the presence of people who offer hope, understanding, and support; who encourage self-determination; and who promote self-actualization. Recovery is best understood as a process, not an outcome. The psychologist assists in this process by supporting the person's life choices and by working in partnership with the person to help him or her better cope with the challenges of an ongoing and serious illness. Psychologists embrace a recovery framework when they assist a person in realizing his or her potential as a unique human being who is not defined by an illness.

As psychologists, we have been influenced by the stigma and hopelessness that accompany a diagnosis of serious mental illness. We have been exposed to theories that hold individuals and families accountable for the development of these disorders and that describe them in pejorative and stigmatizing language. We have been taught that a person with serious mental illness will probably require long-term, intensive care that usually involves hospitalization. In addition, we each bring to our work a set of personal experiences, assumptions, and beliefs that influence our approach to working with people who have been psychiatrically labeled.

Mental health professionals who experience mental illness themselves are likely to find themselves reevaluating their earlier assumptions and beliefs. For example, one of us (Wendy Walker Davis) had the following experience:

> I was given the opportunity to examine my own preconceived notions of mental illness when I was hospitalized. Suddenly, I was very interested in my chances of recovery. I sought out people who were doing well. I was alarmed and devastated when my husband and I were told by psychiatrists that I would have to accept my illness and that there was no hope of recovery. In fact, I have fully recovered from my difficulties. I consider the problems that led to hospitalization as in remission.

We believe that it is important for therapists and clients to know that some people do fully recover. We also realize that complete remission is not possible for every client. However, the stigma associated with mental illness inhibits those who recover from disclosing their positive outcomes. It is easier to distance ourselves from the past. This leaves the impression that there really is no hope for people to go forward with their lives. The silence of those of us who fully recover reinforces the prejudices that exist.

CONSUMER–PROFESSIONALS

At a preconference institute of the annual meeting of the National Alliance for the Mentally Ill (Marsh & Johnson, 1995), one of us (Frederick J. Frese) spoke about the increasing role of *prosumers*, a term that describes people with mental illness who are also mental health professionals (professionals–consumers). The consumer movement strongly supports the need for prosumers. Prosumers model a vision of participatory treatment and recovery that includes people with mental illness as full partners and collaborators in their individual treatment and rehabilitation and in the design, delivery, and evaluation of mental health services. Indeed, all stakeholders (consumers, family members, and service providers) must be involved in addressing such pressing contemporary concerns as managed care, state hospital future planning, and employment and housing for people with mental illness.

At that conference, professional practice in the area of substance abuse, where the personal experience of providers is valued, was contrasted with practice in the area of mental illness, where such experience has traditionally been discounted. Fortunately, the field is increasingly acknowledging the contributions that can be made by those who have developed special expertise through their own experiences with mental illness; those people should be encouraged to pursue careers as mental health professionals. In turn, psychology needs to increase the access of people with mental illness to graduate programs, to offer essential support during their training, and to facilitate their credentialing and employment.

Prosumers face unique challenges, including the vulnerability that attends their disclosure, the risk that their credibility will be lessened by their status as clients, and the backlash that may accompany a request for reasonable accommodations. On the other hand, prosumers bring greater motivation to their professional work, find it easier to empathize with those who receive their services, have a wealth of practical advice and insight, and serve as constructive role models for other clients.

Psychology could make a major contribution to the recovery of people with serious mental illness by sensitizing itself and the public about pejorative stereotypes, by valuing those people's experiences and insights, by defending their rights and needs for quality services, by supporting their education and training at both the undergraduate and graduate levels, by seeking their input on relevant issues, and by advocating their causes and needs before Congress, the courts, and the public.

References

Anthony, W. A. (1993). Recovery from mental illness: The guiding vision of the mental health service system in the 1990s. *Psychosocial Rehabilitation Journal, 16,* 11–23.

Felton, C. J., Carpinello, S. E., Massaro, R., & Evans, M. (1996, May). *Multiple stakeholders: Perceptions of outcomes.* Paper presented at the meeting of the National Conference on Mental Health Statistics, Washington, DC.

Marsh, D. T., & Johnson, J. R. (1995). *The emerging collaborative paradigm: Implications for policy, training, research, and practice* (Report of the NAMI pre-conference institute). Rockville, MD: Center for Mental Health Services.

Source: Federick J. Frese and Wendy Walker Davis. 1997. "The Consumer-Survivor Movement, Recovery, and Consumer Professionals." *Professional Psychology: Research and Practice* 28(3):243–245.

CONSEQUENCES OF THE RECONFIGURED CONSUMER/EX-PATIENT MOVEMENT

The consumer/ex-patient movement has experienced both gains and setbacks for its constituency. Its actions and the consequences of its reform efforts can be understood only within a broader political context.

Gains Initiated through Consumer/Ex-Patient Reform Efforts

Unlike NAMI, which provided an organizational base and professional and economic support for membership development, the consumer/ex-patient movement, with its significantly less privileged membership base, lacked a centralized national organization and machinery for recruitment. Instead, its spokespersons became active participants at various levels of government. Their efforts, supported by the CSP, set in motion a variety of initiatives to raise the consumer voice in policymaking and to open doors for self-help alternatives. As ex-patients and consumers gained increasing presence and voice at the national CSP Learning Conferences between 1978 and 1987, their issues and perspectives began to penetrate the thinking of CSP staff and became instrumental in shaping its philosophical direction and mission. Through their participation at these conferences, ex-patients and consumers also made additional contacts and allies that helped promote their advocacy efforts, which allowed them to extend the consumer movement to a broader base of participants.

Asserting Their Voices; Gaining CSP Support. Consumers and survivors who attended these conferences made two major points: (a) their experiences as patients offered unique insight into the mental health system; and (b) the CSP should no longer collapse their interests with those of families as part of a single group of "consumers" (34, p. 35). Ex-patients in particular argued that the experiences, goals, and ideologies of the two groups—ex-patients and families—were often irreconcilable (e.g., NAMI's support for involuntary commitment and forced treatment versus ex-patient's keen objection to these).

Despite their differences with respect to the medical model and forced treatment, both consumers and ex-patients agreed on the debilitating effects of institutionalization and of control by fatalistic service providers. Both also valued self-determination over one's life and treatment as central to recovery (35, 36), and both endorsed consumer-controlled self-help alternatives as a necessary component of community support.

CSP officials valued this input. By 1984, the CSP identified "self-determination" as a guiding principle of its Community Support Systems (37, p. 11), and "consumer empowerment" was declared one of the CSP's fundamental goals (38, p. 94). The guiding principles of the Community Support Service System were also shaped by consumer/ex-patient ideas: basing services on the client's not the provider's or the service system's needs, leaving the determination of desired services to the consumers themselves, and providing services that reinforce dignity and self-esteem rather than pathology (35, pp. 21–22). The CSP provided legitimacy to consumer-controlled alternatives by endorsing them as a key model of community support programs (36) and by providing federal seed funding to initiate them. The CSP also provided funding for the annual Alternatives Conferences, which began in 1985, to bring consumers/survivors together to share their knowledge. Finally, the CSP also pushed legislation mandating states that received federal mental health funding to adopt services such as consumer-operated alternatives that "empower clients" (35, pp. 21–22).

The consumer/survivors' insistence on maintaining independence from families served them well after consumer representation on policy and decision-making boards became mandated. As the result of their advocacy, federal guidelines suggested that states' Mental Health Planning Councils include a "balanced representation" of primary consumers and family members (35).

Developing Professional Contacts and Alliances. Consumers/survivors who attended national CSP conferences made valuable contacts with lawyers, researchers, state mental health directors, and policymakers at various levels of government. These contacts sometimes resulted in alliances that promoted consumers' causes. For example, alliances with lawyers, such as those from the Mental Health Law Project, helped establish a patients' rights and advocacy network, which promoted patients' rights not only to *receive* treatment but to *refuse* it (39).

Consumer contacts with state mental health commissioners and state CSP directors familiarized administrators with the basis of consumer demands and introduced them to articulate, often compelling ex-patient and consumer spokespersons. Their exchanges helped validate consumer/survivor perspectives and led to their inclusion in state mental health plans (40).

By participating on various committees, consumers/survivors became acquainted with a variety of mental health policymakers who were receptive to their ideas. By 1992, as the result of support from various mental health policy administrators, program directors, and researchers at the national level, a group of consumers who were also researchers initiated the Consumer/Survivor Research and Policy Workgroup. Like NAMI before them (22), these consumer researchers attempted to take charge of the processes of knowledge production by engaging their supporters in a discourse about their concerns, values, perceptions, and desires. By working to restructure the way in which mental health professionals and policymakers conceptualize consumer needs, outcomes (41), and services, they have worked to redirect the national mental health agenda. Perhaps most important, consumers and ex-patients came to know the leaders of the CSP, who became some of their staunchest supporters (42, p. 1).

Expanding the Consumer Movement. The most important outcome of consumers/survivors' negotiations with the mental health system may have been the creation of a larger, broad-based movement. Owing to the successful advocacy for consumer-controlled alternatives, people who had never heard of "consumer empowerment" (1, p. 1062) came to rely on these alternative facilities. Federal seed money to initiate alternatives and legal mandates encouraging states to fund their projects promoted the growth of these programs (37). As "consumer" became a familiar term and consumer alternatives received endorsement from local mental health authorities, providers came to see consumer programs as working *with* the mental health system rather than against it, and began informing their clients about new alternatives. The highly publicized Alternatives Conferences also made more consumers aware of the movement. The 1990 Alternatives Conference in Pittsburgh, Pennsylvania, for example, attracted some 1,300 participants, 43 of them on passes from state hospitals.

Although some ex-patients found their way into consumer programs through consumer outreach efforts, most were referred from within the mental health system. Many newcomers had not heard of the consumer movement, and despite considerable dissatisfaction with the conditions of their lives and their psychiatric treatment, they had been resigned to accepting them.

The Alternatives Conferences temporarily revived the liberation vision of the movement, and their collective spirit evoked feelings of empowerment in many initiates. As consumer-run alternatives mushroomed throughout the country, increasing numbers of new mental health consumers became involved in self-help programs and consumer advocacy activities, and gained more information—both positive and negative—about the mental health system. This produced more consumers who were informed about treatment, medication, and their rights within the mental health system. Primary consumers began to show a marked presence on local mental health boards and committees. New consumer advocates learned to articulate their views about community and mental health system needs; some also participated in efforts to close down psychiatric hospitals as a continuation of deinstitutionalization. Increasing numbers of consumers were proactively confronting undesirable conditions.

Through opportunities to become engaged in advocacy activities, several talented individuals joined efforts to reform the mental health system. With the CSP's encouragement, many of them were hired to fill newly developed consumer offices at both local and state levels of the mental health system. Many of these new leaders gained respect for their energy, dedication, intelligence, and competence.

Setbacks to Reform and the Specter of Co-optation

Everything was not rosy in the consumer/survivor movement, however. Indeed, activism led to some developments that contradicted the movement's initial goals, resulting in setbacks both for new consumers and for the original ex-patient agenda.

"Inadequate Bite" of Federal Legislation. Consumers had made apparent gains with the passing of federal legislation in 1986 (P.L. 99–600, Title 5, The State Comprehensive Mental Health Plan Act of 1986). States were mandated to provide comprehensive mental health plans—promoting consumer representation on planning councils and supporting consumer-run alternatives—before

they were entitled to receive federal dollars. Legal penalties, however, lacked sufficient muscle to force compliance (43). In addition, family representatives continued to provide the dominant consumer voice on planning and policy-making committees in many states. In some cases, primary consumers on committees were simply tolerated, not taken seriously. Even when consumers/survivors were successful in gaining support for their ideas, inadequate budgets limited how much they could actually accomplish.

Vulnerability to Government Funding Trends, Ideology, and Politics. Reliance on government funding to support a movement has a more fundamental disadvantage: government funding trends change as different ideologies gain or lose political favor. Consumer projects were promoted by the CSP—a marginalized agency whose federal funding was subject to the vagaries of political trends. Under such sponsorship, consumer projects, while apparently gaining legitimacy, became vulnerable to political manipulation. The following example illustrates this process. In 1988, the CSP (still part of NIMH) funded 13 consumer-run demonstration services projects to develop and implement innovative programs. Evaluations were considered a necessary but secondary part of the grant (44); indeed, evaluations of demonstration projects are typically concerned with administrative feasibility, not outcomes (45). During this time, Congress, stimulated by NAMI, demanded that NIMH provide evidence that its projects were worthy of funding. To do this NIMH placed new demands for stronger evaluations on projects that it had funded under different terms. Consumer demonstration projects were pressured to initiate more rigorous, standardized evaluations. Many projects were not equipped to do so, and most had not planned or budgeted for this. Even more problematic, rigorous standardized evaluations were methodologically inappropriate and should not have been taken as valid measures of the success (46) of the demonstration projects, given their preliminary nature. Because of the compromised quality of the evaluations, the consumer projects as a whole were perceived as weak, despite exceptional successes, and the CSP lost its authorization to fund similar projects.

Funding Constraints on Consumer-Run Alternatives. Some of the worst fears of ex-patients who had dropped out of the movement in 1986 were realized after other ex-patients decided to accept government funding for their alternatives: dependence on government funding for continued operations; demands for greater accountability to funders than to program users; pressure to redefine program goals in terms meaningful to government agencies; diminished control over program content; and, for some, a lost vision of the liberationist mission.[2]

Funding structures also created language, pay scales, and staff distinctions that challenged egalitarian ideologies. The greatest challenge for many

---

[2] Such continuing constraints have led some activists who had for many years relied on government funds for consumer-run programs to break away and set up their own foundations to support their work (48).

seasoned activists was, in the words of one, to work within those confines "without bending our own principles" (47).

Consumer programs tended to be poorly funded and understaffed, and both the paid and the volunteer staff were overworked. Pay scales for the staff consumer centers were considerably lower than those for staff working in traditional mental health programs (48). This discrepancy "devalues our work," explained one project director. "The expectation is that consumers should work for peanuts" because "we have all the time in the world and nothing better to do with it" (48). Extensive paperwork required by funding agencies further burdened program staff and cut into their time with users. Working under these conditions created extraordinary stress that sometimes resulted in emotional breakdown, even in individuals who had been stable for years.

Internal Problems with Consumer-Run Alternatives. Consumer alternatives were intended to *empower* consumers to gain control over their lives and to restore the self-esteem, independence, and hope many had lost through debilitating experiences in the mental health system (49). These alternative programs deliberately hired only consumers and ex-patients as staff so that they alone—without interference from professionals—would be responsible for determining the direction of their programs. Decisions were to be made through inclusive democratic processes. They also attempted, by these hiring practices, to eliminate a staff–user hierarchy. In actual practice, however, some consumer alternatives fell drastically short of these empowering principles (1, 50). Abuse of power by consumer program directors was not uncommon. Some leaders were dominating and controlling to the point of oppressiveness (1, p. 1063). Power hierarchies developed in which, contrary to participatory democratic principles, decisions were made only by the consumer staff (49). Consciousness-raising sessions, formerly seen as essential for empowering users, were regarded as archaic or irrelevant by many of the new consumer leaders. They were replaced with "services" not that different from those offered by the local clinic. Finally, the power differential between consumer staff and users was so great in some places that "consumer-controlled" came to mean "consumer *staff*–controlled."

Alternatives that departed significantly from the empowering ideals of their founders were generally run by a new breed of consumer who fully accepted the medical model of mental illness but knew very little about the roots of the movement. These consumers often carried impressive professional credentials but lacked an appreciation for the political basis of the consumer movement (1, p. 1067). Worries about hierarchical structures and an oppressive social system were irrelevant to private paying consumers who, through the work of earlier advocates, had experienced a more responsive mental health system. Some of these new consumers had themselves been providers and continued to see themselves in this way in their staff positions in these alternative programs. Others had lost previous jobs because of illness and saw the consumer position as an opportunity to empower themselves personally on a new career ladder, while lacking an understanding of or commitment to the movement. Finally, many of the newer consumer programs were funded by grants written, without any input from consumers, by state mental health administrators hoping to tap available federal funds (46, p 51). They had little understanding of the roots of the consumer movement and of the relevance of empowerment, and they hired consumers, as was required by the grant, simply to staff their programs.

Transformation in the Concept of "Empowerment." The concept of consumer empowerment appealed to many government program leaders. However, the conception they adopted was based on the power of the *consumer* to exercise choice *within* the mental health system, not the personal and political empowerment derived from one's independence from that system (1, 51). Thus, in being tied to the system and the hierarchical structure of which it was a part, the emancipatory values originally associated with empowerment gave way, to various degrees, to the more traditional values embodied by the treatment system.

Discussion: Co-optation and Beyond

Beyond the marginalized and underfunded CSP, consumers have lacked the strong government backing necessary for gaining security for their projects, yet they have been economically unable to run their programs without it. The anarchists of the ex-patient movement, recognizing this dilemma, opted to drop out of the movement rather than risk co-optation of their political cause by accepting government funds. Those who remained tied to the movement elected to accept some level of compromise to achieve some gains. Such has also been the plight of ex-patients in other countries (52, 53) and of activists in other movements (54).

Ex-patients who continued to work for reform accepted significant compromises. Activists have witnessed developments that have blurred their emancipatory vision. They have been particularly disturbed by the perpetuation of abuses to consumers by other consumers (55). Hiring only consumers to run these alternative projects has been an insufficient deterrent to reproducing oppression and abuses of power (1). The programs have too often resembled the traditional mental health programs to which they were intended to be "alternatives." Under such circumstances, the "consumer empowerment" they intended to promote became a far cry from the empowering processes that ex-patients had originally envisioned when they came together for mutual support (20).

Co-optation as a General Problem in Alternative Health Movements. These problems were by no means unique to the ex-patient movement. Wherever health reform movements have acquired legitimacy, there has been a tendency, albeit of a more limited sort, for health planners and providers to usurp control from activists under the guise of promoting the reform (5). Invariably the outcome has been the demise of the political dimensions of the movement. Given its interest in adopting certain products of these movements (generally, the service innovations), the State does not overtly intend to destroy them. Rather, it attempts to promote certain aspects (services) while discouraging others (e.g., collectivist control, nonhierarchical structures, nonprofessional ideology) (56, p. 207) and converting the meaning of still others (e.g., "empowerment") (1, pp. 1055–59). It does this by shaping the "actions and beliefs" of movement participants "through control of political and economic resources" (56, p. 207). These strategies were seen in the free clinic (57), the mental health free clinic (2, p. 10), the feminist health (56), and the battered women (58) movements.

As Morgen (56) explains, the State's funding mechanisms work to support the aspects of movements that it favors by setting funding limits and conditions that undermine their adversarial aspects. For example, by limiting funds in alternative centers to the provision of services, and by placing heavy demands on staff energy and time for documentation and accountability, it diverts attention from larger oppositional movement goals. And the addition of paid staff to an existing voluntary one introduces potential conflict (56). Funding demands for hiring a paid director and administrative or specialized clerical staff can further transform egalitarian organizational structures into hierarchical ones. The new staff may have political ideologies not consonant with those of the movement. Yet overworked staff are unlikely to spend much time familiarizing the newcomers with the movement's political roots (56, p. 203). Indeed, the newcomers often perceive these ideologies as a threat to continued funding (56, p. 206), and dependence on such funding provides a disincentive for challenging established health systems (57, p. 8).

Voluntarism—arguably the "heart" of alternative movements (2, p. 12)—is itself undermined by government support. The "warm, human contact" (2, p. 13), consciousness-raising (2, p. 13; 56, p. 203), advocacy, and anti-authoritarian self-help willingly shared in a local group can be undercut by funding intent on extending indigenous "expertise" to a wider net of "consumers." Such promotion of services has in many cases worked only to reproduce "professional chauvinism" (57, p. 3) and "alienated patterns of interactions" (59).

Despite these problems, ex-patients and activists in other alternative health movements have shared a common dilemma: to remain small, pure, and autonomous, thus limiting their help to a smaller ring of persons, or to accept government funding, at the risk of co-optation, in an effort to reach larger numbers of those in need (2, p. 12; 29; 56, p. 202; 60, p. 5). Many activists, after opting to collaborate with professionals they have come to know in the traditional sector, have had greater difficulty actively opposing the system (2, 57).

Undeniable Strides. At the same time, ex-patients and consumers have also achieved notable strides in gaining admission to the mental health discourse and policy debates. Consumer advocates have given voice to consumers/ survivors throughout the United States, familiarizing them with their rights while working to extend these rights. The presence of mental health consumers on boards side by side with providers and policymakers represents significant strides, but it is a stretch to call it, as did one researcher, "nothing short of a revolution!" (61). This ignores the differential power of elites on such boards (14, pp. 164–65) and the all too frequent reports of "token" consumer board members who are not taken seriously.

Nonetheless, extraordinary personal life successes have resulted from opportunities to participate in self-help alternatives (18, 62, 63). Equally important, consumers/survivors (many of them researchers) have been driving a research agenda and participating in the development of proposal requests that, despite recent setbacks (64), could have greater relevance and meaning in services for a wide range of consumers (46, pp. 11–13). Consumers/ survivors have been directly involved in rewriting state mental health laws (65) and have been major players on national councils and advisory groups, such as the President's National Council on Disability. Thus, despite departures from movement activists' initial dreams, these early activists have had a significant impact on the lives of consumers, even those unaware of the movement.

DISCUSSION: CONSUMERISM AND MENTAL HEALTH IN THE UNITED STATES

In addition to the principal consumer/survivor organizations in the United States (the National Mental Health Consumers' Association and the National Association of Psychiatric Survivors), many other self-help and educational organizations, occupying a broad political and ideological spectrum (e.g., GROW (66) and the National Depressive and Manic Depressive Organization), are independent parts of a larger, noncohesive and unstructured self-help movement. In contrast to the Netherlands and England, the United States has no central organization from which consumers/ex-patients could be drawn as representatives for mental health meetings (46). Government officials have come to rely on individual spokespersons, sometimes on the basis of their postures on specific issues, to represent "the consumer perspective." Their repeated reliance on the same consumers and ex-patients has led to some consumer burnout, limited representation of consumer interest (67, p. 2), and potential political manipulation of consumers on the basis of their views. It has also predisposed those "regulars" to develop an "institutional mind set" and to forget their independent perspective (68, p. 8).

Comparisons with European Consumer Movements

The situation in the United States is unique in several ways: the greater power of the family movement relative to the primary consumer movement, the intense disagreement among factions of consumers/ex-patients (4), and the high priority assigned to self-help alternatives. Neither the Netherlands nor England has a family movement of the size and influence of the National Alliance for the Mentally Ill. Families in England are less organized than the ex-patient group and less integrated into policymaking (52). The ideological differences among consumers in England and the Netherlands never led to the severe personal and ideological rifts that have impeded organizational unity in the United States (4). And consumer groups in the two European countries have limited their activities to system reform rather than promoting support for their self-help alternatives (55, p. 2).

Reflecting on the consumer movement worldwide, one consumer researcher observed how it "is most developed in the United States and tends to be confined to western style democracies that accommodate liberation politics and the individual pursuit of fulfillment" (55, p. 29). Indeed, in the United States, the movement was initiated against psychiatric oppression and in favor of individual human rights. And as Harriet Lefley rightly pointed out (69), activists who insist on individual rights, despise dependency and paternalism, and seek their own self-help alternatives are espousing uniquely Western values, consistent with a capitalist market economy.

Preexisting tensions between professional mental health knowledge and marginalized oppositional self-help knowledge have become intensified as the latter have gained legitimacy. Such tensions further articulate with the realities of the market. Given these realities, dominant medical power has become more inclusive of somewhat alternative ideologies (54, p. 246; 70), particularly as they are increasingly seen as working in conjunction with the mental health system rather than against it. Under the pressure of managed care (71), the dominance of medical professionals has also diminished as cost-cutting alternatives are explored (72, 73) and economically burdened states invite private corporations to manage their service delivery.

Precedents in other countries suggest that self-help may be seen as a potential means for the state to reduce its financial burden (54, p. 250; 74; 75). However, while health maintenance organizations (HMOs) may use individually oriented self-help technologies as part of cost-saving ventures, the continuous nature and community orientation of most self-help services are incompatible with HMOs' preference for cost-cutting, time-limited, individually oriented approaches (76). In addition, recent reports are confirming suspicions that HMOs are far more concerned with making a profit than with providing the services consumers want (26, 77, 78).

Consumerism as a Means to Legitimize and Institutionalize Self-Help Alternatives

In a democratic society subject to these market pressures, consumerism provides a convenient banner under which the state can admit oppositional self-help perspectives. Self-help alternatives are implicitly critical of professional clinical options (79), and many are even antipsychiatric in philosophy (3). However, when reframed as one of many legitimate *consumer options* for which consumers can exercise choice, they lose their oppositional threat (51). They become legitimized and institutionalized as one of many options, in conjunction with—rarely independent of—more traditional services (80).

Thus self-help approaches that may have appeared antithetical to mental health services can now be incorporated in a nonthreatening way as simply one in a menu of consumer options. However, the rhetoric of consumer choice notwithstanding, services—both traditional and consumer alternatives—are being slashed under the cost-saving logic that is driving managed care (26, 28).

Consumerism as a Political Force in Mental Health Services in the United States

The origin of the modern consumer movement in the United States has been dated to the mid-1920s (81, p. 73). In a historical period that abruptly transformed self-reliant producers into consumers dependent on household products, increasing responsibility was being placed on the individual consumer to make adequate choices. Debates fluctuated between educating the consumer to make better choices and restructuring the market system to make choices less demanding—a position that lost out (81). Consumerism in the United States thus put the onus of choice on the individual.

The Community Mental Health Reconstruction Act of 1963 provided for input from consumers (mainly families) on citizen boards, the major early opportunity for consumer input. Under deinstitutionalization and the community mental health movement that followed, a burgeoning market of mental health services developed (62, p. 72). During this period of the 1960s and 1970s, primary and family consumers became involved as critics of existing health services and spawned a new age of self-help (82). They soon monitored the quality of human services as well. By the late 1970s, the Community Support Program was actively recruiting family consumer support to convince Congress to fund its programs. Thus the CSP nurtured consumerism as part of a political process to launch its programs. Ironically, only because of residual support from that family constituency has Congress allowed the CSP to survive (16).

CONCLUSION

Consumerism, in its unique form in the United States, has provided the central link among social, ideological, and political systems to sustain the ex-patient movement, despite the numerous compromises it also necessitated. In becoming transformed into a *"consumer*/ex-patient" (or *"consumer*/survivor") movement, the ex-patient *reform* movement was forced to weaken its oppositional political thread. In the process, the *individualistic* consumerism fostered by this broader movement appealed to a wider group of stakeholders in the mental health system (e.g., families; the mental health industry; federal, state, and local mental health administrators).

At the same time, the language of consumerism masked the blatant *social* differences between private- and public-sector consumers in exercising true market choice and participating as partners in quality treatment. Consumers not only receive ("consume") treatment, they also select and pay for it. The irony of using this term to describe public-sector consumers was captured by one astute "consumer" (83). He was amused at being called a consumer when he was receiving services he would never have chosen if he had held the *actual* power to choose them, and never saw one penny of the funds used to pay for them! At the same time, he was quick to point out how the illusory term *consumer*, given its economic implications, had afforded him his only source of recognition and power within the mental health system.

Managed care, which requires client review of services, has similarly held out the promise of greater consumer power and control in the provider market. Current reports, however, suggest that these promises have been unmet (26–28, 77, 78). Even if consumer control over services were to improve under managed care, this power, as *consumer power*, can be exercised only within a restricted set of options (84) ultimately determined by the bottom line. Propelled by consumerism, the once marginalized ex-patient self-help alternatives, developed as *political opposition to* the mental health system, became institutionalized as *consumer options within* that system. As such, they are subject to the same vagaries of logic under managed care as are any other consumer options. But the social values that have driven these alternatives are likely to place them at a disadvantage compared with the more individually oriented options favored by managed care. This is where the seeds of dissent may stir—particularly in the public sector, most severely affected by these developments—to activate new players to preserve the gains made by ex-patient/consumer activists over the years.

ACKNOLEDGMENTS

The author thanks all the ex-patients and consumers, former and current federal, state, and local mental health officers, and countless others for their forthcoming remarks and generous time during her interviews with them. She also thanks David Mechanic, Jacqueline Parrish, Frances Randolf, Rae Unzicker, and Norman Dain for sharing relevant materials.

Part of the research for this article was supported by National Institute of Mental Health Grant No. 5T32MH16242 and was conducted when the author was a postdoctoral fellow at the Institute for Health, Health Care Policy and Aging Research, New Brunswick, New Jersey. Additional work was supported by NIMH contract No. 92MF03814201D.

References

1. McLean, A. Empowerment and the psychiatric consumer/ex-patient movement: Contradiction, crisis and change. *Soc. Sci. Med.* 40: 1053–1071, 1995.
2. Dain, N. Critics and dissenters: Reflections on "anti-psychiatry" in the United States. *J. Hist. Behav. Sci.* 23: 3–25, 1989.

3. Chamberlin, J. The ex-patients' movement: Where we've been and where we're going. *J. Mind Behav.* 11: 323–336, 1990.
4. Kauffman, C. An introduction to the mental health consumer movement. In *A Handbook for the Study of Mental Health: Social Contexts, Theories and Systems*, edited by A. Horwitz et al., pp. 493–507. Cambridge University Press, New York, 1999.
5. Brown, P. The mental patients' rights movement and mental health institutional change. *Int. J. Health Serv.* 11(4): 523–540, 1981.
6. Starkman, M. The Movement. Unpublished manuscript, n.d.
7. The Radical Therapist/Rough Times Collective (eds.). *The Radical Therapist.* Penguin Books, Harmondsworth, England, 1974.
8. Talbott, J. Radical psychiatry: An examination of the issues. *Am. J. Psychiatry* 131(2): 121–128, 1974.
9. Unzicker, R. Interview with the author, October 8, 1999.
10. Unzicker, R. Mental health advocacy, from then to now. *Rights Tenet,* 1997.
11. Brown, P. The right to refuse treatment and the movement for mental health reform. *J. Health Polit. Policy Law* 9(2): 291–313, 1984.
12. NARPA Mission Statement. *Rights Tenet,* Fall 1999.
13. Turner, J., and TenHoor, W. The NIMH Community Support Program: Pilot approach to a needed social reform. *Schizophr. Bull.* 4: 319–349, 1978.
14. Kenig, S. *Who Plays? Who Pays? Who Cares? A Case Study in Applied Sociology, Political Economy and the Community Mental Health Centers Movement.* Baywood, Amityville, N.Y., 1992.
15. Levine, M. *The History and Politics of Community Mental Health.* Oxford University Press, New York, 1981.
16. Sharfstein, S. Interview with the author, February 27, 1992.
17. Hecker, G. Comment: Involving families of clients in CSS planning. In *A Network for Caring: The Community Support Program of the National Institute of Mental Health. Proceedings of Four National Conferences 1978–1979,* pp. 33–35. DHHS Publication No. (ADM)81–1063. U.S. Government Printing Office, Washington, D.C., 1982 [1979].
18. Schneir, M. Comment In *A Network for Caring: The Community Support Program of the National Institute of Mental Health. Proceedings of Four National Conferences 1978–1979.* DHHS Publication No. (ADM)81–1063. U.S. Government Printing Office, Washington, D.C., 1982 [1979].
19. Shifren-Levine, I. Interview with the author, March 5, 1992.
20. Chamberlin, J. *On Our Own: Patient Controlled Alternatives to the Mental Health System.* Hawthorne Books, New York, 1978.
21. Mosher, L., and Burti, L. *Community Mental Health: Principles and Practice.* Norton Press, New York, 1989.
22. McLean, A. Contradictions in the social production of clinical knowledge: The case of schizophrenia. *Soc. Sci. Med.* 30: 969–985, 1990.
23. Johnson, D. Schizophrenia as a brain disease: Implications for psychologists and families. *Am. Psychol.* 44: 553–555, 1984.
24. Weisborg, D. Personal communication, July 7, 1999.
25. Scull, A. *Decarceration: Community Treatment and the Deviant—A Radical View,* Ed. 3. Rutgers University Press, New Brunswick, N.J., 1977.
26. Mandersheid, R. From many into one: Addressing the crisis of quality in managed behavioral care at the millennium. *J. Behav. Health Serv. Res.* 25(2): 233–237, 1998.
27. Peck, R. Report care woes: NAMI vs. the behavioral HMCO's. *Behav. Health Manag.* December 1997, pp. 30–33.

28. Backlar, P. Ethics in community mental health care. *Community Mental. Health J.* 35(2): 109–113, 1999.

29. Mack, J. Power, powerlessness and empowerment in psychiatry. *Psychiatry* 57: 178–198, 1994.

30. Deegan, P. Recovery: The lived experience of rehabilitation. *Psychosoc. Rehabil. J.* 11(4): 11–19, 1988.

31. Fisher, D. Thoughts on recovery. *Resources: Workforce Issues in Mental Health Systems,* 4: 7–8, 1992.

32. Robbins, H. Influencing mental health policy: The MHA Approach. *Hosp. Community Psychiatr.* 31(9): 610–613, 1980.

33. Brown, P. Attitudes towards the rights of mental patients. *Soc. Sci. Med.* 16: 2025–2039, 1982.

34. Chamberlin, J. Comment: Consumer perspectives on community support systems. In *A Network for Caring: The Community Support Program of the National Institute of Mental Health. Proceedings of Four National Conference 1978–1979,* pp. 33–35. DHHS Publication No. (ADM)81-1063. U.S. Government Printing Office, Washington, D.C., 1982 [1979].

35. U.S. Department of Health and Human Services. *Towards a Model Plan for a Comprehensive, Community-Based Mental Health System.* Administrative document. Washington, D.C., 1987.

36. Stroul, B. *Models of Community Support Service Approaches to Helping Persons with Long-Term Mental Illness,* pp. 49–62. Prepared for the National Institute of Mental Health Community Support Program, Boston University, Boston, 1986.

37. Stroul, B. *Toward Community Support Systems for the Mentally Disabled: The NIMH Community Support Program.* Center for Rehabilitation Research and Training in Mental Health, Boston, 1984.

38. Chamberlin, J., Rogers, J., and Sneed, C. Consumers, families and community support systems. *Psychosoc. Rehabil. J.* 12: 93–106, 1989.

39. Scallet, L. Mental health law and public policy. *Hosp. Community Psychiatr.* 31: 614–616, 1980.

40. National Association of State Mental Health Program Directors. *Position Paper on Consumer Contributions to Mental Health Service Delivery Systems.* Alexandria, Va., December 3, 1989.

41. Trochim, W., Dumont, J., and Campbell, J. *Mapping Mental Health Outcomes from the Perspective of Consumers/Survivors: A Report for the State Mental Health Agency Profiling System.* Technical report. National Association of State Mental Health Program Directors, Alexandria, Va., 1993.

42. Parrish, J. The consumer movement: A personal perspective. *Community Support Network News* 5: 1, 3, 1988.

43. Leiberman, M. Personal communication, April 1992.

44. National Institute of Mental Health. *Developing an NIMH Community Support Research Demonstration Project for Persons with Severe and Persistent Mental Illness.* Arlington, Va., n.d.

45. Williams, W. The organization of the volume and some key definitions. In *Evaluating Social Programs,* edited by P. Rossi and W. Williams, pp. 5–8. Seminar Press, New York, 1972.

46. McLean, A. *The Role of Consumers in Mental Health Services Research and Evaluation.* Report and Concept Paper No. 92MF03814201D. Prepared for the Community Support Program, Center for Mental Health Services, Substance Abuse and Mental Health Services Administration, Rockville, Md., 1994.

47. Zinman, S. Interview with the author, July 15, 1991.

48. Thomas, N. Interview with the author, May 21, 1996.
49. Zinman, S., Howie the Harp, and Budd, S. (eds.). *Reaching Across: Mental Health Clients Helping Each Other.* California Network of Mental Health Clients, Sacramento, 1987.
50. Zinman, S. Issues of power. In *Reaching Across: Mental Health Clients Helping Each Other,* edited by S. Zinman, Howie the Harp, and S. Budd, pp. 126–127. California Network of Mental Health Clients, Sacramento, 1987.
51. Grace, V. The marketing of empowerment and the construction of the health consumer: A critique of health promotion. *Int. J. Health Serv.* 21(2): 329–343, 1991.
52. Chamberlin, J., and Unzicker, R. Psychiatric Survivors, Ex-patients, and Users: An Observation of Organizations in Holland and England. Unpublished manuscript, n.d.
53. Rogers, A., and Pilgrim, D. 'Pulling down churches': Accounting for the British mental health users' movement. *Sociol. Health Illness* 13: 129–148, 1991.
54. Papadakis, E. Interventions in new social movements. In *The Politics of Field Research,* edited by J. Gubrium and D. Silverman, pp. 236–257. Sage, London, 1989.
55. O'Hagan, M. *Stopovers on My Way Home from Mars.* A Winston Churchill Fellowship Report on the Psychiatric Survivor Movement in the USA, Britain and the Netherlands. 1991.
56. Morgen, S. The dynamics of cooptation in a feminist health clinic. *Soc. Sci. Med.* 23(2): 201–210.
57. The selling of the free clinics. *Health/Pac Bull.* 38: 1–8, 1972.
58. Tierney, K. The battered women movement and the creation of the wife beating problem. *Soc. Probl.* 29(3): 207–219, 1982.
59. Seem, M., and Parkin, J. Mental health, normalization and resistance: Two statements. *State and Mind* 6: 16–17, 1977.
60. Editorial: Neighborhood health centers. *Health/Pac Bull.* 42: 1–13, 1972.
61. Estroff, S. Comment at the symposium The Understanding of Mental Illness and Dealing with the Mentally Ill in Western Cultures, Berlin, June 4, 1994.
62. Leete, E. The Role of the Consumer Movement and Persons with Mental Illness. *Switzer Monogram of the National Rehabilitation Association,* 1988, pp. 65–72.
63. Lovejoy, M. Expectations and the recovery process. *Schizophr. Bull.* 8:605–609, 1982.
64. McLean, A. Are Psychiatric Populations "Natural" Populations or Socially Constituted? The Problem of Random Assignment in Self Help Research. Paper presented at the Annual Meeting of the American Anthropological Association, Philadelphia, December 3, 1998.
65. Cichon, D. The Ignored Population: Children and the Mental Health System. Paper presented at the Thomas M. Cooley Law Review Meeting, Individuals with Disabilities: Legal and Treatment Issues, Lansing, Mich., October 29, 1999.
66. Rappaport, J. The power of empowerment language. *Soc. Policy* 15: 12–24, 1985.
67. Peller, B. Primary consumer issues for the future. *InSites,* IV(2). The Robert Wood Johnson Foundation Program on Chronic Mental Illness, 1991.
68. Cox, D. Consumer advocates call others to action. *InSites,* IV(2): 8–9. The Robert Wood Johnson Foundation Program on Chronic Mental Illness, 1991.
69. Lefley, H. Families' Experience of Mental Illness: Constructing New Realities. Paper presented at the symposium The Understanding of Mental Illness and Dealing with the Mentally Ill in Western Cultures, Berlin, June 4, 1994.

70. Arney, W., and Bergin, B. *Medicine and the Management of Living*. University of Chicago Press, Chicago, 1984.
71. Mandersheid, R., et al. Contemporary mental health systems and managed care. In *A Handbook for the Study of Mental Health: Social Contexts, Theories and Systems*, edited by A. Horwitz et al., pp. 412–426. Cambridge University Press, New York, 1999.
72. Wilkerson, J., Devers, K., and Given, S. (eds.). *Competitive Managed Care: The Emerging Health Care System*. Jossey-Bass, San Francisco, 1997.
73. Clement, J. Managed care and recovery: Opportunities and challenges for psychiatric nursing. *Arch. Psychiatr. Nurs.* 11(5): 231–237, 1997.
74. Grunow, D. Debureaucratization and the self-help movement. In *Comparing Welfare States and their Futures*, edited by E. Oyer. Gower, London, 1986.
75. Erasaari, R. The new social state. *Acta Sociol.* 29: 225–241, 1986.
76. McLean, A. Consumer-run Programs and Social Support in the United States in the Age of Managed Mental Health Care: Positioning them for Survival and Competition. Submitted for publication, July 1999.
77. Stout, M. Impact of Medicaid managed mental health care on delivery of services in a rural state: An AMI perspective. *Psychiatr. Serv.* 49(7): 961–963, 1998.
78. Elliott, R. Mental health reform in Georgia, 1992–1996. *Psychiatr. Serv.* 47(11): 1205–1211, 1996.
79. Gartner, A., and Reissman, F. *Self-help in the Human Services*. Jossey-Bass, San Francisco, 1977.
80. Williams, X. "Consumer empowerment" vs. "bundling of services": Why bundling of services is counterproductive. *Consumer Connection* 3(2): 1, 1994.
81. Grahame, P. The construction of a sociological consumer. In *The Politics of Field Research*, edited by J. Gurbrium and D. Silverman, pp. 70–93. Sage, London, 1989.
82. Hatfield, A. The organized consumer movement: A new force in service delivery. *Community Support Serv. J.* 2: 3–7, 1981.
83. Ewing, D. Interview with the author, October 1992.
84. Hopper, K. Regulation from without: The shadow side of coercion. In *Coercion and Aggressive Community Treatment: A New Frontier in Mental Health Law*, edited by D. Dennis and J. Monahan, pp. 197–212. Plenum Press, New York, 1996.

DISCUSSION

1. What is the consumer/ex-patient movement? What is the relationship between the consumer/ex-patient movement and the family movement and more professionally-focused advocacy efforts? What led to the establishment of the various components of this social movement?

2. What has been the impact of this movement on the mental health system? How has the movement changed the way services are provided? What does McLean mean by "consumerism"? What do you see as the strengths and weaknesses of the growth of this view point within the mental health care system?

The Future of the Mental Health Care System

E. Fuller Torrey

Fixing the System

E. Fuller Torrey, a psychiatrist, is one of the most outspoken and controversial critics of our society's response to mental illness. In this chapter of his recent book, The Insanity Offense: How American's Failure to Treat the Seriously Mental Ill Endangers Its Citizens (New York: W. W. Norton, 2008), Torrey offers concrete recommendations for improving the societal response to mental illness. As in much of his early writing, he argues that society has failed people with mental illness. In this chapter, he proposes several specific policy changes that he believes will improve the care and treatment of mental illness and improve the quality of life in society.

> The opposition to involuntary committal and treatment betrays a profound misunderstanding of the principle of civil liberties. Medication can free victims from their illness—free them from the Bastille of their psychoses—and restore their dignity, their free will and the meaningful exercise of their liberties.
>
> Herschel Hardin. 1993

The present treatment system for people with severe psychiatric disorders in the United States is, by any measure, a disaster. The deinstitutionalization movement, implemented half a century ago with the best of intentions and the worst of plans, effectively emptied the nation's public psychiatric hospitals without ensuring that patients would receive care once they left the hospitals.

The disaster is continuing to worsen. In Florida in 1990, there were still 56 state psychiatric beds per 100,000 population; in 2006, this number had been reduced from 56 to 8.[1] In Florida, as in every other state, for those most

Torrey, E. Fuller. 2008. "Fixing the System." Pp. 177–196 in *The Insanity Offense: How America's Failure to Treat the Seriously Mental Ill Endangers Its Citizens.* New York: W.W. Norton and Company.

seriously ill, there are very few beds for treatment as an inpatient and very few resources for treatment as an outpatient.

Clearly, it is time to fix the system. This will require major changes, most of which will not come easily. Civil libertarians will continue to oppose attempts to impose treatment on mentally ill individuals, regardless of how disabled they appear to be, although such opposition is now not as strong as it was in the past. A for-profit system of hospitals and residential settings that has grown skilled at making money by neglecting the most seriously ill patients will also oppose change. And many mental health professionals and administrators simply do not care enough about the problem to work for change. The status quo is always a formidable opponent.

Fixing the system will involve at least the following steps: modification of the laws; identification of the target population; provision and enforcement of treatment; and assessment and research.

MODIFICATION OF THE LAWS

The laws governing the treatment of mentally ill individuals were modified beginning in the late 1960s. Through a series of state legislative changes and judicial decisions, the hospitalization and treatment of individuals with severe psychiatric disorders became very difficult to virtually impossible, depending on the state.

Since 1998, the Treatment Advocacy Center (TAC) in Arlington, Virginia, where I am on the board, has led an effort to modify state laws and make them more consistent with what is now known about severe psychiatric disorders. TAC has helped pass assisted outpatient treatment (AOT) laws, which permit the involuntary treatment of seriously mentally ill individuals who are potentially dangerous in the community, in New York (Kendra's Law), California (Laura's Law), and Florida and has helped modify the treatment laws in Maryland, West Virginia, Illinois, Michigan, Minnesota, North Dakota, South Dakota, Montana, Idaho, Wyoming, Utah, Nevada, and Washington. For example, in West Virginia, the criterion for involuntary treatment was broadened so that the person's past history could be considered; in Maryland, the criterion was broadened so that the person no longer had to be "imminently" dangerous.

Despite these successes, much work remains to be done in modifying states laws. Eight states still do not even have a statute allowing AOT: Maine, Massachusetts, Connecticut, New Jersey, Maryland, Tennessee, Nevada, and New Mexico. Most other states that have effective laws are not utilizing them properly.

IDENTIFICATION OF THE TARGET POPULATION

In order to fix the system, we must identify the target population. Anecdotally, most people involved in community psychiatric services, jails, and homeless shelters can identify that small group of seriously mentally ill individuals who cause the most problems and regularly rotate among these facilities. They are the "regulars" among hospital readmissions, the "frequent flyers," in the jail system, and the "trouble makers" in the homeless shelters. Many of them are well known to local police, who are often on a first-name basis with them.

Surprisingly little research has been done to precisely quantify this group. In Virginia, 14 percent of psychiatric hospital admissions were said to account for 40 percent of the total hospital costs. In North Carolina, among 1,906 individuals with schizophrenia, "about 20 percent" were reported to be disproportionately responsible for psychiatric hospitalizations, use of emergency psychiatric services, arrests, violence, and victimization. In Massachusetts, among 13,816 individuals receiving psychiatric services from the state, 14 percent were responsible for all "serious violence against persons," and less than 2 percent were responsible for 20 percent of arrests.[2] Another useful study was the previously cited one carried out in England, which determined that, among all individuals with schizophrenia, 10 percent were responsible for 80 percent of the total costs.[3]

The number of seriously ill individuals who are homeless or incarcerated could approach 400,000, which is 10 percent of the estimated total of 4 million seriously mentally ill individuals. Until better data become available, it seems reasonable to use 10 percent as the size of the target population on which to focus attempts to fix the system. Within that 10 percent, an estimated 10 percent of those—or 1 percent of all individuals with serious psychiatric disorders—have likely committed homicides or other violent crimes and have therefore clearly demonstrated a propensity for violent behavior.

The best indicators to use in identifying the potentially most problematic individuals with severe psychiatric disorders are found in studies of violent behavior. Seven identifying factors are most frequently cited: past history of violence: substance abuse; anosognosia with medication noncompliance; antisocial personality disorder; paranoid symptoms; neurological impairment; and gender.

1. *Past history of violence.* A person's past history of violence is the most important predicator of future violence among all people, whether mentally ill or not. In addition, the younger people are when they initially become violent, the more likely they are to be violent later.

2. *Substance abuse.* As has been known for centuries, alcohol makes some people more aggressive. Among individuals with severe psychiatric disorders, alcohol abuse is especially pernicious. In a Finnish study, for example, persons with schizophrenia who abused alcohol were seven times more likely to commit violent crimes than those who did not abuse alcohol. Drugs other than alcohol, especially amphetamines, cocaine, and PCP, may also exacerbate violent tendencies. In an Australian study of individuals with schizophrenia, substance abusers, compared to non-substance abusers, were seven times more likely to be convicted of violent offenses and four times more likely to be convicted of homicides.[4]

3. *Anosognosia with medication noncompliance.* Many individuals who are not aware of their illness refuse medication and are liable to become homeless or incarcerated. They are also more apt to become violent, as at least ten separate studies show. For example, in a study of male inpatients with psychosis, "participants who did not generally take their medication engaged in significantly more severe violence." A study of 63 inpatients with schizophrenia reported that "patients who later became violent were, on admission, less compliant [with medication] and had less insight into the necessity for treatment." A study of individuals with schizophrenia found that "treatment noncompliance was ubiquitous among violent patients." Among 133 outpatients with schizophrenia in another study, those who "had problems with medication compliance" were four times more likely to become violent. A three-year study of almost 2,000 outpatients with schizophrenia-related diagnoses reported that those who refused to take medication were twice as likely to be rehospitalized, arrested, or victimized or to become violent.[5]

4. *Antisocial personality disorder.* Severe psychiatric disorders are equal-opportunity diseases that can affect anyone. They may affect people with a kind and generous personality, but they may also affect people with a preexisting antisocial personality disorder. This condition, which in the past was referred to as sociopath, is defined as "a pervasive pattern of disregard for, and violation of, the rights of others" and is exhibited by lying, impulsivity, criminal acts, and lack of remorse, among other acts. The combination of a severe psychiatric disorder in an individual with these personality characteristics leads, as would be expected, to more frequent incarceration and violent behavior. The psychologist Sheilagh Hodgins, a prominent English researcher, and her colleagues have shown that individuals with schizophrenia who are violent can be divided into those with an antisocial personality disorder, in which case they became violent prior to developing schizophrenia, and those without an antisocial personality disorder, in which case they became violent only after developing schizophrenia.[6]

5. *Paranoid symptoms.* Multiple studies have suggested that seriously mentally ill individuals who believe that people are following them or trying to hurt them (i.e., are paranoid) are more likely to commit acts of violence, especially against individuals they believe are persecuting them. If you truly believe someone is trying to harm you, it may seem logical to try to harm the other person first. Some researchers have also suggested that a belief that outside forces are controlling your mind, which clinicians refer to as control override, is associated with increased violent behavior. Similarly, claims have been made that command hallucinations—voices that tell you what to do—increase violent behavior, but other studies have not been able to replicate these findings.[7]

6. *Neurological impairment.* Violent behavior is associated with both specific neurological impairment involving brain structures, such as the amygdala, and brain chemistry, such as the serotonin system. It therefore is not surprising that neurological impairment has been found to be a predictor of violent behavior in individuals with schizophrenia. In one study, inpatients

who were persistently violent had more neurological impairment than either those who were transiently violent or those who were not violent or those who were not violent. In another study, individuals with schizophrenia who were violent were distinguished by multiple differences in brain function, measured by neuroimaging.[8] For example, in a functional MRI study of violent individuals with schizophrenia compared to nonviolent individuals with schizophrenia, the two groups differed in areas of activation in the frontal and temporal brain areas.

7. *Gender.* Men are responsible for 85–90 percent of violent behavior everywhere in the world; women, for only 10–15 percent. Women with severe psychiatric disorders are the exception to this rule. Two studies of inpatients with psychosis reported that men and women were equally assaultive. Studies of homicides committed by mentally ill individuals have almost uniformly found women to be overrepresented. For example, in Austria women accounted for 31 percent of such homicides, and in New Zealand for 32 percent.[9] Mentally ill women are therefore more likely than would be expected to be included in any list of problematic patients.

Although each of these seven factors may operate independently to help identify mentally ill individuals who are problematic, they also influence each other. Individuals with antisocial personality traits are more likely to abuse drugs, and people who are paranoid are less likely to take medication. The maximum predictive value of these seven factors is achieved when they are used together. In a study of violent acts among seriously mentally ill outpatients in North Carolina, neither substance abuse nor medication noncompliance alone predicted which patients would become violent, but a combination of the two factors did.[10] It seems likely that four of these factors—history of violence; substance abuse; anosognosia with medication noncompliance; and antisocial personality disorder—will identify the vast majority of the most problematic patients when considered together.

Attempts are underway to develop systems to predict which seriously mentally ill individuals are most likely to become violent. Several violence risk assessment scales have been developed and have shown promise, an effort led by the MacArthur Foundation's Violence Risk Assessment Network, John Monahan and Henry Steadman of the MacArthur network have suggested that, by means of predictive factors, mentally ill patients can be classified into four categories of violence risk: low, moderate, high, and very high. It should be remembered, however, that predictors are merely that. As summarized by two researchers in this field, "Like a good weather forecaster, the clinician does not state with certainty that an event will occur... [but rather] the likelihood that a future event will occur."[11]

Identifying the target population is useful, of course, only insofar as mental health professionals and police officers are aware of who has been identified. Currently, privacy laws in most states preclude the exchange of critical information. As a result, physicians in emergency rooms often must evaluate psychotic individuals without the benefit of their past history. Similarly,

RED-FLAGGING VIOLENT PATIENTS

At the Veterans Administration Medical Center in Portland, Oregon, hospital staff identified 48 psychiatric patients who had a history of violent behavior. The hospital computer system red-flagged these individuals so that whenever they appeared for treatment, clinicians and administrative personnel were made aware of their status. Some red flags included specific instructions, such as "hospital police should be asked to stand by until released by examining clinician." During the year prior to the implementation of this system, the 48 patients had been responsible for 47 violent incidents in the hospital; during the year following its implementation, the number of violent incidents was only four, a 92 percent reduction. The hospital periodically reviews the red-flag status of each patient, and the flag may be removed "if there is clear evidence of cooperative behavior."

D. J. Drummond, L. F. Sparr, and G. H. Gordon, "Hospital violence reduction among high-risk patients," *Journal of the American Medical Association* 261 (1989): 2531–34.

police officers and sheriffs are often called to homes where a seriously mentally ill individual is threatening family members, yet the officer cannot access information regarding the persons' propensity toward violence or other history.

The solution to this problem is to develop a database listing those individuals with severe psychiatric disorders who have proven dangerous. Names would be added to the list only by judicial order, and it would be restricted to the highest-risk patients. The list undoubtedly would include many of the forty thousand individuals who are the most dangerous. Password-protected, the database would be made available only to authorized mental health professionals, law enforcement officers, and firearms dealers to prevent the sale of guns to at-risk individuals.

In order to be effective, such a list must be available across state lines and would therefore require national legislation. Many severely mentally ill persons migrate from state to state. Officials in each state know some things about them, but nobody knows the person's entire history. An example was Henry Brown, diagnosed with schizophrenia, who was killed in 2004 by officers in California after he shot three people. For 20 years, Brown had migrated across many states, including Mississippi, Georgia, South Carolina, Texas, Ohio, Illinois, and California, in response to voices. He was intermittently hospitalized, jailed, and homeless in most of these states and committed "bizarre crimes that grew increasingly violent" during periods when he was not taking his medication.[12]

PROVISION AND ENFORCEMENT OF TREATMENT

Once state laws governing treatment have been modified and the target population identified, it is then necessary to provide treatment and, if needed, enforce it. The treatment of severe mental illnesses involves, first and foremost, the use of antipsychotic medication.

But medication is only part of the treatment plan. An effective system must also include a sufficient number of psychiatric beds for the admission of acutely ill patients and sufficient funding to allow patients to remain long enough to achieve control of their symptoms, normally a period of 2 to 4 weeks. Such a system must also include a small number of beds for severely and chronically ill individuals for whom existing medications are not effective. In the past, such beds were provided by state psychiatric hospitals, and some similar provision should be available in every state, both to provide humane care and to function as an asylum, in the best sense of the word, for individuals who are too disabled to protect themselves.

Outpatient psychiatric services must also be readily available. The PACT model, started in Madison, Wisconsin, and described in chapter 6, is both clinically effective and cost-effective and should be implemented nationwide.[13] Outpatient care also includes rehabilitation, vocational training, and housing, all of which can be effectively provided by the much lauded clubhouse model. In clubhouses, mentally ill individuals congregate for socialization and to learn job skills; most clubhouses also contract with businesses to provide jobs for their members and have a housing program. The first clubhouse was Fountain House, which opened in New York City half a century ago and which is still considered to be an excellent program.[14] Like PACT programs, clubhouses should be a common ingredient in psychiatric services nationwide.

But outpatient, rehabilitation, vocation, and housing services are not effective for individuals with severe psychiatric disorders unless such individuals are receiving adequate medication to ameliorate their symptoms. The efficacy of medications to treat severe psychiatric disorders is well established. Medications do not *cure* these disorders, but they can help control the symptoms.

The major types of medications available for use are antipsychotics (such as risperidone), mood stabilizers (such as lithium), and antidepressants (such as fluoxetine). Their effectiveness derives, at least in part, from their ability to affect specific brain chemicals, especially neurotransmitters, which carry information between brain cells. Insofar as a patient's violent behavior is caused by psychotic symptoms such as paranoid delusions, the reduction of those symptoms usually produces a reduction in violent behavior. A 2-year study of aggression in individuals with schizophrenia found that "the day-by-day decline of aggressive incidents after the start of neuroleptic [antipsychotic] treatment was highly significant.... The results support the assumption that neuroleptics [antipsychotics] are not only effective in controlling violent outbursts ... but also in preventing violence in schizophrenia."

Similarly, a study of adolescents with bipolar disorder reported that those who did not take medication committed criminal acts almost five times more frequently than those who did take medication.[15]

In addition to being effective in controlling psychotic symptoms, some medications have been claimed to specifically reduce aggressive behavior. Evidence is strong to support this claim for clozapine (Clozaril), an antipsychotic used widely in Europe and China but less widely in the United States. Its lower use in this country is related both to the fact that patients' blood must be regularly monitored to prevent side effects and to the fact that in recent years clozapine has been off-patent and thus available generically, thereby decreasing interest in the pharmaceutical industry in pushing its use. But it is effective. In one study, for example, "the patients [with psychosis] who received clozapine had lower rates of arrest than the patients who never received cloxapine"; in addition, "the arrests rates of the patients taking clozapine were significantly lower while they were taking the drug than before they were given the drug."[16] Clearly, clozapine should be the antipsychotic of choice for severely mentally ill individuals who exhibit violent behavior.

Claims have been made that other drugs have specific anti-aggressive effects, but evidence to support these claims is much weaker than is the evidence for clozapine. These drugs include other antipsychotics, mood stabilizers, and a class of drugs called beta-blockers. Many studies of the antiaggression effects of these drugs are of questionable validity because the pharmaceutical companies that made the drugs funded the studies.

Given the role of substance abuse in exacerbating violent behavior in individuals with severe psychiatric disorders, it is important to utilize all possible treatment methods to minimize such abuse. Disulfiram (Antabuse), which leads to unpleasant side effects when alcohol is ingested; naltrexone (Revia, Vivitrol): and methadone, which blocks the effects of heroin, are moderately effective and should be used. In addition, given the importance of anosognosia as a cause of not taking medication, it would be extremely useful if there were effective treatments for this problem. Approximately one-third of individuals with anosognosia regain some insight into their illness in the course of being treated with antipsychotic or mood-stabilizing drugs, but the other two-thirds do not. Efforts to improve insight in such individuals have failed, including the use of videotapes to show recovering patients what they looked like when they were acutely psychotic.[17]

Although effective medications are available, they work only if people take them. Malcoum Tate, Herb Mullin, Bryan Stanley, and other seriously mentally ill persons who have little or no insight into their illness see no need to take medication. In such cases, involuntary treatment is the only solution.

Involuntarily treating individuals with severe psychiatric disorders is adamantly opposed by some civil libertarians, lawyers, and mental health professionals, who argue that coercion is rarely, if ever, justified. By contrast, members of the general public recognize the need for such involuntarily treatment. A national survey reported that 87 percent of public respondents

UNCIVIL LIBERTIES

The remedy is treatment—most essentially, medication. In most cases, this means involuntary treatment because people in the throes of their illness have little or no insight into their own condition. If you think you are Jesus Christ or an avenging angel, you are not likely to agree that you need to go to the hospital.

Anti-treatment advocates insist that involuntary committal should be limited to cases of imminent physical danger—instances where a person is going to do serious bodily harm to himself or to somebody else. But the establishment of such "dangerousness" usually comes too late—a psychotic break or loss of control, leading to violence, happens suddenly. And all the while, the victim suffers the ravages of the illness itself, the degradation of life, the tragic loss of individual potential.

The anti-treatment advocates say: "If that's how people want to live (babbling on a street corner, in rags), or if they wish to take their own lives, they should be allowed to exercise their free will. To interfere—with involuntary committal—is to deny them their civil liberties." As for the tragedy that follows from this dictum, well, "That's the price that has to be paid if society is to maintain its civil liberties."

Whether or not anti-treatment advocates actually voice such opinions, they seem content to sacrifice a few lives here and there to uphold an abstract doctrine. Their intent, if noble, has a chilly, Stalinist justification—the odd tragedy along the way is warranted to ensure the greater good.

Herschel Hardin, op-ed, Vancouver Sun, *July 22, 1993.*

"said that mentally ill homeless should be sent to mental hospitals even when they don't want to go." Another national survey found the public willing to involuntarily commit a person with schizophrenia to a hospital if that person was a danger to self (91 percent said yes) or a danger to others (95 percent said yes).[18]

There are many methods for ensuring that people with severe psychiatric disorders take medications, and almost all of them are effective. Informal methods include using a person's disability payments as leverage. The vast majority of individuals with severe psychiatric disorders receive monthly disability benefits through Social Security or the Veterans Administration. For those who are disabled, the court can appoint a "representative payee," who can insist that the person follow a specific treatment plan, including taking medication, as a condition for receiving part of the money. Studies have shown that the use of representative payees decreases alcohol and drug abuse and markedly decreases psychiatric readmissions to hospitals.[19]

A second method of informal leverage involves making access to good housing conditional on following a treatment plan. Housing for mentally ill individuals living on disability payments is grossly inadequate throughout the United States, so being able to access the limited supply of special housing is a strong incentive. A survey of five cities found that housing had been used as leverage for approximately one-third of mentally ill persons.[20] Until an adequate supply of housing is available, this method of leverage is likely to be used.

A third method of informal leverage is used for mentally ill individuals charged with crimes, usually misdemeanors. Individuals who meet the criteria are assigned to specialized courts known as mental health courts. These courts are now available in at least thirty-four states, and one study found that 92 percent of them "reported using jail as a sanction for noncompliance" with treatment. The judge, in effect, says, You can either comply with your treatment plan, or you can go to jail—your choice. As would be expected, this method of enforcing treatment is effective. A study of a mental health court in Washington State reported that, among participants, arrests decreased from 119 to 34, and arrests for assault or other violent crimes decreased from 12 to 2, over a 6-month period. A study of a mental health court in Pittsburgh reported that it not only reduced jail time but also saved taxpayers $3.5 million over a 2-year period.[21]

There are also formal mechanisms for compelling treatment. One method makes use of conservatorships, under which a court appoints a person to make decisions for a legally incompetent individual. These are often used for individuals with mental retardation or dementia but have not been widely used for individuals with mental illness.

Conditional release, under which persons who have been committed to psychiatric hospitals can be released on the condition that they continue taking medication and otherwise follow their treatment plan, is much more common. If they do not comply, they can be involuntarily hospitalized. A study in New Hampshire, where conditional release has been widely used, found that the program led to markedly increased medication compliance, decreased rehospitalization, and decreased substance abuse, as well as a reduction in violent episodes by half.[22]

A variant form of conditional release widely used in Oregon is the Psychiatric Security Review Board (PSRB), which has legal jurisdiction over mentally ill individuals charged with crimes. The PSRB has been rightfully praised as a cost-effective way to reduce violence and other criminal behavior. In one study, mentally ill individuals were reported to have only one-quarter as many contacts with the police when under the jurisdiction of the PSRB compared with when they were not under the board's jurisdiction.[23]

The most widely-publicized method of compelling treatment is the use of assisted outpatient treatment (AOT). In other countries, AOT is referred to as a community treatment order. Like conditional release, AOT allows mentally ill persons to live in the community only if they follow their treatment plan, including taking their medications. If they do not, in most states the person can be involuntarily hospitalized. The main difference between conditional release and AOT is that the former must follow a hospitalization, whereas the latter can be initiated for an individual currently living in the community. The criteria for implementing AOT vary by state; forty-two states have some AOT provision, but only a minority use it. At the Treatment Advocacy Center we have developed a model AOT law; it is available on our website. www.treatmentadvocacycenter.org.

Assessments of AOT have found it to be remarkably effective. The most detailed studies were conducted in North Carolina and New York. In the latter, a provision for AOT was implemented in 1999 and called Kendra's Law after Kendra Webdale, who was killed by a man with untreated schizophrenia.[24]

The effect of AOT on medication compliance has been to double it. In New York, for example, 34 percent of patients regularly took medication prior to AOT, but 69 percent did so after being placed on AOT. This level of compliance produced a marked decrease in psychiatric hospital readmissions and total hospital days. AOT's reduction of psychiatric admissions and hospital days is evident in the six studies summarized in Table 1. Another well-designed study, in North Carolina, carried out by Drs. Marvin Swartz and Jeffrey Swanson at Duke University and their colleagues, randomized patients with psychosis to either AOT or services as usual; those maintained on AOT for more than six months had fewer hospital admissions (0.3 vs. 1.2) and fewer hospital days (5 vs. 33) per year.[24-29]

AOT has also been shown to decrease other adverse effects of deinstitutionalization. In New York, AOT reduced homelessness among severely mentally ill persons from 19 percent to 5 percent.[30] In North Carolina, AOT decreased the chances of being victimized, from 42 percent to 24 percent. The researchers speculated on possible reasons for this:

> By facilitating adherence and ensuring more consistent follow-up, outpatient commitment may lead to reduced symptoms, better functioning in social relationships, and improved judgment. In turn these changes should lessen a

Table 1 Effects of Assisted Outpatient Treatment (AOT) on Psychiatric Admissions

	Number of Psychiatric Admissions Per Year		Number of Hospital Days Per Year	
	Before AOT	On AOT	Before AOT	On AOT
New York[24]	3.1	N/A	100	44
District of Columbia[25]	1.8	1.0	55	38
North Carolina[26]	1.4	0.3	22	14
Ohio[27]	1.5	0.4	133	44
Iowa[28]	1.3	0.3	33	5
North Carolina[29]	1.2	0.3	33	5

person's vulnerability to abuse by others and lower the probability of becoming involved in dangerous situations where victimization is more likely.[31]

Two studies have also assessed the effect of AOT on arrest rates. In North Carolina, a randomized study reported that patients "with a prior history of multiple hospitalizations combined with prior arrests and/or violent behavior" had a reduction in arrests from 45 percent to 12 percent in one year while participating in AOT.[32] In New York, the percentage of mentally ill individuals arrested decreased from 30 percent to 5 percent, and the percentage of those incarcerated decreased from 23 percent to 3 percent while on AOT.[33] In both studies, AOT was also accompanied by a major reduction in alcohol and drug abuse.

Finally, two studies have assessed the effect of AOT on violent behavior. In a randomized trial in North Carolina, subjects with a history of serious violence had a reduction in violence from 42 percent to 27 percent when the AOT was continued for at least six months.[34] In New York, AOT reduced the proportion of individuals who "physically harmed others" from 15 percent to 8 percent, and the proportion who "threatened physical harm" from 28 percent to 16 percent.[35]

The consistency of findings regarding the effectiveness of AOT is impressive. Only one U.S. study, in fact, did not find significant effects. In that study, there were no consequences for patients who did not take their medication, so it would seem it was not a true test of AOT.[36]

Despite its success, AOT is still not widely used. In New York State, for example, AOT was implemented on only 6,013 individuals between its inception in 1999 and mid-2007.[37] Resistance to using all forms of involuntary treatment remains high among mental health professionals. In addition, opponents of involuntary treatment have written extensively about its purported adverse effects on individuals forced to undergo it. Multiple studies, however, have shown that the majority of patients forced to take medication will, in retrospect, acknowledge that it was necessary. In one study, for example, 17 of 24 involuntarily medicated patients "felt that their treatment refusal had been correctly overridden by staff and that they should be treated against their will again if necessary.[38] In the analysis of AOT under Kendra's Law in New York, "62 percent of AOT recipients reported that, all things considered, being court-ordered into treatment has been a good thing for them."[39]

So we know how to identify individuals with severe psychiatric disorders who are most in need of treatment, including those who are most dangerous

VIOLENCE COMES TO NAMI

On June 29, 1986, Don Richardson was in Washington, DC, being installed as president of the National Alliance for the Mentally Ill, now called NAMI. At home in Los Angeles, his son Bill had just finished dinner with his mother. Bill, diagnosed with schizophrenia, had had twenty-six psychiatric admissions in the preceding seven years and had stopped taking his medication six weeks before. Bill heard command hallucinations telling him to kill his mother, so he walked behind her and hit her with a hammer, fracturing her skull in three places. She was not expected to live but did.

Don Richardson then attempted to get NAMI to speak out on the problem of violence. "To say the mentally ill are no more dangerous than the general population is a statement all of us family members have been parroting for years because we try hard to break the stigma....In our intensity to reduce stigma NAMI is also losing a lot of credibility....Out of the mentally ill population there is no question that there is a segment that is much more violent and to deny that is just reducing the credibility of our movement....I believe it is time for NAMI members to come all the way out of the closet."

Don Richardson, "On violence and forgiveness; A father confronts his fears," NAMI Advocate, *May/June 1992; Real Jean Isaac and Virginia Armat,* Madness in the Streets: How Psychiatry and the Law Abandoned the Mentally Ill *(New York: Free Press, 1990), pp. 270–78.*

to themselves and others. We have effective medications to treat them, and we have mechanisms, both formal and informal, to compel treatment. One major problem remains: How can we be sure these people actually take their medication?

One simple, but labor-intensive, means for ensuring treatment compliance is to observe the person taking the medication. This is widely used for patients with tuberculosis who are unable to, or refuse to, take their anti-tuberculous medication regularly. Inconsistent medication encourages the emergence of treatment-resistant strains of the tuberculous bacteria as well as the exposure of the public to persons who may spread the disease. This has led to the widespread use of directly observed therapy (DOT), which has been shown to be cost-effective. Patients with tuberculosis who still refuse to take medication under DOT can be involuntarily hospitalized and treated for several months until they are no longer infectious.[40]

A less expensive but highly effective means of ensuring medication compliance is to give the medication by long-acting injection. Three antipsychotics with a long-acting form are available in the United States, and others are available in Europe. They need to be given by injection every 3 or 4 weeks. Attempts are also underway to develop a small medication capsule that can be placed beneath the skin, where it will slowly release antipsychotic medication over several months.

Finally, means are available, and can be further developed, to measure medications in a person's blood or urine to ensure they are being taken. Many mood stabilizers and antipsychotics can already be measured. For those that cannot, it is possible to add to the pills a substance such as riboflavin, which is then detectable in the person's urine.[41] Similar measures have been used to monitor medication compliance for tuberculosis and could be instituted to monitor the treatment of severe psychiatric disorders.

GUARANTEED MEDICATION?

On July 12, 1976. Edward Allaway, a janitor at Cal State Fullerton, walked into the university library with a rifle and opened fire, killing seven people and injuring two others. Allaway, suffering from paranoid schizophrenia, feared that people were trying to put a bomb in his car and kill him. Five years earlier, he had been hospitalized for delusions. Allaway was found not guilty by reason of insanity and hospitalized. Since 1999, his attorney has claimed that he has been in full remission while not on medication and should therefore be released. Many have opposed his release under any circumstances. Others have argued that patients like Allaway should be released only on medication and under circumstances in which it is guaranteed that he will always have to take his medication.

S. Pfeifer, "Mass killer says he's no longer mentally Ill," Los Angeles Times, June 5, 2001

ASSESSMENT AND RESEARCH

The final ingredient in fixing the system is assessment and research. Mental health programs at the local and the state levels should collect regular data on the number of seriously mentally ill individuals who are homeless, jailed, victimized, and violent. These data should then be used to assess the effectiveness of their treatment programs. The federal government could require data as a condition for the annual federal grants given to each state or for eligibility for Medicaid reimbursement. The data could also be used to hold public mental health officials responsible when programs fail.

The federal government should play an important role in research on these issues. More research is needed to determine the best methods for identifying the target population; improved methods for assessing anosognosia; predictors of violent behavior; better pharmacological treatments for reducing violent behavior; and the relative effectiveness of assisted outpatient treatment (AOT) versus other methods of leveraging treatment. Funding for these types of research has been virtually nonexistent among federal agencies. A rare exception occurred in early 2007, when the National Institute of Mental Health announced a $2 million award to the Nathan Kline Institute for Psychiatric Research to study brain changes in individuals with schizophrenia who become violent. This is an excellent example of the kind of research the federal government should be supporting.

Ultimately, the question is not whether we have the means to identify and treat the subgroup of mentally ill individuals who are most problematic. We clearly do. The question, rather, is whether we have the will to do so. And if we do not have the will now, how much worse must the disaster become before we acquire the will?

Endnotes

1. M. B. Pfeiffer, "Let's care for the weakest among us," *Miami Herald*, November 29, 2006.
2. B. McKelway, "Va. chief justice leads the start of effort to revise state's laws," *Richmond Times-Dispatch*, September 2, 2006; H. Ascher-Svanum, D. E. Faries, B. Zhu, et al., "Medication adherence and long-term functional outcomes in the treatment of schizophrenia in usual care," *Journal of Clinical Psychiatry* 67 (2006): 453–60; W. H. Fisher and K. M. Roy-Bujnowski, "Patterns and prevalence of arrest in a statewide cohort of mental health care consumers," *Psychiatric Services* 57 (2006): 1623–28.
3. L. M. Davies and M. F. Drummond, "Economics and schizophrenia: The real cost," *British Journal of Psychiatry* 165, suppl. 25 (1994): 18–21.
4. P. Rasanen, J. Tiihonen, M. Isohanni, et al., *Schizophrenia Bulletin* 24 (1998): 437–41; C. Wallace, P. Mullen, P. Burgess, et al., "Serious criminal offending and mental disorder," *British Journal of Psychiatry* 172 (1998): 477–84.
5. N. Alia-Klein, T. M. O, Rourke, R. Z. Goldstein, et al., "Insight into illness and adherence to psychotropic medications are separately associated with violence severity in a forensic sample." *Aggressive Behavior* 33 (2007): 86–96; P. F. Buckley, D. R. Hrouda, L. Friedman, et al., "Insight and its relationship to violent behavior in patients with schizophrenia," *American Journal of Psychiatry* 161 (2004): 1712–14; D. Hrouda, P. J. Resnick, L. Friedman, et al., "Violence and schizophrenia: Further observations on standards of care" (abstract), *Schizophrenia Research* 60 (2003): 40; S. J. Bertels, R. E. Drake, M. A. Wallach, et al., "Characteristic hostility in schizophrenic outpatients," *Schizophrenia Bulletin* 17 (1991): 163–71; H. Ascher-Svanum, D. E. Faries, B. Zhu, et al., "Medication adherence and long-term functional outcomes in the treatment of schizophrenia in usual care," *Journal of Clinical Psychiatry* 67 (2006): 453–60. See also S. Strand, H. Belfrage, G. Fransson, et al., "Clinical and risk management factors in risk prediction of mentally disordered offenders—More important than historical data?" *Legal and Criminological Psychology* 4 (1999): 67–76; P. Woods, V. Reed, and M. Collins, "The relationship between risk and insight in a high-security forensic setting," *Journal of Psychiatric and Mental Health Nursing* 10 (2003): 510–17; M. Grevatt, B. Thomas-Peter, and G. Hughes, "Violence, mental disorder and risk assessment: Can structured clinical assessments predict the short-term risk of inpatient

violence?" *Journal of Forensic Psychiatry and Psychology* 15 (2004): 278–92; S. R. Foley, B. D. Kelly, M. Clarke, et al., "Incidence and clinical correlates of aggression and violence at presentation in patients with first episode psychosis," *Schizophrenia Research* 72 (2005): 161–68; M. S. Swartz, J. W. Swanson, V. A. Hiday, et al., "Violence and severe mental illness: The effects of substance abuse and nonadherence to medication," *American Journal of Psychiatry* 155 (1998): 226–31; L. D. Smith, "Medication refusal and the rehospitalized mentally ill inmate." *Hospital and Community Psychiatry* 40 (1989): 491–96; J. A. Yesavage, "Inpatient violence and the schizophrenic patient: An inverse correlation between danger-related events and neuroleptic levels," *Biological Psychiatry* 17 (1982): 1331–37; K. E. Weaver, "Increasing the dose of antipsychotic medication to control violence." (letter) *American Journal of Psychiatry* 140 (1983): 1274; J. A. Kasper, S. K. Hoge, T. Feucht-Haviar, et al., "Prospective study of patients' refusal of antipsychotic medication under a physician discretion review procedure." *American Journal of Psychiatry* 154 (1997): 483–89; T. Steinert, T. Sippach, and R. P. Gebhardt, "How common is violence in schizophrenia despite neuroleptic treatment?" *Pharmacopsychiatry* 33 (2000): 98–102.

6. A. Tengstrom, S. Hodgins, and G. Kullgten, "Men with schizophrenia who behave violently: The usefulness of an early- versus late-start offender typology." *Schizophrenia Bulletin* 27 (2001): 205–18. See also K. A. Nolan, J. Volavka, P. Mohr, et al., "Psychopathy and violent behavior among patients with schizophrenia or schizoaffective disorder." *Psychiatric Services* 50 (1999): 787–92.

7. S. Bjorkly, "Psychotic symptoms and violence toward others—A literature review of some preliminary findings: Part I. Delusions," *Aggression and Violent Behavior* 7 (2002): 617–31; B. G. Link, J. Monahan, A. Stueve, et al., "Real in their consequences: A sociological approach to understanding the association between psychotic symptoms and violence," *American Sociological Review* 64 (1999): 316–32; K. Hersh and R. Borum, "Command hallucinations, compliance, and risk assessment." *Journal of the American Academy of Psychiatry and the Law* 26 (1998): 353–59.

8. M. Krakowski, P. Crobor, and J. C.-Y. Chon, "Course of violence in patients with schizophrenia: Relationship to clinical symptoms," *Schizophrenia Bulletin* 25 (1999): 505–17; K. Naudis and S. Hodgins, "Neurological correlates of violent behavior among persons with schizophrenia," ibid., 32 (2006): 562–72; M. Das, V. Kumari, I. Barkataki, et al., "Anticipatory fear in violent schizophrenia and personality disorder subjects: A functional MRI study (abstract)," *Biological Psychiatry* 55 (2004): 70S.

9. M. Krakowski and P. Czobor. "Gender differences in violent behaviors: Relationship to clinical symptoms and psychosocial factors," *American Journal of Psychiatry* 161 (2004): 459–65; J. N. Lain, D. E. McNiel, and R. L. Binder, "The relationship between patients' gender and violence leading to staff injuries," *Psychiatric Services* 51 (2000): 1167–70; H. Schanda, G. Knecht, D. Schanda et al., "Homicide and major mental disorders: A 25-year study," *Acts Psychiatrica Scandinavia* 110 (2004): 98–107; A. I. R. Simpton, B. McKenna, A. Moskowitz, et al., "Homicide and mental illness in New Zealand, 1970–2000," *British Journal of Psychiatry* 185 (2004): 394–98.

10. M.S. Swartz, J.W. Swanson, V.A. Hiday, R. Borum, H.R. Wagner, and B.J. Burns., "Violence and severe mental illness: The Effects of Substance Abuse and Nonadherence to Medication." *American Journal of Psychiatry* 155 (1998):226–231.

11. J. Monahan and H. J. Steadman, eds., *Violence and Mental Disorder. Developments in Risk Assessment* (Chicago: University of Chicago Press, 1994); J. Monahan, H. J. Steadman, E. Silver, et al., *Rethinking Risk Assessment: The MacAnhur Study of Mental Disorder and Violence* (New York: Oxford University Press, 2001); J. Monahan and H. J. Steadman, "Violent storms and violent people: How meteorology can inform risk communication in mental health law," *American Psychologist* 51 (1996): 931–38; C. L. Scott and P.J. Resnick, "Violence risk assessment in persons with mental illness." *Aggression and Violent Behavior* 11 (2006): 598–611.

12. M. Tran, K. Pang, and H. G. Reza, "Sniper's family recalls him as a 'sweetheart'; His mother and son say Henry Lee Brown was a caring man when he took his schizophrenia medication." *Los Angeles Times*, June 16, 2004.

13. D. J. Allness and W. H. Knoedler, *The PACT Model of Community-Based Treatment for Persons with Severe and Persistent Mental Illness* (Arlington, Va.: NAMI, 1998).

14. Mary Flannery and Mark Glickman, *Fountain House: Portraits of Lives Reclaimed from Mental Illness* (Center City, Minu, Hazelden, 1996).

15. Steinert et al., "How common is violence in schizophrenia"; L. F. Dailey, S. W. Townsend, M. W. Dysken, et al., "Recidivism in medication-noncompliant serious juvenile offenders with bipolar disorder." *Journal of Clinical Psychiatry* 66 (2005): 477–84.

16. L. Citrome, J. Valavka, P. Czobor, et al., "Effects of clozapine, olanzapine, risperidone, and haloperidal on hostility among patients with schizophrenia," *Psychiatric Services* 52 (2001): 1510–14; M. I. Krakowski, P. Czobor, L. Citrome, et al., "Atypical antipsychotic agents in the treatment of violent patients with schizophrenia and schizoaffective disorder," *Archives of General Psychiatry* 63 (2006): 622–29; J. Volavka, "Treatment approaches to aggressive behavior in schizophrenia," in Adrian Raine, ed., *Crime and Schizophrenia: Causes and Cures* (Hauppauge, N.Y.: Nova Science Publishers, 2006), pp. 301–14; W.G. Frankel, D. Shera, H. Berger-Hershkowitz, et al., "Clozapine-associated reduction in arrest rates of psychotic patients with criminal histories," *American Journal of Psychiatry* 158 (2001): 270–74; L. Citrome, "The psychopharmacology of violence with emphasis on schizophrenia: Part 2. Long-term treatment." *Journal of Clinical Psychiatry* 68 (2007): 331–32.

17. R. Jorgensen, "Recovery and insight in schizophrenia." *Acts Psychiatrist Scandinavian* 92 (1995): 436–40; M. A. Weiler, M. H. Fleisher, and D. McArthur-Campbell. "Insight and symptom change in schizophrenia and other disorders," *Schizophrenic Research* 45 (2000): 29–36; C. Henry and S. N. Ghzemi, "I might in psychosis: A systematic review of treatment interventions." *Psychopathology* 37 (2004): 194–99; G. M. Gharabawi, R.A. Lasser, C. A. Bossie, et al., "Insight and its relationship to clinical outcomes in patients with schizophrenia or schizoaffective disorder receiving long-acting risperidone," *International Clinical Psychopharmacology* 21 (2006): 233–40.

18. M. Sherrill, "Out There: They are homeless, hopeless, wretched, heartbreaking, cunning, grungy, needy, greedy, idle, hungry, angry, aggravating. And ours," *Washington Post*, January 19, 1992; B. A. Pescosolido, J. Monahan, B. G. Link, et al., "The public's view of the competence, dangerousness, and need for legal coercion of persons with mental health problems," *American Journal of Public Health* 89 (1999): 1339–45.

19. D. J. Luchins, P. Hanrahan, K. J. Conrad, et al, "An agency-based representative payee program and improved community tenure of persons with mental illness." *Psychiatric Services* 49 (1998): 1218–22; K. J. Conrad, G. Lutz, M. D. Matters, et al.,

"Randomized trial of psychiatric care, with representative payeeship for persons with serious mental illness." ibid., 57 (2006): 197–204; P. S. Applebaum and A. Redlich, "Use of leverage over patients' money in promote adherence to psychiatric treatment," *Journal of Nervous and Mental Disease* 194 (2006): 294–302.

20. P. C. Robbins, J. Petrila, S. LeMelle, et al., "The use of housing as leverage to increase adherence to psychiatric treatment in the community." *Administration and Policy in Mental Health and Mental Health Services Research* 33 (2006): 226–36.

21. A. D. Redlich, H. J. Steadman, J. Monahan, et al., "Patterns of practice in mental health courts: A national survey." *Law and Human Behavior* 30 (2006): 347–62; H. Hermcks, S. Swart, S. Ama, et al., *The Clark County Mentally Ill Re-Arrest Prevention (MIRAP) Program, Final Evaluation Report* (Portland, Ore: Regional Research Institute for Human Services. Portland State University, 2003); M. S. Ridgely, J. Engberg, M. D. Greenberg, et al., "Justice, treatment, and cose—An evaluation of the fiscal impact of Allegheny County Mental Health Court," RAND Technical Report, available at www.rand.org/pubs/technical_reports/TR 439, accessed August 2, 2007.

22. C. O'Keefe, D. P. Potenza, and K. T. Mueser, "Treatment outcomes for severely mentally ill patients on conditional discharge to community-based treatment," *Journal of Nervous and Mental Disease* 185 (1997): 409–11.

23. D. A. Bigelow, J. D. Bloom, and M. H. Williams, "Costs of managing insanity acquittees under a Psychiatric Security Review Board system." *Hospital and Community Psychiatry* 41 (1990): 613–14; Joseph D. Bloom and Mary H. Williams, *Management and Treatment of Insanity Acquittees: A Model for the 1990s* (Washington, D.C.: American Psychiatric Press, 1994); K. Heilbrum and L. Peters, "The efficacy and effectiveness of community treatment programmes in preventing crime and violence among those with severe mental illness in the community," in Sheilagh Hodgins, ed., *Violence among the Mentally Ill: Effective Treatments and Management Strategies* (Dordrecht: Khrwer Academic Publishers, 1999), pp. 341–58.

24. *Kendra's Law: Final Report on the Status of Assisted Outpatient Treatment* (New York State Office of Mental Health, March 2005).

25. G. Zanni and L. deVeau, "Inpatient stays before and after outpatient commitment." *Hospital and Community Psychiatry* 37 (1986): 941–42.

26. G. A. Fernandez and S. Nygard, "Impact of involuntary outpatient commitment on the revolving-door syndrome in North Carolina," *Hospital and Community Psychiatry* 41 (1990): 1001–04.

27. M. R. Munetz, T. Grande, J. Kleist, et al., "The effectiveness of outpatient civil commitment," *Psychiatric Services* 47 (1996): 1251–53.

28. R. M. Rohland, *The Role of Outpatient Commitment in the Management of Persons with Schizophrenia* (Iowa Consortium for Mental Health, Services, Training, and Research, May 1998).

29. M. S. Swartz, J. W. Swanson, H. R. Wagner, et al., "Can involuntary outpatient commitment reduce hospital recidivisms?: Findings from a randomized trial with severely mentally ill individuals," *American Journal of Psychiatry* 156 (1999): 1968–75.

30. See note 24 above.

31. V. A. Hiday, M. S. Swartz, J. W. Swanson, et al., "Impact of outpatient commitment on victimization of people with severe mental illness," *American Journal of Psychiatry* 159 (2002): 1403–11.

32. J. W. Swanson, R. Borum, M. S. Swartz, et al., "Can involuntary outpatient commitment reduce arrests among persons with severe mental illness?" *Criminal Justice and Behavior* 28 (2001): 156–89.

33. See note 24 above.

34. J. W. Swanson, M. S. Swartz, R. Borum, et al., "Involuntary out-patient commitment and reduction of violent behaviour in persons with severe mental illness." *British Journal of Psychiatry* 176 (2000): 324–31.

35. See not 24 above.

36. B. Bursten, "Posthospital mandatory outpatient treatment." *American Journal of Psychiatry* 143 (1986): 1255–58.

37. See note 24 above.

38. H. I. Schwartz, W. Vingiano, and C. Bezirganian Perez., "Autonomy and the right to refuse treatment: Patients' attitudes after involuntary medication." *Hospital and Community Psychiatry* 39 (1988): 1049–54; N. H. S. Adams and R. J. Hafner, "Attitudes of psychiatric patients and their relatives to involuntary treatment." *Australian and New Zealand Journal of Psychiatry* 25 (1991): 231–37; H. Variainen, O. Vuorio, P. Halonen, et al., "The patients' opinions about curative factors in involuntary treatment," *Acta Psychiatrics Scandinavic* 91 (1995): 163–66; A. Lucksted and R. D. Coursey., "Consumer perceptions of pressure and force in psychiatric treatments," *Psychiatric Services* 46 (1995): 146–52; W. M. Greenberg, L. Moore-Duncan, and R. Herron, "Patients' attitudes toward having been forcibly medicated," *Bulletin of the American Academy of Psychiatry and the Law* 24 (1996): 513–24.

39. See note 24 above.

40. L. O. Gostin, "Controlling the resurgent tuberculosis epidemic," *Law and Medicine* 269 (1993): 255–61; M. R. Gasner, K. L. Maw, G. E. Feldman, et al., "The use of legal action in New York City to ensure treatment of tuberculosis," *New England Journal of Medicine* 340 (1999): 359–66.

41. G. A. Ellard, P. J. Jenner, and P. A. Downs, "An evaluation of the potential use of isoniazid, acetylisoniazid, and isonicottinic acid for monitoring the self-administration of drugs," *British Journal of Clinical Pharmacology* 10 (1980): 369–81; P. M. Edelbrook, F. G. Zitman, J. N. Schreinder, et al., "Amitriptyline metabolism in relation to antidepressant effect," *Clinical Pharmacology and Therapeutics* 35 (1984): 467–73.

DISCUSSION

1. From Torrey's perspective, what do we need to do to "fix the system?" What specific legal and policy changes does he believe are essential to improve the care and treatment of people with mental illness? Why are they essential? To what extent do his suggestions strike a new balance between the individual rights of people with mental illness and the right of society to protect its members from violence and disruptive behavior?

2. How easy do you think it would be to implement the reforms Torrey proposes? How likely is it that we will be able to transform the mental health system in the way he suggests?

Excerpts from the Executive Summary of the President's New Freedom Commission on Mental Health's Final Report

Presidents Kennedy and Carter were the first U.S. Presidents to attempt to seriously address mental health policy and the needs of people with mental illness in a systematic way. In 2002, President George W. Bush announced the formation of the "New Freedom Commission on Mental Health" (http://www.mentalhealth-commission.gov/). Much like Mental Health: A Report of the Surgeon General, published in 1999 (available at: http://www.surgeongeneral.gov/library/mental-health/home.html), the New Freedom Commission's final report represents a formal call to improve our mental health system and how our society responds to the needs of people with and affected by mental illness. With this excerpt from the Executive Summary of the final report, we conclude this reader with a vision for the future and six broad goals for transforming the mental health system in the United States.

VISION STATEMENT

We envision a future when everyone with a mental illness will recover, a future when mental illnesses can be prevented or cured, a future when mental illnesses are detected early, and a future when everyone with a mental Illness at any stage of life has access to effective treatment and supports—essentials for living, working, learning, and participating fully in the community.

In February 2001, President George W. Bush announced his New Freedom Initiative to promote increased access to educational and employment opportunities for people with disabilities. The Initiative also promotes increased access to assistive and universally designed technologies and full access to community life. Not since the Americans with Disabilities Act (ADA)—the landmark legislation providing protections against discrimination—and the Supreme Court's *Olmstead v. L.C.* decision, which affirmed the right to live in community settings, has there been cause for such promise and opportunity for full community participation for all people with disabilities, including those with psychiatric disabilities.

New Freedom Commission on Mental Health, *Achieving the Promise: Transforming Mental Health Care in America. Final Report.* DHHS Pub. No. SMA-03-3832. Rockville, MD: 2003.

On April 29, 2002, the president identified three obstacles preventing Americans with mental illnesses from getting the excellent care they deserve:

- Stigma that surrounds mental illnesses,
- Unfair treatment limitations and financial requirements placed on mental health benefits in private health insurance, and
- The fragmented mental health service delivery system.

The President's New Freedom Commission on Mental Health (called *the Commission* in this report) is a key component of the New Freedom Initiative. The president launched the Commission to address the problems in the current mental health service delivery system that allow Americans to fall through the system's cracks.

In his charge to the Commission, the president directed its members to study the problems and gaps in the mental health system and make concrete recommendations for immediate improvements that the federal government, state governments, local agencies, as well as public and private health care providers, can implement. Executive Order 13263 detailed the instructions to the Commission. (*See the Appendix.*)

The Commission's findings confirm that there are unmet needs and that many barriers impede care for people with mental illnesses. Mental illnesses are shockingly common; they affect almost every American family. It can happen to a child, a brother, a grandparent, or a coworker. It can happen to someone from any background—African American, Alaska Native, Asian American, Hispanic American, Native American, Pacific Islander, or White American. It can occur at any stage of life, from childhood to old age. No community is unaffected by mental illnesses; no school or workplace is untouched.

In any given year, about 5 percent to 7 percent of adults have a serious mental illness, according to several nationally representative studies.[1-3] A similar percentage of children—about 5 percent to 9 percent—have a serious emotional disturbance. These figures mean that millions of adults and children are disabled by mental illnesses every year.[1,4]

President Bush said,

"Americans must understand and send this message: mental disability is not a scandal—it is an illness. And like physical illness, it is treatable, especially when the treatment comes early."

Over the years, science has broadened our knowledge about mental health and illnesses, showing the potential to improve the way in which mental health care is provided. The U.S. Department of Health and Human Services (HHS) released *Mental Health: A Report of the Surgeon General*,[5] which reviewed scientific advances in our understanding of mental health and mental illnesses. However, despite substantial investments that have enormously increased the scientific knowledge base and have led to developing many effective treatments, many Americans are not benefiting from these investments.[6,7]

Far too often, treatments and services that are based on rigorous clinical research languish for years rather than being used effectively at the earliest opportunity. For instance, according to the Institute of Medicine (IOM) report, *Crossing the Quality Chasm: A New Health System for the 21st Century*, the lag between discovering effective forms of treatment and incorporating them into routine patient care is unnecessarily long, lasting about 15 to 20 years.[8]

In its report, the Institute of Medicine described a strategy to improve the quality of health care during the coming decade, including priority areas for refinement.[9] These documents, along with other recent publications and research findings, provide insight into the importance of mental heath, particularly as it relates to overall health.

MENTAL ILLNESSES PRESENTS SERIOUS HEALTH CHALLENGES

Mental illnesses rank first among illnesses that cause disability in the United States, Canada, and Western Europe.[10] This serious public health challenge is under-recognized as a public health burden. In addition, one of the most distressing and preventable consequences of undiagnosed, untreated, or under-treated mental illnesses is suicide. The World Health Organization (WHO) recently reported that suicide worldwide causes more deaths every year than homicide or war.[11]

In addition to the tragedy of lost lives, mental illnesses come with a devastatingly high financial cost. In the United States, the annual economic, indirect cost of mental illnesses is estimated to be $79 billion. Most of that amount—approximately $63 billion—reflects the loss of productivity as a result of illnesses. But indirect costs also include almost $12 billion in mortality costs (lost productivity resulting from premature death) and almost $4 billion in productivity losses for incarcerated individuals and for the time of those who provide family care.[12]

In 1997, the latest year comparable data are available, the United States spent more than $1 trillion on health care, including almost $71 billion on treating mental illnesses. Mental health expenditures are predominantly publicly funded at 57 percent, compared to 46 percent of overall health care expenditures. Between 1987 and 1997, mental health spending did not keep pace with general health care because of declines in private health spending under managed care and cutbacks in hospital expenditures.[13]

THE CURRENT MENTAL HEALTH SYSTEM IS COMPLEX

In its *Interim Report to the President*, the Commission declared, "the mental health delivery system is fragmented and in disarray…lead[ing] to unnecessary and costly disability, homelessness, school failure and incarceration."

The report described the extent of unmet needs and barriers to care, including:

- Fragmentation and gaps in care for children,
- Fragmentation and gaps in care for adults with serious mental illnesses,
- High unemployment and disability for people with serious mental illnesses,
- Lack of care for older adults with mental illnesses, and
- Lack of national priority for mental health and suicide prevention.

The *Interim Report* concluded that the system is not oriented to the single most important goal of the people it serves—the hope of recovery. State-of-the-art treatments, based on decades of research, are not being transferred from research to community settings. In many communities, access to quality care is poor, resulting in wasted resources and lost opportunities for recovery. More individuals could recover from even the most serious mental illnesses if they had access in their communities to treatment and supports that are tailored to their needs.

The Commission recognizes that thousands of dedicated, caring, skilled providers staff and manage the service delivery system. The Commission does not attribute the shortcomings and failings of the contemporary system to a lack of professionalism or compassion of mental health care workers. Rather, problems derive principally from the manner in which the nation's community-based mental health system has evolved over the past four to five decades. In short, the nation must replace unnecessary institutional care with efficient, effective community services that people can count on. It needs to integrate programs that are fragmented across levels of government and among many agencies.

Building on the research literature and comments from more than 2,300 consumers,[c] family members, providers, administrators, researchers, government officials, and others who provided valuable insight into the way mental health care is delivered, after its yearlong study, the Commission concludes that traditional reform measures are not enough to meet the expectations of consumers and families.

To improve access to quality care and services, the Commission recommends fundamentally transforming how mental health care is delivered in America. The goals of this fundamental change are clear and align with the direction that the President established.

THE GOAL OF A TRANSFORMED SYSTEM: RECOVERY

To achieve the promise of community living for everyone, new service delivery patterns and incentives must ensure that every American has easy and continuous access to the most current treatments and best support services.

Advances in research, technology, and our understanding of how to treat mental illnesses provide powerful means to transform the system. In a transformed system, consumers and family members will have access to timely and accurate information that promotes learning, self-monitoring, and accountability. Health care providers will rely on up-to-date knowledge to provide optimum care for the best outcomes.

When a serious mental illness or a serious emotional disturbance is first diagnosed, the health care provider—in full partnership with consumers and families—will develop an individualized plan of care for managing the illness. This partnership of personalized care means basically choosing *who*, *what*, and *how* appropriate health care will be provided:

- Choosing which mental health care professionals are on the team,
- Sharing in decision making, and
- Having the option to agree or disagree with the treatment plan.

The highest quality of care and information will be available to consumers and families, regardless of their race, gender, ethnicity, language, age, or place of residence. Because recovery will be the common, recognized outcome of mental health services, the stigma surrounding mental illnesses will be reduced, reinforcing the hope of recovery for every individual with a mental illness.

As more individuals seek help and share their stories with friends and relatives, compassion will be the response, not ridicule.

Successfully transforming the mental health service delivery system rests on two principles:

- **First, services and treatments must be consumer and family centered,** geared to give consumers real and meaningful choices about treatment options and providers—not oriented to the requirements of bureaucracies.
- **Second, care must focus on increasing consumers' ability to successfully cope with life's challenges, on facilitating recovery, and on building resilience,** not just on managing symptoms.

Built around consumers' needs, the system must be seamless and convenient.

Transforming the system so that it will be both consumer and family centered and recovery-oriented in its care and services presents invigorating challenges. Incentives must change to encourage continuous improvement in agencies that provide care. New, relevant research findings must be systematically conveyed to front-line providers so that they can be applied to practice quickly. Innovative strategies must inform researchers of the unanswered questions of consumers, families, and providers. Research and treatment must recognize both the commonalities and the differences among

Americans and must offer approaches that are sensitive to our diversity. Treatment and services that are based on proven effectiveness and consumer preference—not just on tradition or outmoded regulations—must be the basis for reimbursements.

The Nation must invest in the infrastructure to support emerging technologies and integrate them into the system of care. This new technology will enable consumers to collaborate with service providers, assume an active role in managing their illnesses, and move more quickly toward recovery.

The Commission identified the following six goals as the foundation for transforming mental health care in America. The goals are intertwined. No single step can achieve the fundamental restructuring that is needed to transform the mental health care delivery system.

GOALS

In a Transformed Mental Health System...

GOAL 1   Americans Understand that Mental Health Is Essential to Overall Health.

GOAL 2   Mental Health Care Is Consumer and Family Driven.

GOAL 3   Disparities in Mental Health Services Are Eliminated.

GOAL 4   Early Mental Health Screening, Assessment, and Referral to Services Are Common Practice.

GOAL 5   Excellent Mental Health Care Is Delivered and Research Is Accelerated.

GOAL 6   Technology Is Used to Access Mental Health Care and Information.

Achieving these goals will transform mental health care in America.

The following section of this report gives an overview of each goal of the transformed system, as well as the Commission's recommendations for moving the Nation toward achieving it. In the remainder of this report, the Commission discusses each goal in depth, showcasing model programs to illustrate the goal in practice and providing specific recommendations needed to transform the mental health system in America.

GOAL 1 AMERICANS UNDERSTAND THAT MENTAL HEALTH IS ESSENTIAL TO OVERALL HEALTH.

In a transformed mental health system, Americans will seek mental health care when they need it—with the same confidence that they seek treatment for other health problems. As a Nation, we will take action to ensure our health and well being through learning, self-monitoring, and accountability. We will continue to learn how to achieve and sustain our mental health.

The stigma that surrounds mental illnesses and seeking care for mental illnesses will be reduced or eliminated as a barrier. National education initiatives will shatter the misconceptions about mental illnesses, thus helping more Americans understand the facts and making them more willing to seek help for mental health problems. Education campaigns will also target specific audiences, including:

- Rural Americans who may have had little exposure to the mental health service system,
- Racial and ethnic minority groups who may hesitate to seek treatment in the current system, and
- People whose primary language is not English.

When people have a personal understanding of the facts, they will be less likely to stigmatize mental illnesses and more likely to seek help for mental health problems. The actions of reducing stigma, increasing awareness, and encouraging treatment will create a positive cycle that leads to a healthier population. As a nation, we will also understand that good mental health can have a positive impact on the course of other illnesses, such as cancer, heart disease, and diabetes.

Improving services for individuals with mental illnesses will require paying close attention to how mental health care and general medical care systems work together. While mental health and physical health are clearly connected, the transformed system will provide collaborative care to bridge the gap that now exists.

Effective mental health treatments will be more readily available for most common mental disorders and will be better used in primary care settings. Primary care providers will have the necessary time, training, and resources to appropriately treat mental health problems. Informed consumers of mental health service will learn to recognize and identify their symptoms and will seek care without the fear of being disrespected or stigmatized. Older adults, children, and adolescents, individuals from ethnic minority groups, and uninsured or low-income patients who are treated in public health care settings will receive care for mental disorders.

The transformed mental health system will rely on multiple sources of financing with the flexibility to pay for effective mental health treatments and services. This is a basic principle for a recovery-oriented system of care.

To aid in transforming the mental health system, the Commission makes two recommendations:

1.1 Advance and implement a national campaign to reduce the stigma of seeking care and a national strategy for suicide prevention.
1.2 Address mental health with the same urgency as physical health.

GOAL 2 MENTAL HEALTH CARE IS CONSUMER AND FAMILY DRIVEN

In a transformed mental health system, a diagnosis of a serious mental illness or a serious emotional disturbance will set in motion a well-planned, coordinated array of services and treatments defined in a single plan of care. This detailed roadmap—a personalized, highly individualized health management program—will help lead the way to appropriate treatment and supports that are oriented toward recovery and resilience. Consumers, along with service providers, will actively participate in designing and developing the systems of care in which they are involved.

An individualized plan of care will give consumers, families of children with serious emotional disturbances, clinicians, and other providers a valid opportunity to construct and maintain meaningful, productive, and healing relationships. Opportunities for updates—based on changing needs across the stages of life and the requirement to review treatment plans regularly—will be an integral part of the approach. The plan of care will be at the core of the consumer-centered, recovery-oriented mental health system. The plan will include treatment, supports, and other assistance to enable consumers to better integrate into their communities; it will allow consumers to realize improved mental health and quality of life.

In partnership with their health care providers, consumers and families will play a larger role in managing the funding for their services, treatments, and supports. Placing financial support increasingly under the management of consumers and families will enhance their choices. By allowing funding to follow consumers, incentives will shift toward a system of learning, self-monitoring, and accountability. This program design will give people a vested economic interest in using resources wisely to obtain and sustain recovery.

The transformed system will ensure that needed resources are available to consumers and families. The burden of coordinating care will rest on the system, not on the families or consumers who are already struggling because of a serious illness. Consumers' needs and preferences will drive the types and mix of services provided, considering the gender, age, language, development, and culture of consumers.

To ensure that needed resources are available to consumers and families in the transformed system, States will develop a comprehensive mental health plan to outline responsibility for coordinating and integrating programs. The state plan will include consumers and families and will create a new partnership among the Federal, State, and local governments. The plan will address the full range of treatment and support service programs that mental health consumers and families need.

In exchange for this accountability, states will have the flexibility to combine federal, state, and local resources in creative, innovative, and more efficient ways, overcoming the bureaucratic boundaries between health care, employment supports, housing, and the criminal justice systems.

Increased flexibility and stronger accountability will expand the choices and the array of services and supports available to attain the desired outcomes. Creative programs will be developed to respond to the needs and preferences of consumers and families, as reflected in their individualized plans of care.

Giving consumers the ability to participate fully in their communities will require a few essentials:

- Access to health care,
- Gainful employment opportunities,
- Adequate and affordable housing, and
- The assurance of not being unjustly incarcerated.

Strong leadership will need to:

- Align existing programs to deliver services effectively,
- Remove disincentives to employment (such as loss of financial benefits or having to choose between employment and health care), and
- Provide for a safe place to live.

In this transformed system, consumers' rights will be protected and enhanced. Implementing the 1999 *Olmstead v. L.C* decision in all states will allow services to be delivered in the most integrated setting possible—services in communities rather than in institutions. And services will be readily available so that consumers no longer face unemployment, homelessness, or incarceration because of untreated mental illnesses.

No longer will parents forgo the mental health services that their children desperately need. No longer will loving, responsible American parents face the dilemma of trading custody for care. Families will remain intact. Issues of custody will be separated from issues of care.

In this transformed system, stigma and discrimination against people with mental illnesses will not have an impact on securing health care, productive employment, or safe housing. Our society will not tolerate employment discrimination against people with serious mental illnesses—in either the public or private sector.

Consumers' rights will be protected concerning the use of seclusion and restraint. Seclusion and restraint will be used only as safety interventions of last resort, not as treatment interventions. Only licensed practitioners who are specially trained and qualified to assess and monitor consumers' safety and the significant medical and behavioral risks inherent in using seclusion and restraint will be able to order these interventions.

The hope and the opportunity to regain control of their lives—often vital to recovery—will become real for consumers and families. Consumers will play a significant role in shifting the current system to a recovery-oriented one by participating in planning, evaluation, research, training, and service delivery.

To aid in transforming the mental health system, the Commission makes five recommendations:

2.1 Develop an individualized plan of care for every adult with a serious mental illness and child with a serious emotional disturbance.

2.2 Involve consumers and families fully in orienting the mental health system toward recovery.

2.3 Align relevant Federal programs to improve access and accountability for mental health services.

2.4 Create a Comprehensive State Mental Health Plan.

2.5 Protect and enhance the rights of people with mental illnesses.

GOAL 3 DISPARITIES IN MENTAL HEALTH SERVICES ARE ELIMINATED

In a transformed mental health system, all Americans will share equally in the best available services and outcomes, regardless of race, gender, ethnicity, or geographic location. Mental health care will be highly personal, respecting and responding to individual differences and backgrounds. The workforce will include members of ethnic, cultural, and linguistic minorities who are trained and employed as mental health service providers. People who live in rural and remote geographic areas will have access to mental health professionals and other needed resources. Advances in treatments will be available in rural and less populated areas. Research and training will continuously aid clinicians in understanding how to appropriately tailor interventions to the needs of consumers, recognizing factors such as age, gender, race, culture, ethnicity, and locale.

Services will be tailored for culturally diverse populations and will provide access, enhanced quality, and positive outcomes of care. American Indians, Alaska Natives, African Americans, Asian Americans, Pacific Islanders, and Hispanic Americans will not continue to bear a disproportionately high burden of disability from mental health disorders.[1] These populations will have accessible, available mental health services. They will receive the same high quality of care that all Americans receive. To develop culturally competent treatments, services, care, and support, mental health research will include these underserved populations. In addition, providers will include individuals who share and respect the beliefs, norms, values, and patterns of communication of culturally diverse populations.

In rural and remote geographic areas, service providers will be more readily available to help create a consumer-centered system. Using such tools as videoconferencing and telehealth, advances in treatments will be brought to rural and less populated areas of the country. These technologies will be used to provide care at the same time they break down the sense of isolation often experienced by consumers.

Mental health education and training will be provided to general health care providers, emergency room staff, and first responders, such as law enforcement personnel and emergency medical technicians, to overcome the uneven geographic distribution of psychiatrists, psychologists, and psychiatric social workers.

To aid in transforming the mental health system, the Commission makes two recommendations:

3.1 Improve access to quality care that is culturally competent.

3.2 Improve access to quality care in rural and geographically remote areas.

GOAL 4 EARLY MENTAL HEALTH SCREENING, ASSESSMENT, AND REFERRAL TO SERVICES ARE COMMON PRACTICE

In a transformed mental health system, the early detection of mental health problems in children and adults—through routine and comprehensive testing and screening—will be an expected and typical occurrence. At the first sign of difficulties, preventive interventions will be started to keep problems from escalating. For example, a child whose serious emotional disturbance is identified early will receive care, preventing the potential onset of a co-occurring substance use disorder and breaking a cycle that otherwise can lead to school failure and other problems.

Quality screening and early intervention will occur in both readily accessible, low-stigma settings, such as primary health care facilities and schools, and in settings in which a high level of risk exists for mental health problems, such as criminal justice, juvenile justice, and child welfare systems. Both children and adults will be screened for mental illnesses during their routine physical exams.

For consumers of all ages, early detection, assessment, and links with treatment and supports will help prevent mental health problems from worsening. Service providers across settings will also routinely screen for co-occurring mental illnesses and substance use disorders. Early intervention and appropriate treatment will also improve outcomes and reduce pain and suffering for children and adults who have or who are at risk for co-occurring mental and addictive disorders.

Early detection of mental disorders will result in substantially shorter and less disabling courses of impairment.

To aid in transforming the mental health system, the Commission makes four recommendations:

4.1 Promote the mental health of young children.

4.2 Improve and expand school mental health programs.

4.3 Screen for co-occurring mental and substance use disorders and link with integrated treatment strategies.

4.4 Screen for mental disorders in primary health care, across the lifespan, and connect to treatment and supports.

GOAL 5 EXCELLENT MENTAL HEALTH CARE IS DELIVERED AND RESEARCH IS ACCELERATED

In a transformed mental health system, consistent use of evidence-based, state-of-the art medications and psychotherapies will be standard practice throughout the mental health system. Science will inform the provision of services, and the experience of service providers will guide future research. Every time any American—whether a child or an adult, a member of a majority or a minority, from an urban or rural area—comes into contact with the mental health system, he or she will receive excellent care that is consistent with our scientific understanding of what works. That care will be delivered according to the consumer's individualized plan.

Research has yielded important advances in our knowledge of the brain and behavior, and helped develop effective treatments and service delivery strategies for many mental disorders. In a transformed system, research will be used to develop new evidence-based practices to prevent and treat mental illnesses. These discoveries will be immediately put into practice. Americans with mental illnesses will fully benefit from the enormous increases in the scientific knowledge base and the development of many effective treatments.

Also benefiting from these developments, the workforce will be trained to use the most advanced tools for diagnosis and treatments. Translating research into practice will include adequate training for front-line providers and professionals, resulting in a workforce that is equipped to use the latest breakthroughs in modern medicine. Research discoveries will become routinely available at the community level. To realize the possibilities of advances in treatment, and ultimately in prevention or a cure, the Nation will continue to invest in research at all levels.

Knowledge about evidence-based practices (the range of treatments and services of well-documented effectiveness), as well as emerging best practices (treatments and services with a promising but less thoroughly documented evidentiary base), will be widely circulated and used in a variety of mental health specialties and in general health, school-based, and other settings. Countless people with mental illnesses will benefit from improved consumer outcomes including reduced symptoms, fewer and less severe side effects, and improved functioning. The field of mental health will be encouraged to expand its efforts to develop and test new treatments and practices, to promote awareness of and improve training in evidence-based practices, and to better finance those practices.

The nation will have a more effective system to identify, disseminate, and apply proven treatments to mental health care delivery. Research and education will play critical roles in the transformed mental health system. Advanced treatments will be available and adapted to individual preferences and needs, including language and other ethnic and cultural considerations. Investments in technology will also enable both consumers and providers to find the most up-to-date resources and knowledge to provide optimum care for the best outcomes. Studies will incorporate the unique needs of cultural, ethnic, and linguistic minorities and will help ensure full access to effective treatment for all Americans.

To aid in transforming the mental health system, the Commission makes four recommendations:

5.1 Accelerate research to promote recovery and resilience, and ultimately to cure and prevent mental illnesses.

5.2 Advance evidence-based practices using dissemination and demonstration projects and create a public-private partnership to guide their implementation.

5.3 Improve and expand the workforce providing evidence-based mental health services and supports.

5.4 Develop the knowledge base in four understudied areas: mental health disparities, long-term effects of medications, trauma, and acute care.

GOAL 6 TECHNOLOGY IS USED TO ACCESS MENTAL HEALTH CARE AND INFORMATION

In a transformed mental health system, advanced communication and information technology will empower consumers and families and will be a tool for providers to deliver the best care. Consumers and families will be able to regularly communicate with the agencies and personnel that deliver treatment and support services and that are accountable for achieving the goals outlined in the individual plan of care. Information about illnesses, effective treatments, and the services in their community will be readily available to consumers and families.

Access to information will foster continuous, caring relationships between consumers and providers by providing a medical history, allowing for self-management of care, and electronically linking multiple service systems. Providers will access expert systems that bring to bear the most recent breakthroughs and studies of optimal outcomes to facilitate the best care options. Having agreed to use the same health messaging standards, pharmaceutical codes, imaging standards, and laboratory test names, the Nation's health system will be much closer to speaking a common language and providing superior patient care. Informed consumers and providers will result in better outcomes and will more efficiently use resources.

Electronic health records can improve quality by promoting adoption and adherence to evidence-based practices through inclusion of clinical reminders, clinical practice guidelines, tools for clinical decision support, computer order entry, and patient safety alert systems. For example, prescription medications being taken or specific drug allergies would be known, which could prevent serious injury or death resulting from drug interactions, excessive dosages or allergic reactions.

Access to care will be improved in many underserved rural and urban communities by using health technology, telemedicine care, and consultations. Health technology and telehealth will offer a powerful means to improve access to mental health care in underserved, rural, and remote areas. The privacy of personal health information—especially in the case of mental illnesses—will be strongly protected and controlled by consumers and families. With appropriate privacy protection, electronic records will enable essential medical and mental health information to be shared across the public and private sectors.

Reimbursements will become flexible enough to allow implementing evidence-based practices and coordinating both traditional clinical care and e-health visits. In both the public and private sectors, policies will change to support these innovative approaches.

An integrated information technology and communications infrastructure will be critical to achieving the five preceding goals and transforming mental health care in America. To address this technological need in the mental health care system, this goal envisions two critical technological components:

- A robust telehealth system to improve access to care, and
- An integrated health records system and a personal health information system for providers and patients.

To aid in transforming the mental health system, the Commission makes two recommendations:

6.1 Use health technology and telehealth to improve access and coordination of mental health care, especially for Americans in remote areas or in underserved populations.

6.2 Develop and implement integrated electronic health record and personal health information systems.

CONCLUSION

Preventing mental illnesses remains a promise of the future. Granted, the best option is to avoid or delay the onset of any illness, but the Executive Order directed the Commission to conduct a comprehensive study of the delivery of mental health services. The Commission recognizes that it is better to prevent an illness than to treat it, but unmet needs and barriers to services must first be identified to reach the millions of Americans with existing mental illnesses who are deterred from seeking help. The barriers may exist for a variety of reasons:

- Stigma,
- Fragmented services,

- Cost,
- Workforce shortages,
- Unavailable services, and
- Not knowing where or how to get care.

The Commission—aware of all the limitations on resources—examined realigning federal financing with a keen awareness of the constraints. As such, the policies and improvements recommended in this *Final Report* reflect policy and program changes that make the most of existing resources by increasing cost effectiveness and reducing unnecessary and burdensome regulatory barriers, coupled with a strong measure of accountability. A transformed mental health system will more wisely invest resources to provide optimal care while making the best use of limited resources.

The process of transforming mental health care in America drives the system toward a delivery structure that will give consumers broader discretion in how care decisions are made. This shift will give consumers more confidence to require that care be sensitive to their needs, that the best available treatments and supports be available, and that demonstrably effective technologies be widely replicated in different settings. This confidence will then enhance cooperative relationships with mental health care professionals who share the hope of recovery.

References

1. United States Public Health Service Office of the Surgeon General (2001). *Mental Health: Culture, Race, and Ethnicity: A Supplement to Mental Health: A Report of the Surgeon General.* Rockville, MD: Department of Health and Human Services, U.S. Public Health Service.
2. Department of Health and Human Services: Substance Abuse and Mental Health Services Administration (2002). *National Household Survey on Drug Abuse: Volume I. Summary of National Findings; Prevalence and Treatment of Mental Health Problems.*
3. Kessler, R. C., Berglund, P. A., Bruce, M. L., Koch, J. R., Laska, E. M., Leaf, P. J. et al. (2001). The prevalence and correlates of untreated serious mental illness. *Health Services Research, 36,* 987–1007.
4. Farmer, E. M. Z., Mustillo, S., Burns, B. J., & Costello, E. J. (2003). The epidemiology of mental health programs and service use in youth: Results from the Great Smoky Mountains Study. In M.H. Epstein, K. Kutash, & A. Duchnowsk (Eds.), *Outcomes for Children and Youth with Behavioral and Emotional Disorders and Their Families: Programs and Evaluation Best Practices 2nd ed., [in press]*
5. United States Public Health Service Office of the Surgeon General (1999). *Mental Health: A Report of the Surgeon General.* Rockville, MD: Department of Health and Human Services, U. S. Public Health Service.
6. Lehman, A. F. & Steinwachs, D. M. (1998). Patterns of usual care for schizophrenia: Initial results from the Schizophrenia Patient Outcomes Research Team (PORT) Client Survey. *Schizophrenia Bulletin, 24,* 11–20.
7. Wang, P. S., Demler, O., & Kessler, R. C. (2002). Adequacy of treatment for serious mental illness in the United States. *American Journal of Public Health, 92,* 92–98.

8. Balas, E. A. & Boren, S. A. (2000). Managing clinical knowledge for health care improvement. In *Yearbook of Medical Informatics* (pp. 65–70). Bethesda, MD: National Library of Medicine.

9. Institute of Medicine Committee on Quality of Health Care in America (2001). *Crossing the Quality Chasm: A New Health System for the 21st Century.* Washington, DC: National Academies Press.

10. World Health Organization. (2001). *The World Health Report 2001 - Mental Health: New Understanding, New Hope.* Geneva: World Health Organization.

11. World Health Organization. (2002). *World Report on Violence and Health.* Geneva: World Health Organization.

12. Rice, D. P. & Miller, L. S. (1996). The economic burden of schizophrenia: Conceptual and methodological issues and cost estimates. In M. Moscarelli, A. Rupp, & N. Sartorius (Eds.), *Schizophrenia* (pp. 321–334). Chichester, UK: Wiley.

13. Coffey, R. M., Mark, T., King, E., Harwood, H., McKusick, D., Genuardi, J. et al. (2000). *National Estimates of Expenditures for Mental Health and Substance Abuse Treatment, 1997* (Rep. No. SAMHSA Publication SMA-00–3499). Rockville, MD: Substance Abuse and Mental Health Services Administration.

DISCUSSION

1. To what extent are the vision and goals of the President's New Freedom Commission informed by the sociological perspective on mental illness? Based on what you have learned about the sociology of mental health and illness, what changes would you make to the Commission's recommendations and why?

2. What has been the outcome of the Commission's recommendations to date? Given the current social and political climate, to what extent do you think the vision and goals are achievable? What changes will be necessary in order to transform the mental health system in the ways desired by the Commission?

LaVergne, TN USA
25 February 2011
217990LV00001B/3/P

9 780195 381719